The Medical Management of the Critically Ill

The Medical Management of the Critically Ill

Edited by

GILLIAN C. HANSON
and P. L. WRIGHT

*Whipps Cross Hospital
Leytonstone, London*

1978

ACADEMIC PRESS · LONDON

GRUNE & STRATTON · NEW YORK

U.K. edition published and distributed by
ACADEMIC PRESS INC. (LONDON) LTD.
24/28 Oval Road
London NW1 7DX

United States Edition published and distributed by
GRUNE & STRATTON INC.
111 Fifth Avenue
New York, New York 10003

Library of Congress Catalog Card Number: 77-85102
ISBN (Academic Press): 0-12-323650-9
ISBN (Grune & Stratton): 0-8089-1066-3

Text set in 11/12 pt Monophoto Baskerville
Printed and bound at William Clowes & Sons Limited
Beccles and London

List of Contributors

E. D. BENNETT, Consultant Physician, St George's Hospital, Blackshaw Road, London SW17 0QT

J. P. BLACKBURN, Consultant in Clinical Measurement, Westminster Hospital, Dean Ryle Street, Horseferry Road, London SW1P 2AP

A. M. BOLD, Consultant Chemical Pathologist, Clinical Chemistry Department, The Queen Elizabeth Hospital, Queen Elizabeth Medical Centre, Edgbaston, Birmingham B15 2 TN

B. CHATTOPADHYAY, Director of Public Health Laboratory, Whipps Cross Hospital, Leytonstone, London E11 1NR

R. D. COHEN, Director, Academic Unit of Metabolism and Endocrinology, The London Hospital, Whitechapel E1 1BB

D. L. COPPEL, Consultant Anaesthetist, Royal Victoria Hospital, Grosvenor Road, Belfast BT12 6BA

J. W. L. DAVIES, Medical Research Council, Industrial Injuries and Burns Unit, Birmingham Accident Hospital, Bath Row, Birmingham B15 1NA

M. A. DENBOROUGH, Department of Clinical Science, The Australian National University, Canberra Community Hospital, Canberra, A.C.T. 2601, Australia

J. S. GEDDES, Consultant Physician, Cardiac Department, Royal Victoria Hospital, Grosvenor Road, Belfast BT12 6BA

F. ST. C. GOLDEN, MOIC Survival Medicine, Institute of Naval Medicine, Alverstoke, Hants PO12 2DL.

D. S. GORDON, Consultant Neurosurgeon, Royal Victoria Hospital, Grosvenor Road, Belfast BT12 6BA

GILLIAN C. HANSON, Consultant Physician in charge of the Intensive Therapy Unit, Whipps Cross Hospital, Leytonstone, London E11 1NR

G. R. HERVEY, Head of Department of Physiology, The University, Leeds LS2 9JT

P. JOHNSON, Consultant Orthopaedic Surgeon, Frimley Park Hospital, Portsmouth Road, Frimley, Surrey GU16 5UJ

P. JONES, Director, Newcastle Haemophilia Centre, Department of Haematology, Royal Victoria Infirmary, Newcastle-upon-Tyne NE1 4LP

J. H. KERR, Consultant Anaesthetist, Nuffield Department of Anaesthetics, The Radcliffe Infirmary, Oxford OX2 6HE

DAPHNE KAYTON, Consultant Gynaecologist and Obstetrician, Whipps Cross Hospital, Leytonstone, London E11 1NR

H. A. LEE, Department of Metabolic Medicine, University of Southampton, Consultant Physician, Wessex Regional Renal Unit, Portsmouth PO3 6AD

M. W. McNICOL, Consultant Chest Physician, Cardio-Thoracic Department, Central Middlesex Hospital, Acton Lane, London NW10 7NS

M. N. MAISEY, Director, Department of Nuclear Medicine, Guy's Hospital, St. Thomas Street, London SE1 9RT

G. W. ODLING-SMEE, Senior Lecturer in Surgery, The Queen's University of Belfast, Institute of Clinical Science, Grosvenor Road, Belfast BT12 6BJ

J. M. OXBURY, Consultant Neurologist, The Radcliffe Infirmary, Oxford OX2 6HE.

M. PANETH, Consultant Cardio-Thoracic Surgeon, Brompton Hospital, Fulham Road, London SW3 6HP

J. S. PEGUM, Senior Physician, Skin Department, The London Hospital, Whitechapel, London E1 1BB

J. S. PORTNOY, Consultant Radiologist, Whipps Cross Hospital, Leytonstone, London E11 1NR

A. J. REES, Senior Registrar to D. K. Peters, Hammersmith Hospital, 150 Du Cane Road, London W12 0HS

KEITH D. ROBERTS, Consultant Paediatric Cardiothoracic Surgeon, The Children's Hospital, Ladywood Middleway, Ladywood, Birmingham B16 8ET

J. S. ROBINSON, University Department of Anaesthetics, Queen Elizabeth Hospital, Birmingham B15 2TH

H. F. SEELEY, Consultant Anaesthetist and Honorary Senior Lecturer, St George's Hospital, Hyde Park Corner, London SW1X 7EZ.

J. M. K. SPALDING, Consultant Neurologist, Department of Neurology, The Radcliffe Infirmary, Oxford OX2 6HE

J. C. STODDART, Consultant in Charge, Intensive Therapy Unit, Royal Victoria Infirmary, Queen Victoria Road, Newcastle-upon-Tyne NE1 4LP

PATRICIA STONE, Principal Pharmacist, Whipps Cross Hospital, Leytonstone, London E11 1NR

J. E. TRAPNELL, Consultant Surgeon, Royal Victoria Hospital, Shelley Road, Bournemouth BH1 4HG

P. N. TREWBY, Senior Registrar, West Middlesex Hospital, Isleworth, Middlesex TW7 6AF

ROGER WILLIAMS, Director of the Liver Unit, King's College Hospital, Denmark Hill, London SE5 9RS

R. S. WINWOOD, Consultant Physician, Whipps Cross Hospital, Leytonstone, London E11 1NR

P. L. WRIGHT, Consultant Physician, Whipps Cross Hospital, Leytonstone, London E11 1NR

M. YACOUB, Consultant Cardiac Surgeon, Harefield Hospital, Harefield, Uxbridge, Middlesex UB9 6JH

Preface

The book was undertaken in response to pressure from colleagues and junior staff who were unable to find a text which described the working and administration of an Intensive Therapy Unit, and the emergency management of the majority of disorders encountered therein. The book is not intended to include patient management in a specialist Intensive Therapy Unit, but problems generally encountered in a unit serving a General Hospital.

The book is divided into four parts, the first gives the medical management of general problems which may arise during the treatment of a patient with a specific illness. We have here tried to base treatment on physiological principles. The second part describes the treatment of more specific aspects of acute illness, particular attention has been paid to the more controversial aspects of management. Chapters have been included on disorders which are only occasionally encountered in the Intensive Therapy Unit and where information on management is not readily available. The third part gives the ancillary facilities required for an Intensive Therapy Unit and describes the investigative and therapeutic aspects of patient care. The final part describes monitoring, instrumentation and organ support systems and, we hope, will both help the clinician to set up an Intensive Therapy Unit and to achieve a more rational approach towards patient monitoring. The chapter on organ support systems gives a guide to the techniques available for support of failing vital organs and describes trends.

Because of the specialism involved we felt only a contributed work could do justice to the aims and the scope of the book. We have tried to smooth out any possible disjointedness and to give a cross-reference system. Some chapters and sections are brief, usually where patient management is non-controversial. All authors were urged to give extensive references for those wishing to read more deeply.

It is hoped that the book will prove useful to doctors and ancillary personnel devoting most of their time to the management of the critically ill; to specialists interested in certain aspects of intensive care and as a reference manual for doctors who rarely encounter critical illness, but want guidance on management. Nurses and technicians working in the intensive therapy unit may also find the book valuable.

We wish to thank all our contributors and hope that the completed manual will do justice to their hard work. We are also indebted to many secretaries at Whipps Cross Hospital who retyped most of the manuscripts and in particular to Mrs Rosemary Selby who worked all hours in order to submit the manuscript as quickly as possible. Nor can we leave unmentioned the constant encouragement, support and expert advice of the publishers, Academic Press.

September 1978   GILLIAN C. HANSON
                                                    P. L. WRIGHT

Contents

Part 2: Specific Management

Part 3: Investigative Facilities and Drug Requirements in the I.T.U.

Part 4: Monitoring, Computer Applications and Instrumentation in the Intensive Therapy Unit

Glossary of Terms

RESPIRATORY SYMBOLS

A	Alveolar gas
A-aDO$_2$	Alveolar-arterial gradient for oxygen
a-ADCO$_2$	Arterial alveolar gradient for carbon dioxide
a	Arterial blood
A-V shunting	Arterio-venous shunting
A-VO$_2$	Arterio-venous oxygen content difference
A.T.A.	Atmospheres absolute
C	Lung compliance
C.P.P.V.	Continuous positive pressure ventilation
D.L.C.O.	Diffusion capacity for carbon monoxide
E	Expired gas
F$_I$O$_2$	Fractional concentration of oxygen in inspired gas
F.R.C.	Functional residential capacity
F.E.V.	Forced expiratory volume
G.A.	General anaesthetic
I	Inspired gas
I.P.P.B.	Intermittent positive pressure breathing
I.P.P.V.	Intermittent positive pressure ventilation
I.M.V.	Intermittent mandatory ventilation
P.E.E.P.	Positive end expiratory pressure
P$_{oes}$	Intra-oesophageal pressure
P$_{aw}$	Airway pressure
PaO$_2$	Arterial pressure of oxygen
PaCO$_2$	Arterial pressure of carbon dioxide
P.C.W.P.	Pulmonary capillary wedge pressure
P$_{50}$	PaO$_2$ at 50% saturation under standard conditions
P.A.P.	Pulmonary artery pressure
Q	Volume of blood
Q̇	Lung perfusion per unit time
R	Airways resistance
R.I.	Respiratory index
R/Q	Respiratory exchange ratio

RESPIRATORY SYMBOLS *(contd)*

V	Volume of gas
$\dot{V}$	Gas flow
V_D	Dead space gas volume
V_T	Tidal gas volume
V_A	Volume of alveolar gas
$\dot{V}_A$	Ventilation reaching the alveoli per unit time
$\dot{V}_{A/\dot{Q}}$	Ratio of alveolar ventilation to pulmonary perfusion per unit time.

OTHER SYMBOLS

ATP	Adenosine triphosphate
ATP-ase	Adenosine triphosphatase
ADH	Antidiuretic hormone
A.C.D.	Acid citrate dextrose
A.I.P.	Acute intermittent porphyria
A.R.F.	Acute renal failure
A.H.F.	Anti haemophilic factor
A.T.G.	Human antitetanus globulin
A.R.M.	Artificial rupture of the membranes
A.H.G.	Antihaemophilic globulin
B.D.	Base deficit
B.E.	Base excess
B.U.	Blood urea
C.S.S.D.	Central sterile supplies department
C.V.P.	Central venous pressure
CPK	Creatinine phosphokinase
C.P.D.	Citrate phosphate dextrose
C.P.P.	Cerebral perfusion pressure
C.T. scan	Computerised tomographic scan
C.O.	Cardiac output
C.A.B.G.	Coronary artery by-pass graft
d.c.	Direct current
D.I.C.	Disseminated intravascular coagulation
2,3-D.P.G.	2,3-Diphosphoglycerate
DHT	Dehydrotachysterol
D.K.A.	Diabetic ketoacidosis
D.T.P.A.	Diethylene triaminepentacetic acid
E.A.C.A.	Epsi-amino caproic acid
E.C.M.	External cardiac massage
E.C.P.	External counterpulsation
E.E.G.	Electroencephalogram

E.C.F.	Extracellular fluid
E.D.	Exfoliative dermatitis
E.M.	Erythema multiforme
F.F.P.	Fresh frozen plasma
F.T.I.	Free thyroxine index
F.D.P.	Fibrin degradation products
G-6-PD	Glucose-6-phosphate dehydrogenase
G.P.P.	Generalised pustular psoriasis
G.B.M.	Glomerular basement membrane
$HBsA_g$	Hepatitus B surface antigen
H.B.O.	Hyperbaric oxygen
Hct	Haematocrit
I.T.U.	Intensive therapy unit
I.C.F.	Intracellular fluid
I.A.D.H.	Inappropriate antidiuretic hormone secretion
I.T.P.	Idiopathic thrombocytopenic purpura
I.C.P.	Intracranial pressure
I.T.P.	Intrathoracic pressure
I.A.B.C.	Intra-aortic ballon counterpulsation
ki/ke	Intracellular/extracellular potassium ratio
kPa	Kilo pascal
LAO	Left anterior oblique
M.A.B.P.	Mean aortic blood pressure
N.K.H.	Non-ketotic hyperglycaemia
$1\alpha(OH)D_3$	1α-Hydroxytachysterol
P.A.T.B.	Paroxysmal atrial tachycardia with block
pH	Refers to arterial blood pH unless specifically stated
pH_a	Arterial pH
P.P.F.	Human plasma protein fraction
P.P.H.	Post-partum haemorrhage
P.R.P.	Platelet rich plasma
P.T.T.K.	Partial thromboplastin time with kaolin
P.T.	Prothrombin time
P.C.V.	Packed cell volume
P.V.	Plasma volume
R.E.S.	Reticulo endothelial system
T.E.N.	Toxic epidermal necrolysis
T_4	Serum thyroxine
T.T.	Thrombin time
T_3	Tri-iodothyronine
T.T.P.	Thrombotic thrombocytopenic purpura

OTHER SYMBOLS (*contd*)

T.B.W.	Total body water
U/P ratio	Urine plasma osmolality ratio
U.V.R.	Ultraviolet radiation
V.F.	Ventricular fibrillation
V.M.A.	4-Hydroxy-3-methoxymandelic acid
V.P.B.s	Ventricular premature beats

PART 1

The General Management of the Critically Ill

I

Introduction: The Function of an Intensive Therapy Unit

GILLIAN C. HANSON

The B.M.A. Working Party on Intensive Care, commented as early as 1967 that the establishment of an Intensive Therapy Unit in a General Hospital was an 'economic arrangement for the treatment of grave illness' and would 'not only improve the chances of a patient with a desperate illness, but was also likely to promote an improvement in the general level of medical and nursing care'.

Three types of patient make extra demands on the traditional ward system; those requiring heavy nursing, those requiring continuous or frequent observation and/or investigation and those requiring complicated, often mechanical, treatment. The nursing profession (Intensive Therapy Nursing Group, 1969) and the British Medical Association Planning Unit (1967) have adopted the term Intensive Care for the former and Intensive Therapy for the latter two groups of patients. An Intensive Therapy Unit was defined (B.M.A., 1967) as a special unit providing a 'facility available to the medical staff for the care of patients who are deemed recoverable but who need continuous supervision and need, or are likely to need, prompt use of specialised techniques by skilled personnel'.

An Intensive Therapy Unit in a General Hospital generally accepts all types of emergency and it is rarely necessary to form several units with specialist divisions. The Intensive Therapy Unit should be separate from but close to the operating theatres and postoperative recovery rooms; and should be sited as close as possible to the Accident Centre and X-ray department. The Coronary Care Unit should be adjacent to, or form part of, the General Intensive Therapy Unit.

It is commonly estimated that 1–2 per cent of patients admitted to an acute hospital will need intensive therapy at some time. A unit of less

3

than six beds is uneconomical to run, staff and equip, and a unit of greater than 10 beds unwieldy. The bed occupancy for an I.T.U. must be lower than that of the general wards because of a wide variation in work load – an occupancy of 60% is considered acceptable.

It is not proposed to discuss the design of an Intensive Therapy Unit since this has been mentioned in detail elsewhere – (D.H.S.S. 1970; Verner, 1974).

REFERENCES

B.M.A. (1967). Planning Unit Report No. 1. Report of the Working Party on Intensive Care. *Publ. Brit. Med. Assoc.*

Intensive Therapy Nursing Group (1969). The Function and Staffing of Intensive Therapy Units and the Preparation of Nurses to Work in the Units. *Publ. Royal Coll. Nursing and Nat. Council of Nurses of the U.K. October 1969.*

D.H.S.S. (1970). Intensive Therapy Unit. *Hosp. Building Note 27.*

Verner, I. R. (1974). The organisation, design and staffing of Intensive Therapy Units. *Brit. J. Hosp. Med.* **II** (6), 828.

II

Respiratory Care and the Principles of Ventilation

J. S. ROBINSON

THE AIRWAY

The necessity for the careful control of the airway in patients in whom its twin prime functions of patency and protection are in any way impaired has been recognised for very many years, furthermore the indications for its artificial control, either by tracheostomy or endotracheal intubation are well established as:

　1. obstruction to the upper respiratory tract;

　2. inability to void secretion from the respiratory tract;

　3. failure of co-ordinated swallowing and/or loss of both; intrinsic and extrinsic laryngeal reflexes; and

　4. maintenance of artificial ventilation of the lungs.

What has not been so well established are the relative merits and demerits of long-term endotracheal intubation or tracheostomy and these might be usefully described.

TRACHEOSTOMY

It is probably true to say that in the I.T.U. tracheostomy is less

5

frequently undertaken perhaps because, as McClelland (1970) suggests, we have had a period of rationalisation following the enthusiasm for the technique, characteristic of the early days of intensive therapy.

Tracheostomy reduces anatomical dead space by approximately 46%, but this has no therapeutic value particularly because patients who require ventilation usually have V_D/V_T ratios of at least 0.5. The complication rate from tracheostomy varies from 50% in a general hospital to 100% for emergency tracheostomy (McClelland, 1970). Complications range from erosion of the tracheal mucosa, or trachea, and surrounding structures to even fatal haemorrhage from erosion into the innominate artery. However, the commonest, the most insiduous and often fatal complication is the introduction of infection into the respiratory tract. The inspired air in the normal respiratory tract reaches the carina at a temperature of 37°C with a relative humidity of 100%, but tracheostomy or endotracheal intubation effectively decreases this protection.

Infection

The importance of preventing the introduction of infection during tracheo-bronchial toilet in the debilitated patient is well recognised and aseptic or no touch techniques should be universal.

Ventilators may be a source of infection and many solutions to the problem have been advocated, ranging from sterilisation of the ventilator with ethylene oxide or ultrasonically nebulised hydrogen peroxide to isolating the ventilator with bacterial filters. This latter method has found the most ready acceptance particularly as some ventilators defy attempts at sterilisation of the gas delivery passages. The bacterial filter on the inspiratory limb of the ventilator does not require changing more frequently than 2 or 3 times per month but that on the expiratory limb should be changed every 48 h and between each patient use. The expiratory filter needs to be heated because the content of water vapour in the expired gas, if deposited on the filter, would raise the resistance of the patient generated expired gas flow through the filter to unacceptable levels. Respiratory hoses to the patient from the machine should be changed for a sterile set each day. Patients have been shown to eliminate a pulmonary infection only to be re-infected with the same organism by the ventilator.

Even though the ventilator is isolated with bacterial filters, the ventilator should be sterilised every three months because where this has been done, the incidence of chest infection with hospital pathogens such as *pseudomonas pyocyaneus* has been shown to decrease.

Humidification

The need to humidify inspired gases during artificial ventilation of the lungs is unquestioned, but the methods for accomplishing this are numerous (Robinson, 1974a) and some are dangerously inefficient (Hayes and Robinson, 1970). Water can exist in two forms in the inspired gas, as water vapour or as droplets.

Water vapour
The heated water 'blow over' type of humidifier (Marshall Spalding, Cape, East etc.), in which *all* the water is in the vapour phase, are surprisingly efficient producing 31 to 40 g of H_2O per cubic metre of air (saturation at 37°C is 44 g/m³); however, most such instruments have a large exchange area (by providing a large liquid water surface) and thus contain a big compressible gas volume. This compressible volume degrades any set inspiratory gas flow pattern delivered into them which may be quite undesirable (*vide infra*). This has been overcome in instruments such as the Fisher Pakell in which a huge heated surface area obtained by the use of absorbent material is presented to the gas flow and this is thermostatically controlled from the temperature of the inspired gas. The compressible gas volume of such instruments is very small.

Aerosol of water droplets
Mists of microdroplets in the inspired gas can be produced by many energy sources, the commonest are the gas driven nebulisers and the ultrasonic nebulisers. The satisfaction of seeing dense clouds of mist issuing from a nebuliser may be misplaced since the carrier gas may not be saturated with water vapour nor are there sufficient droplets to produce saturation when these evaporate. It should be remembered that a visible fog can exist in the atmosphere when the relative humidity is less than 78%. Humidifiers which combine heated water and nebuliser principles are therefore much more efficient both in performance and clinical use (e.g. Ohio).

Another factor that must be considered is the stability of the droplets themselves; this and their site of precipitation in the airways is dependent upon their diameter. Droplets of approximately 10 μm are all deposited in the upper respiratory tract and particles below 1 μm

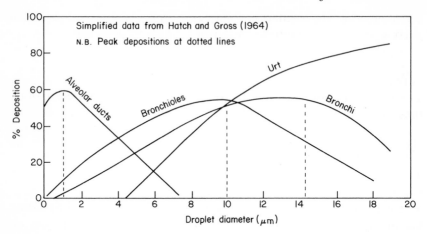

Fig. 1. The site of deposition of droplets expressed as percentage. The dotted lines are the sites of peak deposition of the droplets. (This diagram is simplified from the data of Hatch and Gross, 1964.)

tend to go in and out of the lungs without precipitation at all. A theoretical study of the deposition of droplets is given in Fig. 1, taken from the data of Hatch and Gross, 1964. It can be seen that if droplet deposition is desired throughout all airways, droplet sizes from 2 to 10 μm are required, but if droplets are required to be deposited in the alveoli, a particle size of 2 μm is needed. This fact must be remembered if it is intended to use nystatin suspension for pulmonary monilial infection. The measurement of particle size is difficult and therefore has been attempted by few workers. It should be realised that the statement of the spectrum of particle size delivered by most cheap gas driven nebulisers is but a euphoric estimation by the manufacturers.

The droplet size produced by ultrasonic nebulisers is capable of more precise estimation using energy equations (Robinson, 1970), but the ultrasonic nebulisers have not gained the clinical acclaim that their producers expected. This is because little of the inspired water is in the vapour phase and the necessary cooling of the respiratory tract to produce vapour has deleterious effects on cilial action; furthermore, there is an increase in airways resistance (Cheyney and Butler, 1969), and there is always the danger of water intoxication (particularly in infants). In addition it has proved difficult to obtain precise control over the output of ultrasonic nebulisers. However, there is good clinical evidence that the deposition of particulate water may act as a solvent for viscid sputum retained in the airways, particularly during the early phase of artificial ventilation, but care should be taken if the use of particulate water is continued after this initial phase. If aerosols are to be used for medicaments it should be remembered that often their deposition is required in an area of the lung where there is no ventilation so that patient triggered ventilators with nebulisation therapy may be advantageous. The so-called 'puff therapy' may increase ventilation in those areas of low $\dot{V}_A/\dot{Q}$ where the aerosol is required.

ENDOTRACHEAL INTUBATION

The introduction of plastic endotracheal tubes which are relatively non-irritant coupled with an increasing awareness of the complications of tracheostomy has favoured the use of long-term endotracheal intubation. The incidence of complications with such methods is less and those that occur are usually less severe. Oral endotracheal intubation is simple, reliable and quick, but in some patients is less well tolerated than tracheostomy, the need for sedation being increased. The introduction of prolonged nasal endotracheal intubation (Deane and Mills, 1970) has overcome many of these disadvantages but it should be remembered that tracheal toilet is more difficult via a nasal endotracheal tube. However, prolonged oral endotracheal intubation is finding increasing favour, particularly now that nursing staff are becoming more skilled in managing patients thus intubated so that sedative requirements are decreasing and bronchial toilet is more efficient.

TRAUMA FOLLOWING INTUBATION OR TRACHEOSTOMY

The trachea and larynx seem to suffer injury from tracheostomy or prolonged endotracheal intubation for many reasons, but surprisingly, the duration of intubation or the presence of a cuffed tracheostomy tube do not appear to be major factors (provided these are not of the red rubber variety). Most physicians are now prepared to use prolonged nasotracheal or orotracheal intubation for periods of up to three weeks.

Apart from traumatic intubation there appear to be two main reasons for tracheal erosions and strictures.

Trauma and infection

Tube fixation is most important and movement by the weight of the ventilator tubes or by the energy released by the inflating action of the ventilator, must be minimised. The trachea above the cuff of the tube should be regularly aspirated in order to prevent accumulation of secretions and the attendant risk of secondary infection.

Regular cuff deflation is not effective in preventing tracheal damage and its use is now being abandoned. The size of the tube is important, in one study a permanent tracheostomy appeared to be necessary exclusively in women who had large bore tubes inserted. There is some theoretical evidence that large low pressure cuffs may be an advantage but controlled clinical evidence is lacking.

Trauma during endotracheal toilet has been greatly decreased by suction catheters using a hovercraft principle so that the mucosal damage does not occur (Aero-Flow Sherwood Medical Industries). These catheters are very expensive.

The metabolic state of the patient

The incidence of tracheal erosion is greater in the oedematous patient and in the debilitated. Recent work suggests that the metabolism of trace elements in debilitated patients is altered and there is evidence that such patients are in a negative zinc balance (Editorial, 1973). Metabolic balance studies for such trace elements are difficult to perform and have been little studied. However, the role of zinc in preventing mucosal damage has been established and it is interesting to note that certain manufacturers of amino acids and fat emulsion preparations for parenteral nutrition now include or make available trace elements as supplements (see Part 1, ch. IX, p. 254).

BRONCHOSCOPY

Certain patients when admitted to the I.T.U. have large amounts of retained secretions which are best removed by bronchoscopy, this rarely needs to be repeated. Bronchoscopy may be valuable in the therapeutic management of collapse of a major pulmonary segment. It allows removal of secretions from the relevant bronchus, and if the broncho-scope can be inserted into that bronchus, the segment can often be reinflated. Reinflation can be best achieved by inserting an en-dotracheal tube into the end of the Negus bronchoscope attached to a Mapleson 'C' circuit and by applying a prolonged inspiratory pressure (*vide infra*). This form of therapeutic bronchoscopy has not found much clinical favour because of the danger of producing acute hypoxaemia. The use of a fibre optic bronchoscope which does not require the removal of the tracheostomy or endotracheal tube obviates this difficulty and is being increasingly used (Milledge, 1976).

ARTIFICIAL LUNG VENTILATORS

Introduction

Before reading this section, it is assumed that the reader has a working knowledge of the mechanical and physiological principles involved. (Robinson, 1974b.)

Since the appearance of the new generation of servo ventilators (Elema Servo 900 and Pneumotron 80), it is no longer true that there is no universal ventilator; that is, one which is maximally efficient at treating all forms of respiratory failure (Robinson, 1967). A servo mechanism is a closed loop system in which a small input power controls a large output power in a strictly proportional manner. Servo mechanisms must have two dominant features, firstly control is actuated by a quantity that is affected by the result of the control operation, and secondly a lower power unit controlling a high power operation at a distance.

The control can be mechanical, electrical, pneumatic or a combination, but the servo ventilators are predominantly electrically controlled. In these ventilators the closed loop control is by a negative feedback system, since a positive feedback mechanism would lead to fatal instability. Thus, tidal volume is actually measured and compared with the desired volume, any difference causing an error signal to occur which adjusts the volume of gas delivered during inspiration until the desired volume is achieved. The complete respiratory cycle includes expiration so that, although servo ventilators cycle from inspiration to expiration from a control function (obtained by measuring the volume of gas passing to the patient), the system is not a completely closed loop servo mechanism because the machine is time cycled from expiration to inspiration. All servo ventilators measure the expired tidal volume, compare it with the inspired volume, display the signal, and activate an error alarm if the difference is significant.

The older generation of ventilators have control systems but these are not servo mechanisms because no closed loop exists.

The primary purpose of a lung ventilator is to deliver a set tidal volume into the lungs. This tidal volume is produced indirectly by many ventilators by interpreting the volume of gas delivered into the lungs from parameters effected by the delivery of this volume of gas.

Thus ventilators are cycled from inspiration to expiration by pressure, time, and flow. Ventilators may also be cycled when a volume of gas held as a reservoir has been discharged, usually by the closing of electrical contacts on a bellows (Ohio marketed U.K. Monaghan M228). This system does not represent true volume cycling because even if the set volume is not discharged into the patient the machine will still cycle. It is therefore a volume *preset* device and is no better in this respect than piston/cylinder or bellows machines such as the Cape Ventilator. True volume cycling systems must monitor the volume of gas delivered by the machine at some point in the patient circuit and compare this with the volume expired. A warning device or display should inform the user if there is any discrepancy in these volumes (other than that expected from the respiratory quotient of the patient). True volume cycled machines will probably become universally accepted but because the older types of ventilators are still in use, this chapter seeks to suggest how the best performance can be obtained from these ventilators in the particular type of respiratory failure being treated.

Should monitoring of the inspiratory and expiratory volume be *a primary function of the machine* then it is possible to alter inspiratory flow and pressure patterns and also the expiratory flow and pressure patterns by P.E.E.P. (positive end expiratory pressure), expiratory resistance and the application of a negative phase. Should the volume delivered be used as a control function, i.e. negative feedback, then the control of other primary functions of the machine, I/E ratio, flow pattern, flow rate, type of expiratory phase, etc, will not interact with each other when one is changed. This cannot be true if one of these other functions is used to cycle the ventilator from inspiration to expiration, but we have learnt how to get the best out of the ventilator we are using by a detailed knowledge of the interactions of the controls, so that allowances can be made for any degradation in the performance when the settings are altered. Thus has grown the mystique of the 'ventilator expert' who could get the performance required because of his knowledge of the inadequacy of the behaviour of the machine. The author once considered it necessary to have a detailed knowledge of the workings of ventilators being used but now believes this view was mistaken. We have tended to lose sight of the purpose for which a ventilator was being employed, namely to correct a lung defect. It might be thought that ventilators that allowed the user to independently control most of the functions of the instrument are dreadfully complicated, this is true but does it matter? It does, but only if one persists in believing that the user should know how the machine works. The author is now convinced that the user should know what the ventilator does, not how it does it.

It has been usual to look at the pressure patterns produced during inspiration and expiration for two reasons, firstly they were easier to obtain than other ventilatory indices, and secondly, most ventilators generated a fixed inspiratory flow pattern.

Although it is customary practice to use the airway pressure patterns to analyse the flow and volume traces, in this chapter it is the flow patterns that are used for the primary description of the traces produced.

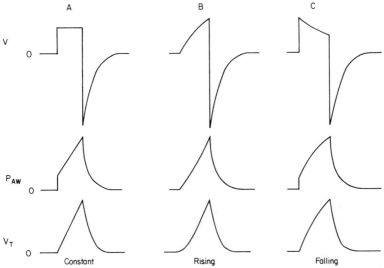

Fig. 2. The three flow modes of ventilation with their resultant airway pressure and tidal volume patterns. $\dot{V}$, flow; P_{aw}, airway pressure; V_T, tidal volume.

There are only three basic inspiratory flow patterns (see Fig. 2). There can be slight modifications of these patterns, e.g. the constant flow pattern can be modified to produce the half sine wave of flow produced by a piston type of ventilator, e.g. the Cape.

Ventilators may be classified according to the method of presenting a volume of gas to the airway, either by pressure generation (Barnet, Phillips, East Radcliffe, etc.) or flow generation (Bird, Loosco, Sheffield, Pneumotron and Servo 900). It is easier, however, to understand the action of a ventilator according to the patterns of flow no matter how they are produced.

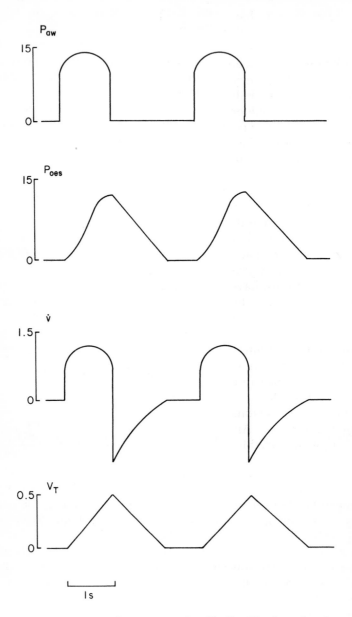

Fig. 3. Half sine wave inspiratory flow pattern produced by Cape Ventilator. P_{aw}, airway pressure (cm H_2O); P_{oes}, oesophageal pressure (cm H_2O).

Inspiratory flow patterns (see Fig. 3)

Over the years there have been conflicting views expressed about the relative effectiveness of various inspiratory flow patterns on the distribution and uptake of the inspired gas. As early as 1956, Otis and his workers observed in analogue models and patient studies that when the breathing frequency was increased, that the 'pulmonary compliance' decreased. Pulmonary compliance was measured by the equation, tidal volume/end inspiratory pressure. The changes observed ought to have been expected because the time constants in the lungs must have remained the same or even slightly greater during the short period of observation when the frequency of ventilation was increased. At the higher respiratory frequencies insufficient time would have been allowed for the gas to enter the alveoli and distribute throughout the lungs, thus the tidal volume would have decreased; and since there was insufficient time for full expiration, the functional residual capacity must have increased. This is partly the explanation for the increase in physiological dead space noted by Watson (1962), and Fairley et al. (1967) when the inspiratory time was shortened to less than 0.5 s. Another factor must have been the maldistribution of inspired gas due to the increase in its velocity when the inspiratory time was shortened (so that the same volume of gas could be given over a shorter time period).

Thus, unless one considers the factor 'time' one cannot to be precise about the characteristics of the flow wave forms used during inspiration and expiration nor can one assess the conflicting work of the various authors in this field.

In order to understand 'time constant' it is necessary to consider exponential function. An exponential function is one in which the rate of change of one variable 'y' is proportional to the magnitude of its own variable 'x' or in mathematical terms $dy/dx = ky$.

Where k is a constant. In our work the first variable is usually time so that

$$\frac{dy}{dt} = ky \quad \text{or} \quad \frac{dy}{dt} = -ky \quad \text{if the quantity decreases with time}$$

It can be shown, in a 'wash out' function that after 1 time constant, the quantity will have fallen to 37% of its initial value or increased to 63% if it is a 'wash in' function.

After 2 time constants, y will have fallen to 13.5% of its initial value (or increased to 86.5%) and after 3 time constants, y falls to 5% of its initial value or (increased to 95%). It can easily be shown that an exponential function will never reach completion but for most physiological functions 95% completion (or 3 time constants) is considered the minimum adequate for near maintenance of physiological homeostasis. (A lucid explanation of the physiological importance of exponential function is to be found in Nunn, 1969.)

When air enters a distending or contracting lung the time constant is governed by two variables, the compliance and airways resistance of the subject. Surprisingly, the product of compliance and resistance is time.

$$\text{Compliance } (C) = l/\text{cm H}_2\text{O}$$
$$\text{Airways resistance } (R) = \text{cm H}_2\text{O}/l/\text{s}$$
$$C \times R = l/\text{cm H}_2\text{O} \times l/\text{cm H}_2\text{O}/\text{s}$$
$$\therefore \text{ the product } CR = \text{seconds}$$

During artificial ventilation a typical compliance is $0.2 l/\text{cm H}_2\text{O}$ and airways resistance 3 cm $\text{H}_2\text{O}/l/\text{s}$.

Thus one time constant: $0.2 \times 3 = 0.6$ s.

It is not surprising therefore that Watson (1962) found an increase in physiological dead space when the inspiratory time was shortened below 0.6 s because his patients must have had only 63% of the inspired gas distributed and taken up by their lungs.

There is now general agreement on the importance of allowing sufficient time for distribution, uptake and excretion of gas in the lungs during artificial ventilation, but little agreement as to whether this distribution, uptake and excretion can be changed by variation of the character or profile of the gas flow into or out of the lungs.

The importance of the shape of the inspiratory wave form has not been firmly established. The opinions of the various authors (Cournard et al., 1948; Otis et al., 1956; Watson, 1962, Herzog and Norlander, 1968; Lygger, 1968; Bergman, 1963, 1967 and 1969) are divided between theoretical considerations derived from analogue models and experimental clinical observations which have frequently produced contrary results. The discrepancies may be due to many factors but are probably related to the difficulty in finding a ventilator which is able to change the inspiratory wave form without changing any other respiratory parameter.

Some workers used different ventilators to produce different wave forms and others used specifically designed pumps which generated a specific pressure pattern. The author believes it more correct to generate a specific flow pattern so that the pressure profile is the resultant of this flow acting upon the patient's compliance and airways resistance. The tidal volume can thus remain constant when these values alter.

When a ventilator which is flow regulated, and volume cycled is assessed in patients with normal respiratory function, it was shown (Johansson, 1975; de Almeida, 1976), that when the 3 inspiratory flow patterns (falling, rising and constant) were studied that the falling or decelerating flow was superior, producing better gas distribution and uptake as measured by alveolar/arterial gradients for oxygen and carbon dioxide and physiological dead space.

These results suggest that in normal patients the decelerating inspiratory flow pattern is marginally better implying that the inspiratory flow pattern is of little importance for approximately 90 per cent of patients treated in an I.T.U. However, this recent work shows the importance of considering the *flow* patterns when considering the effects of artificial ventilation of the lungs, furthermore in the remaining 10% of patients with respiratory failure, the analysis of flow patterns during the 4 phases of action of a ventilator (inspiratory, cycling from inspiration to expiration, expiratory and cycling from expiration to inspiration) allows one to predict the behaviour of the ventilator when used in the various clinical situations posed by the types of respiratory failure requiring ventilator support.

Inspiratory phase – the falling inspiration flow pattern
If the ventilator produces a falling flow pattern into the patient's airways then the pressure must be nearly constant because as the flow declines a lesser volume of gas enters the lungs so the intrathoracic pressure does not rise (Fig. 2). Thus ventilators which produce a nearly constant pressure during inspiration (e.g. the East Radcliffe, East Freeman, Barnet and Phillips AV1, and Manley), give a decelerating flow pattern. The mechanical principles used to produce this pattern are beyond the scope of this chapter, and are described in detail by Mushin and co-workers (1969).

Advantages of the decelerating respiratory flow pattern
Recent work, already referred to, has shown that the falling flow pattern produces the best distribution and uptake of the inspired gas, which probably accounts for the continued popularity of the very early constant pressure generators such as the Radcliffe and Barnet. Although

the basic flow patterns remain the same, these ventilators (as in the East Freeman and Phillips) have been considerably updated.

However, the decelerating flow pattern produces an almost constant pressure in the thorax and this pressure may reduce blood pressure by decreasing cardiac output. In fact, the constant pressure pattern must be approximately twice the form of the pressure pattern produced by the constant flow instruments which have been found by Cournand and his colleagues (1948) to have the least effect on cardiac output. Cardiac embarrassment during institution and artificial ventilation of the lungs is a common phenomenon and this is particularly so in the critically ill patient who commonly has some form of haemodynamic failure. The haemodynamic deficit must be treated either before or concurrently with the institution of artificial ventilation.

Except in an extreme emergency, intubation and ventilation should not be started before ensuring that the dynamic blood volume is adequate (as measured by the right atrial pressure) and that facilities are available for monitoring pulse volume, blood pressure and E.C.G. during the procedure. Should factors be present which have precipitated cardiogenic shock, these should be treated prior to, or during intubation. The management of cardiac dysrhythmias and cardiogenic shock is described in Part 1, ch. III.

Patients who have a normal haemodynamic state should show no cardiovascular response to artificial ventilation other than a slight increase in heart rate (10–15/mm) and a rise in C.V.P. of 5 to 7 cm H_2O. A sudden fall in C.V.P. should be treated immediately by volume replacement with the solution appropriate to the clinical situation and by reducing the pressure transmitted to the thorax either by using a constant inspiratory flow pattern (i.e. rising inspiratory pressure pattern) or by the use of a subatmospheric expiratory phase on the ventilator (*vide infra*). It is axiomatic that whatever pharmacological means are used to institute artificial ventilation these should not of themselves embarrass the cardiovascular system. Far too often drugs are given in doses greater than are required. The dose of drugs or drugs given must be just sufficient to sedate the patient and enable intubation and ventilation to be performed without difficulty.

The decelerating flow pattern produces the best respiratory gas exchange in patients with healthy lungs but such circumstances are not common in the I.T.U. Moreover, this benefit can be achieved only if the constant pressure pattern does not cause a cardiovascular deficit which cannot be overcome by volume 'top up' or the use of drugs to improve cardiac output. The continued use of subatmospheric expiratory phase to overcome a cardiovascular deficit cannot be recommended (*vide infra*).

The decelerating inspiratory flow produces an almost constant inspiratory pressure pattern and the application of a constant pressure is far more efficient at overcoming viscous forces such as those present in lung collapse or consolidation. The re-expansion of such areas depends upon the *rate* at which the strain (force) is applied, that is, a small force applied for a lengthy period is far superior to a large force exerted briefly (Robinson, 1967). This rule also applies to the treatment of the severe crushed chest injury, where not only the deformity of the thoracic wall may be stabilised but the inspiratory atelectasis which is thought to occur in lung segments below the damaged chest wall may be expanded (Robinson, 1968). This probably accounts for the popularity of constant pressure generators in the treatment of chest injuries.

A common problem met during respiratory therapy is the presence of gas leaks in the patient portion of the circuit, e.g. an uncuffed endotracheal tube in young infants or a leak from a broncho-pleural fistula. Little attention appears to have been given to methods of minimising this leak by the control of the inspiratory phase. It can easily be shown that if a constant pressure is applied to such a leak (by the use of a decelerating flow) and sufficient time allowed, then the pressure across the leak will almost equalise. It is surprising, therefore, that constant pressure generators have not been used for ventilating infants. This is probably because it is far easier to design and make a constant flow instrument, whereby the inspiratory flow can be adjusted to a low value, and the tidal volume being given by timing and cycling this flow to give the inspiratory period (Loosco and Sheffield infant ventilators). The recent popularity of the Phillips AV1 as an infant ventilator may be partly because it is a constant pressure generator (decelerating flow) and partly because such a flow pattern is maximally efficient for gas distribution and hence exchange, in the relatively inefficient infant lung. It is not possible to measure the loss of gas at the leak around the endotracheal tube in infants particularly as it occurs both during inspiration and expiration. Gas loss from a broncho-pleural fistula can be measured at the water seal drain, if the gas exit from the bottle is directed through an electronic or mechanical respirometer. A particularly elegant method can be done with the Pneumotron 80, the difference between the inspired tidal volume measured with one transducer and the expired measure with another transducer is displayed *during expiration* as the leak volume on the tidal volume meter which fails to return to its zero setting. It is then possible to adjust the

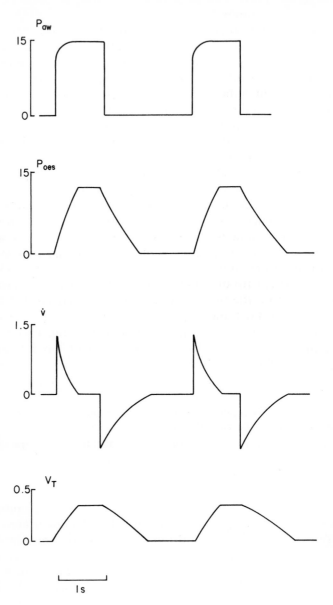

Fig. 4. Pressure flow and volume traces obtained from a patient being ventilated with an East Radcliffe ventilator in which the inspiratory period has been extended for too long a period. Note the unnecessary plateau of intra thoracic pressure seen on the oesophageal pressure trace.

tidal volume and peak flow (keeping a decelerating flow pattern) until the leak is the minimum commensurate with an acceptable inspired oxygen concentration, arterial oxygen and carbon dioxide tensions (*vide infra*).

The decelerating flow pattern appears to have many advantages provided the instrument which delivers it can be adjusted so that the inspiratory phase suits the patient's needs. Emphasis must therefore be placed on the method of cycling from inspiration to expiration.

Sometimes it is the practice to adjust the length of the inspiratory period longer than that necessary to achieve the desired tidal volume; this has the advantage that if there is any change in airways resistance the machine is so set that it will cope with it. However, it must be realised that this will produce a pressure plateau in the thorax after the tidal volume for that particular inspiratory pressure has been produced (Fig. 4). This will occur particularly if the compliance of the patient is lowered because completion (i.e. V_T) will be earlier since reducing the compliance reduces the time constant. It is wise, therefore, unless constant pressure is required to overcome viscous forces, to reduce the inspiratory period with decelerating flow ventilators to the minimum necessary to obtain the best gas exchange (as measured by the tidal volume), the alveolar/arterial gradient for oxygen (Table 1) and the arterial carbon dioxide tension. It is possible to shorten the actual

Table 1. Calculation of the alveolar arterial gradient for oxygen (A-aDO$_2$)

Rapid bedside calculations of the alveolar PO_2 can be made by using a simple form of the equation suggested by Benzinger (1937) and modified by Rossier and Mean (1943).

$$\text{Alveolar } PO_2 = \text{inspired } PO_2 - \frac{\text{arterial } PCO_2 \ (PaCO_2)}{\text{respiratory exchange ratio}}$$

R/Q is usually 0.85 (Nunn *et al.*, 1965) but varies with metabolic rate.

$$\text{Inspired } PO_2 = \frac{(\text{Barometric pressure} - \text{partial pressure of water vapour}) \times \text{inspired oxygen }\%}{100}$$

Barometric pressure 760 mm Hg
Partial pressure water vapour 47 mm Hg

$$\text{Thus inspired } PO_2 = 713 \times \frac{\text{inspired } O_2\% \ (F_IO_2\%)}{100}$$

$$\text{Alveolar } PO_2 = (713 \times F_IO_2) - \frac{PaCO_2 \ (\text{mm Hg})}{\text{Respiratory exchange ratio}}$$

$\therefore$ A-aDO$_2$ = alveolar PO_2 – arterial PO_2

respiratory phase in some decelerating inspiratory flow machines (Phillips and Manley) by setting the machine pressure applied during inspiration higher than that necessary to achieve the desired tidal volume; the length of the inspiratory phase is then decreased so that in the inspiratory time available the desired tidal volume is obtained. This technique of overpressure (Nunn, 1969) has several advantages, the main one being that the inspiratory phase can be shortened so that the ventilator cycles when gas is still entering the chest at a fast rate. This avoids the slow achievement of equilibrium which is taken between the 2nd and 4th time constants. A quite small increase in applied pressure can achieve this object and a working rule is to restrict the overpressure to twice that necessary to achieve the tidal volume if sufficient respiratory time were to be allowed. This technique should not be used if there is an increased airways resistance which greatly extends the time constants. There is also a great danger of over-inflating the lungs if the cycling mechanism fails (because the tidal volume will be doubled) and furthermore an inspiratory pressure limiting safety valve cannot be used because it will prevent the generation of the desired over-pressures. It should also be remembered that the inspiratory phase must not be shortened below 3 time constants (usually 1–2 s) otherwise severe gas distribution and uptake abnormalities become evident. Because of the dangers in the use of overpressure, it is wise to assess its effect on the alveolar/arterial gradient for oxygen (Table 1).

The procedure should be abandoned if the PaO_2 cannot be maintained at 9.3 kPa (70 mm Hg) or greater with an F_IO_2 of not more than 0.5. The Manley ventilator cannot be used in this way because the length of the inspiratory phase is dependent on the rate of fresh gas flow into the storage or cycling bellows. Other true time cycled, decelerating flow (or constant pressure) generators such as the Barnet or Phillips AV1 are suitable.

It is evident that a decelerating flow instrument cannot be used successfully without monitoring tidal volume (V_T) expired by the patient. This should be displayed constantly and in this respect mechanical respirometers are at a disadvantage since the volume reading requires timing or mathematical division by respiratory frequency to obtain V_T. The electronic respirometers do not have this defect (Cox et al., 1974) and must be recommended. It is noteworthy that one time cycled pressure generator, the Phillips AV1, includes such an electronic respirometer.

Even in the early Barnet ventilators the manufacturer produced a flow control and in their later model Phillips AV1 this flow control is simply an adjustable restrictor in the inspiratory limb. This control reduces the flow of gas generated by the machine thus changing the flow pattern from that of decelerating flow to that of an almost constant flow. The ability to change the peak flows and flow profile generated by the ventilator has many theoretical advantages but at the moment little clinical work has assessed the advantages or disadvantages of the various patterns achieved in the management of different types of respiratory failure. If the airways resistance is pathologically high or is so normally (as in infants), then the time constants in the lung are long and considerable advantages can be gained by reducing the peak flows produced by such machines thus enabling a lower pressure to be applied to achieve the required tidal volume. No rules can yet be given for this form of usage, but if the alveolar/arterial oxygen gradient, the arterial carbon dioxide tension, the pressures applied and the tidal and minute volumes achieved are measured, it is possible to find flow and ventilator settings which give the largest improvement in these parameters.

One warning should be given, the restriction to gas flow by such flow controls as on the Phillips AV1 causes the storage bellows on these machines to fill at the end of the inspiratory phase and each successive cycle refills the bellows until the machine cycles from inspiration to expiration with minimal change in the gas volume with the bellows. This is particularly likely to occur if only small tidal volumes are to be delivered, as in paediatric practice. The flow control is relatively coarse and a small change in the position of the flow control limit may suddenly release a large volume of gas from the storage bellows into the infant with possible disastrous results. This problem may soon be overcome but will remain an inherent disadvantage of any ventilator which has a flow control achieved by adding a flow restrictor to the gas delivery line of a storage bellows for inspiratory gas.

The constant flow inspiratory flow generator
This type of machine is common since it is relatively easy to design an instrument which takes the flow of gas from the piped gas supply and delivers it, after suitable reduction in pressure, to the patient. The gas flow must be constant because of the enormous reserve of the piped gas supply and the trivial flow required by the machine. In such ventilators the inspiratory phase is terminated either by timing the inspiratory period or by cycling when the patient's airway pressure reaches a particular value.

The flow patterns produced by such machines (Fig. 2) appears in itself to have no particular advantages but the inspiratory pressure pattern is only half the general shape of the decelerating flow instruments and approximates to that pattern suggested by Cournand and his colleagues (1948) as having the least detrimental effect on cardiac output. Such instruments also have the facility for reduction of the flow values so that it is possible to find a particular flow volume which gives the best distribution and uptake of inspired gas. It must be emphasised that the matching of the flow to the lung mechanics of the patient or his pulmonary time constants requires constant attention because these time constants will alter as treatment proceeds and as the pulmonary defects are overcome, particularly if the machine is pressure cycled. In a pressure cycled machine a disastrous increase in tidal volume can occur as the patient's compliance increases. However, such ventilators (e.g. the Bird) have been deservedly popular for the post-operative respiratory support of patients who have had cardio-pulmonary bypass procedures because they have minimal effects on cardiac output.

If a constant flow generator is time cycled, then the product of the length of the inspiratory period and the flow will give the delivered tidal volume. Because there is great difficulty in measuring the small tidal volumes delivered to infants, constant flow machines which are time cycled from inspiratory to expiration are much in demand (Sheffield, Loosco) since the delivered tidal volume is so readily calculated. However, such a flow pattern is probably not ideal for distribution of inspired gas in infant lungs with their prolonged time constants and certainly it is inefficient at controlling leakage of the inflating gas. Furthermore, such constant flow machines use piped oxygen as their motive power which should not be used as the inflating gas for anything but short periods. The use of air or air/oxygen mixtures to prevent the toxic effects of oxygen on the lung can be achieved with these instruments by driving them with compressed air of medical quality. The clinical use of an injector driven by oxygen to entrain air (e.g. Bird) is fraught with difficulty because such devices do not have a constant entrainment ratio when subjected to back pressure so that the F_IO_2 alters during the inflation cycle. Because of the unreliable F_IO_2 the effectiveness of respiratory therapy cannot be based on calculation of the alveolar/arterial gradient for oxygen. In addition, the use of an injector completely alters the flow characteristics of the ventilator so that it changes from a constant flow to a falling flow generator.

Some ventilators such as the classic Blease Pulmoflator, series of ventilators, accomplish a constant flow pattern by applying the continuous flow of gas from a high frequency displacement pump to a bellows or bag in bottle. However, most of the advantages of these ventilators come from their cycling and/or expiratory phase mechanisms. Another series of ventilators produce a non-constant flow by driving the gas into the patient from a concertina bellows or piston in cylinder, driven from an electric motor (Emerson and Cape ventilators). This flow pattern approximates to that of a constant flow generator (Fig. 3) and has no particular advantages for distribution of inspired gas. Furthermore, as the inspiratory phase is usually limited to produce an inspiratory/expiratory ratio of 1 to 2, these instruments are not as effective at overcoming lung collapse or consolidation as are the decelerating flow generators. The Cape ventilator has an unfortunate characteristic in that to achieve the I/E ratio of 1 : 2 using mechanically timed valves, the first part of inspiration must occur against a closed inspiratory valve so that when the valve does open there is an initial high gas flow into the patient. This cannot be considered helpful in distributing the inspired gas because it must fill the most compliant areas and not enter those areas with long time constants (increased airways resistance). Some patients so ventilated (and the author recalls his own experiences) are distressed by this initial jerk particularly when large tidal volumes are used. Even so, the Cape ventilator has an enviable reputation for reliability and ease of use which becomes evident later when cycling mechanisms are discussed.

The rising flow pattern
Few ventilators produce this flow as their basic inspiratory flow pattern (Fig. 2). The Engstrom ventilator is probably the best example. In this instrument a bag in a bottle is compressed by the flow of air from a piston/cylinder whose volume displacement is greatly in excess of the required tidal volume. This is probably a historical accident because the early Engstrom ventilators need such large volume displacements to power a cuirass type ventilator. The configuration was retained when direct pulmonary ventilation was introduced, the excess gas had to be blown to waste through an adjustable orifice, but the gas escape through this orifice could be relatively small in comparison to that delivered via the bag as tidal volume. As a consequence of this mechanism, as the piston accelerates up the cylinder so does the flow to the patient increase. Attempts have been made to justify this flow and pressure pattern (Herzog and Norlander, 1968). If the time constant in parts of the lung is increased due to high airways resistance this accelerating flow pattern will tend to overcome the resistance because the airway pressure will have risen at the end of inspiration; however, this airways

resistance will still be overcome if the pressure is kept constant and sufficient time is allowed for lung inflation as would occur with the decelerating flow generator. The theoretical justification for this system therefore appears nebulous, nor has any clinical advantage for this system been found.

Inspiratory/expiratory cycling

In the author's view, the most important parameter to consider during artificial ventilation of the lungs is 'time' and this is most readily controlled by the cycling method.

Simple and reliable means of measuring the tidal volume have not previously been available so that many methods of terminating the inspiratory phase were used. A logical consideration of the circumstances requires that the ventilator should cycle when a known volume of gas passes into the patient's airways, and so that leaks may be detected, this volume must be compared with that expired by the patient. This is true volume cycling (Cox and Chapman, 1974). Machines in which a known volume of gas is delivered to the patient and the inspiratory phase terminated when a storage bellows trips a pair of electrical contacts are not volume-cycled but volume-preset (Monaghan M228). Ventilators which have such power that they deliver the set tidal volume no matter what the compliance or airways resistance can be regarded as volume preset machines although they are actually time cycled (e.g. Cape, Engstrom). These machines are able to cope with changes in lung mechanics by increasing the airway pressure which is the resultant of the force generated by the flow acting on the patient's compliance and/or airways resistance (Fig. 5). These machines are deservedly popular with I.T.U. staff because monitoring the airway pressure demonstrates changes in pulmonary mechanics and the machine requires little or no adjustments during use.

Machines which are time cycled from inspiration to expiration and so deliver the fresh gas flow supplied in the set inspiratory period are more difficult to use. Those in which tidal volume can be readily monitored (Phillips AV1) or assessed (Manley) require no further explanation other than to remind the reader of the remarks made on 'overpressure'. However, those in which the tidal or minute volume is estimated from the fresh gas flow (Sheffield, Loosco and Barnet) require some little time to be spent in finding the gas flow settings and inspiratory time to produce the best alveolar/arterial gradient for oxygen.

A simple and cheap method of cycling is to set the peak airway

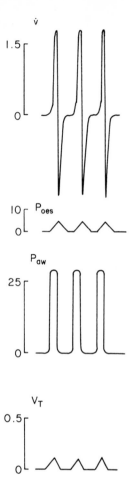

Fig. 5. Pressure flow and volume traces obtained from a patient being ventilated with a volume preset machine (the Cape). The patient had a greatly increased airways resistance, but the ventilator could cope with this load, note that the high airway pressure generated by the machine does not reach the oesophagus (P_{oes}), being lost in overcoming airway resistance.

pressure as the trigger and this requires a constant inspiratory flow (i.e. rising pressure pattern). This system is adequate for brief periods, particularly in patients who are not expected to change their respiratory mechanics, but is hopelessly inadequate for patients with changing compliance or airways resistance when the pressure set may be far too low to produce an adequate tidal volume (Fig. 6). Such machines require the tidal volume to be monitored at frequent intervals

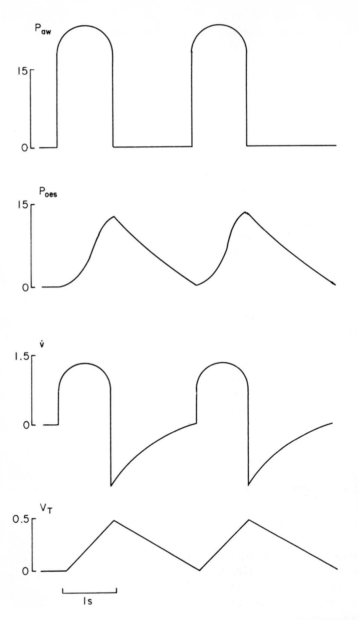

Fig. 6. Pressure flow and volume traces obtained from a patient being ventilated by a pressure cycled Bird ventilator. Although the cycling pressure is set at 30 cm H_2O this is quite inadequate to ventilate the patient, so that the tidal volume is less than 0.1l.

and the advantage of being able to control the flow values to cope with the huge airways resistance is minimal when set against the constant attention the machine requires.

The expiratory phase

Most ventilators open a valve and allow the patient's airways to vent to atmosphere. It is important to realise that in this form of expiration if the lung compliance is reduced, so is the time constant, and emptying will occur more quickly. Conversely, if the patient has an increased airways resistance the time constant is increased and a longer period must be allowed for expiration. Almost *all* ventilators are time cycled at the end of expiration so that the expiratory period should be alterable: the optimum ratio between the length of the inspiratory period to the expiratory period is usually 1:2. Certain ventilators such as the Cape have this ratio fixed. However, if the compliance is greatly reduced then the ratio can be reduced (even approaching 1:1) remembering if the minute volume is to be kept the same the tidal volume must be reduced because the respiratory frequency will be increased.

The consequent elevation in mean intrathoracic pressure this manoeuvre creates, must not cause deterioration in cardiovascular performance. Thus, alteration in gas exchange must be assessed by calculation of the alveolar arterial gradient for oxygen. Conversely the I/E ratio may be increased if the airways resistance is pathologically high but conversely the tidal volume must be increased to maintain the same minute volume because the respiratory frequency falls.

Subatmospheric expiratory phase
It was originally suggested (Esplen, 1952), that if the ventilator generated a negative pressure during expiration, this might assist expiratory gas flow. Later it was realised that the application of a negative expiratory phase could reduce the mean intrathoracic pressure during the whole of one respiratory cycle: the negative phase is now commonly used for this purpose. Should cardiac output fall as a consequence of starting artificial ventilation, a negative phase can be applied to correct this but should be used as a temporary measure only. The cardiovascular deficit must be corrected and not masked by the use of the negative phase. The use of a negative phase may produce intra-alveolar pulmonary oedema and any tendency towards this condition is a contraindication for its use.

Although the negative phase was suggested as a means of increasing

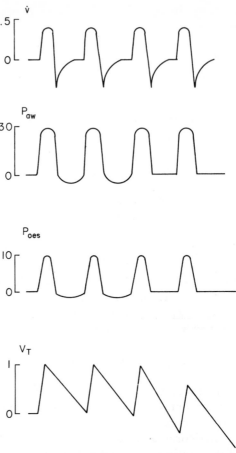

Fig. 7. Pressure flow and volume from a patient being ventilated with a negative expiratory phase from a Cape ventilator. The volume trace shows an increase in expired to inspired volume, which is due to 'trapping'.

lung emptying, in those patients whose closing volume is near to their functional residual capacity (Sutherland *et al.*, 1968), the application of a subatmospheric phase may cause 'trapping' (that is excess gas remaining in the lung at the end of expiration) (Fig. 7). The negative phase should be avoided in such patients and never used routinely in most patients. A similar example of the same phenomena is the increased airways resistance which occurs with the use of a negative phase (Fig. 8), the inverse shows that that component of the airway pressure due to an increase in airways resistance is very striking, *vide infra* (Fig. 10).

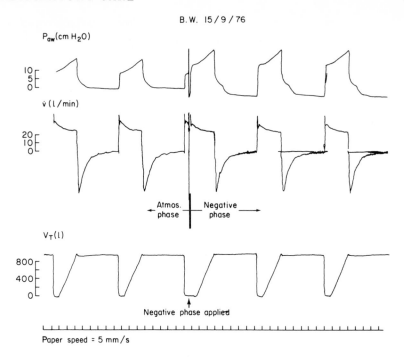

B.W. 15/9/76

P_{aw}(cm H$_2$O)

10
5
0

v̇ (l/min)

20
10
0

Atmos. | Negative
phase | phase

V_T(l)

800
400
0

Negative phase applied

Paper speed = 5 mm/s

Fig. 8. When a negative phase is applied, the vertical component of the airways pressure pattern *falls* until the flow proceeds from the *lungs* and causes the usual compliance slope.

The various methods employed for generating this negative phase have many varying and complex effects on expiratory flow patterns. This complexity is increased by the addition of flow and pressure relief valves. It is therefore impracticable to attempt to analyse the mechanism of production of the negative phase in various ventilators but some general rules can be given. Those ventilators which produce a subatmospheric phase by re-directing the inflating gas to power an entrainment device may actually impede expiratory flow, since the injector acts as a series resistance, its entrainment ratio being insufficient to take the high initial gas flows generated during passive expiration. This becomes evident if the gas supply to the injector can be controlled and reduced (Pneumotron 80, Bird and Blease). The reduction in expiratory gas flow is then similar to that obtained with an expiratory resistance which may be an unwanted and unexpected effect. If the negative phase is generated by an expanding bellows (Cape, Barnet, East Radcliffe, etc.) the flows generated may be very high and 'trapping' becomes probable.

Two other types of expiratory phase modification have recently been introduced, the application of an expiratory resistance and the application of an end expiratory pressure.

End expiratory resistance

The passively generated expiratory flow from the patient is made to pass through an adjustable orifice which impedes flow by acting as a resistance. The designs available, range from a series of holes of varying size to a continually adjustable hole using an iris diaphragm. Such devices greatly reduce the peak expiratory flow and may well prevent 'trapping' in those patients with easily collapsible minor airways, such as those with generalised obstructive lung disease. If an expiratory resistance is effective in preventing trapping, the physiological dead space is reduced so that the arterial carbon dioxide tension falls even though the tidal volume and frequency of the ventilator remains the same as before the application of the resistance. When flow ceases there will be no pressure applied to the airways so that an expiratory resistance has no effect on lung volumes. The clinical benefit of end expiratory resistance is measured by the fall in $PaCO_2$ when V_T and min $\dot{V}$ remain the same as before its use.

Positive end expiratory pressure (P.E.E.P.)

The functional residual capacity falls in patients being artificially ventilated. This may be raised by never allowing the intrathoracic pressure to reach atmospheric during expiration by applying a continuous and constant pressure to the expired gases. P.E.E.P. is generally achieved by directing a flow of gas against the expiratory gas stream (Blease, Pneumotron 80). Examination of the compliance curve reveals that altering the airway pressure range over which the tidal volume is obtained will raise the volume of gas in the lungs at the end of expiration (the F.R.C.) and as inflation takes place higher up the compliance curve, the lungs are more compliant and hence less pressure is required to achieve the desired tidal volume. A decrease in F.R.C. has been suggested as one of the causes of the increased alveolar/arterial oxygen gradients seen during anaesthesia (Nunn et al., 1965a) and during artificial ventilation of the lungs. If arterial hypoxaemia is a problem, the use of an end expiratory pressure is sometimes beneficial although care should be taken not to degrade cardiovascular performance which of itself will produce hypoxaemia.

The end expiratory pressure applied should not exceed 5–10 cm H_2O because higher values will certainly affect cardiac output in patients who have haemodynamic instability. The method by which the end expiratory pressure is applied should be known because certain devices allegedly produce a positive end expiratory pressure by the use of a spring loaded disc valve in the expiratory gas passages. This is not a true pressure generating device since the gas flows through an orifice thereby generating a resistance to flow before it produces an end expiratory pressure. An end expiratory pressure can simply be obtained by placing the outlet of the expiratory limb of the ventilator below the level of an open container of water, the depth of the end of the hose below the level of water being the elevated end expiratory pressure.

The benefit of end expiratory pressure in correcting arterial hypoxaemia complicating a ventilation/perfusion disturbance as in intra-alveolar pulmonary oedema, and blast injuries of the lung has been well established. One feature of this technique which is sometimes overlooked is that because the patients are being ventilated in a more compliant range, i.e. at higher lung volumes, the peak expiratory flow may be increased. The total expiratory gas flow is unchanged because the range of pressures applied over the whole of a respiratory cycle must remain the same, inspiration starting at the elevated end expiratory pressure (Fig. 11).

Increased peak expiratory flows may have adverse effects on regional lung emptying $(A-aDO_2)$ and $(a-ADCO_2)$, and if the application of P.E.E.P. results in no improvement in the alveolar/arterial oxygen gradient, particularly if this is accompanied by some elevation of $PaCO_2$ (tidal volume and frequency being kept constant) then the addition of a minimal expiratory resistance should be tried (Fig. 9). In such a situation it is often helpful to use both an end expiratory pressure and an end expiratory resistance.

Although the various types of ventilators can be used successfully if these attributes and defects are known, the author firmly believes that if a ventilator is truly volume cycled from inspiration to expiration by the use of a volume transducer and if this value is compared with the expired volume, then the delivered flow can be easily adjusted to that desired by the operator (Cox and Chapman, 1974; Johansson, 1975). Thus, the new so-called servo ventilators must become the ventilators of choice. Once inspired and expired volumes can be measured it is a simple matter to change flow patterns, inspiratory and expiratory time, and minute volume which will result in a change in respiratory frequency. The important factor is that none of these controls will

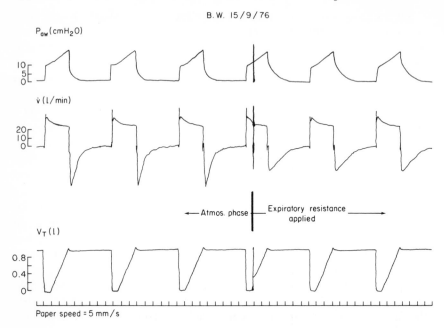

B.W. 15/9/76

Fig. 9. Use of end expiratory resistance in same patient as in Fig. 8. Note the use of a resistance has slowed the expiratory flow. V_D/V_T estimations indicating a reduction in 'trapping'.

interact and thus the ventilator can be set in whatever manner the operator requires without the necessity for a knowledge of the working of the control functions and their interaction.

If a constant inspiratory flow pattern is used to inflate the patient and the patient's airways pressure (x) is displayed as an oscilloscope trace against time base (Y), then the display gives a very good indication of the forces required to overcome compliance and airways resistance. A complete explanation is given by Don and Robson (1965). Referring to Fig. 10, a,b, is the pressure required to overcome airways resistance and is seen to rise vertically because no flow occurs into the lung until airway resistance is overcome. The slope of the pressure rise from b to c is that due to compliance. The constant flow inspiratory pattern when displayed as a pressure trace on an oscilloscope enables a ready appreciation to be made of the various components of the resistance to inflation of the lungs. This type of oscilloscope display is increasingly used and is offered by several ventilator manufacturers. An example of its use is shown in Fig. 8. It can be seen that the use of a negative phase in this elderly man with chronic obstructive lung disease doubled his

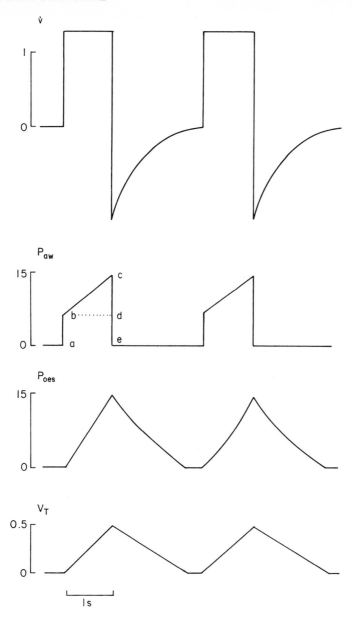

Fig. 10. Pressure flow and volume traces obtained from a patient using a constant flow generator. The separation of the pressure pattern components due to airways resistance and compliance can easily be seen (Don and Robson, 1965). See also Fig. 8.

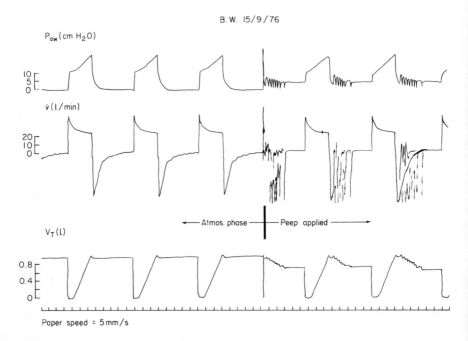

B.W. 15/9/76

Paper speed = 5mm/s

Fig. 11. Application of P.E.E.P. to the same patient as Fig. 8. The application of the P.E.E.P. valve in this ventilator (Pneumotron 80) gives an oscillating flow and pressure pattern because the solenoid operated valve opens or closes as the set P.E.E.P. pressure is reached. However, the estimated expiratory flow trace drawn in over the final flow curve does show that the application of P.E.E.P. increases the rate of expiratory flow although not its total volume.

airways resistance. A simple airway pressure display on an oscilloscope, with the facility to alter the flow pattern (both inspiratory and expiratory) on the ventilator may give answers to many clinical problems posed during ventilator therapy. Similarly, as such ventilators in effect meter the compressed fresh gas flow, the concentration of oxygen delivered to the patient can be easily altered.

Once ventilators have accurate means of measuring flow, volume and airway pressure then by using an inspiratory hold, total thoracic compliance can be measured. The hold is necessary to allow the airway pressure to equilibrate with alveolar pressure (i.e. 3 + time constants). If the compliance is measured and the expiratory flow from a pneumotachograph trace is recorded, then from this trace, the time taken for 63% of the expiratory volume to occur is measured. As expiration occurs exponentially this must equal one respiratory time constant, but as the product of compliance and airways resistance is one time constant and compliance is already known, simple division of the time constant by the compliance value will give the airways resistance. Thus the airways resistance can be calculated. One manufacturer of a servo ventilator is already offering a digital readout from electrical calculation of such values which gives surprisingly accurate results. The advantage of knowing these values and any changes in them is very obvious.

Control of ventilation

Most patients, after an initial period, comply easily with the imposed pattern of the ventilator. If a patient begins to 'fight' the ventilator it is wise to find out why, rather than controlling the situation pharmacologically. Patients with severe ventilation/perfusion disturbances can seldom be ventilated without pharmacological control but this should cease as soon as sufficient correction of the abnormality is achieved.

Weaning

Once a patient has been ventilated for some time it is often difficult to establish adequate spontaneous ventilation. A number of ventilators have the facility for terminating the expiratory phase when the patient generates a subatmospheric phase i.e. patient triggering. This can be used to wean patients from ventilators, the respiratory muscles can be given increasing work to do by increasing the subatmospheric pressure necessary to trigger the machine so that eventually the patient is glad to breathe spontaneously. Sometimes, minor changes in lung mechanics or sheer terror causes patients to trigger the ventilator at such a fast rate that the physiological dead space rises alarmingly. Such patients responded remarkably well to small doses of narcotics and often maintain an adequate breathing pattern once this is established. Patient triggering is not to be recommended during actual ventilator therapy particularly when treating severe pulmonary failure since the consequent pressure swings make the ventilation/perfusion abnormalities very much worse.

A much more elegant method of re-establishing spontaneous ventilation is by the technique of intermittent mandatory ventilation.

Originally I.M.V. was achieved by setting a minimal minute volume (usually obtained by using a preset tidal volume and respiratory frequency) and allowing the patient to breathe spontaneously through a separate breathing circuit.

If the machine is a servo ventilator then the operator can decide on the required minute volume and if the volume monitors on the machine do not show the patient has reached this value spontaneously, the machine then ventilates his lungs at a preset tidal volume and frequency until the desired minute volume is reached. Obviously such machines require an accurate volume monitor but it is difficult to see how any judgement of ventilator performance can be made without one.

Servo ventilators do have an accurate expiratory volume meter so that this form of I.M.V. is easily achieved. Such a system has been developed for one instrument using the expiratory volume controls and its alarm circuits. It seems likely that other manufacturers will finally attempt to close the second part of the control loop by using negative feedback to terminate expiration. The author believes this further development of servo ventilators will be slow.

I.M.V. can be used in patients who only require respiratory support i.e. not total control of ventilation and the technique has been enthusiastically received by most of those who have used it.

The same cannot be said for the sigh mechanism the claims for which have never been substantiated by others.

CONCLUSION

This chapter would have been considerably shorter and more comprehensible if only the newer 'servo' ventilator were discussed, but so many of the other generations of ventilators are still in use that some guide to their operation must be given.

It must not be forgotten that if control of inspiratory flow patterns proves as important as seems likely, then certain plenum type humidifiers (i.e. hot water) will need to be discarded since the compressible gas volume is so large as to effectively change whatever flow pattern is introduced to them by the ventilator.

REFERENCES

Benzinger, T. (1937). Untersuchungen über die Atmung und den Gasstoffwechsel insbesondere bei Sauerstoffmangel und Unterdruck, mit fortlaufend unmittelbar aufzeichenden Methoden. *Ergeb. Physiol.* **40**, 1.

Bergman, N. A. (1963). Effect of different pressure breathing patterns on alveolar-arterial gradients in dogs. *J. App. Physiol.* **18**, 1049.

Bergman, N. A. (1967). Effect of varying wave form on gas exchange. *Anaesthesiology* **28**, 290.

Bergman, N. A. (1969). Effects of varying respiratory wave forms on distribution of inspired gas during artificial ventilation. *Am. Rev. Resp. Dis.* **100**, 518.

Cheyney, F. W. and Butler, J. (1969). The effect of ultrasonically produced aerosols on airway resistance in Man. *Anaesthesiology* **29**, 1099.

Cournand, A., Motley, H. L., Werko, L. and Richards, D. W. (1948). Physiological studies of the effects of intermittent positive pressure breathing on cardiac output in Man. *Am. J. Physiol.* **152**, 162.

Cox, L. A., de Almeida, A. P., Robinson, J. S. and Horsley, J. K. (1974). An electronic respirometer. *Brit. J. Anaesth.* **45**, 302.

Cox, L. A. and Chapman, E. D. W. (1974). A comprehensive volume cycled lung ventilator embodying feedback control. *Med. Biol. Enging.* 160.

De Almeida, A. P. (1975). Some effects on inspiratory flow patterns on blood gas exchange in artificial ventilation during anaesthesia. Ph.D. Thesis.

Deane, R. S. and Mills, E. L. (1970). Prolonged naso tracheal intubation in adults. *Anaes. and Anal. Curr. Res.* **49**, 89.

Don, H. R. and Robson, J. G. (1965). The mechanics of the respiratory system during anaesthesia. *Anaesthesiology* **26**, 168.

Editorial (1973). *Brit. Med. J.* **4**, 313.

Esplen, J. R. (1952). A new apparatus for intermittent pulmonary inflation. *Brit. J. Anaes.* **24**, 305.

Fairley, H. B. and Blenkarm, G. D. (1966). Effect on pulmonary gas exchange of variations in inspiratory flow rate during intermittent positive pressure ventilation. *Brit. J. Anaesth.* **38**, 320.

Hatch, T. F. and Gross, P. (1964). *In* 'Pulmonary Deposition and Retention of Inhaled Aerosols'. Academic Press, New York.

Hayes, B. and Robinson, J. S. (1970). An assessment of methods of humidification of inspired gas. *Brit. J. Anaesth.* **42**, 94.

Herzog, P. and Norlander, O. P. (1968). Distribution of alveolar volumes with different types of positive pressure gas flow patterns. *Opuscula Medica* **13**, 27.

Johansson, H. (1975). Effects on breathing mechanics and gas exchange of different inspiratory gas flow patterns in patients undergoing respiratory treatment. *Acta Anaesth. Scand.* **19**, 19.

Lygger, S. (1966). Influence of flow pattern on the distribution of respiratory air during intermittent positive pressure ventilation. *Acta Anaesth. Scand.* **12**, 191.

McClelland, R. N. A. (1970). 'History of Tracheostomy'. Proc. of 4th World Congress of Anaesthesiology, 195. Amsterdam, Excerpta Medica.

Milledge, J. S. (1976). Therapeutic fibre optic bronchoscopy in intensive care. *Brit. Med. J.* **2**, 142.

Mushin, W. W., Rendell Baker, L., Thompson, P. W. and Mapleson, W. W. (1969). *In* 'Automatic Ventilation of the Lungs'. Blackwell, Oxford.

Nunn, J. F. (1969). 'Applied Respiratory Physiology with Special Reference to Anaesthesia'. Butterworth, London.

Nunn, J. F., Bergman, N. A. and Cleman, A. J. (1965a). Factors influencing the arterial oxygen tension during anaesthesia with artificial ventilation. *Brit. J. Anaes.* **37**, 898.

Nunn, J. F., Coleman, A. J., Sachithanadan, T., Bergman, N. A. and Laws, J. W. (1965). Hypoxaemia and atelectasis produced by forced expiration. *Brit. J. Anaesth.* **37**, 3.

Otis, A. B., Mekerrow, C. B., Bartlett, R. A., Mead, J., Mellroy, M. B., Selverstone, N. J. and Radford, E. P. (1956). Mechanical factors in distribution of pulmonary ventilation. *J. App. Physiol.* **8**, 427.

Robinson, J. S. (1967). The Choice of a Ventilator, p. 190. *In* 'Modern Trends in Anaesthesia III' (Ed. F. T. Evans and J. C. Gray). Butterworth, London.

Robinson, J. S. (1968). The critically crushed chest. *Proc. R.S.M.* **6**, 218.

Robinson, J. S. (1974a). Humidification, p. 488. *In* 'Scientific Foundations of Anaesthesia' (Ed. C. Scurr and S. Feldman). Heineman, London.

Robinson, J. S. (1974b). Automatic Lung Ventilators, p. 469. *In* 'Scientific Foundations of Anaesthesia' (Ed. C. Scurr and S. Feldman). Heineman, London.

Russier, P. H. and Mehr, H. (1943). L'insulfiaire pulmonaire ses diverses formes. *J. Suisse Med.* **11**, 327.

Sutherland, P. W., Katsura, T. and Milic Emili, J. (1968). Previous volume history of the lung and regional distribution of gas. *J. App. Physiol.* **25**, 566.

Watson, W. E. (1962). Observations on physiological dead space during intermittent positive pressure respiration. *Brit. J. Anaesth.* **34**, 502.

III

Cardiac Care

R. S. WINWOOD

THE MANAGEMENT OF CARDIAC DYSRHYTHMIAS
Introduction

Abnormalities in cardiac rhythm occur frequently in the critically ill; their management is an important part of I.T.U. work.

The treatment of cardiac dysrhythmias has been improved by greater accuracy in diagnosis and by advances in electrophysiology. Nevertheless, in many cases treatment necessarily remains pragmatic (Krikler, 1974) and one treatment may be more appropriate than another in individual cases of a given dysrhythmia.

A few general points are worth mentioning before considering the management of specific dysrhythmias.

1. The mere occurrence of a dysrhythmia does not constitute an indication for treatment. Asymptomatic dysrhythmias, causing no significant haemodynamic impairment, are often initially best left alone. Even these merit treatment, however, if they are of a kind which frequently herald a more serious rhythm disturbance.

2. If the dysrhythmia is secondary to severe haemodynamic impairment, it is likely to be abolished only by successful treatment of the latter, which therefore takes precedence.

41

3. Factors which promote dysrhythmias include pain, fear and other causes of excessive sympathetico-adrenal discharge, hypoxia, metabolic acidosis, electrolyte disturbances and drugs, especially digitalis glycosides.

4. All antidysrhythmic drugs can, in high dosage, cause myocardial depression.

Of contributors to this subject, Julian (1968), Oliver and Julian (1970) and Aber (1973) deal particularly with arrhythmias following acute myocardial infarction. Krikler and Goodwin (1975) concern themselves with fundamental and investigative aspects of rhythm disturbances and with certain specific dysrhythmias and treatments.

Sinus tachycardia, bradycardia and atrial extrasystoles

Sinus tachycardia

Causes include pain, emotion, fever and thyrotoxicosis. Apart from attention to the underlying condition, no therapy is usually required.

Sinus bradycardia

Causes include athleticism, digitalis intoxication, beta-blockade, opiates and the 'sick sinus' syndrome.

After acute myocardial infarction, treatment is probably advisable if (a) the sinus rate is less than 50/min or (b) it is less than 60/min and associated with ventricular premature beats or hypotension. Elevation of the legs may alone increase the heart rate. If this simple measure is inadequate, atropine may be given intravenously or intramuscularly and repeated as necessary. The value of increasing the heart rate in this way cannot, however, be uncritically accepted (Epstein *et al.*, 1972 and Lie *et al.*, 1974). It has been suggested that ventricular extrasystoles associated with bradycardia, in contrast to those associated with tachycardia, are mostly benign and unlikely to herald ventricular fibrillation. Even hypotension, in the absence of pallor and sweating, may be well tolerated. It has also been suggested that an increased heart rate could be inimical to ischaemic heart muscle which is tolerating bradycardia.

The intravenous dose of atropine usually lies between 0.3 mg and 1.2 mg but should be titrated slowly in increments of not more than 0.3 mg. An excessive increase in heart rate (to above 110/min) after acute myocardial infarction is undesirable as it may cause myocardial oxygen requirements to exceed supplies, resulting in extension of the infarct. Atropine occasionally causes ventricular fibrillation, by inducing a state of unopposed sympathetic activity.

If sinus bradycardia does not respond to atropine, pacing (which can be atrial) may be necessary.

Atrial extrasystoles
No treatment is usually required, but if very frequent digitalisation might be considered.

Supraventricular tachycardia, atrial flutter and atrial fibrillation

Treatment should be given if the ventricular rate exceeds 120/min. The following measures may be tried, although not necessarily in the order given.

1. *Carotid sinus pressure* may terminate supraventricular tachycardia. An electrocardiogram should be recorded during the procedure since a period of asystole occasionally occurs.

2. A *beta-blocker* by slow intravenous injection may abolish supraventricular tachycardia. Examples are practolol ('Eraldin') and acebutolol ('Sectral') up to 25 mg, and Sotalol ('Beta-Cardone') 10–20 mg, repeated if necessary.

3. *Digoxin* 0.5 mg orally, intramuscularly or intravenously, depending on urgency, provided the patient has not had a digitalis preparation in the previous two weeks. This may be followed by 0.25 mg orally every 6 h until the patient is digitalised. The initial dose is usually given intravenously if the ventricular rate exceeds 140/min or if there is pulmonary oedema. Digitalis glycosides are of most use in cases of atrial fibrillation.

Intravenous digoxin may cause a lethal dysrhythmia if the patient has recently received a cardiac glycoside or has renal impairment or electrolyte abnormalities. Digitalis induces enhanced ventricular automaticity which is potentiated by low potassium or high calcium concentrations.

4. *Verapamil* ('Cordilox') is very effective in the treatment of AV nodal tachycardia and in the reciprocating tachycardia of the Wolff-Parkinson-White (WPW) syndrome (Krikler and Spurrell, 1974). 5–10 mg should be given by slow intravenous injection. If this promptly terminates the tachycardia, an 8-hourly oral dose of 40–120 mg may be given prophylactically.

5. *Disopyramide* ('Rhythmodan') produces little effect on the AV node (Spurrell, 1976) and is therefore unlikely to terminate nodal

tachycardia. However, the drug may suppress atrial and ventricular premature beats and may terminate tachycardias due to a re-entrant mechanism in either the atria or the ventricles. The intravenous dose is 2 mg/kg B.W. (max 150 mg) injected over 5 min, followed by 0.4 mg/kg hourly by i.v. infusion. Oral dosage is 300–800 mg daily in divided doses. In the treatment and prophylaxis of reciprocating tachycardias associated with the WPW syndrome, disopyramide may be the drug of choice. However, identification and section of the anomalous pathway may be more satisfactory in some cases and mandatory in patients with refractory tachycardias.

6. *Electroversion (d.c. cardioversion)*. The whole subject of electroversion has been helpfully reviewed by Resnekov (1973). He emphasises the importance of the correct choice of patients and meticulous attention to detail, including the correction of electrolyte imbalance if present, the postponement of treatment in the presence of over-digitalisation, proper synchronisation and correct choice of anti-dysrhythmic agents. He urges the clinician to beware of the tachycardia of the sick sinus syndrome. Electroversion in these patients should be preceded by the insertion of a pacing electrode into the right ventricle for there is a very high risk of profound bradycardia or asystole immediately after the shock. The clinician is also urged to beware of digitalis-induced dysrhythmias, for which electroversion is contraindicated except under the most exceptional circumstances. Always it is wise to start with low-energy settings (e.g. 5 J) in digitalised patients and to stop if showers of ventricular premature beats are induced.

It is important to ensure that the patient's skin is isolated from the metal of the bed, trolley or operating table during electroversion. The physician and assisting personnel must not touch the patient or bed during the electric discharge and *it is the physician's duty to give a clear and adequate warning before he presses the button.*

Synchronised electroversion should be considered for the treatment of supraventricular dysrhythmias if the ventricular rate exceeds 140/min or if drugs are ineffective. For atrial flutter it is often the treatment of choice because it is generally better for a patient to be in sinus rhythm or controllable atrial fibrillation than in atrial flutter variably blocked by digitalis. Atrial flutter is an unstable rhythm. Remarkably small energy outputs, sometimes as small as 5 J and commonly less than 40 J may be successful in its conversion. Such small doses of electrical energy can usually be tolerated by the conscious patient, with minimal sedation, if he or she is warned to expect a sudden jerk.

Electroversion may be the first line of treatment in supraventricular dysrhythmias if there is great urgency because of, for example, associated heart failure or shock.

Diazepam amnesia is usually satisfactory for electroversion; an anaesthetist should be in attendance. The initial energy loading, except in atrial flutter and in digitalised patients, should be 50 J. If even 300 J is unsuccessful, it is worth repeating the procedure after intravenous injection of 10 mg of practolol, acebutalol or sotalol.

A digitalised patient requiring electroversion should have any potassium deficit corrected by an intravenous infusion (never a direct intravenous injection) of potassium chloride. An intravenous injection of a beta-blocker (e.g. sotalol 10 mg) or phenytoin 100 mg may also be wise if there is any doubt about possible digitalis toxicity or if there is no time to estimate the serum potassium level.

After electroversion, oral digitalis, disopyramide (Rythmodan, 100 mg 6-hourly) or other appropriate drug is given to prevent recurrences of the dysrhythmia. Occasionally, troublesome recurrences occur in spite of prophylactic drugs. Atrial pacing should then be considered.

7. *Atrial pacing.* Atrial and AV junctional tachycardias and atrial flutter can be effectively treated by 'overdrive' atrial pacing i.e. pacing the atrium at a rate faster than the ectopic tachycardia. When control of the heart has been captured, the pacing rate can be reduced and pacing discontinued, leaving the electrode *in situ*. The process can be repeated as often as necessary. If the problem is one of recurrences of dysrhythmia, pacing at a rate faster than the sinus rate may prevent them.

Refractory atrial tachycardias can be treated by very rapid atrial pacing (rate 3000/min), thereby inducing atrial fibrillation which is amenable to control.

Atrial pacing avoids the disadvantages of electroversion and cardiodepressant doses of antidysrhythmic drugs. Furthermore, it can be used even when an excess of digitalis has been given.

8. Drugs which are occasionally successful in refractory arrhythmias include edrephonium, phentolamine and procainamide.

Edrephonium is given in doses of 2.5 mg intravenously, repeated at 2 min intervals up to a total of 10 mg. If this slows the ventricular rate, 0.25–2.0 mg per minute may be infused continuously until reversion occurs spontaneously or as the result of electric countershock.

Phentolamine is given in 5 mg doses intravenously.

Procainamide is given as for ventricular tachycardia.

Paroxysmal atrial tachycardia with AV block

This is characterised by long PR intervals or dropped beats.

Provided that the patient has not been taking a digitalis glycoside, the dysrhythmia is treated like other atrial arrhythmias. If, however, digitalis has been taken recently, no more should be given, but potassium chloride should be administered, preferably by mouth (e.g. 'Slow K' 1.8 g, 3 tablets, 8 hourly). If there is great urgency, potassium chloride may be given by intravenous infusion of 50 mmol in 500 ml 5% dextrose at a rate not exceeding 15 mmol/h. Phenytoin or a beta-blocker may be given intravenously if tachycardia merits it.

AV junctional rhythm

Often this requires no treatment but occasionally, after acute myocardial infarction, ventricular pacing is required if the rate is less than 60/min.

Ventricular dysrhythmias

Ventricular premature beats (VPBs)

Digitalis should be considered as a possible cause, particularly if VPBs are multiform. Phenytoin is probably the best drug for treating digitalis-induced arrhythmias but potassium chloride and beta-blockers are often effective.

Unifocal VPBs in an otherwise normal electrocardiogram are nearly always benign.

If VPBs, after acute myocardial infarction, are associated with bradycardia, treatment of the latter with atropine will often abolish them (but see p. 42).

Ventricular extrasystoles are common after acute myocardial infarction and are usually benign but may herald ventricular tachycardia or ventricular fibrillation. The traditional indications for suppressing them are probably too wide (Campbell, 1975), but it is generally agreed that the R on T type and multiform ventricular extrasystoles should be suppressed. This is done with lignocaine or one of the other drugs used in the treatment of ventricular tachycardia.

Ventricular tachycardia

Unless the cause is digitalis, lignocaine is the treatment of choice.

Lignocaine ('Xylocard') is given over 1–2 min intravenously in a bolus dose of 100 mg followed by a continuous intravenous infusion of 1–4 mg/min. The infusion is prepared by adding 1 g of lignocaine to 500 ml of dextrose (5%) solution. It is continued for a minimum of 36 h.

Further bolus doses of 50–100 mg lignocaine may be given if ventricular ectopic beats reappear.

Therapeutic plasma levels of lignocaine lie between 1 and 6 μg/ml.

If, in spite of lignocaine, ventricular tachycardia persists and is associated with hypotension or heart failure, *electroversion* is used. If countershock fails, it should be repeated after a further intravenous bolus of 100 mg lignocaine. After electroversion, suppressive therapy is necessary using lignocaine or one of its alternatives.

Excessive doses of lignocaine may cause central nervous or cardiovascular effects such as drowsiness, disorientation, tremor, convulsions, respiratory depression, hypotension and bradycardia. The risk of overdosage is increased, and lower doses are therefore advisable, in patients with severely impaired hepatic or renal function.

Mexiletine ('Mexitil') is an amine with some structural similarity to phenytoin. It is given in a dose of 100–250 mg intravenously over five to ten minutes, followed by an intravenous infusion of 250 mg over one hour and a further 250 mg over two hours. The infusion rate should then be adjusted to 1 mg/min. Therapeutic plasma concentrations are in the range 1–2 μg/ml.

The most common side effect of the bolus is vomiting, but hypotension, with or without bradycardia, may also occur. The rate of injection or infusion is appropriately reduced and atropine is given for bradycardia.

Mexiletine is of most value in its oral form and provides useful oral prophylaxis when infusions of lignocaine or other drugs are discontinued. An initial loading dose of 400–600 mg is followed after two hours by a regime of 200–250 mg three or four times a day. If the patient is already receiving the drug intravenously, a loading dose is not required provided that oral treatment is commenced before the infusion is discontinued.

Oral prophylaxis may alternatively be provided by quinidine after a lignocaine infusion. 'Kinidin Durules' 1–3 (250–750 mg) twice daily are suitable. The therapeutic range of plasma levels is 2– 8 μg/ml.

Long-term prophylaxis with oral procainamide carries the risks of agranulocytosis and a lupus erythematosus-like syndrome. If, however, this drug is considered necessary it must either be given in adequate dosage every three hours throughout the day and night or as a slow-release preparation ('Procainamide' Durules 1–1.5 g thrice daily).

Beta-adrenoreceptor blocking agents and disopyramide (100–200 mg three or four times a day) are alternative prophylactic drugs.

Beta-adrenoreceptor blocking agents may be effective, as in supraventricular tachycardias.

Phenytoin is given intravenously at the rate of 50 mg per minute up to 250 mg, with blood pressure and E.C.G. checks between aliquots. It can cause ventricular fibrillation or respiratory arrest. It cannot be given as an infusion because of precipitation.

If it is successful, the drug may be given in a six-hourly oral dosage to a total of 1 g/diem for the next one to three days. It is thereafter gradually reduced to 3–6 mg/kg B.W./diem to maintain plasma levels of 10–20 μg/ml.

Procainamide ('Pronestyl') is given by intravenous injection as aliquots of 50 mg every minute to a total of 1 g. The blood pressure and E.C.G are checked between aliquots. If this treatment terminates the dysrhythmia, an infusion may be given to maintain plasma levels of 4–8 μg/ml. As soon as possible a change should be made to oral prophylaxis with 375 mg (250–500 mg) 3-hourly or 'Procainamide Durules' 2–3 t.d.s. Alternatively, 'Kinidin Durules' 250–750 mg b.d. may be given. Prophylaxis is usually continued for six weeks.

Bretylium tosylate is given in a dose of 5 mg/kg body weight intramuscularly or by slow intravenous injection, followed by 3 mg/kg intramuscularly twice or thrice daily with the patient supine.

If drug therapy fails, *overdrive ventricular pacing* should be considered. 'Overdriving' consists of driving the heart at a rate greater than that of the tachycardia.

Torsade de pointes

This dysrhythmia consists of paroxysms of an atypical ventricular tachycardia with undulation and definite changes of direction of the QRS axis over runs of 5–20 beats. It is therefore characterised by the twisting complexes so elegantly implied by its French name (Dessertenne, 1966; Krikler, 1974). It differs from ordinary ventricular tachycardia not only in its morphology but also in its initiation by a late ventricular premature beat rather than an early one. It is usually preceded by a long Q–T interval (Fig. 1).

Electroversion has only a temporary effect. Attention should be given to the possible causes: hypokalaemia should be corrected and suspected drugs (e.g. quinidine, prenylamine, phenothiazines and tricyclic antidepressants) should be withdrawn.

Krikler and Curry (1976) recommend initial treatment with an

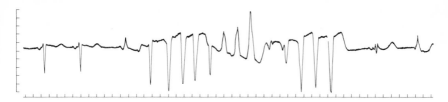

Fig. 1. Torsade de pointes. (Reproduced by permission of R. A. J. Spurrell.)

intravenous infusion of isoprenaline to shorten repolarisation time. This allows time to institute cardiac pacing which should be ventricular if there is underlying atrioventricular block but may otherwise be right atrial at a rate of 100–120/min. The increased rate shortens re-polarisation and diminishes the opportunities for re-entry.

Accelerated idioventricular rhythm
This looks like ventricular tachycardia but the rate is less than 100/min. It usually requires no treatment but should be carefully watched for progression to ventricular tachycardia. Talbot and Greaves (1976) found that idioventricular rhythm only progressed to ventricular tachycardia if the rate exceeded 75/min. They therefore suggested that the heart rate provided the basis of a useful distinction between idioventricular rhythms. Those that only became manifest with sinus slowing would be classified as benign or slow idioventricular rhythms (rate less than 75 beats per minute) and the term rapid idioventricular rhythm would be used for faster rhythms (75–100 beats per minute). The treatment of the two might differ, atropine eliminating those associated with sinus slowing but lignocaine being better for those associated with a sinus rate of over 75/min.

Ventricular fibrillation (see also Part 2, ch. I, p. 281)
The treatment for this is *electrical defibrillation*. The chances of success are greatest if it is done immediately; hence the value of teaching the technique to coronary care nurses and ambulance personnel. An initial shock of 200 J is followed by one of 400 J if the first is ineffective. If countershock is unsuccessful, it should be tried again after the intravenous injection of either (*a*) 100 mg lignocaine or 100 mg phenytoin intravenously or (*b*) isoprenaline 0.01–0.10 mg or adrenaline 10 ml of a 1 in 10 000 solution to coarsen 'fine' ventricular fibrillation. External cardiac massage (E.C.M.) is, of course, given during and after the intravenous injections.

Any delay in administering electrical countershock (preferably d.c.) must be covered by E.C.M. and artificial ventilation through an endotracheal tube.

If the patient has required artificial ventilation, or if there has been delay in defibrillation, or if the fibrillation is refractory to d.c. countershock, 100 mmol of sodium bicarbonate are given intravenously. Further doses of bicarbonate are given to correct the arterial pH every 5–10 min if necessary.

Antidysrhythmic drugs are given as for ventricular tachycardia.

On resumption of co-ordinate contraction, there may be a need for 5–10 ml of 10% calcium chloride intravenously to enhance myocardial contractility.

Asystole (see also Part 2, ch. 1, p. 283)

This may occasionally respond to:

1. a sharp blow to the precordium;
2. mechanical pacing, using light taps over the precordium with the side of the hand sixty times per minute;
3. E.C.M. and artificial ventilation;
4. internal cardiac massage (I.C.M.) if necessary in viable cases – especially if cardiac rupture is suspected;
5. isoprenaline infusion, 2 mg in 500 ml dextrose or laevulose solution, at 12–20 drops/min;
6. adrenaline and calcium as above;
7. large d.c. countershocks;
8. electrical pacing.

Heart block

Pacing may be required for sinoatrial block and atrioventricular block and occasionally for sinus bradycardia.

First degree atrioventricular block following acute myocardial infarction requires no treatment. If, however, it is associated with left bundle branch block or bifascicular block, it is wise to insert a prophylactic pacing electrode.

Atrioventricular block associated with *inferior myocardial infarction* is usually benign. If, however, there is associated hypotension, syncope or cardiac failure, intravenous atropine should be tried and, if that is ineffective, a pacing electrode should be inserted.

The development of second or third degree atrioventricular block after acute *anterior myocardial infarction* indicates extensive cardiac damage and mortality is high. Demand pacing should be instituted.

Patients with chronic heart block, who are having Adams-Stokes attacks, also require emergency pacing, until an implanted unit can be provided.

ACUTE CARDIAC PACING. INDICATIONS AND TECHNIQUE

Few would disagree with the indications formulated in the Coronary Care Unit of the Royal Infirmary, Edinburgh (Julian, 1974) for inserting a pacing electrode. They are:

1. Any bradyarrhythmia, unresponsive to atropine, if associated with syncope, hypotension, cardiac failure or ventricular ectopic rhythm.

2. First degree heart block if associated with bifascicular block or with complete left bundle branch block.

3. Second or third degree heart block associated with acute anterior infarction. A further indication for insertion of a pacing electrode in cases of anterior infarction is right bundle branch block, particularly when associated with anterior or posterior hemiblock (Joint Working Party, 1975).

4. Atrioventricular block complicating inferior myocardial infarction if it is associated with hypotension, syncope, cardiac failure or ventricular ectopic rhythm and is unresponsive to atropine.

5. Overdrive for ventricular arrhythmias (as reviewed by De Sanctis and Kastor, 1968).

6. Asystole.

It is important after acute myocardial infarction to keep the pacemaker in the demand mode to avoid competition, which might induce ventricular fibrillation.

The pacing electrode is inserted percutaneously into the subclavian vein (Macauley and Wright, 1970) or by 'cut-down' into a medial antecubital vein. The electrode is advanced to the apex of the right ventricle with the help of an X-ray image intensifier. The operator should wear a protective lead apron and reduce the screening time as much as possible. If bedside fluoroscopy is not available and the patient is too ill to move, a standard unipolar or bipolar electrode may be introduced transvenously into the right ventricle using intracavitary electrocardiography as described by Chatterjee *et al.* (1969). A properly earthed electrocardiograph is essential because of the possible induction of ventricular fibrillation by current leakage through the intracavitary electrode.

The threshold for pacing should be less than 1 volt initially and should not subsequently be allowed to rise above 1.5 v. The threshold should be measured twice daily and the pacing voltage generally adjusted to twice the threshold value.

THE MANAGEMENT OF THE HYPERTENSIVE CRISIS

A high blood pressure accompanying acute left ventricular failure, caused by hypertensive heart disease, usually responds to vigorous antifailure measures (Finnerty, 1974) but acute antihypertensive therapy is occasionally necessary. Hypertensive encephalopathy always demands immediate treatment with rapidly-acting antihypertensive agents. It is now uncommon but may occur in cases of acute glomerulonephritis, eclampsia, essential or secondary hypertension, and drug interaction. Another hypertensive emergency, requiring immediate reduction of blood pressure, is aortic haematoma (aortic dissection).

Agents given intravenously in hypertensive emergencies are the vasodilators diazoxide ('Eudemine'), sodium nitroprusside and hydrallazine ('Apresoline'), and the ganglion-blocker trimetaphan ('Arfonad'). Intravenous methyldopa and intramuscular reserpine are less often used, partly on account of their delayed onset of action and the drowsiness they frequently produce.

Sheps and Kirkpatrick (1975) emphasize that the physician should familiarise himself with the side effects, doses and contraindications of these agents before using any of them. They also stress that the particular treatment selected should reflect the nursing care and medical supervision available. Some of the agents necessitate constant monitoring in an intensive therapy unit because frequent adjustments are necessary.

Diazoxide
Ninety-five per cent of adult patients respond to an intravenous dose of 300 mg but the dose for a child or very large adult (over 90 kg) should be calculated on the basis of 5 mg/kg. The full dose must be given in one bolus injected as rapidly as possible. The effect is almost immediate and lasts for 3 to 12 hours or longer. The dose may, however, be repeated after one hour if necessary.

Because diazoxide causes sodium retention and a reduction in urinary output, Finnerty (1974) regularly injects 40 mg frusemide intravenously with it. This addition commonly results in postural hypotension and the patient should therefore remain supine.

The blood glucose level should be closely monitored if the drug is administered for more than 48 h.

Sodium nitroprusside

This has a prompt and evanescent hypotensive action. It is given as an intravenous infusion in a concentration of 60 mg/l, commencing with 10 drops/min and adjusting the drip-rate appropriately. It is light-sensitive and the drip bottle should be covered to inhibit degradation. Until recently, sodium nitroprusside infusion was not available commercially and had to be freshly prepared by the pharmacy, following special instructions (Palmer and Lasseter, 1975). ('Nitride' (Roche) is now available.)

Nitroprusside therapy requires constant supervision and frequent small adjustments in order to prevent extremes of blood pressure, which should be monitored every 2–3 min.

Trimetaphan

This drug is also administered as an intravenous infusion requiring constant monitoring and titrating the drip-rate against the blood pressure. The other main disadvantage is that drug resistance frequently develops rapidly.

An infusion with a concentration of 500 mg/ml is commenced at a rate of 1 mg/min and titrated. The effect is immediate and transient.

Hydrallazine

This may be given intravenously or intramuscularly in a dose of 10–20 mg, or up to 60 mg i.m. Its onset of action is in 30–40 min and its duration of action is 2–8 h. It is less potent than the other agents and its side effects (e.g. tachycardia, flushing and headache) limit its usefulness. The reflex tachycardia and increase in cardiac output can (in the absence of left ventricular failure) be inhibited with a β-adrenergic blocking agent, which potentiates the hypotensive action.

The above drugs are listed in their usual order of preference. However, the most appropriate one must be selected in any given case. Any one of them might be suitable in hypertensive encephalopathy. However, if aortic dissection or myocardial infarction has occurred, it would generally be wiser to withhold agents such as diazoxide and hydrallazine which stimulate the heart. Agents such as nitroprusside and trimetaphan, with minimal reflexive cardiac effects, might be preferable (Frohlich, 1973).

Diazoxide is probably the hypotensive agent of choice in the treatment of acute hypertension related to pregnancy.

Sodium nitroprusside and trimetaphan should, if possible, be avoided in pregnancy.

Phentolamine, 5–30 mg intravenously, has an immediate and transient action in cases of catecholamine hypersecretion or release (e.g. phaeochromocytoma and cheese reaction) but is ineffective in all other hypertensive crises.

Parenteral hypotensive therapy with these drugs should be tapered off as control is gained with oral antihypertensive agents; these may be started with or shortly after the parenteral agent.

THE MANAGEMENT OF CARDIAC TAMPONADE

This condition of critical cardiac compression must always be considered when one is called to a patient with circulatory collapse.

The clinical setting may be one of pericarditis (from any cause), myocardial infarction, aortic dissection or trauma (blunt or penetrating) to the chest or upper abdomen. Except in the case of abrupt haemopericardium, the shock-like state is attended by a high dominant venous pressure, with a systolic descent (Gibson, 1960) in the wave form. There is pulsus paradoxus with an inspiratory fall in systolic arterial pressure exceeding 15 mm Hg or 50% of the pulse pressure. No third heart sound is audible. The E.C.G. may show marked electrical alternans (Kumar and Dayhem, 1974; Friedman *et al.*, 1974).

As Cortes and McDonough (1971) usefully reiterate, Beck's acute cardiac compression triad consists of (*a*) a falling arterial pressure, (*b*) a rising venous pressure and (*c*) a small quiet heart.

When practicable, investigations to confirm the presence of a pericardial effusion might be echocardiography (preferably), radio-isotope scanning or right heart catheterisation, with injection of carbon dioxide or aqueous contrast medium into the right atrium and radiography. In tamponade, the right atrial, right ventricular end-diastolic, pulmonary diastolic and pulmonary artery wedge pressures are all elevated and are within 5 mm Hg of each other.

The immediate treatment is pericardiocentesis, usually with the patient sitting propped up. A suitable needle has a length of 7.5 cm and a short bevel. A bore of 1 mm diameter is usually adequate but a 2 mm bore may be required for thick effusions. It is attached to a three-way stop cock (with attached drainage tube) and a 20 ml or 50 ml syringe.

A needle with a 'Teflon' sleeve may be preferred so that, when the pericardial sac has been entered, the needle can be removed and the cannula left in place, thus minimising the danger of trauma to the heart and coronary vessels. With the subcostal approach, the risk of trauma can also be diminished before the needle is advanced, by asking the patient to take a deep breath, as this causes the fluid to collect between the heart and diaphragm (Cortes and McDonough, 1971).

Davila and Palmer (1971) draw attention to the important anatomical relationships. The internal mammary arteries lie 1 cm lateral to the sternal borders. The anterior descending branch of the left coronary artery lies very close to the left border of the heart. The left pleural reflection to the anterior chest wall leaves a small area to the left of the lower half of the sternum where the pericardium can be aspirated without crossing the pleura.

Spodick (1967) illustrates eight 'standard' sites for pericardiocentesis but the subxiphoid-subcostal and the apical are the commonest approaches.

The subxiphoid-subcostal approach, preferred by Davila and Palmer (1971) utilises the angle between the xiphisternum and the left costal margin, through which the needle passes directly into the anterior mediastinum, avoiding the pleural spaces and the internal mammary vessels. After raising a wheal of 1% lignocaine with a fine hypodermic needle, infiltration is continued with a 7.5 cm needle advanced at about a 45° angle to the anterior abdominal wall, directed cephalad and towards the spine. The plunger of the syringe is withdrawn frequently to avoid intravascular injection of the local anaesthetic and to detect the effusion. The depth of the parietal pericardium from the skin surface is about 3.8 cm. When the region has been adequately anaesthetised, the aspirating needle assembly is advanced along the same track, with slight negative pressure created by traction of the plunger of the syringe.

The apical approach is preferred by Gold (1967) who contends that it is less likely to result in cardiac damage or to cause confusion due to aspiration of blood from the right atrium.

The apical impulse does not necessarily disappear with effusion and may be palpable well within the area of cardiac dullness. In this case, the needle is inserted into the fifth intercostal space 1–2 cm to the left of the apical impulse. Otherwise it is introduced about 2 cm inside the left border of percussion dullness. The needle is directed posteriorly, slightly cephalad and slightly mesially. Continued suction on the syringe is made as the needle is introduced. Forcible pulsations are felt if the needle touches the heart, when it should immediately be withdrawn slightly to avoid damaging a coronary vessel. The chest wall thickness in adults averages 3–4 cm.

Continuous monitoring of the electrocardiogram is advisable during pericardiocentesis. The V lead of a properly grounded electrocardiograph is connected to the exploring needle by a sterile wire with attached alligator clips. Contact of the needle with the epicardium results in elevation of either the S–T segment or the P–R segment, depending on whether it is a ventricle or the right atrium which is touched. Ventricular or atrial premature beats may appear. If bloody fluid is aspirated, its haematocrit can be compared with that of peripheral venous blood to determine whether the heart has been penetrated.

Dramatic improvement is usual after only 50–100 ml of fluid have been aspirated. If, on the other hand, needle exploration fails to yield fluid but there is good evidence for tamponade, pericardiotomy or pericardiectomy is indicated.

If there is unavoidable delay in evacuating the pericardium, *supportive measures* should be applied. These may include oxygen, intravenous fluids (dextrose, saline or, in the case of haemopericardium or severe anaemia, blood) and isoprenaline or noradrenaline. I.P.P.V. is contraindicated because it raises both intrapleural and intrapericardial pressures and thereby reduces venous return to the heart.

When tamponade is a recurrent problem, as in some uraemic patients undergoing chronic intermittent haemodialysis, pericardiectomy may be the best solution (Wray *et al.*, 1974; Singh *et al.*, 1974; Hällgren *et al.*, 1974).

ACUTE HEART FAILURE: INDICATIONS FOR ARTIFICIAL VENTILATION

Intermittent positive pressure ventilation (I.P.P.V.) increases the intrathoracic pressure and thereby diminishes the effective right atrial filling pressure and reduces the cardiac output. This effect is accentuated by excessive inflation pressures and inadequate expiratory duration (Kelman, 1971a).

However, I.P.P.V. can be life-saving in severe acute left ventricular failure. Hypoxia decreases myocardial efficiency and increases pulmonary vascular resistance (Kelman, 1971b). Mechanical ventilation is indicated if there is severe hypoxaemia with increasing hypercarbia i.e. $PaO_2 < 8$ kPa (60 mm Hg) and $PaCO_2 > 6.7$ kPa (50 mm Hg).

Application of a positive end expiratory pressure (P.E.E.P.) of 5–15 cm H_2O widens small airways and reduces alveolar collapse, thus improving the distribution of ventilation and correcting ventilation-perfusion abnormalities (Leftwich *et al.*, 1973). Problems may arise, however, in assessing the best level of P.E.E.P. to apply in individual cases (Lenfant, 1975) and even a level of 2 cm or less may impair cardiac output. P.E.E.P. in such cases, should therefore be applied with extreme caution. The changes encountered during its use and following withdrawal are enumerated and discussed in Part 2, p. 327.

INDICATIONS FOR CARDIAC SUPPORT

The heart may need support in the following acute conditions:

Cardiogenic shock
Pump failure
Ruptured papillary muscle, causing acute severe mitral regurgitation and left ventricular failure
Perforation of the interventricular septum
Penetrating wounds of the heart

In the first two conditions, support may be provided pending investigation and operation for a surgically correctable lesion. In the absence of such a lesion, mechanical assistance usually fails to improve the outlook.

Adequate management demands bedside monitoring of arterial pressure, left ventricular filling pressure (or pulmonary capillary wedge pressure, P.C.W.P.), hourly urine output and arterial blood gases (Cohn, 1975). The balloon of the catheter used for measurement of the P.C.W.P. must be deflated between measurements lest it causes pulmonary infarction.

THE MANAGEMENT OF CARDIOGENIC SHOCK

It would be surprising if the high mortality and lack of any consistently effective treatment in cardiogenic shock did not engender therapeutic nihilism. This would seem to be further justified by the extent of muscle damage found at necropsy (Hanarayan *et al.*, 1970 and Page *et al.*, 1971) in patients dying of cardiogenic shock complicating myocardial infarction. It is tempting to believe that shock is simply a manifestation of massive myocardial destruction which is irreversible. This view would not, however, take account of secondary changes and other aggravating factors which might be ameliorated to improve the prognosis. Nor should the picture be entirely coloured by acute myocardial infarction. Cardiogenic shock resulting from acute myocardial depression associated with general anaesthesia and with cardiopulmonary bypass, for example, has a far more favourable prognosis.

The diagnosis of shock must be based on the demonstration of inadequacy of tissue blood flow (Cohn, 1975). It is characterised by hypotension (systolic blood pressure 80 mm Hg or less), oliguria (urine output less than 20 ml/h), pale cold clammy skin, mental lethargy and confusion.

'Pump failure' implies severe left ventricular failure but not necessarily hypotension or failure of organ perfusion in a patient with acute myocardial infarction. Supportive measures at this stage should have a greater chance of success than treatment delayed until the patient is in frank cardiogenic shock.

Circulatory collapse, particularly if occurring several days after acute myocardial infarction, should not automatically be diagnosed as cardiogenic shock due to power failure. A grossly elevated jugular venous pressure may lead to the diagnosis of subacute cardiac rupture, amenable to surgical repair (O'Rourke et al., 1975; Mahoney et al., 1976).

Therapy in pump failure and in cardiogenic shock may be considered under three main headings, viz.

(a) General measures
(b) Drugs
(c) Circulatory-assist devices

(a) *General measures*
Attempts should be made to correct hypoxia, metabolic acidosis and significant arrhythmias. As antidysrhythmic drugs are myocardial depressants, however, they should be used only for serious dysrhythmias and in minimal effective doses.

For hypoxia, assisted ventilation is provided through an endotracheal tube if oxygen by mask proves inadequate.

Intravenous fluids may be helpful especially if there is hypovolaemia or if vasodilator therapy is instituted, but careful haemodynamic monitoring is required. It may be beneficial to raise the left ventricular filling pressure (or P.C.W.P.) to above 20 mm Hg in cardiogenic shock. It should not, however, be raised above 25 mm Hg, for fear of inducing pulmonary oedema.

(b) *Drugs*

The principal drugs used in cardiogenic shock fall into one or more of the following categories: 1. *inotropic* agents, 2. *vasopressors* and 3. *vasodilators*:

Inotropic agents include digitalis, noradrenaline, metaraminol, isoprenaline, dopamine, dobutamine and glucagon. Digitalis glycosides are probably better avoided unless required for the treatment of supraventricular tachyarrhythmias.

Vasopressors include noradrenaline, metaraminol and angiotensin.

Vasodilators include isoprenaline, corticosteroids, chlorpromazine, phentolamine, phenoxybenzamine, nitroglycerine, sorbide nitrate and sodium nitroprusside. Vasodilators are commonly used in combination with volume expansion. This may be satisfactorily achieved by monitored challenges with aliquots of dextran 70 solution or other fluids which are retained in the circulation. The left ventricular filling pressure (or P.C.W.P.) should be measured after each aliquot.

Inotropic agents

A continuous intravenous infusion of *isoprenaline*, preferably by infusion pump, is often used for the treatment of acute haemodynamic impairment, especially with bradycardia and in the absence of dysrhythmias. The ideal dose for myocardial impairment *after open-heart surgery* was found by Goenen *et al.* (1976) to be between 0.8 and 2.0 micrograms per minute. This gave the maximum inotropic effect but limited bathmotropic and chronotropic effects. Above 2 µg/min, the cardiac output decreased and the frequency of arrhythmias increased. The same authors note that glucagon may be preferable in situations of tachycardia, arrhythmia or beta-blockade. The dose is 2 mg by slow intravenous injection, repeated every 30 min. However, Hamer *et al.* (1973) found no convincing inotropic response in the diseased heart and argued that the regional redistribution of blood flow produced by the drug must considerably limit its therapeutic value in cardiology.

After acute myocardial infarction, inotropic agents may have detrimental effects. Following experimental coronary artery occlusions, the intravenous administration of isoprenaline increases the extent and severity of myocardial ischaemia (Maroko *et al.*, 1971). This is partly due to the inotropic effect and partly due to the vasodilator action of the drug. The inotropic effect unfavourably alters the balance of myocardial oxygen demand and supply. The vasodilator action of isoprenaline reduces coronary collateral blood flow to the acutely ischaemic zone. It does this by two mechanisms (Cohen *et al.*, 1976). One is coronary steal, in which vasodilatation in normal areas induces reduction of blood flow in ischaemic myocardium. The other is a reduction of coronary perfusion pressure, in which coronary collateral flow is reduced by a decrease in aortic diastolic pressure secondary to peripheral vasodilatation.

Infarct size is an important determinant of power failure of the heart and the aim of therapeutic measures should be to attempt to limit the extent of myocardial necrosis after acute coronary occlusion. As inotropic agents may, under certain circumstances, aggravate an ischaemic injury and actually increase the size of an infarct, their use must be examined critically. Lesch (1976), reviewing the problem, rejects a general condemnation of all inotropic agents in all situations but condemns the use of isoprenaline in pump failure complicating myocardial infarction. He would not, however, withhold the drug if it reversed bradycardia-induced hypotension, unresponsive to atropine, when pacing was either unavailable or necessarily delayed.

Dopamine is a naturally occurring catecholamine. Like noradrenaline it is an alpha and beta-adrenergic agonist which causes peripheral vasoconstriction and augments heart rate and myocardial contractility. Unlike noradrenaline, however, it dilates renal and mesenteric vascular beds and does not therefore compromise renal blood flow and urine output. It may be used alone or in combination with other pressor agents or with diuretic agents. Karliner (1973) notes that the combination of isoprenaline and dopamine may be particularly useful in selected patients by minimising excessive vasoconstriction produced by dopamine and excessive vasodilatation produced by isoprenaline. The combination may augment cardiac output and urine flow beyond that produced by either drug alone.

Dopamine hydrochloride is diluted in 5% dextrose solution to a concentration of 800 µg/ml for intravenous administration. Infusion is begun at a rate of 1–2 µg/kg B.W./min. Every 15–30 min, the dose is increased by 1–4 µg/kg/min until the optimal effect is achieved as judged by urine output and systemic arterial pressure.

Unfortunately, the catecholamines, including isoprenaline and dopamine, used for their vasoactive and inotropic properties, may induce an excessive tachycardia or dysrhythmias.

Dobutamine is an inotropic agent with lesser chronotropic and dysrhythmogenic effects. These properties and the haemodynamic profile of the drug in chronic congestive cardiac failure (Beregovich *et al.*, 1975) suggest that dobutamine will prove of value in acute cardiac insufficiency.

Vasopressors

Vasopressor agents are frequently used in hypotensive states but have the disadvantage that they further diminish tissue perfusion. They also increase left ventricular afterload. Unfortunately all drugs with inotropic and vasoconstrictor properties increase myocardial oxygen consumption. This may be counterbalanced, as in the case of noradrenaline, by a rise in coronary blood flow because of the restoration of aortic diastolic pressure. However, shock is rarely reversed by agents which reduce regional blood flow.

Lesch (1976) regards noradrenaline as the drug of choice following acute myocardial infarction when shock is due to inadequate vasoconstriction rather than to intrinsic pump failure. Direct blood pressure recordings via a central arterial line are required to justify this treatment, however, in patients who appear less ill than sphygmomanometry suggests, as cuff pressure readings may be spuriously low.

Vasodilators

Left ventricular failure complicating acute myocardial infarction may respond favourably to vasodilator therapy, which reduces the impedance to left ventricular ejection. The benefits are not, however, confined to cases of myocardial infarction. Vasodilator therapy is based on consideration of the physiological mechanisms operative in shock (Dietzman and Lillehei, 1968) and is directed towards restoration of visicerocutaneous perfusion by volume replacement when necessary (infrequently after myocardial infarction) and reduction of vasoconstriction. Vasodilators are used in the 'pre-shock' ('pump failure') stage of reduced peripheral blood flow, whilst the patient is still normotensive.

Sodium nitroprusside is a well known vasodilator, which is given by intravenous infusion at a rate of 30–150 μg/min.

Perret *et al.* (1975) obtained very favourable haemodynamic effects with phentolamine infused intravenously in a dose of 10 mg/h. Although no adverse effects were noted, such a therapeutic procedure should, as the authors point out, be employed only where haemodynamic monitoring facilities (especially for measurement of the P.C.W.P.) are available.

Phentolamine has a variety of applications in clinical practice (Gould and Reddy, 1976).

Orally administered sorbide nitrate is a vasodilator of therapeutic value in the treatment of left ventricular failure caused by acute myocardial infarction. It produces a significant decrease in left

ventricular filling pressure. In patients in whom this is initially high
(>20 mm Hg), a pronounced increase in cardiac output occurs. The
effect is maintained for 4–5 h after a 30 mg oral dose (Bussman *et al.*,
1977).

It should be appreciated that the optimal left ventricular filling
pressure in patients with acute myocardial infarction is not in the
normal range but higher i.e. between 14 and 18 mm Hg (Crexells *et al.*,
1973).

Haemodynamic monitoring is essential for the proper drug therapy of
cardiogenic shock. It is vital to know quickly whether the treatment is
having a beneficial or a deleterious effect. Hourly measurements of
urine output (via an indwelling catheter) are helpful but the more
immediate response to a drug, or other therapeutic intervention, can
often be adequately assessed only by measurement of the left ventricular filling pressure, intra-arterial pressure and perhaps right
ventricular filling pressure (or central venous pressure). The pulmonary
capillary wedge pressure (P.C.W.P.) usually suffices as a measure of left
ventricular filling pressure and can be measured using a balloon-tipped
flotation catheter (Swan and Ganz, 1970), a strain-gauge transducer
and a visual display. This unfortunately demands facilities and
personnel denied to most district general hospitals. For further details of
haemodynamic monitoring refer to Part 2, chapter II.

Mechanically assisted circulation
If moderate doses of catecholamines or other agents fail to produce
sustained improvement (e.g. if drugs are required for more than 4 hours
to maintain a systolic pressure of 80 mm Hg), mechanical cardiac
assistance is considered. Intra-aortic balloon counter-pulsation
(I.A.B.C.), otherwise known as intra-aortic balloon pumping is now
well known (Editorial, *Lancet*, 1972; Braunwald and Maroko, 1972)
and is principally used to stabilise the condition of patients prior to
evaluation for emergency surgical procedures. I.A.B.C. is able to
decrease myocardial oxygen consumption, increase coronary flow and
relieve shock (Lefermine *et al.*, 1962 and Hahnloser *et al.*, 1966). It
favourably influences both coronary collateral flow (Jacobey *et al.*, 1963
and Gundell *et al.*, 1970) and cardiac metabolism (Leinbach *et al.*,
1971). The increased coronary blood flow and the decreased myocardial work and oxygen consumption help to minimise the myocardial
injury. I.A.B.C. was designed to treat severe refractory cardiogenic
shock but better results may ensue from its earlier use. The technique of
insertion is described in Part 4, chapter IV.

By decreasing myocardial work, and improving oxygen demand and supply relationships, balloon pumping may minimise myocardial necrosis. The eventual amount of infarcted muscle may not then be so great as to exclude recovery.

One plan of action (Jackson, 1976) in medically refractory cardiogenic shock is as follows: if it has been present for more than 12 h, I.A.B.C. is not commenced. Patients who have had refractory cardiogenic shock for at least 2 h, but less than 12 h, are accepted. If I.A.B.C. for 12 to 24 h results in improvement, the patient is placed in one of two categories, 'balloon dependent' and 'balloon independent'. Balloon dependent patients are those who have, for example, a recurrence of cardiac pain, further E.C.G. changes or a raised P.C.W.P. These patients undergo emergency investigation and surgery if feasible. 'Balloon independent' patients are weaned over twenty-four hours and proceed to interval investigation and surgery if necessary.

As used to date, I.A.B.C. alone marginally improves hospital survival. Perhaps more importantly it improves a patient's condition sufficiently to permit transport to a cardiac surgical centre for treatment of a mechanical problem such as a ruptured interventricular septum. The results of others (e.g. O'Rourke et al., 1975) support the view that I.A.B.C. and cardiac surgery have a definite role in the management of the mechanical complications of myocardial infarction, but further point to counterpulsation having an important preventive role in limiting infarct size. I.A.B.C. and its potential value in various forms of inodine failure is discussed in greater detail by Yacoub in Part 4, chapter IV.

Assisted circulation may also be achieved by E.C.G.-synchronised external counterpulsation (E.C.P.), in which the lower limbs are compressed during diastole, so augmenting diastolic pressure, and released or subjected to negative pressure during systole.

Soroff et al. (1974) approach the problem of cardiogenic shock with adequate fluid loading (in an attempt to increase the preload of the left ventricle), vasodilators and external counterpulsation. This type of solution has the appeal of aiming to assist the sick ventricle whereas inotropic and vasoconstrictor agents increase its workload and oxygen consumption.

Other possible mechanical means of cardiac support are cardiopulmonary bypass (possibly transarterial closed-chest left ventricular bypass), whole body acceleration, and implantable left-ventricular assist pumps.

INDICATIONS FOR EMERGENCY CARDIAC SURGERY

(a) *Complications of myocardial infarction*

Aortocoronary saphenous vein bypass grafting is of established value as an elective operation for the relief of angina. As an emergency operation, its use in evolving myocardial infarction is controversial but for acute coronary insufficiency (Lawson *et al.*, 1975) it is proposed as the treatment of choice (Yacoub, 1975).

Rupture of a papillary muscle causes left ventricular failure which is intractable unless emergency surgery is performed. Chatterjee *et al.* (1973) found sodium nitroprusside helpful in the management of patients with acute mitral regurgitation complicating acute myocardial infarction. It increases forward cardiac output and forward stroke volume and reduces systemic vascular resistance and regurgitant flow.

Perforations of the interventricular septum require surgical repair but the operative mortality is high in the first six weeks after infarction. Often, cardiac function is severely compromised and intractable biventricular failure makes early operation necessary. Surgical repair is safer and easier, however, if cardiac function can be supported for six weeks, by which time the margins of the infarct and of the perforation contain a sufficiency of fibrous tissue. Intensive drug treatment or intra-aortic balloon-pumping (I.A.B.C.) may tide the patient over the waiting period.

Tecklenberg *et al.* (1976) concluded that afterload reduction with either intravenous sodium nitroprusside or sublingual sorbide nitrate was a potentially useful adjunct in the medical management of septal perforation, pending surgical repair. Systemic blood flow (cardiac index) is improved and shunt flow is reduced. In contrast, inotropic agents often increase the afterload and shunt flow as well as increasing left ventricular work and myocardial oxygen demands. In view of these adverse haemodynamic consequences, inotropic agents should, if possible, be avoided.

Excision of a *ventricular aneurysm* should be considered if it is complicated by refractory heart failure, refractory arrhythmias or thromboembolism.

(b) *Aortic dissection (dissecting haematoma of the aorta)*

Hypotensive therapy must give way to surgery if: (*i*) pain is not alleviated, (*ii*) the blood pressure cannot be brought under control, (*iii*) there is aortic regurgitation, (*iv*) X-rays show continuing enlargement of the aorta or (*v*) leakage or imminent rupture are suspected (Brockman, 1975).

(c) *Infective endocarditis*

Emergency aortic valve replacement is the patient's only hope if there is torrential aortic regurgitation, causing refractory cardiac failure. In other cases, surgery may be the only way of reaching and eliminating the infected tissue.

(d) *Cardiac trauma*

Non-penetrating trauma often causes myocardial contusion, requiring only rest and observation. It may, however, cause laceration of the walls of cardiac chambers, rupture of the interventricular septum and disruption of valves, and necessitate surgery.

Penetrating trauma requires pericardiocentesis, attention to non-cardiac complications (e.g. pneumohaemothorax) and early thoracotomy (Naclerio, 1964 and Carrasquilla *et al.*, 1972).

Emergency cardiopulmonary bypass may be lifesaving.

(e) *Some cases of cardiac tamponade* either cannot be relieved by pericardiocentesis or recur very rapidly and require pericardiotomy or pericardiectomy. Pyopericardium, like any other abscess, requires surgical drainage.

(f) In infants, palliative or curative procedures are urgently required for congenital cardiac anomalies complicated by congestive cardiac failure or cyanosis.

REFERENCES

Aber, C. (1973). *In* 'Recent Advances in Cardiology.' Sixth Edition (Ed. J. Hamer) p. 84. Churchill Livingstone, Edinburgh and London.

Beregovich, J., Bianchi, C., D'Angelo, R., Diaz, R. and Rubler, S. (1975). Haemodynamic effects of a new inotropic agent (dobutamine) in chronic cardiac failure. *Brit. Heart J.* **37**, 629.

Braunwald, E. and Maroko, P. R. (1972). Intra-aortic balloon counterpulsation: an assessment. *Ann. intern. Med.* **76**, 659.

Brockman, S. K. (1975). *In* 'Cardiac Emergency Care' (Ed. E. K. Chung) p. 308. Lea and Febiger, Philadelphia.

Bussman, W. D., Löhner, J. and Kaltenbach, M. (1977). Orally administered isosorbide dinitrate in patients with and without left ventricular failure due to acute myocardial infarction. *Am. J. Cardiol.* **39**, 91.

Campbell, R. W. F., Dolder, M. A., Prescott, L. F., Talbot, R. G., Murray, A. and Julian, D. G. (1975). Comparison of procainamide and mexiletine in prevention of ventricular arrhythmias after acute myocardial infarction. *Lancet* **1**, 1257.

Carrasquilla, C., Wilson, R. F., Walt, A. J. and Arbulu, A. (1972). Gunshot wounds of the heart. *Ann. Thorac. Surg.* **13**, 208.

Chatterjee, K., Parmley, W. W., Swan, H. J. C., Berman, G., Forrester, J. and Marcus, H. S. (1973). Beneficial effects of vasodilator agents in severe mitral regurgitation due to dysfunction of subvalvar apparatus. *Circulation* **48**, 684.

Chatterjee, K., Sutton, R., Layton, C. A. and Edwards, A. (1969). The cavity electrocardiogram in emergency artificial pacing. *Post Grad. Med. J.* **45**, 713.

Cohen, M. V., Sonnenblick, E. H. and Kirk, E. S. (1976). Coronary steal: its role in detrimental effect of isoproterenol after acute coronary occlusion in dogs. *Am. J. Cardiol.* **38**, 880.

Cohn, J. N. (1975). *In* 'Cardiac Emergency Care' (Ed. E. K. Chung) p. 35. Lea and Febiger, Philadelphia.

Cortes, F. M. and McDonough, M. T. (1971). *In* 'The Pericardium and its Disorders' (Ed. F. M. Cortes) p. 215. Charles C. Thomas, Springfield, Illinois, U.S.A.

Crexells, C., Chatterjee, K., Forrester, J. S., Dikshit, K. and Swan, H. J. C. (1973). Optimal level of filling pressure in the left side of the heart in acute myocardial infarction. *New Engl. J. Med.* **289**, 1263.

Davila, J. A. and Palmer, T. E. (1971). *In* 'The Pericardium and its Disorders' (Ed. F. M. Cortes) p. 263. Charles C. Thomas, Springfield, Illinois, U.S.A.

De Sanctis, R. W. and Kastor, J. A. (1968). Rapid intracardiac pacing for treatment of recurrent ventricular tachyarrhythmias in the absence of heart block. *Am. Heart J.* **76**, 168.

Dessertenne, F. (1966). La tachycardie ventriculaire a deux foyers opposes variables. *Archs. Mal. Cœur* **59**, 263.

Dietzman, R. H. and Lillehei, R. C. (1968). The nature and treatment of shock. *Brit. J. Hosp. Med.* **1**, 300.

Editorial (1972). Intra-aortic balloon pumping. *Lancet* **2**, 1938.

Epstein, S. E., Redwood, D. R. and Smith, E. R. (1972). Atropine and acute myocardial infarction. *Circulation* **45**, 1273.

Finnerty, F. A. (1974). Hypertensive crisis. *J. Am. Med. Ass.* **229**, 1479.

Friedman, H. S., Gomes, J. A., Tardio, A. R. and Haft, J. I. (1974). The Electrocardiographic features of acute cardiac tamponade. *Circulation* **50**, 260.

Frohlich, E. D. (1973). The hypertensive crisis. *In* 'Clinician' (Ed. H. P. Dustan) p. 78. Searle, Puerto Rico.

Gibson, R. (1960). The significance of the systolic descent in the jugular venous pulse in constrictive pericarditis and cardiac tamponade. Proceedings of the Third European Congress of Cardiology, Part A, p. 279. Excerpta Medica.

Goenen, M., Jaumin, P., Raveau, A. and Tremouroux, J. (1975). Comparative haemodynamic effects in glucagon and isoprenaline in the early postoperative period in cardiac surgery. *Scand. J. Thorac. & Cardiovasc. Surg.* **9**, 206.

Gold, R. G. (1967). Acute non-specific pericarditis. *Post. Grad. Med. J.* **43**, 534.

Gould, L. and Reddy, C. V. R. (1976). Phentolamine. *Am. Heart J.* **92**, 397.

Gundel, W. D., Brown, B. G. and Gott, V. L. (1970). Coronary collateral flow studies during variable aortic root pressure waveforms. *J. Appl. Physiol.* **29**, 579.

Hahnloser, P. B., Gallo, E. and Schenk, W. G. Jr. (1966). The hemodynamics of counterpulsation. *Scand. J. Thorac. & Cardiovasc. Surg.* **51**, 366.

Hällgren, R., Fjellström, K.-E., Wibell, L. and Åberg, T. (1974). Treatment of uraemic haemopericardium by pericardectomy. *Scand. J. Thorac. & Cardiovasc. Surg.* **8**, 192.

Hamer, J., Gibson, D. and Coltart, J. (1973). Effect of Glucagon on left ventricular performance in aortic stenosis. *Brit. Heart J.* **35**, 312.

Harnarayan, C., Bennett, M. A., Pentecost, B. L. and Brewer, D. B. (1970). Quantitative study of infarcted myocardium in cardiogenic shock. *Brit. Heart J.* **32**, 728.

Jackson, G. (1976). The use of circulatory support by balloon pumping in the treatment of acute myocardial infarction. Ciba Symposium, 'Cardiovascular Medicine', England, Jan 24–25.

Jacobey, J. A., Taylor, W. J., Smith, G. T., Gorlin, R. and Harken, D. E. (1963). A new therapeutic approach to acute coronary occlusion. II. Opening dormant coronary collateral channels by counterpulsation. *Am. J. Cardiol.* **2**, 218.

Joint Working Party of the Royal College of Physicians of London and the British Cardiac Society (1975). The care of the patient with coronary heart disease. *J. Roy. Coll. Phycns.* (Lond.) **10**, 5.

Julian, D. G. (1968). The management of dysrhythmias in cardiac infarction. *J. Roy. Coll. Phycns.* (Lond.) **3**, 54.

Julian, D. G. (1974). Personal communication.

Karliner, J. S. (1973). Dopamine for cardiogenic shock. *J. Am. Med. Ass.* **226**, 1217.

Kelman, G. R. (1971a). *In* 'Applied Cardiovascular Physiology.' pp. 111, 113, 166 and 167. Butterworths, London. Ibid. (1971b) pp. 112 and 152.

Krikler, D. M. (1974). A fresh look at cardiac arrhythmias. 'The Lancet'. London.

Krikler, D. M. and Curry, P. V. L. (1976). Torsade de Pointes, an atypical ventricular tachycardia. *Brit. Heart J.* **38**, 117.

Krikler, D. M. and Goodwin, J. F. (1975). 'Cardiac Arrhythmias; The Modern Electrophysiological Approach.' Saunders, London, Philadelphia and Toronto.

Krikler, D. M. and Spurrell, R. A. J. (1974). Verapamil in the treatment of paroxysmal supreventricular tachycardia. *Post Grad. Med. J.* **50**, 447.

Kumar, S. and Dayhem, M. K. (1974). Electrical alternans. Case report and comments on its mechanism and diagnostic significance. *Illinois Med. J.* **145**, 500.

Lawson, R. M., Chapman, R., Wood, J. and Starr, A. (1975). Acute coronary insufficiency: an urgent surgical condition. *Brit. Heart J.* **37**, 1053.

Lefermine, A. A., Low, H. B. C., Cohen, M. L., Lunzer, S. and Harken, D. E. (1962). Assisted circulation III. The effect of sychronised arterial counterpulsation on myocardial oxygen consumption and coronary flow. *Am. Heart J.* **64**, 789.

Leftwich, E. I., Witorsch, R. J. and Witorsch, P. (1973). Positive end-expiratory pressure in refractory hypoxaemia: a critical evaluation. *Ann. Intern. Med.* **79**, 187.

Leinbach, R. C., Buckley, M. J., Austen, W. G., Petschek, H. E., Kantrowitz, A. R. and Sanders, C. A. (1971). Effects of intra-aortic balloon pumping on coronary blood flow and metabolism in man. *Circulation* **43** (Suppl. I) 77.

Lenfant, C. (1975). Editorial: Practical Method to Regulate PEEP. *New Engl. J. Med.* **292**, 313.

Lesch, M. (1976). Inotropic agents and infarct size: theoretical and practical considerations. *Am. J. Cardiol.* **37**, 508.

Lie, K. I., Wellens, H. J. and Durrer, D. (1974). Characteristics and Predictability of primary ventricular fibrillation. *Eur. J. Cardiol.* **1**, 379.

Macaulay, M. B. and Wright, J. S. (1970). Transvenous cardiac pacing. Experience of a percutaneous supraclavicular approach. *Brit. Med. J.* **4**, 207.

Mahoney, P. G. C., Slesser, B. V., Baigent, D. F., Humber, P. J. B., Slade, P. R. and Lawson, C. W. (1976). Subacute cardiac rupture after myocardial infarction. *Brit. Med. J.* **1**, 747.

Maroko, P. R., Kjekshus, J. K., Sobel, B. E., Watanabe, T., Covell, J. W., Ross, J. and Braunwald, E. (1971). Factors influencing infarct size following experimental coronary artery occlusions. *Circulation* **43**, 67.

Naclerio, E. A. (1964). Penetrating wounds of the heart: experience with 249 patients. *Dis. Chest* **46**, 1.

Oliver, M. F. and Julian, D. G. (1970). 'Manual on intensive coronary care.' WHO Regional Office for Europe, Copenhagen.

O'Rourke, M. F., Chang, V. P., Windsor, H. M., Shanahan, M. X., Hickie, J. B., Morgan, J. J., Gunning, J. F., Seldon, A. W., Hall, G. V., Michell, G., Goldfarb, D. and Harrison, D. G. (1975). Acute severe cardiac failure complicating myocardial infarction: experience with 100 patients referred for consideration of mechanical left ventricular assistance. *Brit. Heart J.* 1975, **37**, 169.

Page, D. L., Caulfield, J. B., Kastor, J. A., De Sanctis, R. W. and Saunders, C. A. (1971). Myocardial changes associated with cardiogenic shock. *New Engl. J. Med.* **285**, 133.

Palmer, R. F. and Lasseter, K. (1975). Sodium nitroprusside. *New Engl. J. Med.* **292**, 294.

Perret, Cl., Gardaz, J.-P., Reynaert, M., Grimbert, F. and Enrico, J.-F. (1975). Phentolamine for vasodilator therapy in left ventricular failure complicating acute myocardial infarction: haemodynamic study. *Brit. Heart J.* **37**, 640.

Resnekov, L. (1973). Electroversion. *In* 'Recent Advances in Cardiology,' Sixth Edition (Ed. J. Hamer) p. 329. Churchill, Livingstone, Edinburgh and London.

Sheps, S. G. and Kirkpatrick, R. A. (1975). Hypertension. *Mayo Clin. Proc.* **50**, 709.

Singh, S., Newmark, K., Tshikawa, I., Mitra, S. and Berman, L. (1974). Pericardiectomy in uraemia. The treatment of choice for cardiac tamponade in chronic renal failure. *J. Am. Med. Ass.* **228**, 1132.

Soroff, H. S., Cloutier, C. T., Birtwell, W. C., Begley, L. A. and Messer, J. V. (1974). External counterpulsation: management of cardiogenic shock after myocardial infarction. *J. Am. Med. Ass.* **229**, 1441.

Spodick, D. H. (1967). Acute cardiac tamponade: pathologic physiology, diagnosis and management. *Prog. cardiovasc. Dis.* **10**, 64.

Spurrell, R. A. J. (1976). The effects of disopyramide on the human heart: an electrophysiological study. *J. Int. Med. Res.* **4**, (Suppl. 1) 31.

Talbot, S. and Greaves, M. (1976). Association of ventricular extrasystoles and ventricular tachycardia with idioventricular rhythm. *Brit. Heart J.* **38**, 457.

Tecklenberg, P. L., Fitzgerald, J., Allaire, B. I., Alderman, E. L. and Harrison, D. C. (1976). Afterload reduction in the management of post infarction ventricular septal defect. *Am. J. Cardiol.* **38**, 956.

Wray, T. M., Humphreys, J., Perry, J. M., Stone, W. J. and Bender, H. W. (1974). Pericardiectomy for treatment of uraemic pericarditis. *Circulation* **50** (Suppl.) 268.

Yacoub, M. (1975). Personal Communication.

IV

The Management of Acute Renal Failure

H. A. Lee

INTRODUCTION, CLASSIFICATION AND PHYSIO-PATHOLOGY

Introduction

Although enormous advances have been made in the management of chronic renal failure over the past 20 years it remains a depressing fact that the mortality from acute renal failure still remains above 50%. A number of reasons has been put forward to explain this persistent high mortality. Firstly, the type of patients being referred with acute renal failure has changed over the past 15 years and secondly the mean age range has increased. However, the mortality amongst obstetric acute renal failure patients remains consistently the lowest at 13% with medical acute renal failure patients occupying a middle position and surgical and post-traumatic cases the highest mortality rates. There is little doubt that increasing age confers a decreasing prognosis on the outcome of acute renal failure. Nowadays increasing numbers of elderly patients have more extensive surgery in the wake of improved medical and surgical concepts.

Perhaps too much endeavour has been directed towards chronic renal failure and it is time to reflect again on the diagnosis and management of acute renal failure. Unless one is constantly aware of

Table 1. Causes of acute renal failure

A   PRE-RENAL (i.e. hypovolaemia and/or hypotension)
- (i) Dehydration e.g. fulminating diarrhoea, heat stroke
- (ii) Blood loss i.e. haemorrhage
- (iii) Plasma loss e.g. burns
- (iv) Septicaemia particularly gram negative organisms
- (v) Cardiogenic shock
- (vi) Hypnotic drug overdosage

B   INTRINSIC (PARENCHYMAL) RENAL FAILURE
(syn. ACUTE TUBULAR NECROSIS)

1   *Ischaemic*
- (i) Any group A cases if corrective measures inadequate or not undertaken soon enough
- (ii) Major vessel obstruction
  - (a) arterial e.g. saddle embolus, bilateral renal artery emboli, bilateral renal artery thrombosis, aortic dissection
  - (b) venous e.g. i.v.c. thrombosis, renal vein thrombosis
- (iii) Small vessel obstruction e.g. malignant hypertensive nephroarteriolosclerosis
- (iv) Neurological reflex e.g. calculus anuria, obstetric emergencies, cross clamping of aorta

2   *Nephrotoxic*
- (i) Pigments
  - (a) Haemoglobinaemia e.g. mismatched blood transfusion, sodium chlorate poisoning, excessive haemolysis e.g. blackwater fever
  - (b) Abnormal haemoglobin e.g. sickle cell disease
  - (c) Myoglobinaemia e.g. crush injuries
- (ii) Chemicals
  - (a) Organic e.g. carbon tetrachloride, ethylene glycol, paraquat
  - (b) Inorganic e.g. heavy metals, phosphorus
  - (c) Drugs e.g. cephaloridine, gentamicin, phenindione, sulphonamides (crystalluria)

3   *Metabolic*
- (i) Hypercalcaemia
- (ii) Hyperuricaemia – primary, secondary
- (iii) Myelomatosis – Bence Jones protein
- (iv) Hepato-renal syndrome

4 *Inflammatory*
  (*i*) Glomerulonephritis – acute GN
      – rapidly progressive GN particularly of the elderly
      – Goodpasture's syndrome
      – Collagenoses e.g. DLE, PAN
      – non-specific vasculitis e.g. drug induced
  (*ii*) Fulminating acute pyelonephritis
  (*iii*) Leptospirosis (Weil's disease)
5 *Altered blood coagulability (DIC)*
  (*i*) Haemolytic uraemic syndrome
  (*ii*) Thrombotic thrombocytopaenic purpura
  (*iii*) Acute pancreatitis
  (*iv*) Endotoxinaemia e.g. *Cl. Welchii*
  (*v*) Other toxins e.g. fungal, insect bites, protein derivatives e.g. horse serum

C POST-RENAL
  (*i*) Calculus obstruction of
    (*a*) solitary kidney or
    (*b*) remaining functioning kidney
  (*ii*) Retroperitoneal fibrosis
    (*a*) benign idiopathic
    (*b*) peri-aneurysmal
    (*c*) malignant
  (*iii*) Malignancy
    (*a*) Primary e.g. prostatic, bladder
    (*b*) Secondary e.g. breast
    (*c*) Involvement e.g. Ca. cervix
  (*iv*) Prostatic hypertrophy
  (*v*) Urethral strictures

this possibility complicating a wide range of medical and surgical problems then its diagnosis will be made late and undoubtedly management becomes more difficult and carries a poorer prognosis. The longer the delay between the onset of acute renal failure and its recognition the higher the number of complications that follow and the poorer the prognosis.

Classification of acute renal failure

Table 1 shows some of the possible causes of acute renal failure. The main merit of having such a table is that it may direct the clinician towards more appropriate investigations and subsequent management. The time-honoured classification of acute renal failure remains basically pre-renal, intrinsic reversible renal and post-renal. Though there may well be an overlap between the first two, nonetheless such a classification has some merits because rapid recognition and correction of the extrinsic renal causes can prevent the development of intrinsic renal failure in many cases.

Pre-renal failure implies hypovolaemia and/or hypotension arising from such diverse conditions as haemorrhage, irrespective of source, plasma loss, e.g. burns, dehydration, e.g. cholera, septicaemia with or without cardiogenic shock and overdosage with certain types of drugs, e.g. aspirin, and paraquat. Rapid correction of the depleted plasma and/or blood volume with restoration of blood pressure can prevent the onset of acute renal failure. It is more important to restore the circulating blood volume than to be overconcerned with the level of blood pressure *per se*. Indeed the over zealous use of vaso-constrictor agents may adversely affect renal blood flow even though improving blood pressure. If delay occurs in correcting the pre-renal elements then the risk of intrinsic reversible or irreversible renal failure increases.

Acute intrinsic reversible renal failure simply describes an acute disturbance of normal renal function which if not quickly corrected results in acute renal failure. The term does not imply any specific aetiology of the renal parenchymal functional disturbance. The syndrome is characterised by a prompt cessation of renal function with associated disturbances in serum biochemistry and diminished urine volume. There are many different possible causes for its occurrence. Over the last 25 years many theories have been suggested and it is quite clear that no one single aetiology is responsible for the onset of all forms of acute renal failure. However, it does seem likely that once renal failure has occurred then the common denominator is a prolonged diminution of glomerular filtration rate.

The old term of acute tubular necrosis was meant to describe this syndrome but it must be emphasised that tubular necrosis is by no means uniformly seen. It has already been shown that in 30% of cases of acute renal failure it is impossible to define with certainty the precise aetiology (Muehrcke, 1969). It seems clear that whilst in some cases a single mechanism may be operative in others the aetiology may be multifactorial. There seems to be general agreement that in most cases of acute renal failure there is an initial situation of shock (hypovolaemia and/or hypotension) resulting in a disturbance of renal perfusion. This results in temporary renal ischaemia and the development of intrinsic reversible renal failure if corrective measures cannot be undertaken quickly enough.

Physio-pathology of acute renal failure (Muehrcke, 1969; Kerr, 1973; Flamenbaum, 1973; Kerr, 1974)

One of the earliest explanations put forward was that of renal tubular blockage by casts and debris. Whilst this explanation may be valid in certain animal experiments it cannot be true in all human cases. The classic form of this type of acute renal failure follows the crush syndrome. Acute renal failure may still be due to this cause in myelomatosis where blockage by Bence Jones protein casts occur. Likewise tubular cast formation may contribute to acute renal failure complicating conditions such as heat stress, marked haemoglobinuria, paroxysmal myoglobinuria, a variety of insect stings, electrical burns and certain poisons.

Renal cortical ischaemia with diversion of the blood flow through the medullary parts of the kidney has gained wide acceptance as a cause of acute renal failure (Hollenberg et al., 1968; Dempster, 1972). What role the renal sympathetic innervation has in this situation remains in doubt for cortical diversion can occur even in the denervated kidney. Similarly it has been found after renal transplantation. However, there must be variation of individual susceptibility for if renal vasoconstriction does follow shock with diversion of blood flow through the medullary areas it is by no means a uniform reaction with uniform consequences. Alternatively there may be a critical time duration effect of such a response to shock. Certainly by no means all patients with severe shock will develop acute renal failure. In spite of large numbers of patients admitted to hospital with severe gastrointestinal haemorrhage or suffering from cardiogenic shock and who subsequently recover, acute renal failure is not a prominent complication.

It has recently been suggested that local renin-angiotensin II mechanisms operate within the kidney in acute renal failure (Brown *et al.*, 1970). It has been postulated that the perfusion disturbances within the kidney result in a release of renin and angiotensin locally which maintain the intensive vasoconstriction and lead to acute renal failure. However, not all such patients have been found to have high renin (peripheral vein measurements) levels although perhaps only the intrinsic changes are important and not the peripheral ones with respect to renin measurements. It is relevant to note that some experiments using antibodies to angiotensin II have shown that the kidney can be protected against myoglobinuric acute renal failure (Powell-Jackson *et al.*, 1972). Such evidence supports the concept of renin/angiotensin II induced acute renal failure.

It has become increasingly evident that intravascular coagulation (DIC) which is known to occur in specific syndromes such as the haemolytic uraemic syndrome in children and adults and in postpartum renal failure, may have an important role in acute renal failure (Clarkson *et al.*, 1970; Ponticelli *et al.*, 1972; Lee, 1976). The role of intravascular coagulation may depend on its severity which in turn may determine whether or not acute renal failure occurs. Furthermore some instances of DIC are instantaneous, may not be severe and thus may not cause acute renal failure. In others there may be a persistent DIC with continuing involvement of the kidney at a time well after the initial insult so that renal failure may develop late. In this context it is noted the associations that have been put forward between endotoxinaemia and DIC and the occurrence and/or persistence of acute renal failure (Wardle, 1975). The diagnosis of DIC can readily, although not always easily, be made. In such cases of acute renal failure the difficulty arises whether to ascribe its occurrence to this aetiology. Investigations have clearly shown the deposition of fibrin-like material within the capillaries of the glomerular tufts at a time when there was little haematological support for the occurrence of DIC. DIC is now widely associated with the various forms of acute renal failure complicating pregnancy, can occur in many shock syndromes, is associated with septicaemia, with acute organ disturbances such as pancreatitis and can complicate certain types of poisoning e.g. mercurial. Finally, the kidney itself possesses a high fibrinolytic activity so that, depending when biopsies are taken, no evidence may be seen of the microthrombi that may have initially developed and caused the acute renal failure. Even though microthrombi may not totally occlude vessels, they may cause sufficient ischaemia to result in the release of certain vasoconstrictor substances. In some cases DIC is an all or none phenomenon whilst in others it may continue at a low grade level. Another difficulty then arises because although blood cultures may be negative particularly in the patients receiving antibiotics, this in no way excludes the possibility of continuing endotoxinaemia with associated DIC. Since the Limulus test is not widely used and is considered by some workers unreliable, the exact prevalence of endotoxinaemia in clinical cases is not known. This may be a very useful avenue of research for the development of anti-endotoxins in the management of these cases.

The cause of the continuing oliguria once developed has been ascribed to various theories such as generalised renal oedema and hence in the early years the concept of decapsulation now abandoned. Leakage of glomerular filtrate across necrotic basement membranes of the renal tubules has had its advocates but then not all patients have this lesion. However, a combination of these factors is a totally plausible explanation for many cases. Whatever the cause of the renal vaso-constriction there is no doubt there is a persistent reduction of the glomerular filtration rate (Sevitt, 1959; Hollenburg et al., 1973).

In spite of the multitude of possibilities for causing acute renal failure the clinician should not be dismayed if he cannot define the precise aetiology. Suffice it to say that a diagnosis of acute intrinsic reversible renal failure having been made sufficiently early, then attempts can be made to eradicate the possible causes and prevent the development of the full syndrome.

It is most important not to overlook causes of post-renal acute renal failure as their prompt correction leads to speedy resolution of the whole problem. Thus in a female a vaginal examination is mandatory to exclude the possibility of a cervical carcinoma obstructing the ureters. Likewise a rectal examination in the male must be part of routine examination. A plain X-ray of the abdomen to exclude the possibilities of renal calculi must not be forgotten. In all cases of total anuria prompt cystoscopy with bilateral ureterograms is indicated to establish (a) that the patient has two kidneys and (b) that a post-renal cause is excluded.

Of the renal parenchymal lesions it must not be forgotten that acute glomerulonephritis particularly of the elderly can occur as acute renal failure presentation (Lee et al., 1966). Also, a large number of nephrotoxins can cause acute renal failure. Thus careful history taking is mandatory in all cases. The possibility of major vessel involvement either arterial or venous must be considered. The fibrillating patient may have shot off a massive embolus obstructing the aorta and both renal arteries. Bilateral renal vein thrombosis remains another rare possibility.

A more difficult situation is to determine whether the current renal failure is an acute episode or whether associated with long-term renal insufficiency.

Helpful pointers suggesting chronic renal disease are the following. Symptoms of micturation difficulties, haematuria, loin pain or dysuria give a duration estimate. The patient may be receiving treatment for hypertension or be known to have had proteinuria. Progressive nocturia with later nausea vomiting and lethargy are suggestive of chronic renal failure. The finding of renal osteodystrophy (on chest X-ray or plain X-ray abdomen), of left ventricular hypertrophy on ECG or small kidneys on nephrotomography may lead to a similar conclusion. Finally in the younger patient retarded growth particularly with a normocytic, normochromic anaemia is very suggestive. However, where doubts remain as to this possibility this should never prevent the clinician in the first instance mounting a full management programme for the patient who may subsequently be found to have chronic irreversible renal failure. Then the appropriate decisions can be made. One must never adopt the attitude that it may be chronic renal failure and therefore not attempt treatment and thus lose all opportunity of renal tissue recovery.

BILATERAL RENAL CORTICAL NECROSIS

This lesion may occur in a minority of patients developing acute renal failure in circumstances indistinguishable from those usually leading to acute tubular necrosis. This is a patchy lesion and in the majority of cases is irreversible. It not infrequently follows the haemorrhagic complications of pregnancy but has been seen after insect bites and recovery from cardiogenic shock.

Clinically, it may be recognised by the abrupt onset of total anuria and the passage of blood-stained urine prior to shutdown. It may be diagnosed later (4 weeks onwards) by observing renal cortical calcification on a plain X-ray of abdomen.

DIAGNOSIS AND MANAGEMENT

Diagnosis of acute renal failure (Eliahou and Bata, 1965; Luke and Kennedy, 1967)

Over the years a vast number of tests has been suggested for making this

Table 2. Suggested diagnostic investigations in acute renal failure

1	Urine microscopy	7	Blood urea concentration
2	Proteinuria	8	Urine/plasma (U/P) urea ratio
3	Urine sodium concentration	9	U/P osmolality ratio
4	Urine sodium/potassium ratio	10	Renal excretory index
5	Urine specific gravity	11	Response to replacement of deficits
6	Urine urea concentration	12	High dose intravenous pyelogram

diagnosis (Table 2). Many of these investigations become less applicable to patients with pre-existing renal disease and in the elderly. Most of these involve a wide range of estimations on the patient's urine e.g. urinary sodium, urinary sodium/potassium ratios, microscopy of the urinary deposit, urinary urea concentration, urinary pH and presence or absence of glycosuria. It is clear from the literature that none of these tests in isolation has proved to be consistently valuable. Nevertheless, any urine should be examined. If proteinuria found then always test for Bence Jones protein. The finding of cellular casts on microscopy may point to a glomerulonephritic lesion. If haematuria present and red cell casts found this immediately indicates a renal parenchymal lesion as opposed to a lower urinary tract one. In making the diagnosis of acute renal failure one must always bear in mind the history, the nature of the onset incident and the time lapse since it occurred. Thereafter one can never dissociate the urinary parameters from blood biochemistry measurements. Basically acute renal failure implies a diminution in urine concentrating ability i.e. a reduced capacity for solute excretion with a concomitant accumulation of solute within the body fluids, i.e. rising blood biochemical values. Such measurements are more readily interpreted the sooner in the patient's illness they are made.

Undoubtedly the most useful measurements for assessing renal function are blood and urine urea concentrations, serum and urine osmolalities and serum creatinine. The range for urine osmolality in normal individuals after modest dehydration is 800–1400 mOsm/kg. This usually falls to 400– 800 mOsm/kg during and after anaesthesia and for 24–36 h after surgery. This fall in concentrating ability is in part related to alterations in glomerular filtration rate. The serum osmolality is 285 mOsm/kg in normal individuals, rising to 300 after moderate dehydration. Thus in normal subjects the U/P osmolality ratio falls in the range 2.7–4.0. The blood urea range in normal subjects is 3–7 mmol/l, with a urine urea concentration in the range 150–660 mmol/l. Therefore a normal U/P urea ratio lies in the range 50–132.

It is thus readily appreciated how a high blood urea will radically alter the interpretation of any such ratio.

Thus attempts must be made to gauge the hourly urine volume, to measure the urinary urea (on fresh urine) and osmolality, to measure serum urea, creatinine and osmolality and then to define ratios. If the urinary urea concentration drops such that the U/P ratio falls below 14:1 in the first 24 h of oliguria, then it is suggestive of acute renal failure, whilst a ratio of 10:1 or less implies it has occurred. Likewise if the U/P osmolality ratio falls below 1.4 and 1.1 respectively in this time similar conclusions may be reached.

Table 3. Modifying influences on interpretation of plasma urea to creatinine ratio (normal range 20–40)

A HIGH RATIO i.e. >60 g e.g. urea 30, creatinine 0.25 mmol/l
1 Protein Catabolism
   (a) High metabolic rate e.g. trauma, fever, sepsis
   (b) Influence of steroids e.g. pulse therapy post renal transplantation
   (c) Increased urea synthesis e.g. tetracycline therapy, gastro-intestinal bleed

2 Salt and Water Depletion
   (a) Salt wasting nephropathy
   (b) Gastro-intestinal losses e.g. diarrhoea, entero-cutaneous fistulae
   (c) Over zealous use of diuretics

3 Pre-renal Failure
   (a) Cardiac failure
   (b) Water depletion e.g. particularly in elderly on high protein, low water feeds

B LOW RATIO <15 g e.g. urea 11, creatinine 0.8 mmol/l
   (a) Low protein (Giovannetti) diet
   (b) Hepatic insufficiency
   (c) Water overloading e.g. excessive intake, inappropriate ADH
   (d) Recent dialysis procedure (urea has better clearance than creatinine)

It is important to note, particularly in the elderly, that the blood urea may rise disproportionately to serum creatinine because of the reduced capacity of the ageing kidney to handle an increased solute load (Table 3). Thus in patients with severe trauma and/or on steroids a rising blood urea may be seen with little change in the serum creatinine and an adequate U/P urea and osmolality ratio maintained.

Additional investigations
In addition to the specific tests referred to in the previous section all acute renal failure patients should have the following. Full serum

electrolytes, serum calcium and phosphate, serum albumin and total proteins and alkaline phosphatase. Haematological investigations should include haemoglobin, W.B.C., platelets, blood film, serum fibrin degradation products, British prothrombin ratio and serum for grouping and cross matching purposes. In pyrexial patients a blood culture is indicated. Urine should also be cultured.

Routine radiology should include a chest X-ray and plain X-ray of abdomen. The latter is an invaluable first-line investigation. This may show the presence of renal calculi and both renal outlines may be seen. Finding two small kidneys may give an immediate clue to pre-existing disease.

A high dose intravenous pyelogram may be of value in making the diagnosis of acute intrinsic renal failure (Fry and Cattell, 1971). Although the occurrence of an immediate, dense, persistent nephrogram is typical of acute renal failure associated with the histological lesion of acute tubular necrosis, it does not occur in all cases. For this reason and because the investigation may be time consuming, it does not rank high in investigational priorities. Whenever an I.V.P. examination is done it should be mandatory to do a 24 h film as this may reveal evidence of an obstructive uropathy.

Renal biopsy should only be undertaken early in the course of acute renal failure if there are good reasons for suspecting a glomerulonephritic aetiology. It has no place in the investigation of acute tubular necrosis. Later if a patient does not enter a diuretic phase after 4 weeks a renal biopsy is justified so as to determine the possibility of renal recovery.

Depending on resources some Units may carry out routine renography. In selected cases renal arteriography or venography may be indicated.

The management of incipient acute renal failure

The therapeutic manoeuvres for preventing acute renal failure are applicable only if carried out within 48 h of the insult. Thus given that restoration of blood and plasma volume together with electrolyte and fluid repletion have been achieved if the urine volume does not improve and the ratios are at the level described above, then a trial of mannitol may be undertaken (Eliahou, 1964; Luke et al., 1970). Only then is it permissible to catheterise such a patient so that an accurate record of hourly urine volumes can be maintained. Once the patient is catheterised he is then given a 25 g bolus of mannitol preferably in a

25% solution. Alternatively 200 ml of a 10% solution may be given. The hourly urine volumes are then measured over the next 2 h when it is hoped that the urine volume will exceed 50 ml/h. If such a urine flow has not been achieved by 2 hours then a second bolus of mannitol may be given. If then, after a further 2 hours, the desired urinary volume is not obtained there is no indication for using further mannitol infusions and it must be assumed that acute renal failure is established.

It is particularly important that these mannitol loads are not exceeded and that preferably hypertonic solutions are used to minimise excess administration of fluids to oliguric patients. In such a way the intravenous fluid volumes are kept within reasonable limits and the danger of giving excessive mannitol averted. Since mannitol is not metabolised, if an excess is given which is then not excreted by the failing kidney, it will stay in the extracellular fluid compartment and cause extracellular fluid volume expansion at the expense of intra-cellular fluid volume depletion. This can have grave consequences in the elderly patient with poor myocardial function where an expansion of the circulating volume may occur.

Considerable controversy surrounds the use of diuretics such as frusemide for reversing acute renal failure (Bailey et al., 1973). There are no reports of good controlled clinical trials having been undertaken to ascertain this point. There are some good theoretical reasons for not using frusemide since this may accentuate renin release within the kidney and intensify the cortical vasoconstriction and reduction in glomerular filtration rate. Most reports on the use of frusemide for reversing incipient acute renal failure do not show good responses (Brown et al., 1974; Brown, 1974). However, many nephrologists would accept the view that having given mannitol and not obtained a response, then a single dose of frusemide e.g. 500–1000 mg is worth a try. The smaller dose may be given intravenously in a total volume of 100 ml using 5% dextrose as diluent over 20 min. The larger dose is usually given over 4 h. This use of frusemide refers only to its application in trying to avert established acute renal failure. The use of daily large doses of frusemide (up to 3 g) to convert oligura into non-oliguria in established acute renal failure is an even more tenuous therapeutic manoeuvre and not without danger from toxic effects e.g. deafness, gastrointestinal disturbance. Others may argue there is more to recommend a 50 mg dose of ethacrynic acid as opposed to frusemide (Kjellstrand, 1973). Whatever the situation frusemide must never be considered the first option and should always follow fluid and electrolyte repletion and a trial of mannitol.

The role of beta-blockade has yet to be explored more fully in this situation but there is some evidence that suggests that propanolol may inhibit the renin/angiotensin II mechanism (Iaina *et al.*, 1975).

Finally a note about the use of prophylactic mannitol infusions in high risk cases for developing acute renal failure. Jaundiced patients requiring operations and others undergoing surgery on the biliary tract (Dawson, 1964), upper gastrointestinal tract and abdominal aorta fall into this group. It is recommended that a 5% mannitol infusion is begun pre-operatively and continued for 12 h post-operatively and the infusion rate kept to maintain a urine flow of >40 ml/min.

The management of established acute renal failure

Such cases are far better managed in acute renal failure units or in combined intensive care units. This is not because of the better dialysis facilities that obtain in such centres but because acute renal failure must be considered as a problem of total body metabolic management and not simply focused on the renal derangement. It is clear in view of the diverse aetiologies of acute renal failure that many aspects of patient care have to be considered.

There is some merit in dividing patients into non-catabolic and hypercatabolic groups. The latter group is usually associated with trauma, major surgery and gross sepsis. Hypercatabolic acute renal failure patients defined as those in whom the blood urea rises by between 10 and 16 mmol/l/day are generally best managed by haemodialysis once the circulation is stabilised. Not infrequently patients require urgent dialysis treatment at a time when they have grossly unstable circulation. This is often a compounded problem of myocardial insufficiency, severely abnormal metabolic environment and a depleted circulating blood/plasma volume. Clearly, such patients are poor candidates for haemodialysis but they can always tolerate immediate peritoneal dialysis. This combined with a glucose–insulin regimen can adequately control hyperkalaemia, contribute significantly towards restoration of normal acid base parameters and allow a time for 'circulation' volume repletion. Later, in a hypercatabolic patient haemodialysis can be resorted to, according to individual requirements. A daily rise of 16 mmol/l of blood urea in a 70 kg man represents 672 mmol urea synthesis equivalent to catabolism of 118 g protein (17 mmol = 1 g urea = 3 g protein). Furthermore, such cases because of their increased nutritional requirements are less well managed by peritoneal dialysis which not only further accentuates their nutritional deficiencies by obligatory losses of amino acids and protein but impairs their eating capacity. Physiotherapy may be the important factor in the rehabilitation of acute renal failure patients and is undoubtedly made easier by the shorter time haemodialysis techniques. In the elderly patient the risk of bilateral basal pulmonary complications is reduced.

Most of so-called medical acute renal failure patients have a daily blood urea increment of 5–6 mmol, which can be reduced to 3–4 mmol by strict metabolic dietary management. The obstetric group of renal failure patients tend to occupy a middle position with daily blood urea rises of anywhere between 10–20 mmol but even here reduction in rate can be achieved (*vide infra*). In all patients there is a tendency for the rate of rise to drop the longer the duration of the oliguric-uraemic state.

In non-catabolic acute renal failure patients the hallmarks of treatment are modest protein restriction with fluid restriction (Berlyne *et al.*, 1967a; Lee, 1975). The time-honoured approach of 500 ml/day plus whatever has been excreted the previous day, i.e. urine, diarrhoea, fistula losses, vomitus, remains appropriate. It must be emphasised that, in the calculation of any fluid requirements, the water of metabolism amounts to 0.4 to 0.5 litres/day in adults. Unless this is taken into account it is readily seen how in a 7 day period a patient can accumulate 3.5 litres of excess water with clinical consequences. The acute Giovannetti dietary regimen has much to recommend it in such patients and the full quantity must be eaten. Such a diet allows of 0.26 g of protein/kg body weight and 0.17 mJ/kg body weight (40 kcals/kg body weight). Sodium is restricted, in the absence of any extra-renal losses, to 40 mmol per day and likewise potassium. More severe restrictions make the diet unpalatable. With such a regimen a diminished rate of rise of blood urea has been noted which is not due to any proven urea recycling processes but due to reduced catabolism. Palatable high energy low fluid volume carbohydrate sources are Hycal a liquid dextrose concentrate with various flavourings and Caloreen a soluble glucose polymer, less sweet than Hycal, which can be made up into ice creams. Four hundred and seventy-five kcals can be gained from 175 ml of Hycal (1 bottle containing 106 ml water).

In patients who cannot or will not take the full diet, then early placement of a nasogastric tube is indicated. Then a complete tube feed 'mix' of the appropriate ingredients can be made up and given in small equal boluses or as a continuous drip throughout the day.

For individuals with associated gastro-intestinal failure there should not be any hesitation in starting an intravenous feeding regimen via a subclavian vein catheter (Lee *et al.*, 1968; Abel *et al.*, 1973). A suggested regimen follows. Give 0.5 litre Vamin-glucose (KabiVitrum), 0.5 litre 20% Intralipid (KabiVitrum) and 0.5 litre 50% glucose (as 21 ml bolus each hour via a metriset or through continuous infusion pump). This regimen yields 9.25 mJ (2200 kcals), 4.7 g nitrogen (35 g amino acid or 29.4 g protein), 25 mmol sodium, 10 mmol potassium and potentially 7.5 mmol phosphorus. The rate of glucose administration is unlikely to warrant large doses of soluble insulin but sufficient should be given to keep the blood sugar below 10 mmol/l. This can be checked by 6 hourly Ames meter blood sugar estimations (nurse operated). The fat emulsion is best given during the first twelve hours of each day to ensure complete bloodstream clearing before blood samples for routine laboratory tests are taken in the morning.

Table 4. Modification of dose schedules of some commonly used drugs in acute renal failure

1	Hypnotics and anti-convulsants	Phenobarbitone Butobarbitone Epanutin	Half normal
	NOTE Short-acting barbiturates, Diazepam and Chlorpromazine – no change		
2	Cardiovascular agents	Digoxin standard initial dose	$\frac{1}{3}$ normal maintenance
		Methyldopa	Usually half normal
	NOTE Diazeoxide, Propranolol, Hydrallazine – no change		
3	Antibiotics	Fusidic Acid, Nalidixic Acid, Carbenicillin, Doxycycline	Normal
		Ampicillin, Flucloxacillin, Lincomycin, Clindamycin, Benzylpenicillin Normal loading dose	Half normal maintenance
		Cephaloridine, Gentamicin, Kanamycin, Streptomycin, Colistin Normal loading dose	Very considerable reduction Check serum levels
		Vancomycin	Major reduction
4	Antimetabolites	Azathioprine	Half normal
		Cyclophosphamide	Check Hb., platelets, W.B.C. daily

The following antibiotics are best avoided: Nitrofurantoin, Tetracycline, Chloramphenicol, Amphotericin.

If all the energy is supplied as glucose then larger requirements for soluble insulin can be anticipated. The advantages of a glucose/insulin–amino acid or glucose/insulin-fat emulsion–amino acid regimens are that they diminish the rate of urea synthesis and therefore blood urea rise, promote protein synthesis, diminish the rate of hyperkalaemia and metabolic acidosis and decrease dialysis requirements. Such are the anabolic effects of these regimens that potassium and phosphorus supplements may have to be given. Depending upon duration, water soluble vitamins and trace elements should be added to these regimens.

The early use of such a regimen even in patients who have normal gastro-intestinal function may be a useful way of delaying the first dialysis procedure where there may be medical contra-indications to an early start.

It cannot be overstressed that these patients require strict attention to pulmonary function, bowel activity and physiotherapy. Modification of drug prescriptions may be required depending on the known renal excretion. Thus lower doses of drugs will need to be given if they are known to be excreted by the kidney (Table 4). Conversely, when such patients are receiving peritoneal dialysis, as is often the case in this group, then further modification of the drug prescription will be required allowing for peritoneal losses.

Daily biochemical investigations are important (i.e. blood urea, sodium, potassium, bicarbonate, phosphate, creatinine, albumin, haemoglobin, P.C.V., W.B.C.) for in this way one can predict, in the absence of increasing urine volume, when the patient's blood parameters will reach certain levels and hence when dialysis will be indicated. Careful daily fluid balance and weight charts must be kept so that appropriate adjustments can be made for excessive sweat losses and dialysis fluid losses. When urine flow recommences it is valuable to do urine urea concentrations for this will help predict the likelihood of further dialysis requirements. The daily urea production rate is known from the daily increment of blood urea. Knowing the urine urea concentration and volume the amount of urine that would need to be voided to prevent further rise of blood urea can be calculated.

e.g. 70 kg man has daily blood urea rise of 8 mmol/l
Total body water = 42 litres
∴ Urea production/day = 256 mmol
Passing 800 ml urine
Urine urea concentration = 102 mmol/l
∴ Excreting 81.6 mmol/day

$\therefore$ his blood urea will continue to rise by approximately 4 mmol/-day unless urine volume trebles at this concentration.

There is general acceptance that prophylactic dialysis is the ideal and frequent measurements allow for this decision to be made. It is recommended that the blood urea should not rise above 40 mmol/l. Likewise, dialysis may be indicated sooner if the serum potassium level is seen to rise quickly. Although peritoneal dialysis can be handled anywhere (Lee, 1964) it is important to stress that it is not the dialysis *per se* that matters but the total management of these patients who have dialysis as part of their treatment. For this reason peritoneal dialysis is best carried out in special units. An appreciable number of complications can arise even with a simple procedure like peritoneal dialysis (see Table 6) such as, perforation of a hollow viscus, peritonitis, trapping of fluids in the wrong tissue layers, fluid retention, protein losses, bilateral basal pneumonia and haemorrhage (Lee, 1967).

When a patient has peritoneal dialysis not only do prescribing habits have to be modified but likewise their nutritional intake. Amino acid losses and protein losses are considerable with peritoneal dialysis and appropriate adjustments have to be made to the nutritional programme. Up to 13 g amino acids and 40 g protein may be lost per 45 litre peritoneal dialysis (Berlyne *et al.*, 1967b). Hypoproteinaemia is a common complication of peritoneal dialysis. The successful conservative management of acute renal failure implies that the full dietary regimen is taken. This is even more important across peritoneal dialysis where extra nutrients i.e. protein, have to be taken. Protein malnutrition (easily measured by serum C3 and transferrin levels) and increased susceptibility to infection are well-known bedmates. It is our policy to make use of the glucose in the peritoneal dialysate as additional energy substrate which may sometimes need the use of concomitant intramuscular insulin. The standard peritoneal dialysis solution has a glucose concentration of 1.36 g/100 ml (75.5 mmol/l) and the blood glucose usually rises to 22–30 mmol/l during peritoneal dialysis. By using appropriate doses of soluble insulin, 1000 kcals of dialysate glucose energy can be utilised daily. Amino acid nitrogen is also added to the peritoneal dialysis fluid e.g. 10 ml of Vamin N (KabiVitrum) per litre of dialysate to obviate losses.

The peritoneal dialysis catheter is never left in for more than 5 days because thereafter there is an increased risk of infection. Furthermore, from a purely comfort standpoint it is to the patient's advantage to have a break between peritoneal dialysis and rarely is it necessary to go beyond 5 days.

Table 5. Indications for dialysis

A BIOCHEMICAL	B CLINICAL
Blood urea >40 mmol/l	Fluid overload
Serum potassium >7 mmol/l	Uraemic nausea and vomiting
Serum bicarbonate <12 mmol/l	Uraemic drowsiness

C   ELECTIVE
Pre-operative
Accommodate blood transfusions
Facilitate i.v. feeding
Prophylactic

Dialysis

Indications for dialysis

These include the time honoured criteria of hyperkalaemia (higher than 7 mmol/l), increasing metabolic acidosis (serum bicarbonate 12 mmol/l or less) and increasing uraemia (blood urea greater than 40 mmol/l). In other patients the indication for dialysis will be that of overhydration and pulmonary oedema arising because inappropriately high amounts of intravenous fluids have been given or the patient allowed too much fluid orally. In the very young or the very old dialysis should be started earlier than normally indicated. In some patients a decreased sense of wellbeing even in the presence of reasonable figures may be an indication for dialysis (Table 5).

The choice between peritoneal dialysis and haemodialysis should not be one of facilities alone (Table 6). All acute hypercatabolic renal failure patients are preferably haemodialysed and this is the method of choice for patients with major abdominal surgery or severe traumatic injuries. For patients with a haemorrhagic diathesis peritoneal dialysis may sometimes be associated with intra-abdominal haemorrhage. Patients with hypercatabolic renal failure and associated gastrointestinal failure (precluding normal oral nutrition) are more easily managed by haemodialysis which allows adequate volume for intravenous feeding.

Management of hyperkalaemia

Hyperkalaemia is the most life-threatening metabolic complication of acute renal failure. In the conservatively managed patient it can be delayed or prevented by routine use of resins which may be taken orally or given rectally. Calcium resins are preferable to sodium resins with

Table 6. Comparison of Haemodialysis and peritoneal dialysis techniques

	Haemodialysis	Peritoneal dialysis
1 TECHNIQUE		
Equipment	Complex	Simple
Expertise required	Considerable	Little
Time to set up	1½ hours	½ hours
Access problems	May be difficult i.e. shunt	Rare
Efficiency	High	Low
Cost per dialysis	Almost equal	
2 SPECIFIC INDICATIONS		
Rapid correction of biochemical abnormality	Yes	No
Poisonings e.g. Paraquat	Yes	No
Hypercatabolism	Yes	Preferably no
Injuries to abdomen ⎫ Burns ⎭	Yes	No
Pancreatitis with shock	No	Yes
Major pulmonary problems	Yes	No
Diabetes with fluid overload	Yes	Preferably no
Heart failure	No	Yes
Haemorrhage and no blood available	No	Yes
Infants	Can be done depending on circumstances	Preferable
Acute on known chronic renal failure	No (usually)	Yes
3 COMPLICATIONS (Lee, 1967)		
Disequilibrium syndrome		
Brain	Yes	No
Heart	May occur	Less so
Circulation disturbances	May occur	Less so
Bleeding problems due to excess heparin	Yes	No
Infection	Very rare	Occ. peritonitis
Perforation of hollow viscus	No	May occur
Dissection of fluid	No	Yes
Loss of protein	No	Yes
Loss of amino acids	Yes	Yes
Respiratory difficulties	No	Yes
Discomfort	No	Yes
Air embolus	May occur	No
Ease of physiotherapy	Good	May be difficult

their associated risk of salt and water overloading. The usual dose is 30 g b.d. which most patients tolerate readily. For the emergency control of hyperkalaemia glucose/insulin regimens are indicated. Here one unit of insulin per 3–4 g of glucose are given. Usual dosage is 50 g of glucose and 15 units of soluble insulin. Such a manoeuvre allows only short-term respite and must be followed by a dialysis procedure. Intravenous sodium bicarbonate 8.4% 100 ml may also be given.

If peritoneal dialysis is used to control hyperkalaemia it is important to remember not to add potassium to the peritoneal dialysate. Usually the potassium can be omitted for at least 24 hours and then the position reconsidered. When potassium is added to an established peritoneal dialysis, the amount should not exceed 3 mmol/l.

Principles of dialysis

1. *Peritoneal dialysis.* Here fluid is put into the peritoneal cavity which when in contact with the large peritoneal surface area comes into equilibrium with the surrounding blood vessels. Two litres of peritoneal dialysate are exchanged per hour. For the sake of patient convenience and to decrease pulmonary complications one litre per half hour is exchanged. For the patient who is not fluid overloaded 1.36% peritoneal dialysate is used. If the patient is overhydrated and fluid removal important then a 6.36% peritoneal dialysate is available. The peritoneal dialysis fluid should be warmed before running into the patient. Sometimes the addition of lignocaine 2 ml to 4 ml 2% lignocaine/litre can alleviate pain. There is little indication for adding heparin or antibiotics to the peritoneal dialysate. The peritoneal catheter is inserted in the midline at the junction of the upper one-third with the lower two-thirds point umbilicus to symphysis pubis. The bladder must always be emptied before insertion of a peritoneal catheter. When a patient is having an abdominal operation and it is known that peritoneal dialysis will be necessary postoperatively, advantage should be taken of placing the peritoneal catheter at operation. Only very rarely, usually because of gross intestinal distension, is it necessary to insert a peritoneal catheter under direct vision. Occasionally when difficulties are encountered with drainage of the peritoneal dialysate from the abdominal cavity, then insertion of a second catheter for drainage alone can resolve the problem. If two catheters are in place, so peritoneo-extra corporeal dialysis can be practised. This procedure has the advantage of not requiring blood for the extra corporeal circuit and avoids protein losses. However, in reality, though a relatively simple procedure, it is very rarely practised and this method is not recommended because it combines the disadvantages of both techniques.

A variety of methods is available for running the peritoneal dialysis fluid into the patient and from 'the patient. Our method is to use a standard Baxter giving set with an outflow limb to a standard collection bag. It is important to accurately measure the input and output and to keep an accurate record of the patient's weight. Peritoneal dialysis is eminently suitable for the management of acute renal failure in neonates and infants. Where it is important that fluid is not removed from a patient then use of a Hartmanns solution (non-glucose containing) is valuable. Since this solution contains potassium it is recommended that one unit of the Hartmanns solution alternates with a standard 1.36% peritoneal dialysate. In this case no potassium additions will be made to the standard peritoneal dialysate. Where indicated additions to the peritoneal dialysate can be made e.g. amino acids. (Further details in Part 4, ch. III, p. 973.) A number of automated dialysis machines is available. Automatic peritoneal dialysis machines have little to recommend them since their functioning still depends primarily on the patency and placement of the peritoneal catheter. The simplicity of the method is also lost with the machine.

2. *Haemodialysis*. Here the principle is for blood to pass through an extra corporeal circuit via some form of cellophane membrane artificial kidney. Access to the circulation is usually via a shunt (teflon tips and silastic rubber extensions) inserted into the radial artery of the forearm and associated vein. Haemodialysis usually lasts for 6–9 h depending upon the efficiency of the kidney used. Most modern types of coil do not require priming with blood, i.e. small extracorporeal volume. The best type of artificial kidney to use is a coil and various types are available according to specific needs. Where considerable fluid needs to be removed, a 1.5 m ultrafiltration coil may be used. For a simple dialysis without fluid removal a 1.0 m coil is available. Where considerable solute needs to be removed but less emphasis on fluid removal then a 1.4 m coil with higher dialysance is available. Heparinisation of the extracorporeal circuit is mandatory. The patient must be dialysed on a weigh bed, an essential piece of equipment in the dialysis unit.

Across haemodialysis various additions to the circulation may be added e.g. plasma, blood, nutritional fluids e.g. soyabean oil emulsion ('Intralipid'). The dialysis fluid usually does not contain any potassium or a low concentration. Subsequently potassium may need to be added to the dialysate. The principle of solute removal is via diffusion gradients whilst fluid removal is on the basis of increased ultrafiltration i.e. increased hydrostatic pressure within the circulation. One now seldom uses the Seldinger method of gaining access to the circulation via the inferior vena cava for the purpose of a veno-venous haemodialysis. Recirculation of peritoneal dialysate through an extracorporeal circuit i.e. kidney coil which obviates protein losses is rarely used.

Hypercatabolic acute renal failure patients. (Overall metabolic care)

These are the more severely ill patients in the surgical and post-traumatic groups. These have the highest mortality rates which is further compounded by the increased age of this group. The sooner overall aggressive metabolic care is taken in these patients the better the outcome. Many of them will have associated gastrointestinal failure and respiratory insufficiency and may need assisted ventilation. Team management is the key theme in the treatment of such cases where multiple organ function has to be considered and not just the kidneys. Planned management should consider individual consideration of cardiovascular, pulmonary, gastro-intestinal, renal, bacteriological, haematological and metabolic requirements.

Although there is some advocacy for mobile haemodialysis units rarely has it been shown that a patient with acute renal failure cannot be moved. Nor is there any real evidence to show that moving such a patient from place A to B impairs the prognosis. Such a policy is, however, compatible with immediate resuscitation at the referring hospital and then subsequent transfer not too long delayed. Occasionally a patient may not be moved because of the orthopaedic or respiratory problems.

An important reminder here is appropriate with respect to those patients given immediate resuscitation and do not develop immediate acute renal failure. One should remain over vigilant of this possibility in such cases, for it was clearly shown that acute renal failure patients presenting after the Vietnam war were different from those of the Korean war (Whelton and Donadio, 1969). During the Korean war the acute renal failure patients presented early whereas in the Vietnam war they were late. This was correlated with the better immediate field resuscitation in the Vietnam war which meant that many patients that would previously have died survived only to develop acute renal failure as a late complication. This may in turn be related to secondary infections and the immunological consequences of later relative malnutrition in such cases. Thus the relevance of DIC and continuing endotoxinaemia and the effects of other possible nephrotoxins becomes all the more important.

Once haemodialysis is indicated it is preferable to plan for alternate

Table 7. Example of a tube feed for acute renal failure patient

	ALBUMAID/CALOREEN[1]
Protein	60 g
Energy	8.4 mJ (2000 kcal)
Sodium	40 mmol
Potassium	25 mmol
Feed composition	CALOREEN[1] 10 g/kg
	ALBUMAID[1] 1 g/kg
	EGG YOLK 1 (for essential fatty acids: or 75 ml
	20% 'Intralipid')
	MINERAL MIX[1] 8 g
	KETOVITE Tabs 2
	KETOVITE MIX 5 ml
	FOLIC ACID 5 mg

[1] Hospital Supplies Ltd.

day haemodialysis since this allows for easier metabolic management and the patient feels generally better. The risk of inducing a disequilibrium syndrome is diminished by avoiding too steep a rise in the blood parameters between dialysis. A further advantage of frequent dialysis particularly for patients with gastrointestinal failure is that it allows of complete intravenous nutrition.

Patients with acute renal failure are no different in the metabolic sense from others without renal failure. They undergo the same tissue catabolism and metabolic consequences as other patients. To deny this concept is bound to lead to inappropriate management of such cases.

Thus the patient with normal gastrointestinal function should be given at least a 60 g protein diet (sometimes more is required) and 10.5 mJ (2500 kcals). Only modest salt (60 mmol) and potassium (60 mmol) restriction should be attempted since frequent dialysis will maintain electrolyte equilibrium. If the patient cannot voluntarily cope with the oral regimen, then a nasogastric tube feed regimen should be started (Table 7). Those who require intravenous nutrition can be given amino acid solutions (synthetic full profile crystalline amino acid solutions only not casein hydrolysates) and intravenous energy substrates in exactly the same way as their non-renal failure counterparts. Any intravenous fluid volume constraints can be met by appropriate dialysis frequency and fluid removal. Furthermore, advantage can be taken of the dialysis procedure to give the patient more energy and nitrogen. One litre of Intralipid 20% (KabiVitrum) can be infused across haemodialysis without interfering with the

Table 8. Example of i.v. nutrition regimen in patient with acute renal failure and gastro-intestinal failure

Source	Volume l	Energy carbo. (mJk cals)	Fat	Nitrogen (g)	Sodium[4] (mmol)	Potassium[3] (mmol)	Phosphorus (mmol)
50% GLUCOSE[1]	0.5	4.2 (1000)	—	—	—	—	—
20% INTRALIPID	0.5	—	4.2 (1000)	—	—	—	7.5
VAMIN-GLUCOSE[5]	1	1.68 (400)	—	9.4	50	20	—
BOOTS PHOSPHATE[2]	0.25	—	—	—	40	5	25
Total	2.25	10.08 (2400)		9.4[6]	90	25	32.5

[1] May need to add soluble insulin; if *all* energy from glucose *will* need insulin.
[2] May not be needed over first 48 h. May require *more* later.
[3] Potassium additions may increase later.
[4] Requirements may be greater if entero-cutaneous fistula present.
[5] Add water soluble vitamins and trace elements solution (Addamel – KabiVitrum).
[6] Equivalent to 58.8 g protein.

efficiency of dialysis and 0.5 litres of, for example, Vamin N (35 g amino acid) over the last 3 hours of dialysis. In this way, for example, per 3 dialyses per week 25.2 mJ (6000 kcals) extra can be given and complete compensation for haemodialysis amino acid losses (2–3 g/h) made. A suggested i.v. feeding regimen is shown in Table 8. The more nearly to normal that the metabolic mileu is maintained the more appropriately utilised are the various nutritional substrates. Many patients with acute renal failure develop severe malnutrition through lack of attention to this aspect of their management. Since malnutrition in turn leads to increased susceptibility to infection and decreased wound healing it is mandatory that nutritional requirements are met. Special compli-cations of intravenous nutrition in these patients may arise e.g. hypophosphataemia, trace element deficiencies, water soluble vitamin deficiencies. This arises because many solutions used for intravenous nutrition are inadequate in phosphate content and when these patients become anabolic, phosphate is taken up into the cells as well as being lost across the dialysis membrane. Water soluble vitamins and trace elements are likewise dialysed out of the patient and not replaced by normal solutions. Appropriate plasma and blood volume replacement must also be met.

When indicated surgical procedures should not be delayed on the mistaken idea that they would be better carried out when the patient has recovered from acute renal failure. It is common experience with such patients that if, for example, there is an intra-abdominal focus of infection or an ischaemic leg that requires amputation then abdominal exploration or amputation must be carried out at the earliest possibility. This requires careful planning between the medical and surgical teams, appropriate timing of the frequency and duration of dialysis and manipulations in metabolic care. Thus a pre-operative haemodialysis with extra corporeal heparinisation may be planned with appropriate blood and plasma replacement. If there is concern about normal coagulation function fresh frozen plasma or platelet transfusions may also be indicated. Steps can also be taken to delay the postoperative dialysis with possible attendant bleeding problems (even with extra corporeal heparinisation). This is achieved by placing a subclavian catheter either pre- or intra-operatively so that a glucose–insulin–amino acid regimen can be started (this applies equally to patients with normal gastro-intestinal function). In this way, I have been able to reduce pre-operative daily blood urea rises of 12–14 mmol to 6 mmol and significantly reduce the hyperkalaemia and metabolic acidosis tendency. Recent evidence has shown that continuing endotoxinaemia is associated with persistent disseminated intravascular coagulation, maybe predominantly within the kidney and makes aggressive surgical procedures mandatory. Thus until the foci of infection are cleared or necrotic tissue removed acute renal failure will not recover.

Early expert respiratory management is an important aspect of the management of many patients with acute renal failure. All acute renal failure units should be well versed in the handling of respiratory problems and ventilators and have an anaesthetist attached to them who has a particular interest in these combined difficulties.

The adequate management of acute renal failure demands attention to all aspects of total patient care. Expertise and knowledge of the handling of certain types of machinery is important e.g. artificial kidneys, ventilators, cardiac monitors, peritoneal dialysis procedures. Although peritoneal dialysis is a simple procedure this alone does not result in the recovery of an acute renal failure patient. Unless total awareness of all aspects of metabolic care is present then disaster can but supervene. Many of the so-called simple procedures have a high complication of themselves.

Why does the mortality of acute renal failure still remain so depressingly high? This may be due to the fact that acute renal failure patients are not referred early enough to acute units where there is sufficient expertise which alone can bring about the increased survival of these patients. Many weeks of hard work are often required with these patients yet even so success will not be uniform. Often an elderly patient can be brought through the acute renal failure syndrome successfully only then to die of pulmonary embolus. This may in part be avoided by using physiotherapy earlier and by employing dialysis techniques that do not make the patient bedbound for so many hours. Again peritoneal dialysis can be conducted with the patient sitting out of bed. Obtaining patient co-operation is an important aspect of the psychological management of these desperately ill elderly patients who often feel they will not be able to make it. The sooner that such patients can be mobilised the more the benefits. For example, they become anabolic more quickly and deep-vein thrombosis incidence is decreased.

PROGNOSIS OF ACUTE RENAL FAILURE (Stott *et al.*, 1972; Lindsay, 1974)

The mortality rate complicating obstetric acute renal failure is 13.2%. Within this sub-group criminal abortions complicated by *Clostridium welchi* infections have the worst chance of survival. Amongst surgical and trauma patients the mortality rate is 59%. In the surgical group lesions of the stomach, small intestine, pancreas and biliary tree are associated with the worst prognosis when the mortality rises to between 65% and 70% whilst patients with urological conditions have a mortality of between 30% and 35%.

Within the medical acute renal failure patients there is considerable variation depending upon the type of patient. The older patients do less well than those with myocardial infarction and those poisoned with nephrotoxins such as paraquat and sodium chlorate do badly. In all patients the occurrence of septicaemia always increases the mortality rate. The occurrence of infection in those dying from acute renal failure varies between 55% and 72%. Reviewing the association of infection with acute renal failure Montgomerie *et al.* (1968) found sepsis was a common cause of death. In spite of the improved therapeutic armamentarium, particularly with antibiotics, the types of infection now being met are changing from common bacteriological ones to fungal infections and rarer types of viral ones.

Both Stott *et al.* (1972), and Lindsay (1974) have noted the importance of age upon the outcome of acute renal failure. The mortality rate rises appreciably after the age of 40 and as Lindsay has pointed out the mortality at 50 years of age is almost double that at 30. Whether peritoneal or haemodialysis methods are used in the management of acute renal failure this appears to have little bearing on the outcome contrary to former opinion.

Perhaps it is not surprising that older patients do not do as well. Often they get through the initial acute renal failure but cannot cope with the physical and mental stress of weeks of debilitating illness. It can be generalised that for acute hypercatabolic renal failure patients that alternate day haemodialysis on *a priori* grounds is a more reasonable method of management than peritoneal dialysis. Thus acute renal failure remains a challenge and demands all that modern medicine can provide to improve the current poor prognosis.

REFERENCES

Abel, R. M., Beck, C. H., Abbott, W. M., Ryan, J. A., Barnett, G. O. and Fischer, J. E. (1973). Improved survival from acute renal failure after treatment with intravenous essential L-amino acids and glucose. *New. Engl. J. Med.* **288**, 695.

Bailey, R. R., Natale, R., Turnbull, D. I. and Linton, A. L. (1973). Protective effect of frusemide in acute tubular necrosis and acute renal failure. *Clin. Sci. Molec. Med.* **45**, 1.

Berlyne, G. M., Bazzard, F. J., Booth, E. M., Janabi, K. and Shaw, A. B. (1967a). The dietary treatment of acute renal failure. *Quart. J. Med.* **36**, 59.

Berlyne, G. M., Lee, H. A., Giordano, C., de Pascale, C., Esposito, R. (1967b). Amino acid loss in peritoneal dialysis. *Lancet* **1**, 1339.

Brown, C. B., Ogg, C. S., Cameron, J. S. and Bewick, M. (1974). High dose frusemide in acute reversible intrinsic renal failure. A preliminary communication. *Scot. Med. J.* (Suppl. 1) 35.

Brown, J. J., Gleadle, R. I., Lawson, D. H., Lever, A. F., Linton, A. L., MacAdam, R. F., Prentice, E., Robertson, J. I. S. and Tree, M. (1970). Renin and acute renal failure: studies in man. *Brit. Med. J.* **1**, 253.

Brown, J. J. (1974). Discussion: 'Acute Renal Failure'. (Ed. C. T. Flynn) p. 135. MTP Co. Ltd., Lancaster U.K.

Clarkson, A. R., Lawrence, J. R., Meadows, R. and Seymour, A. E. (1970). The haemolytic-uraemic syndrome in adults. *Quart. J. Med.* **39**, 227.

Dawson, J. L. (1964). Jaundice and anoxic renal failure: protective effect of Mannitol. *Brit. Med. J.* **1**, 810.

Dempster, W. J. (1972). The nature of renal perfusion in normal, oliguric and anuric states. *Urologia* **39**, 2.

Eliahou, H. E. (1964). Mannitol therapy in oliguria of acute onset. *Brit. Med. J.* **1**, 807.

Eliahou, H. E. and Bata, A. (1965). The diagnosis of acute renal failure. *Nephron* **2**, 287.

Flamenbaum, W. (1973). Pathophysiology of acute renal failure. *Arch. Internal Med.* **131**, 911.

Fry, I. K. and Cattell, W. R. (1971). Radiology in the diagnosis of renal failure. *Brit. Med. Bull.* **27**, 148.

Hollenberg, N. K., Epstein, M., Rosen, S. M., Basch, R. I., Oken, D. E. and Merrill, J. P. (1968). Acute oliguric renal failure in man; evidence for preferential cortical ischaemia. *Medicine* **47**, 455.

Hollenburg, N. K., Sandor, T., Conroy, M., Adams, D. F., Solomon, H. S., Abrams, H. L. and Merrill, J. P. (1973). Xenon transit through the oliguric human kidney; analysis of maximum likelihood. *Kidney International* **3**, 177.

Iaina, A., Solomon, S. and Eliahou, H. E. (1975). Beta-adrenergic blockade reduces the severity of acute renal failure in rats. *E.D.T.A., 1975*, **12**.

Kerr, D. N. S. (1973). Acute Renal Failure. *In* 'Renal Disease'. (Ed. D. A. K. Black) pp. 417–461. Blackwell, Oxford.

Kerr, D. N. S. (1974). The pathogenesis of acute failure. *In* 'Acute Renal Failure'. (Ed. C. T. Flynn) pp. 9–36. MTP Co. Ltd., Lancaster, U.K.

Kjellstrand, C. M. (1973). Ethacrynic acid in acute tubular necrosis. *Nephron* **9**, 337.

Lee, H. A. (1966). Peritoneal dialysis in the management of acute renal failure. Second Symposium in Advanced Medicine. *Roy. Coll. Phys.*, p. 107–121. London.

Lee, H. A. (1967). Evaluation of peritoneal dialysis and haemodialysis in paediatrics. *Israel. J. Med. Sci.* **3**, 28.

Lee, H. A. (1975). Nutritional management of acute and chronic renal failure. *Hospital Update* **1**, 601.

Lee, H. A. (1976). *In* 'The role of heparin in the management of intra-vascular coagulation with renal insufficiency and renal transplantation'. (Ed. V. V. Kakkar and D. P. Thomas) pp. 261–282. Academic Press, London.

Lee, H. A., Hill, L. F., Ginks, W. R. and Pohl, J. E. F. (1968). Some aspects of parenteral nutrition in the treatment of renal failure. *In* 'Nutrition in Renal Disease'. (Ed. G. M. Berlyne) pp. 216–227. Livingstone, London and Edinburgh.

Lee, H. A., Stirling, G. and Sharpstone, P. (1966). Acute glomerulonephritis in middle-aged and elderly patients. *Brit. Med. J.* **2**, 1361.

Lindsay, R. M. (1974). The prognosis of acute renal failure. *In* 'Acute Renal Failure'. (Ed. C. T. Flynn) pp. 103–112. MTP Co. Ltd., Lancaster, U.K.

Luke, R. G., Briggs, J. D., Allison, M. E. M. and Kennedy, A. C. (1970). Factors determining response to mannitol in acute renal failure. *Amer. J. Med. Sci.* **259**, 168.

Luke, R. G. and Kennedy, A. C. (1967). Prevention and early management of acute renal failure. *Postgrad. Med. J.* **43**, 280.

Montgomerie, J. Z., Kalmanson, G. M., Guze, L. B. (1968). Renal failure and infection. *Medicine* (Baltimore) **47**, 1.

Muehrcke, R. C. (1969). Acute Renal Failure. *In* 'Diagnosis and Management'. Mosby, St. Louis.

Ponticelli, C., Imbasciati, E., Tarantino, A., Graziani, G. and Redaelli, B. (1972). Post-partum renal failure with micro-angiopathic haemolytic anaemia. *Nephron* **9**, 27.

Powell-Jackson, J. D., Brown, J. J., Lever, A. F., MacGregor, J., MacAdam, R. F., Titterington, D. M., Robertson, J. I. S. and Waite, M. A. (1972). Protection against acute renal failure in rats by passive immunization against angiotensin. *Lancet* **1**, 774.

Sevitt, S. (1959). Pathogenesis of traumatic uraemia; a revised concept. *Lancet* **2**, 135.

Stott, R. B., Cameron, J. S., Ogg, C. S. and Bewick, M. (1972). Why the persistently high mortality in acute renal failure? *Lancet* **2**, 75.

Wardle, E. N. (1972). Endotoxinaemia and the pathogenesis of acute renal failure. *Quart. J. Med.* **44**, 389.

Whelton, A. and Donadio, J. V. (1969). Post-traumatic acute renal failure in Vietnam. *Johns Hopkins Med. J.* **124**, 95.

V

The Management of Hepatic Failure

P. N. Trewby and Roger Williams

Hepatic coma and precoma are the cardinal signs of hepatic failure, and it is important to establish as early as possible whether their development is a result of fulminant (acute) hepatic failure, or decompensated chronic liver disease. The latter is the more common clinical problem and, fortunately, carries a better prognosis, at least in the short term.

HEPATIC FAILURE IN DECOMPENSATED CHRONIC LIVER DISEASE

Introduction

The progression into coma may be slow and is often preceded by intellectual changes and bizarre psychiatric and personality disorders, including paranoia, depression, violent behaviour and delirium (Table 1). Examination may show the superficial stigmata of cirrhosis with palmar erythema, leuconychia, and spider naevae. Mild jaundice is usually evident and ascites is common. The breath has a characteristic slightly sweetish, faecal odour (fetor hepaticus).

The most obvious neurological sign is a flapping tremor of the outstretched hand, but other abnormalities include slurred speech and difficulty in writing and copying simple diagrams (constructional apraxia). As the encephalopathy progresses, extensor plantar responses,

99

Table 1. Clinical stages in the development of hepatic
coma

Grade	Mental state
I	Euphoria, occasionally depression Fluctuant, mild confusion Slowness of mentation and affect Untidy. Slurred speech Disorder in sleep rhythm
II	Drowsy but responds to simple commands Inappropriate behaviour
III	Sleeps most of the time, but rousable Marked confusion. Incoherent speech
IV	Unrousable. May or may not respond to noxious stimuli

hyperflexia and hyperventilation are found, and decerebrate rigidity
may occur. Hypoventilation and vasomotor instability occur late and
preterminally a flaccid paralysis and respiratory failure supervene.

Investigations and treatment of precipitating factors

Liver function tests, particularly the degree of prolongation of the
prothrombin time, give some indication of the severity of the underlying
liver damage. In addition to serum electrolyte estimation (see later), the
blood sugar is tested on admission as, although dangerous hypoglycaemia is commoner in fulminant hepatic failure, it may sometimes
occur in cirrhotic patients, and may be indicative of an underlying
hepatoma (Kreisberg and Pennington, 1970). Hyperglycaemia is more
commonly seen and carbohydrate intolerance, usually without clinical
diabetes, is well recognised in cirrhosis (Megyeri et al., 1967).

   An electroencephalogram (E.E.G.) (Fig. 1) may show a characteristic and symmetrical rhythm disturbance with slow, high amplitude
delta and theta waves with triphasic waves (Parsons-Smith et al., 1957).
Although these changes may also occur in renal and respiratory failure,
these seldom cause diagnostic difficulties. The E.E.G. is especially
useful in those patients in whom hepatic encephalopathy may present as
a personality disorder and in whom clinical and biochemical signs of
underlying cirrhosis are minimal.

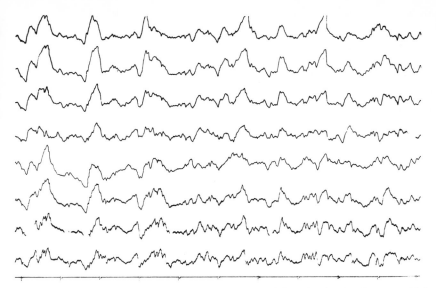

Fig. 1. E.E.G. tracing from patient with fulminant hepatic failure showing low frequency, high amplitude delta and triphasic waves.

Further investigation is aimed at detecting the precipitating factors for hepatic failure, of which the five commonest are:
Gastrointestinal haemorrhage
Misuse of diuretics
Infection
Sedatives, hypnotic drugs or opiates
Progression of the underlying disease

Investigation and control of gastrointestinal haemorrhage
Blood loss is usually self-evident although the onset of melaena may be delayed and haemorrhage only suspected because of the onset of encephalopathy or unexplained hypotension and tachycardia. The site of bleeding must be established by fibreoptic endoscopy, as in 28% of cases acute gastric or oesophageal mucosal erosions or gastroduodenal ulceration, rather than varices, are responsible for the haemorrhage (Waldram *et al.*, 1974). In men under the age of 50, if liver failure is not advanced, this figure falls to 16%, 84% of upper gastrointestinal haemorrhages in these patients being from oesophageal varices (Teres *et al.*, 1976). In 10% of patients bleeding may be from multiple sites.

Bleeding from whatever source may occur without warning and may be recurrent and torrential. For this reason an ante-cubital fossa cut down is normally performed and a 42 cm 8 fg Argyle infant feeding tube inserted into an arm vein with full aseptic precautions, and its position checked by X-ray (Strunin, 1969). This not only allows rapid transfusions to be given, but also allows blood samples to be taken and the C.V.P. to be measured.

If variceal bleeding has been diagnosed, the treatment of choice, in our experience, is variceal compression with a Sengstaken-Blakemore tube (Fig. 2). Two main varieties of this tube are available – a stiff, red rubber tube that must be passed through the mouth which, in our opinion, is easier to use, and a soft rubber tube that will sometimes pass through the nose. Whichever tube is used, it must be carefully tested before use to ensure that the balloons are not punctured. After light anaesthesia of the pharynx (Lignocaine spray 2%), the lubricated tube is passed into the stomach with the patient on his left side. An efficient suction machine supplied with stiff pharyngeal suckers must be near at hand. 150 ml of water containing 10% Hypaque are used to inflate the gastric balloon and the tube is then gently withdrawn until the balloon lodges in the cardia. The tube is fixed to the face under light traction

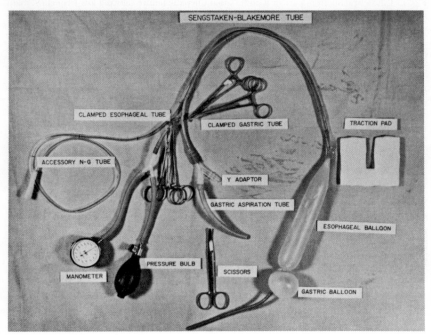

Fig. 2. Red rubber trilumen Sengstaken–Blakemore tube with attached pharyngeal drainage tube (from Pitcher, 1971).

and the oesophageal balloon is then inflated with air to a pressure of 40 mm Hg measured by a Tycos gauge. The position of the gastric balloon is then checked radiologically. External fixation with weights is seldom necessary (Fig. 3).

The major danger of the Sengstaken tube is laryngeal obstruction from upward displacement of the tube and a nurse must remain in constant attention. Should respiration become laboured, the oesophageal balloon is at once deflated, and if there is any doubt about this, the tube is cut across. The nursing staff must be carefully instructed in the mechanics of the tube and asked to deflate the oesophageal balloon for five minutes each hour. The pharynx is kept dry by continuous low pressure suction on the pharyngeal tube and regular gastric aspiration is carried out to keep the stomach empty. With careful management a Sengstaken tube may be used to prevent haemorrhage for 24 to 48 hours on any one occasion, but after that the risks of pressure necrosis of the oesophageal mucosa increase. Variceal bleeding can usually be

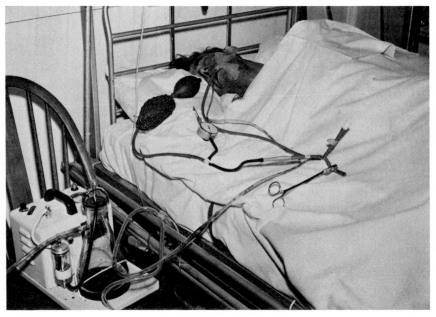

Fig. 3. Sengstaken–Blakemore tube in position in a patient. The gastric balloon has been filled with 50 ml of 10% hypaque and 100 ml water and clamped. Skin traction has then been applied and the oesophageal balloon inflated to 40 mm Hg measured by the Tycos gauge. Continuous suction is being applied to the accessory pharyngeal tube. The gastric tube (spigotted) is drained intermittently. Conscious patients are provided with hand held pharyngeal suckers. Under normal circumstances, the oesophageal balloon should not be left inflated for more than 24 h at a time.

controlled by these means and time allowed for consideration of short-term measures such as oesophageal transection (Pugh *et al.*, 1973) or injection of varices (Raschke and Paquet, 1973), and long-term control of portal hypertension by portacaval anastomosis in selected cases.

If bleeding from peptic ulceration is diagnosed and coma is of mild degree and the patient is considered fit on other grounds (good nutrition, mild jaundice, little ascites), then emergency surgery may be life-saving if bleeding persists.

The management of acute gastric and oesophageal erosions is often a more difficult problem. Gastric lavage and antacids are not often helpful. Perfusion of the coeliac axis with vasopressin (0.02 μ/ml/min), praised in the American literature (Nusbaum *et al.*, 1974), is sometimes of benefit in our experience, but the complication rate (bleeding at the site of insertion, local and generalised infection) is high (Murray-Lyon *et al.*, 1973). More promising is the H_2-receptor antagonist cimetidine. We have demonstrated the effectiveness of cimetidine (150 mg given intravenously over 90 min 6 hourly) in the treatment of active bleeding due to gastric and oesophageal erosions in patients with cirrhosis (Macdougall *et al.*, 1977). Unlike the earlier H_2-receptor antagonist metiamide, cimetidine has not been associated with leukopenia, although at the time of going to press, it is still being evaluated.

Diuretic-induced coma
Misuse of potent diuretics may precipitate coma through electrolyte disturbance, hypokalaemia, alkalosis, or hypovolaemia (Schenker *et al.*, 1974). The latter may occur even though ascites is still present, and the daily weight loss whilst on diuretics should not be allowed to exceed 0.5 kg. Hypovolaemia may also contribute towards the pathogenesis of diuretic-induced uraemia, though this type of renal failure is usually reversible if diuretics are discontinued.

Renal failure in liver disease may develop without a precipitating cause and has been attributed to failure of the liver to clear endotoxins that are absorbed from the gastrointestinal tract (Wilkinson *et al.*, 1974).

Two types are recognised – namely functional renal failure, in which renal tubular function remains intact and is characterised by a very low urine sodium concentration of less than 12 mmol/l, and acute tubular necrosis in which the urine sodium is greater than 12 mmol/l. It is likely, though, that these two varieties of renal failure are part of a spectrum (Wilkinson *et al.*, 1975). Sometimes functional renal failure is followed by evidence of acute tubular necrosis, particularly during the terminal stages of disease. In some instances where acute tubular necrosis occurs earlier there has been a definite precipitating factor, such as haemorrhage or sepsis.

The use of dialysis in cirrhosis is associated with many complications (Parsons *et al.*, 1975). Peritoneal dialysis is the preferred treatment, although in the presence of gross ascites it will result in a large protein loss even though no net removal of ascitic fluid occurs. Haemodialysis, on the other hand, may result in profound hypotension and, in addition, may exacerbate the patient's pre-existing bleeding diathesis. In chronic liver disease neither form of dialysis has been shown to improve survival. This contrasts with renal failure secondary to obstructive jaundice where dialysis is very worthwhile (Parsons *et al.*, 1975). If the biliary obstruction can be relieved, renal function usually returns to normal.

Infection
Even life-threatening infections may be entirely asymptomatic in cirrhotics. Consequently blood, urine, and sputum must always be cultured and a sample of ascitic fluid cultured, as well as examined for cells. Eight per cent of patients presenting to hospital with ascites have spontaneous bacterial peritonitis, gram negative bacilli accounting for two-thirds of these and pneumococci for most of the remainder (Conn and Fessel, 1971). The finding of greater than 1000 cells/mm^3 of ascitic fluid should immediately alert one to this possibility. The possibility of tuberculosis, both pulmonary and ascitic and often silent, must also be considered, particularly in alcoholics and patients on corticosteroids. When antibiotic therapy is thought necessary before bacterial sensitivities are available, Gentamicin and Cephradine are the antibiotics of choice. Normal doses of these should be given if the patient is not in renal failure (Gentamicin 120 mg loading dose, followed by 80 mg 8 hourly, Cephradine 500 mg 6 hourly), but peak gentamicin levels must be measured, and the dose adjusted to produce levels of 10–12 µg of Gentamicin/ml.

Sedatives and hypnotics
Sedatives of all sorts are likely to precipitate hepatic coma in cirrhotics and are to be avoided wherever possible. Physical restraint, although distressing to the patient and attendants, is to be preferred. In the occasional instance where sedatives cannot be avoided, then diazepam (5 mg i.v. slowly), chlormethiazole (0.8% solution i.v.), or phenobarbitone (60 mg i.m.) may be given, but with considerable caution.

Treatment of hepatic coma in cirrhosis

Standard therapy is designed to reduce blood levels of nitrogenous compounds derived from the gut which fail to be metabolised by the damaged liver. With such treatment Benhamou *et al.* (1972) showed in a study of 272 cirrhotics with encephalopathy that the encephalopathy underwent remission in 65.5% of cases when it was a sequel to gastrointestinal haemorrhage, and in 48% of cases when it was not.

Protein restriction and purgation
In early hepatic failure protein should be restricted to 20 g of first class protein daily, but when coma develops it must be withdrawn altogether. Constipation must be avoided and an initial magnesium sulphate enema (80 ml of a 50% solution w/v) should be administered to empty the bowel and lactulose (see below) should be given orally.

Intestinal antibiotics
Neomycin sulphate (1 g orally 6 hourly) is the usual choice. Small amounts of neomycin are absorbed from the gut (normally $< 1\%$) and excreted in the urine, so if large doses are being used there is a risk of nephro- and ototoxicity, especially in the presence of renal failure (Breen *et al.*, 1972).

Lactulose
The starting dose is 60 ml mane and 40 ml midday, and this is adjusted to produce two soft bowel actions a day. Its beneficial effect in hepatic coma has been demonstrated by controlled trial (Elkington *et al.*, 1969), although its precise mode of action is unknown. It is known to produce an osmotic diarrhoea and it may, by reducing the intracolonic pH, favour the formation of the non-absorbable NH_4 and suppress the growth of ammonia-producing bacteria such as bacteroides. It is safe in renal failure and so provides a useful substitute for neomycin, and there is also evidence to suggest the two may act synergistically (Protte *et al.*, 1974).

General supportive measures
When hepatic coma is prolonged, careful fluid and electrolyte balance, nutrition, physiotherapy and nursing care are of critical importance. A non-protein diet such as 'Hycal' containing 2500–3000 calories should be given if necessary via a Ryles tube. If the patient is at risk from inhalation, or if a paralytic ileus develops, then 10% dextrose is given

via a central venous line. Although fresh frozen plasma may partially correct the clotting defect, it does not, in our experience, influence the incidence or severity of haemorrhage and it represents a considerable volume and sodium load. Infusions of salt poor albumin may occasionally be useful in maintaining the colloid osmotic pressure when voluminous ascites is present.

Supplementary vitamins are given in the form of Parentrovite (Forte amps, 1 and 2 i.v. daily), vitamin K (10 mg i.v. daily), and folic acid (5 mg i.v. daily). Vitamin deficiencies are common in all patients with liver disease, especially with respect to thiamine and pyridoxine (Labadarios et al., 1976).

The combination of aspiration pneumonia, a poor respiratory excursion due to ascites, and anatomical intrapulmonary shunts (Berthelot et al., 1966) may sometimes result in marked hypoxaemia. Chest physiotherapy is of fundamental importance and, if carbon dioxide retention is absent, oxygen should be routinely administered.

Corticosteroids are of no benefit in hepatic coma unless the underlying disease process responds to them. Active chronic hepatitis is one such disease and should be suspected if autoantibodies, hyper-gammaglobulinaemia, and raised serum transaminases are present. Prednisolone (initially 30 mg/day) should be given without delay: the subsequent dosage being 10–15 mg/day. Combination treatment with azathioprine (75 mg/day) often allows a lower maintenance dose of prednisone to be used. Alcoholic hepatitis is also often treated with corticosteroids although evidence from controlled trials is conflicting (Helman et al., 1971; Porter et al., 1971). This serious illness may precipitate coma and is suspected wherever a history of alcoholism is obtained and features, including abdominal pain, leukocytosis, fever, a raised aspartate aminotransferase, and jaundice are present.

Other methods of treatment

L-Dopa (Parkes et al., 1970; Lunzer et al., 1974). Administration of relatively large doses (0.5–2 g daily) by nasogastric tube is occasionally followed by arousal both from the coma of cirrhosis and fulminant hepatic failure. Benefit has also been demonstrated in patients who are encephalopathic but not in coma, although no controlled trial has been performed. Side-effects may be severe and persistent nausea and psychiatric disturbances are troublesome.

Surgical exclusion of the colon (Resnick et al., 1967). This should only be considered in patients with chronic encephalopathy resistant to all standard measures. The operative mortality is unacceptable except in those with well-compensated disease and relatively normal liver function tests.

Hepatic homotransplantation. This could soon be the treatment of choice in chronic hepatic failure, and should always be considered when conventional treatment fails. The longest survival to date in the Cambridge/King's College Hospital series was 5 years and, at the time of writing, 8 patients are alive and well up to 2½ years after transplantation.

FULMINANT (ACUTE) HEPATIC FAILURE

Introduction

This condition, fortunately, is rare, for the mortality among those reaching grade IV coma is 80–90% in most series (Benhamou *et al.*, 1972). Early recognition is vital as intensive care, rapidly instituted, may increase survival. The cause is usually fulminant viral hepatitis, although in England hepatic necrosis from paracetamol overdoses are almost as common. Less frequent causes include repeated halothane anaesthesia, hypersensitivity to anti-tuberculous drugs or monoamine oxidase inhibitors, carbon tetrachloride poisoning, mushroom poisoning (*Amanita phalloides*), acute fatty liver of pregnancy, and Reyes syndrome in infancy (Fig. 4).

Acute viral hepatitis	103
HBsAg positive 33	
HBsAg negative 70	
Paracetamol overdose	82
Halothane associated	25
Other drug toxicity	12
Fatty liver of pregnancy	3
Amanita phalloides	2
Leptospirosis	1
Total	228

Fig. 4. Causes of fulminant hepatic failure with grade IV coma seen at the Liver Unit, King's College Hospital between 1966 and 1976.

Diagnosis

The tempo of the whole illness is quicker than in chronic liver disease. The cardinal signs of confusion and drowsiness may precede clinical jaundice and the diagnosis may not be made with certainty until a prolonged prothrombin time (often greater than 2 min) and raised aspartate aminotransferase (usually in the thousands) are found. Once in coma, examination reveals a fetor hepaticus but no cutaneous stigmata of chronic liver disease; ascites is uncommon even late in the disease. The liver is often reduced in size on percussion. Hyperventilation is usual, and decerebrate movements may occur either in response to painful stimuli or spontaneously. The pupils are dilated and react sluggishly to light, and hyperreflexia, sustained ankle clonus and extensor plantar responses are common. As the disease progresses, hypotension, cardiac arrhythmias, and respiratory arrest may occur and preterminally the patient is hypothermic and areflexic with fixed pupils.

Investigations

One of the most important estimations is the blood sugar. Hypoglycaemia is common during the early stages of the patient's illness, but may occur at any time often suddenly and without warning, and if uncorrected will result in irreversible brain damage. 50 ml of 50% dextrose should be given i.v. whenever the dextrostix reading falls below 45 mg% and the patient must be maintained on a 10% dextrose infusion and the blood sugar estimated 2 hourly.

Tests for the hepatitis B virus surface antigen (HBsAg) are carried out on admission and, if present, is tested for again 2–3 times per week, as patients with fulminant hepatic failure often rapidly clear HBsAg.

The blood gases and electrolytes are estimated on admission and at least daily. Although a respiratory alkalosis due to hyperpnea is the most common finding a severe lactic acidosis sometimes predominates especially early in paracetamol overdoses (Record *et al.*, 1975), when correction with sodium bicarbonate may be needed. Hypokalaemia is a very frequent finding, and may require large amounts of potassium for correction. Because urea is manufactured in the liver, the serum creatinine concentration and not the urea is used as the index of renal failure.

As well as a grossly prolonged prothrombin time, thrombocytopenia is common and may be partly the result of increased consumption secondary to disseminated intravascular coagulation (Rake *et al.*,

1971). If this is suspected, the fibrin degradation products and fibrinogen are estimated and a blood film examined. Blood is grouped on admission and two pints always available cross-matched as haemorrhage may be sudden and unexpected, particularly after the patient has been ill for some days.

Patients with fulminant hepatic failure, like other very sick and debilitated patients, are at risk from infection. Daily blood and urine cultures should be taken, sputum cultured whenever possible, and swabs taken from wound and cut-down sites.

Treatment of fulminant (acute) hepatic failure

The patient is transferred without delay to an intensive care unit. At King's College Hospital patients are looked after in a purpose-built liver failure unit with 24-hour medical cover. A urinary catheter, nasogastric tube, and central venous line are inserted, and regular readings of pulse, blood pressure, central venous pressure, and fluid balance are obtained and the patient's E.C.G. monitored.

The same general supportive measures apply in fulminant hepatic failure as in coma complicating cirrhosis, namely protein restriction, purgation, vitamin supplements, neomycin and lactulose adminis-tration, and the avoidance of sedatives. In addition, there are several specific problems.

Fluid and electrolyte balance

This is complex, as in severe cases renal failure almost invariably develops. Unlike the situation in chronic liver disease, the development of renal failure in fulminant hepatic failure is by no means always associated with a fatal outcome (Wilkinson *et al.*, 1975). If the patient survives, renal function returns to normal, although occasionally this may take some weeks and treatment of the renal failure should be vigorous. Once the intravascular volume has been restored frusemide (80–500 mg i.v.) or mannitol (200 ml 20% solution) are only occasion-ally of value in restoring urine output. More frequently dialysis is needed and peritoneal dialysis is the treatment of choice. Haemodialysis is poorly tolerated, often precipitating hypotension and bleeding.

Ten per cent dextrose with added potassium is the standard infusion fluid, and saline is to be avoided unless a genuine sodium depletion is demonstrated, as there is avid re-absorption of sodium by the renal tubule. Amino acid preparations are also avoided as the serum levels of most are greatly elevated and may exacerbate hepatic coma. Fat emulsions are also contraindicated in the presence of severe liver impairment.

Respiratory problems
A major problem is protection of the patient's airway from the risk of aspiration of blood or stomach contents. Early intubation is desirable and is performed as soon as the patient's gag reflex becomes depressed. Unexpected and unheralded respiratory arrest may occur before this

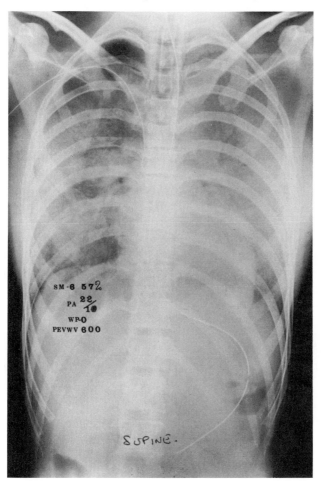

Fig. 5. Chest X-ray of patient with fulminant hepatic failure showing bilateral pulmonary oedema. The pulmonary artery wedge pressure was 0 mm Hg, pulmonary artery pressure 22/10 mm Hg and cardiac output 10 l/min.

stage and facilities for rapid intubation and ventilation must be available (Ward *et al.*, 1977).

The chest is X-rayed at least daily as pulmonary oedema (Fig. 5) (Trewby *et al.*, 1976) and pulmonary consolidation are common and often unsuspected by the clinician. Physiotherapy and adequate humidification are essential at all stages of the patient's illness.

Bleeding

Fifty per cent of patients with fulminant hepatic failure have marked lower oesophageal erosions, and these, together with gastric erosions constitute the major bleeding problems in fulminant hepatic failure. One group (Opolon and Caroli, 1974) have reported that increasing the gastric pH with antacids may decrease the incidence of gastrointestinal bleeding, but these are now being superseded by the H_2-receptor antagonist cimetidine. If continuing experience supports our initial results with cimetidine (Bailey *et al.*, 1976), it should be given prophylactically in fulminant hepatic failure to prevent bleeding from gastric and oesophageal erosions. The standard dose is 150 mg 6 hourly given over 90 minutes when the gastric pH falls below 5. Cimetidine may also be given in the same dose to prevent established bleeding (Macdougall *et al.*, 1976) from acute erosions.

Bleeding into the lungs, retroperitoneal haemorrhage, epistaxis and haemorrhage from peptic ulceration may also occur. The value of fresh frozen plasma in replacing the clotting deficiency is by no means proven, and the considerable sodium load (140 mmol/unit) may restrict its use. Concentrations of coagulation factors are not used as they may precipitate intravascular coagulation.

Only in those patients with unequivocal haematological evidence of DIC should heparin therapy be considered, and then heparin levels must be monitored by protamine sulphate titration, and the dose adjusted to keep levels between 0.5 and 1 mg/100 ml (Rake *et al.*, 1971).

Cardiovascular problems

The cardiac output is raised and transient hypotension is very common, particularly during the later stages of the illness, when it is often accompanied by bradycardia. In most instances it responds to infusions of either blood or plasma, even though no blood loss has occurred. If inotropic agents are needed to maintain the cardiac output the prognosis is very poor. We have found dopamine (10% w/v solution) to be more effective than isoprenaline in this situation.

Cerebral oedema

Cerebral oedema is found at autopsy in approximately 38% of patients dying from fulminant hepatic failure and coning with tonsillar herniation in 13% (Gazzard *et al.*, 1975). It is seldom possible, however, to predict during life which patients have developed cerebral oedema or coned. Papilloedema is rarely seen and bradycardia, pyrexia, and hypertension are uncommon. We have used glycerol (Record *et al.*, 1975), mannitol and dexamethasone in an attempt to lessen the frequency of this complication, but no convincing benefit has been observed.

CONCLUSION

Despite the measures outlined above, the mortality of grade IV hepatic coma remains depressingly high. This has led to the development of specialised techniques for artificial liver support and these are discussed in Part 4, ch. IV, p. 982.

REFERENCES

Bailey, R. J., MacDougall, B. R. D., and Williams, R. (1976). A controlled trial of H_2-receptor antagonists in prophylaxis of bleeding from gastrointestinal erosions in fulminant hepatic failure. *Gut* **17**, 389.

Benhamou, J. P., Rueff, R., and Sicot, C. (1972). Severe hepatic failure: a critical study of current therapy. *In* 'Liver and Drugs' (Ed. F. Orlandi and A. M. Jezequel) p. 213. New York.

Berthelot, P., Walker, J. G., Sherlock, S., and Reid, L. (1966). Arterial changes in the lungs in cirrhosis of the liver – lung spider nevi. *New Engl. J. Med.* **274**, 291.

Breen, K. J., Bryant, R. E., Levinson, J. D., and Schenker, S. (1972). Neomycin absorption in man: studies of oral and enema administration, and effect of intestinal ulceration. *Ann. Intern. Med.* **76**, 211.

Conn, H. O., and Fessel, J. M. (1971). Spontaneous bacterial peritonitis in cirrhosis: variations on a theme. *Medicine* (Baltimore) **50**, 161.

Elkington, S. G., Floch, M. H., and Conn, H. O. (1969). Lactulose in the treatment of chronic portal-systemic encephalopathy. A double blind clinical trial. *New Engl. J. Med.* **281**, 408.

Gazzard, B. G., Portmann, B., Murray-Lyon, I. M., and Williams, R. (1975). Causes of death in fulminant hepatic failure and relationship to quantitative histological assessment of parenchymal damage. *Quart. J. Med.* **176**, 615.

Helman, R. A., Temko, M. H., Nye, S. W., and Fallon, H. J. (1971). Alcoholic hepatitis: natural history and evaluation of prednisolone therapy. *Annals of Internal Medicine* **74**, 311.

Kreisberg, R. A., and Pennington, L. F. (1970). Tumour hypoglycaemia: a heterogeneous disorder. *Metabolism* **19**, 445.

Labadarios, D., Rossouw, J. E., Davis, M., and Williams, R. (1976). Pyridoxine deficiency in severe liver disease. *Proceedings of the Nutrition Society*. **35**, 141A.

Lunzer, M., James, I. M., Weinman, J. and Sherlock, S. (1974). Treatment of chronic hepatic encephalopathy with levadopa. *Gut* **15**, 555.

Macdougall, B. R. D., Bailey, R. J. and Williams, R. (1977). Histamine H_2-receptor antagonists in the prophylaxis and control of acute gastrointestinal haemorrhage in liver disease. *In* 'Cimetidine', pp. 329–336. Excerpta Medica.

Megyeri, C., Samols, E. and Marks, V. (1967). Glucose tolerance and diabetes in chronic liver disease. *Lancet* **2**, 1051.

Megyesi, C., Samols, E. and Marks, V. (1967). Glucose tolerance and diabetes in chronic liver disease. *Lancet* **2**, 1051.

Murray-Lyon, I. M., Pugh, R. N. M., Nunnerley, M. B., Laws, J. W., Dawson, J. L. and Williams, R. (1973). Treatment of bleeding oesophageal varices by infusion of vasopression into the superior mesenteric artery. *Gut* **14**, 59.

Nusbaum, M., Younis, M. T., Baum, S. and Blakemore, W. S. (1974). Control of portal hypertension. Selective mesenteric arterial infusion of vasopressin. *Archs. Surg.* **108**, 342.

Opolon, P. and Caroli, J. (1974). Etudes des facteurs du traitement des atrophies hepatiques aigues d-origine virale. *Medicine et Hygiene*, **32**, 159.

Parkes, J. D., Sharpstone, P. and Williams, R. (1970). Levadopa in hepatic coma. *Lancet* **1**, 1341.

Parsons, V., Wilkinson, S. P. and Weston, M. J. (1975). Use of dialysis in the treatment of renal failure in liver disease. *Postgrad. M. J.* **51**, 515.

Parsons-Smith, B. G., Summerskill, W. H. J., Dawson, A. M. and Sherlock, S. (1957). The electroencephalogram in hepatic coma. *Lancet* **2**, 867.

Pitcher, J. L. (1971). Safety and effectiveness of the modified Sengstaken-Blakemore tube: a prospective study. *Gastroenterology* **61**, 291.

Porter, H. P., Simon, F. R., Pope, C. E. H., Volwiler, W. and Fenster, L. F. (1971). Corticosteroid therapy in severe alcoholic hepatitis. A double blind drug trial. *New Engl. J. Med.* **284**, 1350.

Protte, J., Guffens, J. M. and Devas, J. (1974). Comparative study of basal arterial ammonemia and of orally induced hyperammonemia in chronic portal systemic encephalopathy, treatment with Neomycin, Lactulose and an association of Neomycin and Lactulose. *Digestion* **10**, 435.

Pugh, R. N. H., Murray-Lyon, I. M., Dawson, J. L., Pietroni, M. L. and Williams, R. (1973). Transection of the oesophagus for bleeding oesophageal varices. *Brit. J. Surg.* **60**, 646.

Rake, M. O., Flute, P. J., Shilkin, K. B., Lewis, M. L., Winch, J. and Williams, R. (1971). Early and intensive therapy of intravascular coagulation in acute liver failure. *Lancet* **2**, 1215.

Raschke, E. and Paquet, K. J. (1973). Management of haemorrhage from oesophageal varices using the oesophagoscopic sclerosing method. *Ann. Surgery* **177**, 99.

Record, C. O., Chase, R. A., Hughes, R. D., Murray-Lyon, I. M. and Williams, R. (1975). Glycerol therapy for cerebral oedema complicating fulminant hepatic failure. *Brit. Med. J.* **2**, 540.

Record, C. O., Iles, R. A., Cohen, R. D. and Williams, R. (1975). Acid-base metabolism and metabolic disturbance in fulminant hepatic failure. *Gut* **16**, 144.

Resnick, R. H., Ishihara, A., Schimmel, E. M., Chalmers, T. C. and the Boston

Interhospital Liver Group (1967). A controlled trial of colon exclusion. *Gastroenterology* **52**, 1115.

Schenker, S., Breen, K. J. and Hoyumpa, A. M. (1974). Hepatic encephalopathy: current status. *Gastroenterology* **66**, 121.

Strunin, L. (1969). Intravenous cannula for pressure measurements and prolonged fluid therapy. *Lancet* **1**, 502.

Teres, J., Bordas, J. M., Bru, C., Diaz, F., Brugucia, M. and Rodes, J. (1976). Upper gastrointestinal bleeding in cirrhosis: clinical and endoscopic correlations. *Gut* **17**, 37.

Trewby, P. N., Warren, R., Mackenzie, R., Crosbie, W. A., Laws, J. and Williams, R. (1976). Shock lung in fulminant hepatic failure. *Gut* **17**, 395.

Waldram, R., Davis, M., Nunnerley, H. and Williams, R. (1974). Emergency endoscopy after gastrointestinal haemorrhage in 50 patients with portal hypertension. *Brit. Med. J.* **4**, 94.

Ward, M. E., Trewby, P. N., Williams, R. and Strunin, L. (1977). Acute liver failure. Experience in a specialist unit. *Anaesthesia.* **32**, 228.

Wilkinson, S. P., Arroyo, V., Gazzard, B. G., Moodie, H. and Williams, R. (1974). Relation of renal impairment and haemorrhagic diathesis to endotoxaemia in fulminant hepatic failure. *Lancet* **1**, 521.

Wilkinson, S. P., Hurst, D., Portmann, B. and Williams, R. (1975). Pathogenesis of renal failure in cirrhosis and fulminant hepatic failure. *Post. Grad. Med. J.* **51**, 503.

VI

The Management of Abnormalities in Body Temperature

Section 1: The Physiology of Temperature Control

G. R. Hervey

INTRODUCTION

It is two hundred years since Blagden (1775) described the famous experiment in which a man remained well in a room heated to over 100°C by a red-hot stove, while a beefsteak alongside him cooked. The existence of physiological thermoregulation was thus demonstrated, and a certain tradition of 'do-it-on-yourself' established. The latter may be justified by the wide species differences in thermoregulatory mechanisms, although the actual body temperature regulated varies remarkably little between species (Burton and Edholm, 1955).

PATHOPHYSIOLOGY

Human body temperature in health is popularly considered to be 98.4°F, but in fact varies in space and time. There is a temperature gradient through the superficial layers of the body and along the limbs, reflecting insulation which is an essential part of the mechanism of regulation. Normally the skin is at an intermediate temperature between core and environment, with a further gradient through layers of air trapped in clothes and on the surface (Fig. 1). Body temperature exhibits a diurnal cycle, and rises in exercise, in the luteal phase of the

117

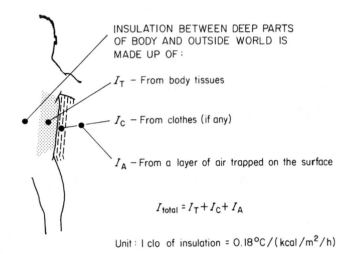

INSULATION BETWEEN DEEP PARTS
OF BODY AND OUTSIDE WORLD IS
MADE UP OF :

I_T – From body tissues

I_C – From clothes (if any)

I_A – From a layer of air trapped on the surface

$$I_{total} = I_T + I_C + I_A$$

Unit : 1 clo of insulation = $0.18°C / (kcal/m^2/h)$

Fig. 1. The insulation available to the body.

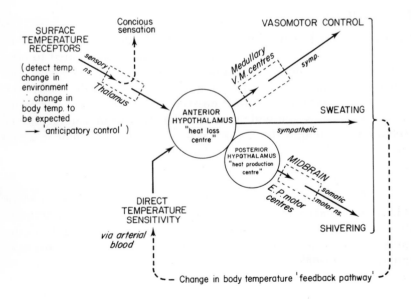

Fig. 2. Flow diagram of human thermio-regulation.

menstrual cycle, and in infections: in these situations the physiological thermostat evidently re-sets. When thermoregulatory responses occur there are variations in temperature which can be interpreted as 'load errors' of the thermostat (i.e. deviations from the ideal set point, which must be allowed to exist to produce the responses).

Man possesses three thermoregulatory effectors: vasomotor control, shivering and sweating (Fig. 2). Sympathetic vasomotor control varies blood flow from core to surface at the extremities, by-passing the insulation to a variable extent. The large surface-to-volume ratio of the extremities makes them efficient radiators (strictly convectors) when well perfused; in the cold the association of the deep arteries and venae comitantes provides a heat exchanger which reduces loss of heat to the surface. Vasomotor control affects a small proportion of the body surface and can only provide a fine adjustment.

Shivering is a special form of muscular exercise, initiated by connections from posterior hypothalamus to mid-brain motor system. It produces heat at up to about four times resting rate, which is about equivalent to brisk walking. Harder exercise can produce more heat but may be less efficient because it increases heat loss more. Shivering is as subject to fatigue as other forms of exercise.

Sweating, the active secretion of water on to the surface of the body, is a mechanism for heat loss which is uniquely developed in man. In favourable circumstances it can dissipate heat at twenty times resting rate, which exceeds the highest possible rate of heat production.

There are two inputs to the physiological thermostat (Fig. 2): the temperature of the hypothalamus, and nervous pathways from surface thermal receptors. The sensitivity to deep body temperature provides the closed-loop feedback which a control system must provide, if it is to maintain a set level. The surface receptors provide an open-loop, i.e. anticipatory or rate-sensitive, input, which improves the response of the system. The exact way in which the hypothalamus responds to the pattern of inputs has not, however, been fully analysed.

Thermoregulation

Thermoregulation can be studied quantitatively in terms of heat balance, and a quite simple approach can yield useful results. The significant channels of gain and loss of heat by the body core are estimated; clearly their algebraic sum, the heat balance, must be zero if core temperature is steady. There are only three important items (Fig. 3): metabolic heat production; exchange with the environment by conduction, convection and radiation (lumped together); and loss by evaporation. Each is expressed per unit of 'surface area' as given by Du Bois' formula. Metabolism can be measured via oxygen consumption, or predicted from knowledge of average metabolic rates at rest and in exercise. Heat flow to or from the environment is most simply found from Newton's Law, which states that the flow of heat per unit area is proportional to temperature difference. Replacing the proportionality

HEAT BALANCE	=	HEAT PRODUCTION (Basal + activity)	$\pm$	EXCHANGE WITH ENVIRONMENT (Radiation + conduction + convection)	$-$	HEAT LOSS BY EVAPORATION (Insensible perspiration + sweating)

= 0, when body temperature is steady.

Exchange with environment obeys Newton's Law of cooling.

So, rearranging:

$$\frac{T_B - T_E}{I_T + I_C + I_A} = M - E$$

where: T_B is body core temperature
T_E is environmental temperature
I_T is insulation due to body tissues
I_C is insulation due to clothing
I_A is insulation due to air
M is metabolic heat production
E is evaporative heat loss

in compatible units, e.g. °C and kcal/m²/h.

Fig. 3. The heat balance equation.

constant by its reciprocal makes it insulation, and produces a formula analogous to Ohm's Law for electricity (Fig. 3). Successive layers of insulation are additive. The clo is a convenient unit which approximates the insulation afforded by an average North American suit (Fig. 1). Evaporation can be predicted adequately for non-shivering conditions from Du Bois' empirical finding that it accounts for a quarter of resting heat production. Average rates of sweating in hot conditions can be predicted from tables such as those of McArdle et al. (1947).

If heat balance is not zero, the rate of change of body temperature can be predicted with the aid of suitable assumptions as to the body's specific heat (0.86) and the proportion to be counted as core (0.64: Burton and Edholm, 1955).

The equation enables such questions to be answered as: 'At what environmental temperature will an average unclothed man, at rest and in comfort, be in heat balance?' T_B is 37°C. T_E is to be found. M is 1 met (50 kcal or 210 kJ . m^{-2} . h^{-1}). E *is* $\frac{1}{4}$ of this. I_C is 0 . I_A in still air is about 0.8 clo. Thermal 'comfort' implies neither sweating nor shivering. If vasomotor control varies over the possible range, for an average man I_T will be 0.15 to 0.75 clo (Burton and Edholm, 1955). Solving gives T_E a

Table 1. Ranges of physiological temperature regulation available from vasomotor control, from sweating and from shivering

	Air temperature at which nude man would be in heat balance (°C)	Temperature at which normally clothed man would be in heat balance (°C)	Effect on heat balance of nude man at 28°C air temperature (kcal/h)	Resulting rate of change of body temperature (°C/h)
Max sweating	150°	(Clothes would interfere with sweating)	− 1200	− 19°
Sweating				
Max vasodilation	30°	22°	− 21	− 0.3°
Vasomotor range	28°	20°	0	0
Max vasoconstriction	26°	18°	+ 13	+ 0.2°
Shivering				
Max shivering	− 10°	− 40°	+ 230	+ 4°

Results of heat balance calculations, demonstrating the ranges of control and effectiveness of the thermoregulatory effector mechanisms.

Notes: All figures are the results of calculations for an assumed average individual. The figures for extreme temperatures should not be taken as practical ones, but as indicating the relative ranges of control available. In practice air movement and humidity will usually make the effective temperature of an environment more unfavourable than the air temperature alone would indicate. Also, tolerance may be limited by local injury to the body surface and not by ability to maintain heat balance. Sweating and shivering at high rates can only be sustained for a limited time.

range of 26.5 to 30.5°C. If the subject were to don 1.2 clo of clothing, T_E would become 20 to 24°C, a result which agrees with everyday experience. Table 1 lists the results of calculations to show the ranges of control of the body's three thermoregulatory effectors.

These simple calculations lead to some interesting conclusions. First, man is a tropical animal. His neutral environmental temperature – that at which heat balance obtains with minimum thermoregulatory effort – is a tropical one. He has an enormous capacity to dissipate heat, but his physiological mechanisms cannot achieve heat balance at temperatures regularly met in cold climates. Secondly, the calculations demonstrate the narrow range of vasomotor control. This may seem paradoxical: common experience suggests that man can exist in a considerable range of environments without sweating or shivering, or even using full vasoconstriction or dilation. The two points, however, demonstrate a key fact of human thermoregulation: it is not for the most part a physiological process, but rather a behavioural and technological one. Situations which would call for thermoregulatory responses cause discomfort: this motivates individuals with any control over their situation toward alterations in behaviour, such as changing clothing, heating or ventilation. On the longer time scale, the behavioural responses are expressed in the technologies of clothing, building, heating and ventilation and so forth. Behavioural thermoregulation can also be described as operating to maintain a constant, neutral (i.e. tropical) micro-climate in immediate contact with the body. The supersession of physiological mechanisms by technological ones has its obverse. Anywhere outside the tropics, man is very dependent on his technology, and on the large energy turnover it entails.

Insulation

Heat balance calculations also bring out the importance of insulation. Most forms of insulation, including clothing and mammalian fur, insulate by trapping air, and provide about 4.7 clo of insulation per inch of thickness. Not all parts of the body can be fully covered, and maximum, arctic-style clothing achieves around 6 clo overall. For a resting man this lowers the calculated T_E for balance only to about $-10°C$. Table 1 shows that changing M, alone, to the $3\frac{1}{2}$ mets characteristic of hard shivering or moderate work has about the same effect. If, however, I_C and M are both increased, the calculation gives the apparently absurd value for T_E of $-170°C$. The qualitative conclusions are sound, however. The tolerance of a heavily clad man working in an arctic environment is limited by local exposure of the skin, not by heat balance. Arctic clothing is very likely to be inadequate at rest; it must be adjustable for insulation, and also permeable to water vapour, to allow for work. In general, the combination of high heat production and high insulation is highly effective in maintaining body temperature in the cold, while either alone is ineffective. If the insulation surrounding the body core is low, thermoregulation is therefore gravely disadvantaged: this is important to the management of babies (even in incubators), the elderly, and victims of trauma or exposure.

The extreme situation for lowered insulation is immersion in water.

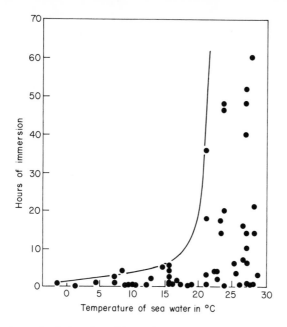

Fig. 4. Molnar's graph relating time of immersion to sea temperature for successful survival incidents. (Re-drawn from Molnar, 1946.)

The high conductivity and heat capacity of water makes trapping on the surface and in clothes – unless specially designed, e.g. the 'wet suit' – so ineffective that I_A and I_C approximate to zero. For a maximally shivering man T_E for balance then works out at 20°C. In water below this temperature the body temperature must fall. This is a most important conclusion for shipwreck survival. It is confirmed by the data of Molnar (1946) (Fig. 4). Only in water above 20°C was survival time independent of water temperature; below, there was a maximum duration, which fell from around 10 hours at 18°C to less than one hour at 0°C. The hazards of sudden immersion in cold water are compounded by the effects of respiratory and cardiovascular reflexes (Keatinge and Evans, 1961). The value of wearing ample clothing and if possible a waterproof outer layer when immersion is possible cannot be overstressed. The rapid flow of heat is also the basis of immersion in hot water as a method of re-warming.

Individuals vary in tissue insulation. Molnar (1946) noticed some exceptions among his subjects, and these in fact include anyone who swims the English Channel. Swimming involves about twice the heat

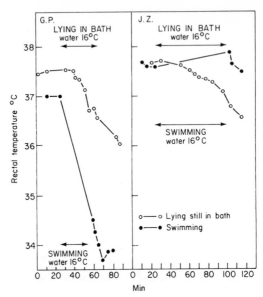

Fig. 5. Deep body temperature in Pugh and Edholm's experiment.

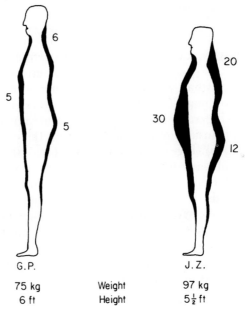

Fig. 6. Diagrammatic representation of subcutaneous fat thickness. Measured by skinfold calipers. Figures are in mm. (Reproduced from Pugh and Edholm, 1955.)

production seen in shivering. Pugh and Edholm (1955) (Figs 5 and 6), however, showed that this is not the whole story. Lying still in water at 16°C, both the swimmer J.Z. and the physiologist G.P. cooled gradually. When they swam, J.Z. maintained a normal temperature, but G.P.'s temperature fell catastrophically. The explanation of J.Z.'s advantage is evident from Fig. 6 and Table 2. Swimming halved tissue insulation, presumably by bringing blood to the limbs and stirring the water. This made G.P.'s insulation so low that his heat loss increased more than his heat production. A subsequent study (Pugh et al., 1960) showed that Channel swimmers are characterised by overweight, which is about half due to extra fat and half to muscle. Such 'fat athletes' are

Table 2. Calculated insulation between body core and water. (Data from Pugh and Edholm, 1955)

| In water at 16°C | Calculated Insulation (clo) | |
	G.P.	J.Z.
Lying still	0.44	0.94
Swimming	0.23	0.42

unusual. Advice to all others accidentally immersed must be not to swim, unless to easily attained safety (Keatinge, 1969). Golden and Hervey (1972) performed some further studies which included the first female subjects. One female, who although below standard weight for her height had a low lean body mass and correspondingly high fat content, cooled at only a fifth of the rate seen in a male classmate, who was an athlete and produced heat much faster (Hervey, 1975). It is possible that some groups, for example professional divers and fast long-distance swimmers, develop adaptations which effectively increase their insulation, possibly by means other than fat accumulation.

HYPOTHERMIA

The very young and the very old are particularly liable to accidental hypothermia, because they have the further disadvantage of less sensitive thermoregulatory mechanisms than those in the prime of life. Their capacity for heat production is relatively low. If, on top of this, malnutrition leads to loss of fat, body temperature becomes virtually dependent upon the environment, and can only be maintained normal if this is in a narrow, unusually warm range. Very rarely, adults of normal build are encountered who appear to have a specific defect of the central thermoregulatory mechanism, leading to the same result.

As in other fields of medicine, the best treatment for hypothermia is undoubtedly prevention. Understanding of the principles of thermoregulation, and the methods of predicting the outcome in specific situations, should help to achieve this. If hypothermia nevertheless occurs, the next section will be concerned with its treatment.

REFERENCES

Blagden, C. (1775). Experiments and observations in a heated room. *Phil. Trans. Roy. Soc.* **65**, 111.

Burton, A. C. and Edholm, O. G. (1955). 'Man in a cold environment'. Edward Arnold, London.

Golden, F. St. C. and Hervey, G. R. (1972). A class experiment on immersion hypothermia. *J. Physiol.* **227**, 35.

Hervey, G. R. (1975). Physiological changes encountered in hypothermia. *Proc. Roy. Soc. Med.* **66**, 1053.

Keatinge, W. R. (1969). 'Survival in cold water'. Blackwell Scientific Publications, Oxford and Edinburgh.

Keatinge, W. R. and Evans, M. (1961). The respiratory and cardiovascular response to immersion in cold and warr water. *Q. J. exp. Physiol.* **46**, 83.

McArdle, B., Dunham, W., Holling, H. E., Ladell, W. S. S., Scott, J. W., Thomson, M. L. and Weiner, J. S. (1947). Prediction of the physiological effects of warm and hot environments. MRC, RNPRC Report RN47/391.

Molnar, G. W. (1946). Survival of hypothermia by men immersed in the ocean. *J. Am. med. Assoc.* **131**, 1046.

Pugh, L. G. C. and Edholm, O. G. (1955). The physiology of channel swimmers. *Lancet* **2**, 761.

Pugh, L. G. C., Edholm, O. G., Fox, R. H., Wolff, H. S., Hervey, G. R., Hammond, W. H., Tanner, J. M. and Whitehouse, R. H. (1960). A physiological study of channel swimming. *Clin. Sci.* **19**, 257.

Section 2: The Management of the Hypothermic Patient

F. St. C. Golden

INTRODUCTION

The normal deep body temperature (core temperature) for man is in the region of 37°C, although variations of 1°C about this level are within physiological limits. When the core temperature falls below an arbitrarily defined limit of 35°C, then the state of 'hypothermia' is said to exist. The lower limits of core temperature compatible with life are in the region of 24–26°C, although survival has been recorded in a patient whose rectal temperature was accidentally lowered to 18°C (Laufman, 1951) and one in whom the core temperature was intentionally reduced to 9°C (Niazi and Lewis, 1958). However, all patients with core temperatures below 30°C should be regarded as being critically ill.

Hypothermia, as the name implies, is just a descriptive term for the state of the core temperature of the body and, as in pyrexia (hyperthermia), should not *per se* be considered synonymous with any definite clinical condition requiring a standard treatment, since the cause may be secondary to some co-existing pathology. The management will therefore be dependent on the aetiology and whether the condition has developed acutely or has been slow in onset. In temperate and arctic climates the majority of cases of hypothermia encountered will be of the primary nature, i.e. without associated causative pathology.

In this section, an attempt will be made to review the problem and suggest guidelines on management, although with the current limitations of good factual scientific knowledge of the subject it is extremely difficult to give any authoritative advice on precise lines of treatment.

127

AETIOLOGY

When body heat loss exceeds heat production then hypothermia is the inevitable consequence. The imbalance may result from simple overwhelming of the normal thermoregulatory mechanisms from exposure to an extreme environment, or to a relatively moderate environment with inadequate body insulation. Hypothermia so caused, may be classified as 'Primary Accidental Hypothermia'. Depending on its rate of onset it may be further subdivided into 'acute' or 'chronic' types. The former term is usually reserved for the condition encountered in fit young adults, following accidental immersion in cold water; chronic accidental hypothermia being classically a geriatric problem.

'Secondary Accidental Hypothermia' is, as its name implies, a complicating condition of some other malady where the body thermoregulatory mechanisms are impaired, partially or totally, resulting in a negative imbalance in the heat balance equation. Thus, any disease process, metabolic disorder or traumatic condition which interferes with either the thermoregulatory control centre, the input or output from that control, or the organs through which such output is effected, could result in secondary hypothermia if the patient is in a cold environment. The management of a patient with hypothermia associated with other pathology (secondary hypothermia) requires appropriate treatment of the primary disorder. Management of the hypothermic state should be largely based on whether it has developed acutely or has been present for some time. Clearly the reader should refer to the relevant chapters regarding other aspects of management in secondary hypothermia.

PATHOLOGY AND CLINICAL FEATURES

The most noticeable effect of hypothermia, and the one which normally brings the condition to attention, is the effect on the central nervous system. Although no precise temperature level can be correlated with the disappearance or reappearance of some particular response; in general the temperature at which symptoms become manifest appears to be related to the rate of loss of body temperature. In acute hypothermia, signs of C.N.S. depression are noticeable at higher core temperatures, whereas in chronic hypothermia the signs and symptoms described below may not become apparent until the body temperature has fallen a further 2°C or so.

In acute hypothermia the patient generally becomes dysarthric and spatially disorientated at core temperatures below 34°C, although pain is still readily appreciated. Below 33°C there is a progressive clouding of consciousness, drowsiness and confusion. The pupils begin to dilate and, along with musculo-skeletal reflexes, reactions become progressively sluggish with diminished slow prolonged responses. Around 30°C, consciousness is normally lost and the muscles become hypertonic often leading to some confusion in diagnosis – neck stiffness simulating that of meningism. At about 28°C the muscles become flaccid and the pupillary light reflex and deep tendon reflexes are lost. Below this level the 'gag reflex' may also be lost.

Table 1. Estimated maximum safe period of cerebral anoxia at varying deep body temperatures around 30°C (after Hunter, A. R., 1975)

Temp. °C	Time (min)
32	3
31	$4\frac{1}{2}$
30	6
29	8
28	10–12

Shivering may or may not be present in the early stages, depending on the rate of change of skin temperature and the absence of fatigue. Shivering will be absent if skin temperature is high, or fatigue or some intoxicating or paralysing condition is present. Shivering when present, will usually wane at around 32°C when the progressive onset of muscle rigidity will diminish its observable intensity, although still giving rise to interference on the E.C.G. tracing. If shivering is present, C.S.F. pressure will be raised.

Oxygen consumption will also be related to shivering but as metabolism progressively declines with deepening hypothermia oxygen consumption is reduced, while respiration is slow, shallow and difficult to detect in profound hypothermia. During rewarming, hypoxaemia may reach dangerous levels, particularly if shivering is present. When circulatory arrest complicates acute hypothermia the interval before cerebral damage occurs is greater than that pertaining to euthermic patients (Table 1).

The most important physiological disturbance produced by hypothermia is that to the cardiovascular system. The cooling of the peripheral tissues is accompanied by vasoconstriction with an associated rise in blood pressure and central venous pressure. However, with time there is a compensatory diuresis resulting in a reduction in circulating blood volume, and a marked haemoconcentration. Again, in the absence of shivering, the direct effect of cold on the atrial pacemaker results in a progressive slowing of the heart rate and, although stroke volume increases, the overall effect is a reduction in cardiac output.

Coronary blood flow is reduced, but both Penrod (1951) and Berne (1959) have shown that it is sufficient for the needs of the hypothermic myocardium. Nevertheless, because of the great relative prolongation of diastole at myocardial temperatures below 28°C, myocardial capillary perfusion will be very poor and at these temperatures there is a tendency to fibrillate, particularly if the heart is irritated or the demands or work load are increased. Death usually results from asystole or ventricular fibrillation at temperatures in the region of 24–26°C.

At temperatures below 33°C the electrocardiogram often shows the presence of atrial fibrillation with associated heart block. Later, the QRS complex may be broadened with a very prolonged Q–T interval. In some cases, a 'J' wave is visible at the junction of the QRS and ST segments. Some regard this as an ominous sign but it may not necessarily be so. Much more portentous is the appearance of frequent ventricular ectopics which may be the forerunner of ventricular fibrillation. In acute accidental hypothermia, however, there is normally a ventricular tachycardia with frequent ectopics, even at core temperatures as high as 30°C. In these cases, such an E.C.G., although alarming, is not necessarily pathological and usually returns to normal without any specific treatment on rewarming (*vide infra*).

The depressant effect of cold on the renal tubule results in a reduction in water and Na^+ reabsorption and excretion of K^+, so although there is an overall reduction in glomerular filtration this is counteracted by an increase in the proportion of the filtrate excreted. The increased loss of Na^+ and retention of K^+ is not significant in acute hypothermia but may be so in the chronic condition.

Interpretation of blood investigations

Caution should be exercised in interpreting blood samples. Because of the disturbances to the peripheral circulation only arterial samples are likely to be of value, and even then the interpretation of many of the results is difficult, as accepted norms apply only to normothermic individuals. Many of the observed 'abnormalities' return to normal levels without treatment, as body temperature rises. Blood gases, analysed automatically at 37°C, should be corrected for temperature before interpretation (*vide infra*).

Raised serum amylase levels are frequently encountered in chronic accidental hypothermia (McClean *et al.*, 1973), but are not necessarily associated with acute pancreatitis. Similarly, hyperglycaemia (<14 mmol/l) may be found in non-diabetic patients. The explanation for this phenomenon is the inability of insulin to assist the passage of glucose across the cell membrane at tissue temperatures in the region of 30°C (Wynn, 1954). Thus a hypothermic diabetic will remain largely unresponsive to insulin therapy until rewarmed above 31°C, and if given large amounts of insulin before rewarming, is in danger of developing hypoglycaemic coma without regaining consciousness on rewarming. Continuous monitoring of blood sugar is therefore essential.

A hypothermic patient may be mistakenly diagnosed as dead, breath and heart sounds being difficult to detect by auscultation, pupils being fixed and dilated and the skin cold. This particularly applies to cases of barbiturate poisoning, complicated by hypothermia. In the absence of confirmatory electrocardiographic evidence the definition of death is failure to revive.

COMPLICATIONS

Complications include erythematous skin patches and a puffy facial appearance. Acute haemorrhage may develop from single or multiple gastric erosions and acute pancreatitis is a well recognised complication. Bronchopneumonia may develop and like the preceding complications, appears to be related to the duration of hypothermia rather than the magnitude. Little information exists as to the underlying mechanisms producing these changes. It is uncertain whether they are a primary consequence of the prolonged tissue cooling below a critical level or secondary to the associated physiological adjustments which occur. None of these complications were found in patients maintained between 29° and 33°C for periods of 1 to 8 days following intracranial surgery (Bloch, 1967) or by Fay and Smith (1941) who maintained patients below 30°C for up to 5 days in an attempt to treat advanced malignancy.

Acute pancreatitis is common in chronic cases of accidental hypothermia; it is usually mild, but even when severe it is not accompanied by signs of an intra-abdominal emergency and does not directly affect the patient's chances of survival (McClean *et al.*, 1973). It is usually only diagnosed on necropsy. Bronchopneumonia is the most frequently encountered complication and the commonest cause of death.

Renal failure is an occasional late complication of chronic hypothermia. It is probable that this is a consequence of concomitant prolonged mild hypoxaemia, hypotension and hypovolaemia rather than a direct effect of cold on the renal tubular tissue.

The E.C.G. trace may give rise to considerable alarm but usually returns to normal within 8 to 12 hours of rewarming without any specific treatment. At core temperatures below 30°C ventricular fibrillation may develop, this may be precipitated by movement of the patient by attending personnel. Patient stimulation (e.g. by movement or nasopharyngeal suction) must therefore be avoided at core temperatures of 30°C or below.

MANAGEMENT

Several controversies exist regarding patient management, viz. should they be rapidly or slowly rewarmed, and how much active interference is necessary. Insufficient good scientific information exists at present to enable categoric advice to be given. Before deciding any course of therapy it will be necessary first to measure deep body temperature to confirm the diagnosis, and thereafter to monitor it and some other parameters during the course of treatment.

Patient monitoring

A variety of systems exist for monitoring core temperature, Part 2, ch. II, p. 312. For monitoring the progress of hypothermic patients during rewarming, rectal temperature, monitored on electric telethermometer, is adequate for most purposes. There are, however, some pitfalls to be aware of, viz. the probe should be inserted at least 10 cm past the anal sphincter and the lead should be taped to the buttock to prevent accidental withdrawal. The temperature recorded will be 0.25–0.5°C below blood temperature and there is a lag of several minutes between the two when blood temperature is changing. A more accurate indication of true blood temperature may be obtained by monitoring oesophageal temperature behind the right heart. Blood temperature can also be recorded accurately from the external auditory meatus using a servo controlled heating pad over the pinna to counter the thermal gradient (Keatinge and Sloan, 1975). Core temperature may also be accurately and conveniently measured by a system developed by the Bioengineering Division of the M.R.C., utilising a pad heated to skin temperature placed over the sternum (Fig. 5, p. 313).

E.C.G. monitoring is essential. Shiver interference may obscure the wave form. The use of electronic filters coupled with the placing of electrodes away from muscle masses, e.g. over the sternum, will markedly improve the trace although making the wave form unconventional. Rate and rhythm will however be discernable.

Arterial blood gases should be frequently monitored, in particular when the patient is being actively rewarmed.

Interpretation of blood gases may produce some difficulty due to their increased solubility at lower temperatures. As most auto analysers are pre-set to measure the blood sample at 37°C, the $PaCO_2$ obtained will be artificially high while the pH will be artificially low. Fig. 1 is an alignment nomogram which gives some indication of their actual values when their values at 37°C and the blood (core) temperature at the time the sample was taken are known. Some caution should be exercised in interpreting the nomogram too literally as the data is calculated assuming a $PaCO_2$ of 40 mm Hg at 37°C, and a normal haemoglobin concentration. If shivering is present, the $PaCO_2$ could be considerably above 40 mm Hg.

A central venous catheter is recommended for both pressure monitoring and the administration of warmed intravenous fluids when necessary. Since these patients are susceptible to cardiac dysrhythmias the catheter must be inserted under E.C.G. monitoring control and care must be taken not to irritate the tricuspid valve with the catheter tip. The bladder should be catheterised and hourly urinary output observed.

Treatment

The incidence of complications in hypothermia is high at core temperatures below 32°C, and appears to be time related, complications increasing with time spent below these temperatures. Death from ventricular fibrillation is possible below 30°C and likely below 28°C.

The first priority of treatment is to stem heat loss from the surface of the body by insulating the patient with a woollen blanket. In ambient temperatures below 30°C the head should also be insulated because of the absence of a cold vasoconstriction response in the blood vessels of the

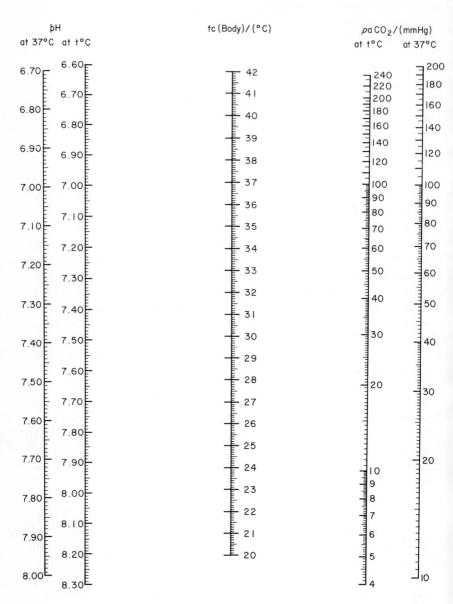

Fig. 1. pH/PaCO$_2$ temperature nomogram for whole blood. (Reproduced, with permission, facsimile from Siggaard–Andersen, 1974.)

head. Even with adequate insulation, because of the temperature gradient between the 'core' and the 'shell', there will be a continued fall in core temperature for a further period of 10–20 min before the core temperature stabilises and begins to increase.

The indications for active rewarming are controversial. In patients in whom core temperature is falling very slowly, an interval of 30 minutes should be allowed after the application of insulation to determine whether active rewarming is called for. Patients in whom the history suggests acute hypothermia, e.g. immersion victims, will benefit from active rewarming early on. Active rewarming should also be instituted in patients with a core temperature on admission of 30°C or below with an associated cardiac dysrhythmia.

Where hypothermia has developed gradually, e.g. in the elderly or in the patient with hypothyroidism, rewarming by simple insulation is probably adequate. Certainly the rate of rewarming in such patients should be gradual and any form of active rewarming instituted, should ensure that the rate of core temperature rise should be no greater than 0.5°C per hour. It should also be noted that rewarming a hypovolaemic patient without volume replacement may be fatal.

Published evidence exists which favours rapid active rewarming with (Ledingham and Mone, 1972; Exton Smith, 1973) and without (Alexander, 1945; Keatinge, 1969) supportive therapy. Other works favour slow passive rewarming (Maclean *et al.*, 1973; Mills, 1974).

Active rewarming

Active rewarming entails the addition of heat to the body to supplement its own metabolic heat production. Such a procedure is necessary when body temperature does not increase following the application of adequate insulation to the surface of the body. Active rewarming can vary in sophistication from extracorporal heating of blood or peritoneal dialysis, to the simpler use of heat cradles.

Heated hot water blankets and heat cradles

Probably the most extensively used methods are electrically heated hot water blankets and heat cradles. These increase the core temperature at a rate of 0.5–1°C/h. Alexander (1945) stated that rewarming with heat cradles was uneven and there was also danger of burns developing in tissues with an impaired circulation. The heat cradle over the torso has added disadvantages, namely by heating a large surface area it increases the demands on blood volume and cardiac output, by extending the area affected by heat vasodilation, and heat transfer being by radiation is less effective than the conductive heat transfer of a hot water blanket.

Immersion in hot water

One of the most widely advocated and controversial methods of active rewarming is to immerse the patient in a bath of hot water without supportive therapy. Both Alexander (1945), who reported on the experiments carried out by the Nazis at Dachau, and Keatinge (1969) referred to acute hypothermia following immersion in cold water in relatively fit young adults. Their evidence, supported by animal work (Zingg, 1969), showed that the optimum treatment for such cases immediately after removal from the cold water is rapid surface rewarming by placing the patient in a hot water bath at a temperature of 42–45°C. No supportive evidence exists to prove the value of hot bath teatment when there has been a time delay of 30 min or more between the time the victim was removed from the cold stress and a hot bath being available.

In view of these findings, immersion in a hot bath has little place in hospital management of hypothermic patients, except in the rare case of complete immersion in a patient known previously to be well, where the victim can be placed in the hot bath within 30 min of being removed from the cold water.

Experience suggests that in immersion accidents the victim is actually more likely to drown before sufficient time has elapsed for cooling to a critical level, unless the airway was supported clear of the surface of the water, as by a life-jacket. The recent upsurge in aquatic recreational activities, coupled with the increasing use of life-jackets, makes it likely that hypothermia, often complicated by partial drowning, will be encountered more frequently. The management of such cases is discussed in Part 2, ch. V, p. 577.

Hot bath immersion has proven however to be the ideal treatment of shipwreck survivors at sea. In such cases it may prove lifesaving in those who appear to be dead on rescue.

Rewarming by immersing an isolated limb in hot water is theoretically feasible, provided the circulation is adequate, but no evidence exists to prove the effectiveness of this technique in profoundly hypothermic patients. Chronic hypothermic patients may in addition be suffering from some degree of peripheral non-freezing cold injury which would contraindicate rapid rewarming of the injured part.

Peritoneal dialysis

Peritoneal dialysis has been used successfully, particularly in those cases where the hypothermia has resulted from barbiturate overdosage. This technique has the advantage of permitting the removal of barbiturate from the blood at the same time as rewarming.

Respiratory rewarming

In recent years, 'respiratory rewarming' by warming (to 41°C) and humidifying (to 100%) the air or oxygen the patient is breathing, has been advocated as a means of actively rewarming hypothermic patients (Lloyd, 1973; Shanks and Marsh, 1973). The success claimed for this technique is unlikely to be attributable to any physical transfer of heat into the body, as the heat capacity of the gases in question is too small and the heat transfer from the latent heat of condensation is also small in relation to the heat input required to increase the body temperature (ca. 100 watts for $1°C\,h^{-1}$). The value must lie in reduction of evaporative heat loss from the respiratory tract. The procedure has been found valuable in patients with cardiac dysrhythmias associated with hypothermia and should certainly be instituted if the patient has to be intubated and ventilated during resuscitation. Limited clinical experience has been supported by the research experience of Lloyd and Mitchell (1974) who claimed an immediate improvement of the E.C.G. of hypothermic sheep when using this technique.

Associated abnormalities

Hypoxia. During rewarming hypoxia may become sufficiently severe to warrant administration of oxygen by intermittent positive pressure ventilation (I.P.P.V.). A pulmonary end-expiratory pressure (P.E.E.P.) may be indicated but should be instituted with care (Part 2, ch. II, p. 327). Endotracheal intubation may precipitate a cardiac dysrhythmia but generally this reverts spontaneously with hand ventilation on oxygen. A profound fall in $PaCO_2$ may easily develop in hypothermic patients on artificial ventilation and should be avoided by the judicious introduction of a dead space.

Acidosis. Metabolic acidosis is likely to become marked during active rewarming and should be corrected by intravenous warmed sodium bicarbonate.

Hypotension during rewarming is generally due to a fall in the dynamic blood volume and is generally corrected by volume replacement with a warmed fluid – the fluid used depending upon electrolyte and acid base analyses. Volume replacement should be gauged according to right atrial pressure readings, pulse rate and volume, and urine output (Part 2, ch. II, p. 362).

Hyperglycaemia. Abnormalities of blood glucose should be noted but do not require any corrective measures until core temperature approaches 33°C when, if still present, routine therapeutic measures should be taken. Insulin should be given intravenously – the initial dose being 16–20 units followed by 4–8 units hourly. Dextrostix monitoring is essential – insulin being stopped once the blood glucose is 8 mmol/l or less.

Arrhythmias

Antiarrhythmic drugs have little, if any, effect on hypothermic cardiac arrhythmias which normally resolve as temperature returns to normal and invariably within 12 hours of doing so. Hypothermic ventricular fibrillation is remarkably resistant to defibrillation but appears to be more susceptible following the administration of magnesium sulphate (Büky, 1970). Ventricular fibrillation is often precipitated by patient interference, e.g. turning.

Drug therapy

Drugs are not of value in the specific management of hypothermia, and if indicated because of some co-existing clinical problem, the efficacy of the drug, in particular its distribution in the tissues and rate of metabolism should be considered. Antibiotics may be indicated if the hypothermic condition is complicated by infection such as bronchopneumonia.

Passive rewarming

Passive rewarming should be conducted where hypothermia has

developed slowly and where there is no cardiac dysrhythmia. It consists of intensive barrier nursing care with the patient being allowed to rewarm spontaneously by his or her own metabolic processes in a room maintained at $30 \pm 2.0°C$. Convective heat loss from the skin is reduced by covering with one or two blankets, usually supported by a cradle. Core temperature is monitored continuously to ensure rewarming is progressing steadily but not too rapidly (i.e. not exceeding 0.5–0.75°C h^{-1}), should this be so insulation must be reduced. A right atrial pressure line should be inserted – fluid being given should the level fall. Urine output and E.C.G. monitoring is essential. Electrolyte, acid base

Table 2. Summary of management of the hypothermic patient

INITIAL ACTION on admission:	1 Monitor – Core temperature E.C.G. Blood gases Electrolytes and blood glucose Right atrial pressure 2 Insulate the patient to prevent further heat loss 3 Place in warm room $(30 \pm 2.0°C)$
REWARM:	ACTIVELY 1 All whose core temperature is static or still falling 30 min after insulation was instituted 2 All who are shivering violently 3 All whose E.C.G. appearance is deteriorating 4 All whose history is suggestive of acute hypothermia e.g. immersion victims PASSIVELY 1 All whose core temperature is rising on being adequately insulated
CONTROL:	1 Rate of rise of temperature to $< 1.0°C$ h^{-1} by regulating temperature of rewarming system or the amount of insulation used. An exception to this advice should be made in acute hypothermia when temperature increase may be as rapid as possible or when the core temperature is $< 30°C$ and cardiac dysrythmias are present 2 PaO_2 by oxygen via a face mask or by I.P.P.V. with or without P.E.E.P. Maintained $PaCO_2$ within normal range ($PaCO_2$ will be artificially raised if analysed at 37°C – see Fig. 1) 3 pH by warmed i.v. $NaHCO_3$ but again avoid over-correction by referring to Fig. 1 4 Hypotension by warmed i.v. fluids under right atrial pressure monitoring control

balance and blood gases should be monitored. Hypoxia is invariably present and should be treated with oxygen via a face mask unless the corrected PaO_2 is 8.0 kPa (60 mm Hg) or less when intubation and ventilation should be considered. Sodium bicarbonate may be required to correct a metabolic acidosis and insulin for hyperglycaemia.

This method of rewarming may encourage shivering and thus hypoxia and acidosis. Shivering may increase oxygen demands and can be reduced by warming the skin by a heat cradle or hot water blanket. As bronchopneumonia is an almost inevitable sequel in chronic hypothermia in geriatric cases, a broad spectrum antibiotic should be given.

Suggested management of the hypothermic patient is summarised in Table 2.

In the intensive care situation, with active rewarming and full supportive therapy, a success rate of 70% has been claimed (Ledingham and Mone, 1974) while a 50% success rate has been reported for similar patients treated by slow passive rewarming and barrier nursing (Mills, 1974).

REFERENCES

Alexander, L. (1945). The treatment of shock from prolonged exposure to cold, especially in water. Combined Intelligence Objectives Sub-committee APO413, CIOS Item 24, HMSO, London.

Berne, R. M. (1959). Cardiodynamics and the coronary circulation in hypothermia. *Ann. N.Y. Acad. Sci.* **80**, 365.

Bloch, M. (1967). Cerebral effects of rewarming following profound hypothermia: significance for the management of severe cranio-cerebral injury in acute pyrexia. *Brain* **90**, 769.

Büky, B. (1970). Effect of magnesium on ventricular fibrillation due to hypothermia. *Br. J. Anaesth.* **42**, 886.

Exton-Smith, A. N. (1973). Accidental hypothermia. *Brit. Med. J.* **4**, 727.

Fay, T. and Smith, G. N. (1941). Observations on reflex responses during prolonged periods of human refrigeration. *Arch. Neurol. Psychiat.* **45**, 215.

Hunter, A. R. (1975). 'Neurosurgical anaesthesia', Second Edition, p. 193. Blackwell Scientific Publications, Oxford, London, Edinburgh and Melbourne.

Keatinge, W. R. (1969). 'Survival in cold water'. Blackwell Scientific Publications, Oxford and Edinburgh.

Keatinge, W. R. and Sloan, R. E. G. (1975). Deep body temperature from aural canal with servo-controlled heating to outer ear. *J. appl. Physiol.* **38**, 919.

Laufman, H. (1951). Profound accidental hypothermia. *J. Am. Med. Assoc.* **147**, 1201.

Ledingham, I. McA. and Mone, J. G. (1972). Treatment after exposure to cold. *Lancet* **1**, 534.

Ledingham, I. McA. and Mone, J. G. (1974). Paper to the First World Conference on Intensive Care, London. Unpublished.

Lloyd, E. L. (1973). Accidental hypothermia treated by central rewarming through the airway. *Brit. J. Anaesth.* **45**, 41.

Lloyd, E. L. and Mitchell, B. (1974). Factors affecting the onset of ventricular fibrillation in hypothermia. *Lancet* **2**, 1294.

Maclean, D., Murison, J. and Griffiths, P. D. (1973). Acute pancreatitis and diabetic ketoacidosis in accidental hypothermia and hypothermic myxoedema. *Brit. Med. J.* **4**, 757.

Mills, G. L. (1974). Paper to the First World Conference on Intensive Care, London. Unpublished.

Niazi, S. A. and Lewis, F. J. (1958). Profound hypothermia in man. *Ann. Surg.* **147**, 264.

Penrod, K. E. (1951). Cardiac oxygenation during severe hypothermia in dogs. *Am. J. Physiol.* **164**, 79.

Shanks, C. A. and Marsh, H. M. (1973). Simple core rewarming in accidental hypothermia: a case treated with heated infusions, endotracheal intubation and humidification. *Brit. J. Anaesth.* **45**, 522.

Siggaard-Andersen, O. (1974). 'The acid-base status of the blood', Fourth Edition, p. 90. Munksgaard, Copenhagen.

Wynn, V. (1954). Electrolyte disturbances associated with failure to metabolise glucose during hypothermia. *Lancet* **2**, 575.

Zingg, W. (1969). Fast and slow rewarming after acute and prolonged hypothermia in rabbits. *J. Trauma* **9**, 250.

Section 3: The Management of Malignant Hyperpyrexia

M. A. DENBOROUGH

INTRODUCTION

The onset of malignant hyperpyrexia is one of the most dramatic events in clinical medicine. An apparently healthy patient, usually having a minor operation, suddenly becomes moribund during, or shortly after, a general anaesthetic. Although rare, the syndrome is of considerable importance as it is associated with a high mortality rate in the region of 70%.

CLINICAL FEATURES

An important early sign of malignant hyperpyrexia is the onset of prolonged fasciculation and generalised muscular rigidity of transient duration following the intravenous injection of succinylcholine (Britt and Kalow, 1970; King and Denborough, 1973a). Because muscles of the neck and jaw are involved this may lead to difficulty with intubation. In the days before malignant hyperpyrexia was well recognised a further dose of succinylcholine was often given in an attempt to achieve relaxation. Later, there is a rapid rise in body temperature, without shivering, in the absence of an obvious cause such as infection or hot and humid environmental conditions. Any temperature rise should be regarded with suspicion as during anaesthesia the temperature usually falls. Generalised muscular rigidity often develops which is most easily detected in the arms or legs. Other clinical features which should be watched for are an unexplained tachypnoea during anaesthesia with rapid exhaustion and heating of the soda-lime canisters, tachycardia with no obvious cause, and cyanosis of the patient with dark blood at the operative site, despite apparently adequate oxygenation. Biochemical investigation at this stage shows acidosis, hypercapnia and hyperkalaemia.

Association with myopathies

Malignant hyperpyrexia occurs in individuals who have an underlying disease of muscle. The observation that muscle rigidity often occurs during malignant hyperpyrexia, led to biochemical estimations of muscle metabolism during an acute episode (Denborough *et al.*, 1970b). Very high serum levels of creatine phosphokinase (CPK), phosphate, and potassium were found. It was concluded that these biochemical changes had resulted from severe muscle damage induced by the anaesthetics in a susceptible individual.

Non-affected relatives were found to have elevated serum CPK levels (Isaacs and Barlow, 1970; Denborough *et al.*, 1970a) and in a later study of the families of 18 patients who had developed malignant hyperpyrexia two clinical myopathies were defined (King *et al.*, 1972). In the commonest myopathy, which was inherited as a Mendelian dominant characteristic, clinical examination of the muscles was usually within normal limits, and evidence of underlying muscle disease was revealed only by finding elevated levels of serum CPK. The affected individuals had little, if any, physical disability and several had been prominent athletes. The second was a progressive congenital myopathy in young boys with a number of physical abnormalities, which included short stature, antimongoloid obliquity of the eyes, ptosis, low-slung ears, crowded lower teeth, pointed chin, cryptorchidism, pectus carinatum, winging of the scapulae, webbing of the neck, kyphosis and lordosis. No evidence of muscle disease was found in the relatives of these boys (King and Denborough, 1973b).

BIOCHEMICAL BASIS OF MALIGNANT HYPERPYREXIA

If an episode of malignant hyperpyrexia is to be managed properly, an understanding of the underlying biochemical abnormality in this syndrome is necessary. It seems that all the clinical features of the syndrome result from an excess of calcium ions in the myoplasm of the affected individual. This knowledge has come from experiments on susceptible individuals and on an animal model, as certain breeds of pig develop a syndrome on exposure to anaesthetics which, if not identical, is very similar to malignant hyperpyrexia in man (Hall et al., 1966; Harrison et al., 1968). When susceptible pigs are anaesthetised with halothane the first major chemical change is a steep fall in blood pH due to a massive production of lactic acid (Denborough et al., 1973). This acidosis precedes both the rise in temperature and the muscular rigidity. All these clinical features could be explained by a raised calcium ion concentration in the myoplasm. The muscular rigidity would result from the excess calcium stimulating and maintaining muscle contraction. Calcium ions also activate phosphorylase and so stimulate glycolysis. The increased formation of lactic acid from glycogen would account for the metabolic acidosis. The precise cause of the hyperpyrexia is yet to be defined, but could be explained by the heat generated by the continued synthesis and utilisation of ATP in muscle and liver during glycolysis. This effect would be compounded by the fact that halothane partly uncouples oxidative phosphorylation in both muscle and liver.

The central role of calcium ions in the development of malignant hyperpyrexia has been confirmed by in vitro studies on human muscle from affected individuals. The strength of a muscle contraction is a function of the concentration of free calcium ions in the myoplasm. Caffeine causes contracture of skeletal muscle in vitro by raising the calcium concentration in the myoplasm, and caffeine contracture is greater in muscle from patients who are susceptible to malignant hyperpyrexia than in controls (Kalow et al., 1970). A characteristic feature of malignant hyperpyrexia muscle is its ability to give an increased contracture, not only in response to caffeine, but also when exposed to a wide variety of stimuli, including the seemingly chemically unrelated stimuli of halothane (Ellis et al., 1971; Moulds and Denborough, 1972), succinylcholine and potassium chloride, and the physical stimulus of a temperature change (Moulds and Denborough, 1974a). These effects are dependent on extracellular calcium concentration, and on temperature (Nelson et al., 1977). These findings suggest that the essential abnormality in malignant hyperpyrexia is an impaired binding of calcium to the calcium storing membranes in the muscle cell. When these membranes are exposed to halothane, succinylcholine and other general anaesthetic agents there is an excessive and rapid release of calcium into the myoplasm, which in turn gives rise to all the clinical features of the syndrome. Recent experiments with dantrolene suggest that the primary lesion in malignant hyperpyrexia may lie in the sarcolemma, and involve a mechanism whereby excitation (depolarisation of the surface membrane) is coupled to calcium release from the sarcoplasmic reticulum (Nelson and Denborough, 1977).

MANAGEMENT OF AN ACUTE EPISODE OF MALIGNANT HYPERPYREXIA

As soon as the diagnosis is made, all offending anaesthetic agents should be stopped immediately and hyperventilation with an oxygen-rich mixture should be substituted. Early diagnosis is most important as there is a direct correlation between mortality and the amount of temperature rise during the reaction (King and Denborough, 1973a).

Specific treatment to lower myoplasmic calcium concentration

As has been pointed out already all the clinical features of malignant hyperpyrexia can be explained by a high calcium ion concentration in the myoplasm, so that the most important therapeutic aim is to restore normal myoplasmic calcium levels.

Because the effect of caffeine on skeletal muscle is blocked by local anaesthetics, procaine hydrochloride has been suggested for the treatment of malignant hyperpyrexia (Strobel and Bianchi, 1971). The use of procaine hydrochloride is supported by evidence that procaine prevents the development of malignant hyperpyrexia in susceptible Landrace pigs *in vivo* (Harrison, 1971), and by the finding that procaine reverses halothane induced contracture of muscle from patients susceptible to malignant hyperpyrexia *in vitro* (Moulds and Denborough, 1972). The concentration of procaine hydrochloride which was used to produce these effects *in vitro*, however, may lead to hypotension in the clinical situation, and this has led to the use of this drug being questioned in malignant hyperpyrexia (Clarke and Ellis, 1975). Other drugs that have been used in the treatment of malignant hyperpyrexia include procainamide (Hall and Lister, 1974), hydrocortisone and dexamethasone (Ellis et al., 1974).

Recent suggestions that the muscle relaxant dantrolene (Fig. 1) might block excitation-contraction coupling without affecting caffeine contractures (Putney and Bianchi, 1974) neuromuscular transmission or electrical properties of muscle (Ellis and Carpenter, 1972; Ellis and Bryant, 1972), raised the possibility that this drug might be useful in the treatment of malignant hyperpyrexia. This possibility has now been

examined in pigs susceptible to malignant hyperpyrexia, and it has
been found that dantrolene can be used to block the initiation of the
syndrome in these animals, and also to reverse the condition once it has
occurred (Harrison, 1975).

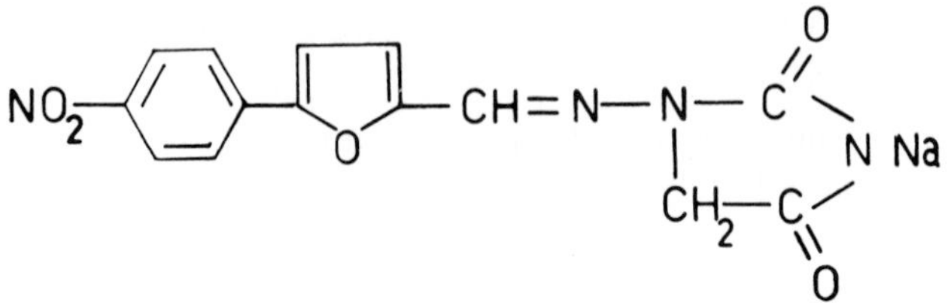

Fig. 1. Dantrolene sodium.

A recent study has compared the effects of the various drugs which
have been suggested for use in malignant hyperpyrexia (Austin and
Denborough, 1977). This investigation showed that dantrolene is the
most effective agent for reversing and inhibiting drug induced
contractures *in vitro*, both in normal muscle and in muscle from patients
who are susceptible to malignant hyperpyrexia. It seems that at present
dantrolene is the drug of choice for specifically lowering the raised
myoplasmic calcium levels in malignant hyperpyrexia.

Concentrations of dantrolene of 3–6 µM completely inhibited and
reversed the abnormal drug induced contractures diagnostic of
malignant hyperpyrexia in human muscle. This concentration appears
to be safe in man (Chyatte and Birdsong, 1971). High doses of
dantrolene given intravenously to pigs (Harrison, 1975) and to dogs
(Ellis *et al.*, 1975) have produced no serious side effects.

The fulminant nature of malignant hyperpyrexia means that an
intravenous preparation of dantrolene is urgently needed for the
treatment of malignant hyperpyrexia. This has still to be approved in
the United Kingdom and America, and dantrolene is not yet available
at all in Australia. A recommended intravenous dose of dantrolene
would be 1 mg/kg body weight, and this could be repeated twice at
10 min intervals if necessary.

In the absence of dantrolene the next most effective drug is procaine
hydrochloride. In an adult procaine hydrochloride should be given
intravenously in a dose of 0.5 mg per kilogram body weight per minute,
with careful monitoring of the electrocardiogram and the blood
pressure so that hypotension does not result. After 0.5 g of procaine has

been given, the efficacy of the infusion should be evaluated before continuing. If the diagnosis of malignant hyperpyrexia has been delayed until the patient is acutely ill, the use of procaine at that late stage may aggravate the circulatory failure. Procaine hydrochloride should be used rather than procainamide, which is less effective. Furthermore, commercial preparations of procainamide may contain a small amount of alcohol as preservative, which increases the release of calcium into the myoplasm and this aggravates the clinical problem (Austin and Denborough, 1975).

TREATMENT OF COMPLICATIONS

Commence active cooling

The temperature should be recorded continuously. Cooling is probably best achieved by packing the patient in ice and using fans. An ice-water bath has been suggested but this might present problems if d.c. shock is needed to revert cardiac arrhythmias. Other suggested methods have been intragastric cooling and cold water enemata (Relton et al., 1972) and when an expert cardiovascular team is available, extra-corporeal cooling (Ryan et al., 1974).

Another suggested method of cooling is peritoneal dialysis using a cold dialysate (Gjessing et al., 1976). Although this method has not yet been used in the treatment of malignant hyperpyrexia, it sounds promising. Peritoneal dialysis is a simple procedure, and cooling can be obtained when 2 litres of either cool (20°C) or cold (9°C) dialysis fluid is used over a 20 min period. Cold dialysis solutions cause discomfort in a conscious patient, but this would not be a problem in the treatment of malignant hyperpyrexia. A further advantage of peritoneal dialysis would be that it would correct the biochemical abnormalities which occur.

Correct electrolyte imbalances

An electrocardiogram should be used to monitor changes in blood levels of potassium and calcium. Arterial blood samples may be required at 10 min intervals for estimation of blood gases. Serum electrolytes should also be measured frequently.

A buffer, such as sodium bicarbonate, should be used promptly to correct the severe lactic acidosis which invariably occurs. Two milli-litres per kilogram body weight of 8.4% sodium bicarbonate should be given at once intravenously, and then repeated according to the blood gas estimations. Central venous monitoring may be helpful to detect fluid overload, which in turn may need correction by intravenous frusemide.

Hyperkalaemia is another early metabolic abnormality which often needs treatment. Correction of the metabolic acidosis may lower the serum potassium to an acceptable level. If not, 100 ml of 50% dextrose and 30 units of soluble insulin should be given intravenously to an adult. The serum potassium should be monitored frequently as hypokalaemia may develop in the recovery phase which may need intravenous potassium supplements.

Frequent ventricular ectopic beats should be treated by procaine rather than procainamide or pronestyl. Ventricular tachyarrhythmias should be treated promptly by d.c. shock and procaine.

Correct late complications

Dialysis may be needed to correct persisting metabolic acidosis and hyperkalaemia and to reverse high serum phosphate levels which may lead to hypocalcaemia. Dialysis may also be needed for renal shut down.

Another late complication which may need treatment is disseminated intravascular coagulation (Colman et al., 1972; Damus and Salzman, 1972).

A summary of the management of malignant hyperpyrexia is shown in Table 1.

PREVENTION

Because malignant hyperpyrexia develops so rapidly, and because the mortality from this anaesthetic complication remains high in spite of advances in its treatment, prevention of the syndrome is most important.

A high index of suspicion for malignant hyperpyrexia should always be maintained in anyone given a general anaesthetic, and a history of any previous abnormal reaction to anaesthesia in the patient or his family should be sought. Relatives of patients who have developed malignant hyperpyrexia should be examined clinically for evidence of a myopathy, and initially serum CPK estimations should be performed. In some families serum CPK levels accurately reflect susceptibility to malignant hyperpyrexia, but in others this is not so, and in these *in vitro* muscle tests (Moulds and Denborough, 1974b) should be carried out in

Table 1. Management of acute episode of malignant hyperpyrexia

1 Stop all offending anaesthetic agents and hyperventilate with an oxygen-rich mixture.

2 *Lower myoplasmic calcium concentration*
Intravenous infusion of dantrolene 1 mg/kg body weight if available. Repeat twice at 10 min interval if necessary.
  If dantrolene not available infuse procaine 0.5 mg/kg body weight per min, with careful monitoring of electrocardiogram and blood pressure to avoid hypotension. Review efficacy of procaine after 0.5 g has been given.

3 *Treat complications*
(*a*) Commence active cooling by packing the patient in ice and using fans. ? Peritoneal dialysis with 2 litres of cool (20°C) or cold (9°C) dialysis fluid.
(*b*) Correct lactic acidosis by intravenous 8.4% sodium bicarbonate, 2 ml/kg of body weight.
(*c*) Correct hyperkalaemia.

4 *Late complications*
(*a*) ? Dialysis
(*b*) ? Treat disseminated intravascular coagulation.

centres where such investigations have been established. In individuals who have been shown to be susceptible to malignant hyperpyrexia operations should be carried out under local, regional or spinal anaesthesia if this is possible. If general anaesthesia is necessary barbiturates such as thiopentone, tranquillisers such as diazepam, narcotics such as the opiates neuroanaleptics such as fentanyl, nitrous oxide, *d*-tubocurarine, and althesin appear to be safe.

Malignant hyperpyrexia, however, usually appears unexpectedly. The only way to prevent the fulminant syndrome in these patients is to pick up the complication at an early stage by monitoring the temperature during general anaesthesia.

REFERENCES

Austin, K. L. and Denborough, M. A. (1975). Treatment for malignant hyperpyrexia: procaine or procainamide? *Clin. exp. Pharmac. Physiol.* **2**, 48.

Austin, K. L. and Denborough, M. A. (1977). Drug treatment of malignant hyperpyrexia. *Anaesth. intens. Care* **5**, 207.

Britt, B. A. and Kalow, W. (1970). Malignant hyperthermia. A statistical review. *Can. Anaesth. Soc. J.* **17**, 293.

Chyatte, S. B. and Birdsong, J. H. (1971). The use of dantrolene sodium in disorders of the central nervous system. *Sth. Med. J.* **64**, 830.

Clarke, I. M. C. and Ellis, F. R. (1975). An evaluation of procaine in the treatment of malignant hyperpyrexia. *Brit. J. Anaesth.* **47**, 17.

Colman, R. W., Robboy, S. J. and Minna, J. D. (1972). Disseminated intravascular coagulation (DIC): An approach. *Am. J. Med.* **52**, 679.

Damus, P. S. and Salzman, E. W. (1972). Disseminated intravascular coagulation. *Archs. Surg.* **104**, 262.

Denborough, M. A., Ebeling, P., King, J. O. and Zapf, P. (1970a). Myopathy and malignant hyperpyrexia. *Lancet* **1**, 1138.

Denborough, M. A., Forster, J. F. A., Hudson, M. C., Carter, N. G. and Zapf, P. (1970b). Biochemical changes in malignant hyperpyrexia. *Lancet* **1**, 1137.

Denborough, M. A., Hird, F. J. R., King, J. O., Marginson, M. A., Mitchelson, K. R., Nayler, W. G., Rex, M. A., Zapf, P. and Condron, R. J. (1973). Mitochondrial and other studies in Australian Landrace pigs affected with malignant hyperthermia. In 'International Symposium on Malignant Hyperthermia'. (Ed. R. A. Gordon, B. A. Britt and W. Kalow) p. 229. Charles C. Thomas, Illinois, U.S.A.

Ellis, F. R., Clarke, I. M. C., Appleyard, T. N. and Dinsdale, R. C. W. (1974). Malignant hyperpyrexia induced by nitrous oxide and treated with dexamethasone. *Brit. Med. J.* **4**, 270.

Ellis, F. R., Harriman, D. G. F., Keaney, N. P., Kyei-Mensah, K. and Tyrrell, J. H. (1971). Halothane-induced muscle contracture as a cause of hyperpyrexia. *Brit. J. Anaesth.* **43**, 721.

Ellis, F. R., Keaney, N. P., Harriman, D. G. F., Sumner, D. W., Kyei-Mensah, K., Tyrrell, J. H., Hargreaves, J. B., Parikh, R. K. and Mulrooney, P. L. (1972). Screening for malignant hyperpyrexia. *Brit. Med. J.* **3**, 559.

Ellis, K. O. and Bryant, S. H. (1972). Excitation-contraction uncoupling in skeletal muscle by dantrolene sodium. *Nauyn-Schmiedebergs Arch. exp. Path. Pharmak.* **274**, 107.

Ellis, K. O. and Carpenter, J. F. (1972). Studies on the mechanism of action of dantrolene sodium. *Naunyn-Schmiedebergs Arch. exp. Path. Pharmak.* **275**, 83.

Ellis, R. H., Simpson, P., Tatham, P., Leighton, M. and Williams, J. (1975). The cardiovascular effects of dantrolene sodium in dogs. *Anaesthesia* **30**, 318.

Gjessing, J., Barsa, J. and Tomlin, P. J. (1976). A possible means of rapid cooling in the emergency treatment of malignant hyperpyrexia. *Brit. J. Anaesth.* **48**, 469.

Hall, G. M. and Lister, D. (1974). Procaine and malignant hyperthermia. *Lancet* **1**, 208.

Hall, L. W., Woolf, N., Bradley, J. W. P. and Jolly, D. W. (1966). Unusual reaction to suxamethonium chloride. *Brit. Med. J.* **2**, 1305.

Harrison, G. G. (1971). Anaesthetic-induced malignant hyperpyrexia: A suggested method of treatment. *Brit. Med. J.* **3**, 454.

Harrison, G. G. (1975). Control of the malignant hyperpyrexic syndrome in MHS swine by dantrolene sodium. *Brit. J. Anaesth.* **47**, 62.

Harrison, G. G., Biebuyck, J. F., Terblanche, J., Dent, D. M., Hickman, R. and Saunders, S. J. (1968). Hyperpyrexia during anaesthesia. *Brit. Med. J.* **3**, 594.

Isaacs, H. and Barlow, M. B. (1970). Malignant hyperpyrexia during anaesthesia: Possible association with subclinical myopathy. *Brit. Med. J.* **1**, 275.

Kalow, W., Britt, B. A., Terreau, M. E. and Haist, C. (1970). Metabolic error of muscle metabolism after recovery from malignant hyperthermia. *Lancet* **2**, 895.

King, J. O. and Denborough, M. A. (1973a). Malignant hyperpyrexia in Australia and New Zealand. *Med. J. Aust.* **1**, 525.

King, J. O. and Denborough, M. A. (1973b). Anesthetic-induced malignant hyperpyrexia in children. *J. Pediat.* **83**, 37.

King, J. O., Denborough, M. A. and Zapf, P. W. (1972). Inheritance of malignant hyperpyrexia. *Lancet* **1**, 365.

Moulds, R. F. W. and Denborough, M. A. (1972). Procaine in malignant hyperpyrexia. *Brit. Med. J.* **4**, 526.

Moulds, R. F. W. and Denborough, M. A. (1974a). Biochemical basis of malignant hyperpyrexia. *Brit. Med. J.* **2**, 241.

Moulds, R. F. W. and Denborough, M. A. (1974b). Identification of susceptibility to malignant hyperpyrexia. *Brit. Med. J.* **2**, 245.

Nelson, T. E., Austin, K. L. and Denborough, M. A. (1977). Screening for malignant hyperpyrexia. *Brit. J. Anaesth.* **49**, 169.

Nelson, T. E. and Denborough, M. A. (1977). Studies on normal human skeletal muscle in relation to the pathopharmacology of malignant hyperpyrexia. *Clin. exp. Pharmac. Physiol.* **4**, 315.

Putney, J. W. Jr. and Bianchi, C. P. (1974). Site of action of dantrolene in frog sartorious muscle. *J. Pharmac. exp. Ther.* **189**, 202.

Relton, J. E. S., Steward, D. J., Creighton, R. E. and Britt, B. A. (1972). Malignant hyperpyrexia: a therapeutic and investigative regimen. *Can. Anaesth. Soc. J.* **19**, 200.

Ryan, J. F., Donlon, J. V., Malt, R. A., Bland, J. H. L., Buckley, M. J., Sreter, F. A. and Lowenstein, E. (1974). Cardiopulmonary bypass in the treatment of malignant hyperthermia. *New Engl. J. Med.* **290**, 1121.

Strobel, G. E. and Bianchi, C. P. (1971). An *in vitro* model of anesthetic hypertonic hyperpyrexia, halothane-caffeine-induced muscle contractures. *Anesthesiology* **35**, 465.

VII

The Acute Metabolic Management of the Critically Ill Patient

Section 1: The Metabolic Response to Acute Stress and Starvation

GILLIAN C. HANSON

The metabolic response to acute stress and starvation is different from that of chronic malnutrition where a form of adaptation takes place. The early depression of metabolism, local and general, following injury, the 'ebb' phase, lasts several hours. This is generally followed by a period of enhanced heat production associated with excess protein catabolism, over anabolism, which is more general than local – the 'flow phase'. This period is generally at its height 5–8 days after injury (Cuthbertson *et al.*, 1972). The maximum daily loss of nitrogen during the flow phase may exceed 20 g and urinalysis suggests that the major source of extra nitrogen excreted is from muscle (Cuthbertson, 1964). The extent of the catabolism of protein is approximately related to the severity of the skeletal injury (Cuthbertson, 1942) or to the extent and depth of the burned area (Davies, 1970). O'Keefe and co-workers (1974) have argued that the 'catabolic' response reflects a predominant fall in protein synthesis and not a rise in breakdown.

Clean anaesthetised surgical trauma is generally associated with no increase in energy expenditure or a maximum increase of 10–15 per cent (Kinney, 1960). Patients with multiple fractures have increases of 10–25% above normal and in major infection there will be an increase of 20–50% (Kinney, 1974). The only clinical situation where the energy expenditure is increased to twice the resting normal level is in major burns (Kinney, 1974). The malnourished patient is found to have a less dramatic response to trauma or infection; maximum nitrogen losses and energy expenditure are seen in the well-built young male.

Kinney (1974) has investigated the composition of tissue lost during weight loss following surgery. He found that protein contributed only 10%, fat 20% and the remainder was assumed to be water. Provided that the initial weight of the patient is known, it is possible to estimate the nitrogen deficit by assuming that 10% of the weight has been lost as protein (1 g nitrogen equals 6.25 g protein).

In health, in addition to the energy required to cover resting metabolism, there must be added the specific dynamic effect of food up to 6% (Swift and Fischer, 1964) and physical activity of 0.0017–0.0058 mJ/min (0.4–1.4 kcal/min) whether sitting or walking. The energy requirements can therefore vary between 0.092–0.13 mJ/kg body weight per day (22 to 31 kcal/kg body weight per day) from the age of 12 years and upwards (Wretlind, 1972). Wretlind (1972) recommends that the basal supply of energy for women on intravenous nutrition should always exceed 0.092 mJ/kg/day (22 kcal/kg/day) and for men 0.125 mJ/kg/day (30 kcal/kg/day).

The approximate daily energy losses in varying situations are summarised in Table 1.

Table 1

	kcal	mJ
Medical patient (no temperature)	1500–2000	6.25– 8.3
Postoperative state (uncomplicated)	2000–4000	8.3–16.7
Hypercatabolic state		
e.g. major burn, multiple trauma	4000–6000	16.7–25.0

The catabolic response to fever has been well documented by Beisel (1972). For each 1°C rise in temperature above normal there has been estimated a 10–12% increase in energy expenditure. The immune response to infection is influenced adversely by protein deficiency.

The effect of the ambient temperature on the metabolic response during the flow phase has been reviewed by Cuthbertson and Tilstone (1969) and Davies and Liljedahl (1970). The nitrogen loss is considerably reduced by keeping the patient in a 30°C environment and this is particularly pronounced in severe burns. Patients with extensive loss of skin surface should therefore be nursed in a 30°C environment in order to reduce the obligatory heat provided by the body to compensate for that lost by evaporation of water from the damaged skin surface.

Because of the increased calorie utilisation after stress from trauma and/or sepsis, carbohydrate is broken down to yield energy. The total carbohydrate stores in the healthy adult do not greatly exceed 100–200 g and therefore in serious illness muscle protein breakdown (in order to provide calories) will occur rapidly if carbohydrate calories are withheld (Peaston, 1968). Blackburn and colleagues (1973) suggested that nitrogen balance can be maintained in the immediate post-operative period by the provision of amino acids without additional energy. His work was done however in surgical patients with minimal nitrogen losses (7 g $\pm$ 2.3 g/day) and should not therefore be related to the average hypercatabolic patient in an intensive therapy unit.

Azar and Bloom (1963) showed that a regime which does not supply carbohydrate calories fails to arrest loss of body weight, and Van Way and co-workers (1975) confirmed that in order to reverse a post-operative negative nitrogen balance, nitrogen and calories were required. Kinney (1974) commented about the uncertainty of our present knowledge in the nutritional management of acute catabolic situations. He felt that in the postoperative state the optimum energy to nitrogen ratio should be approximately 0.2 mJ (150 kcal) to one gram of nitrogen administered and that the total energy given should be 50% more than the patient's measured or estimated resting requirement.

Following stress, various endocrine changes occur which radically affect electrolyte balance and tolerance to administered carbohydrate. Acute stress must be considered as a general imbalance of anabolic hormones such as insulin androgens, and growth hormone and catabolic hormones as glucocorticoids thyroid hormone and oestrogen. Glucagon should be considered catabolic and has been found to be increased in stress (Unger and Lefebure, 1972). Immediately after acute stress there may be a decrease in glucose utilisation associated with a fall in insulin secretion. Following this ebb phase (24–72 h) plasma insulin levels may be high in the presence of continuing glucose intolerance (Allison et al., 1968). There develops a resistance to the action of administered insulin (Editorial, 1965), but in spite of glucose intolerance there is a net increase in glucose utilisation (Allison, 1972–4). Insulin enhances the transport of amino acids into cells and their incorporation into protein. Stress provides a stimulus to increased ACTH and hence cortisol secretion. The quantity of corticosteroid released is proportional to the severity of the stress and is associated with an increased level of aldosterone and antidiuretic hormone. It is probable that the increased level of these three hormones account for the sodium and water retention and potassium loss after acute stress. Catecholamine levels rise following surgery, burns and sepsis (Birke *et al.*, 1967), and by inhibiting insulin secretion and producing fat mobilisation, provide a mechanism for mobilising amino acids from the periphery. The mobilisation of amino acids from the periphery (skeletal muscle) and their utilisation for anabolic processes – especially in the liver – is enhanced by the rise in glucocorticoids (Border, 1970). Thus the metabolic response to stress could be based on the changes that occur in relationship to the anabolic and catabolic hormones – the catabolic hormones predominating. In some patients there is lack of correlation in time with the endocrine and metabolic changes.

REFERENCES

Allison, S. (1972–74). The metabolic response to injury. *Medicine* **II**, 730.

Allison, S. P., Hinton, P. and Chamberlain, M. J. (1968). Intravenous glucose tolerance and free fatty acid levels in burned patients. *Lancet* **2**, 1113.

Azar, G. J. and Bloom, W. L. (1963). Similarities of carbohydrate deficiency and fasting. *Arch. Int. Med.* **112**, 338.

Beisel, W. R. (1972). Interrelated changes in host metabolism during generalised infectious illness. *Am. J. Clin. Nutr.* **25**, 1254.

Birke, G., Duner, H., Liljedahl, S. O., Pernow, B., Plastin, L. O. and Troell, L. (1967). Histamine catecholamines and adrenocortical steroids in burns. *Acta Chir. Scand.* **114**, 87.

Blackburn, G. L., Flatt, J. P., Clowes, J. H. A., O'Donnell, T. F. and Hensle, T. E. (1973). Protein Sparing Therapy during periods of starvation with sepsis and trauma. *Ann. Surg.* **177**, 588.

Border, J. A. (1970). Metabolic response to short-term starvation, sepsis and trauma. *Surg. Annu.* **2**, 11.

Cuthbertson, D. P. (1942). Post-shock metabolic response. *Lancet* **I**, 433.

Cuthbertson, D. P. (1964). Physical injury and its effects on protein metabolism in Mammalian protein metabolism (Ed. H. N. Munro and J. B. Allison) Vol. 2. Academic Press, New York.

Cuthbertson, D. P. and Tilstone, W. J. (1969). Metabolism during the post injury period. *Adv. Clin. Chem.* **12**, 1.

Cuthbertson, D. P., Fell, G. S., Smith, C. M. and Tilstone, W. J. (1972). Nutrition in the post-traumatic period. *Nutr. Metabol.* **14** (Suppl.) 92.

Davies, J. W. L. (1970). Protein metabolism following injury. *J. Clin. Path.* **23** (Suppl. 4) 56.

Davies, J. W. L. and Liljedahl, S. O. (1970). Protein catabolism and energy utilisation in burned patients treated at different environmental temperatures. *In* 'CIBA Foundation Symposium on Energy Metabolism after Injury', p. 43. Churchill, London.

Editorial (1965). Hyperglycaemia and diabetes after burns. *Lancet* **I**, 225.

Kinney, J. M. (1960). A consideration of energy exchange in human trauma. *Bull. N. Y. Acad. Med.* **36**, 617.

Kinney, J. M. (1974). Energy requirements in injury and sepsis. *Acta Anaesth. Scand.* **55** (Suppl.) 15.

O'Keefe, S. J. D., Sender, P. M. and Jones, W. P. T. (1974). Catabolic loss of body nitrogen in response to surgery. *Lancet* **2**, 1035.

Peaston, M. J. T. (1968). Parenteral nutrition in serious illness. *Hosp. Med.* **2**, 708.

Swift, R. W. and Fischer, K. H. (1964–65). A comprehensive treatise. *In* 'Nutrition Medicine' (Ed. G. H. Beaton and B. W. McHenry). Academic Press, New York.

Unger, R. H. and Lefebure, P. J. (1972). Glucagon physiology in Glucagon. *In* 'Molecular physiology, Clinical and Therapeutic Implications' (Ed. Lefebure and Unger) p. 213. Pergamon Press, Oxford and New York.

Van Way, C. W., Meng, H. C. and Sandstead, H. H. (1975). Nitrogen balance in post-operative patients receiving parenteral nutrition. *Archs. Surg.* **110**, 272.

Wretlind, A. (1972). Complete intravenous nutrition. *Nutr. Metabol.* **14** (Suppl.) 1.

Section 2: The Management of Acute Disorders of Fluid and Electrolyte Balance

GILLIAN C. HANSON

ACUTE DISORDERS IN WATER AND SODIUM BALANCE

Introduction

Very rapid changes in weight are generally associated with changes in fluid balance – the exception being in critical illness where rapid breakdown of fat and to a lesser extent of lean tissue, forms part of the metabolic response to severe injury. Losses above 1.0 kg in hypercatabolic patients should be considered to be related to loss of water. Less accurate assessment of fluid balance can be made by measuring fluid intake and output and making allowances for water derived from the oxidation of foods (0.41, 0.60 and 1.07 ml water per gram of protein carbohydrate or fat respectively) and the output from insensible losses from the skin and lungs (Table 1). The insensible loss in an adult is

Table 1. Average insensible losses in an adult at rest in bed. (Reproduced by permission of Taylor, 1967.)

Oral temperature (°C)	Net insensible loss (ml)
NORMAL	500
38	565
39	640
40	720
41	820

158

approximately 500 ml and this loss increases by 13% for each degree rise in centigrade (Hayes *et al.*, 1957). A patient who is being ventilated with warmed humidified gases requires approximately half the estimated insensible losses and the insensible losses should be reduced to approximately 300 ml in mild hypothermia (33–35°C). To the net

Table 2. Average loss of fluid through sweating in an adult patient. (Reproduced by permission of Taylor, 1967.)

	Vol. per day (ml)
Mild intermittent	300
Moderate inter-mittent	600
Severe inter-mittent	1000
Continuous	2–15 litres

insensible loss should be added a volume allowance for visible sweating (Table 2). Mild sweating involves the axilla and pubic region, moderate sweating the scalp and face and in severe cases sweating involves the whole body surface (Taylor, 1967).

The average water requirement in an adult is 20–40 ml/kg body weight daily.

There is a fall in the total body water represented as a percentage of body weight with age – in an infant under one month 77% of the body weight is water, 60% at the age of 16 and 60% and 51% in men and women respectively between the age range of 17–34 years (Black, 1967).

Table 3. Body fluid compartments represented as a percentage of total body weight

Extracellular 20% of body weight		Intracellular 50% of body weight
Plasma 5%	Interstitial 15%	

The intracellular and extracellular compartments of body fluid are separated from one another by cell walls. The extracellular fluid acts as a transport medium and can be divided into intravascular and interstitial compartments (Table 3). An equilibrium is established between the capillary hydrostatic pressure and the colloid osmotic effect of the protein rich plasma vs the protein poor interstitial fluid.

Table 4. Balance of the main cations and anions in plasma and intracellular fluid. (Reproduced by permission of Black, 1967.)

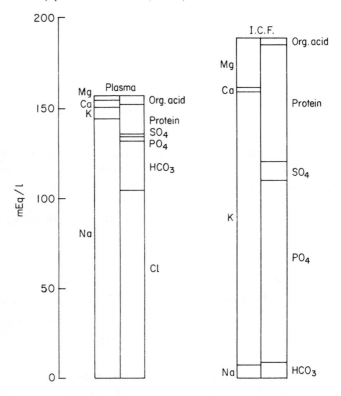

Interchange of small molecules and ions between the two compartments takes place with rapidity. A fall in plasma volume can take place as a result of an intravascular decrease in sodium ions or protein thereby decreasing the serum osmolality, or from a fall in the extracellular fluid volume. The electrolyte structure of the extracellular fluid (E.C.F.) can be determined by analysis of the plasma or serum and reflects the E.C.F. of most tissues. Intracellular fluid electrolyte concentration can be estimated from the erythrocytes but is not representative of the composition of body fluids in general (Black, 1967).

The composition in mEq/l of the intracellular and extracellular electrolytes is shown in Table 4. The E.C.F. is predominantly a sodium containing fluid whereas the intracellular fluid (I.C.F.) contains mainly potassium ions. Potassium is transported into the cell and sodium out of the cell by an electrochemical gradient. When electrolytes are expressed in terms of electrical activity, cations balance anions. The total quantity of anions and cations in plasma is approximately 300 mEq/l and for I.C.F. approximately 400 mEq/l (Table 4). Inside the cells the ions are predominantly polyvalent and the number of particles will therefore be less than their electrical change, as a consequence of this the total osmolality of I.C.F. and plasma is approximately equal.

Abnormalities of sodium and water balance

The term dehydration is commonly used to denote sodium and water depletion when it should be confined to pure water depletion. In pure water depletion the effect is initially distributed evenly throughout all body fluid compartments and the osmolality of these fluid compartments rise. In severe water depletion the diminished intravascular volume stimulates the secretion of aldosterone (Bartter, 1958). Sodium is retained in the extracellular space and because of its osmotic effect, water is removed from the intracellular space. In sodium depletion the extracellular fluid can no longer be maintained and there is a fall in the intravascular volume (Table 5). As a consequence of these alterations in intravascular volume sodium depletion produces clinical signs consistent with a falling intravascular volume relatively early whereas in pure water depletion this only occurs when the depletion is advanced. In clinical practice the diagnosis of water depletion should not only include an absolute deficiency but also relative water deficiency in which the water content of the body may be normal or even increased but the electrolyte content increased to a greater degree.

The comparison between pure water depletion and pure sodium depletion is shown in Table 6.

The diagnosis and management of predominant water depletion

Diagnosis
It is unusual in clinical situations to meet pure water depletion but it is important to differentiate predominant water loss from sodium loss

Table 5. Effect of sodium depletion and of mild and severe water depletion, on the partition of fluid between E.C.F. and I.C.F. The partial preservation of E.C.F. at the expense of I.C.F. in severe water depletion is probably related to secondary aldosteronism. (Reproduced by permission of Black[1], 1967.)

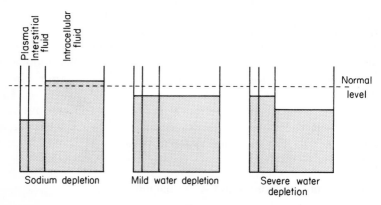

(Table 6). Predominant water depletion may be related to a decreased intake, diarrhoea, or fluid loss from a fever, sweating or hyperventilation. Relative water depletion may also occur where saline solutions have been used to replace lower intestinal losses of low sodium content. The patient with water depletion, if conscious, will complain of severe thirst. The patient is generally noted to be weak and apathetic but the hypotension and low tissue turgor is not seen (as in sodium depletion) until late. Water depletion may be associated with tissue wasting and therefore the differentiation between salt and water depletion cannot be made by the texture of the subcutaneous tissue. The biochemical changes are shown in Table 6.

Acute and dramatic changes in body weight are an excellent guide to the volume of fluid lost from the body – 1 kg of weight lost being equivalent to the loss of 1 litre of water. In mild deficits 2% of the body weight is lost. Thirst is generally noted when 2% or more of the body weight is lost. A moderate fluid deficit is evident when 2–5% of the body weight is lost and a severe deficit when greater than 6% is lost.

Management
The patient with mild water depletion is unlikely to be sufficiently ill to

[1] Professor Black commented that since the plasma contains protein it might be expected that the intravascular volume would be depleted to a lesser extent than the interstitial fluid in pure sodium depletion. Elkington *et al.* (1946) found, however, that the plasma volume was more greatly reduced than was E.C.F. volume and observed loss of serum protein in particular albumin.

Table 6. Comparison between pure water depletion and pure sodium depletion

	Pure water depletion	Pure salt depletion
1 SYMPTOMS		
Thirst	Present	Absent
Headache	Absent	Present
Weakness	Mild, develops late	Early, progressively
Lassitude		severe
Muscle cramps	Absent	Present
2 SIGNS		
Temperature	High	Normal
Skin	Dry flushed, normal elasticity, doughy	Inelastic, loose and wrinkled
B.P.	Normal until late	Low
3 BIOCHEMISTRY		
Urine		
Volume	Diminished	Normal until late
Osmolality	Increased	Decreased
Chloride	Normal	Low except in Addison's disease
Blood		
P.C.V.	Normal until late	Decreased
Osmolality	Normal or increased	Decreased
Sodium	Increased	Normal or decreased
Urea	Slight increase	Moderate to severe increase

require intensive therapy except due to some associated disease. Such patients can generally have fluid volume replaced by mouth, the volume administered should be sufficient to relieve thirst. In more severe deficits the volume can be replaced with 5% dextrose where it is suspected that the fluid loss is predominantly water but where sodium ions have been lost to a lesser degree $-\frac{1}{5}$ normal saline or dextrose saline can be used.

In severe predominant water depletion where the patient is drowsy, generally pyrexial and the blood pressure has begun to fall, a central venous pressure line should be inserted and $\frac{1}{5}$ normal saline infused until the central venous pressure and blood pressure have risen to normal. Urine output should be observed carefully in these patients since in severe predominant water depletion there may be a period of oliguria lasting up to 3 days. During this period it is easy to over-hydrate the patient. Acute renal failure is rare under such circumstances unless there are associated features (e.g. sepsis) which predispose the patient to this condition.

The infusion rate should be approximately 1 litre hourly until the blood pressure and central venous pressure are normal and the rate should then be slowed down so that approximately $\frac{1}{3}$ to $\frac{1}{2}$ of the total estimated loss is replaced over the subsequent 24 hours. Loss can be estimated approximately from the fluid balance charts, the weight loss and the history. The electrolyte content of the fluid lost and of the urine should be analysed and replaced daily together with insensible losses and losses from sweat. The range of electrolyte composition of various gastrointestinal fluids and their maximum losses over 24 hours is shown in Table 7; the approximate insensible fluid losses in relation to temperature and fluid loss through sweating are mentioned in Tables 1 and 2 respectively.

Table 7. Average range of electrolyte concentrations in mmol/l of intestinal fluids in normal adults and the approximate maximum volume loss per 24 h. (Complied from multiple author data.)

	Na^+	K^+	Cl^-	Approx. max fluid loss per 24 h (litres)
Stomach	20–116	5–32	50–154	20
Bile	130–160	3–12	80–120	1.5
Pancreatic juice	110–150	3–10	54–95	1.5
Small bowel (suction)	72–148	2–15	43–137	6.0
Ileostomy (recent)	105–144	6–29	90–136	3.0
Caecostomy	45–115	11–28	35–70	3.0
Formed stool	10	10	15	0.2
Watery diarrhoea	50–100	20–40	40–80	17.0

During replacement careful monitoring of potassium is required and of magnesium and calcium in patients with glycosuria or predominant gastrointestinal losses. Potassium replacement should be started once the serum potassium has fallen to 3.5 mmol/l or less and in the presence of a metabolic acidosis once the level has fallen to less than 3.8 mmol/l. Dextrose 5% should not be used until the serum potassium is 3.5 mmol/l or more and should be infused with 20–40 mmol of potassium ions per litre if the serum potassium is in the range 3.5–4.0 mmol/l. A metabolic alkalosis is rare in the presence of predominant water depletion and if present should suggest a fall in total body potassium – in spite of a serum potassium which may be in the normal range.

Table 8. The causes for a low serum sodium

1. *Loss of total body sodium*

Renal	Osmotic diuretics Diuretic therapy Renal disease Adrenal insufficiency
Gastrointestinal	Vomiting Intestinal fluid loss
Skin	Sweat in particular in mucoviscidosis Burns
Drainage	Pleural Peritoneal Other

2 *Dilutional* (Normal total body sodium)

Water intoxication	Decreased renal perfusion Renal failure Post-stress states Induced following the use of pitressin tannate Inappropriate secretion of ADH
Fluid shift	Mannitol Glucose

3 *Sodium shift* (Normal or increased total body sodium)
   Hypokalaemia
   Sick cell syndrome

Abnormalities in serum sodium concentration

Hyponatraemia

True salt depletion and water intoxication were for many years considered the main causes for a serum sodium level of less than 135 mmol/l. It is now realised that these two causes are relatively rare. Danowski and co-workers (1955) evaluated the clinical diagnosis and probable aetiology of 137 hospitalised patients (including children) with hyponatraemia. Only 37 of these patients were thought to be suffering from pure sodium depletion and only 15 from water intoxication.

The causes for a low serum sodium are summarised in Table 8 and the diagnosis and treatment of hypoatraemic states is summarised in Table 9.

1. *Loss of total body sodium*

The total body sodium amounts to about 5250 mmol in a 70 kg man, a

Table 9. Diagnosis and treatment of hyponatraemic states

DIAGNOSIS	Extra-renal sodium loss	Renal sodium loss	Dilutional states	Sodium shift
History	Evidence of excessive non-renal sodium loss	Evidence of renal disease, or Addison's disease	1 Evidence of decreased renal water clearance. Excessive hypotonic fluid administration in the presence of oliguria. 2 Condition present in which I.A.D.H. syndrome is said to occur (see p. 169). Fluid shift e.g. mannitol glucose.	Oedematous states. Hypokalaemia. Patient suffering from a critical illness, e.g. sepsis, trauma, cardiogenic septic or hypovolaemic shock.
E.C.F. volume	Decreased	Decreased	Increased	Normal or increased
Urine sodium conc.	<30 mmol/l	>30 mmol/l	1 generally >30 mmol/l 2 >30 mmol/l	<30 mmol/l
Treatment	Saline replacement therapy. Corticosteroid for Addison's disease		1 Treatment of renal failure. Restriction of fluid administration. 2 *I.A.D.H. syndrome* – consider corticosteroids. Treatment of factor producing I.A.D.H. syndrome. *Fluid shift* Mannitol consider dialysis if fluid overload and no diuresis. Glucose give insulin.	*Oedematous states* Consider diuretics. Sodium and water restriction. *Hypokalaemia* Potassium replacement. *Sick cell syndrome* Treat the cause. Sodium replacement not indicated.

(see p. 169)

large quantity of this is sequestered in bone leaving approximately 3000 mmol as exchangeable sodium.

Salt depletion may be aggravated by a low intake but cannot occur by dietary restriction alone since the normal kidney can conserve salt almost completely.

The causes of loss of total body sodium are enumerated in Table 8. Alimentary secretions (apart from gastric) are approximately isotonic but sodium depletion may develop if fluid volume is replaced with low sodium containing solutions such as $\frac{1}{5}$ normal saline or dextrose/saline. Large sodium losses from the bowel may occur in severe diarrhoea this may result in hypokalaemia as a result of sodium and potassium exchange in the distal renal tubule. Mucinous discharges are rich in sodium and sodium depletion is well recognised in the mucin-secreting villous tumours of the rectum and colon. In fibrocystic disease, the sodium loss in sweat is higher than usual and such patients are predisposed to sodium depletion and heat exhaustion. Removal of a large volume of ascitic fluid may cause shock from loss of sodium and protein.

Salt loss from the kidney may be the result of an osmotic diuresis or secondary to an increase in filtered urea per nephron as in renal failure. Tubular reabsorption of sodium is impaired in certain renal diseases such as pyelonephritis and polycystic disease, and following the use of certain nephrotoxic drugs. Sodium depletion has also been observed in the diuretic phase of acute renal failure and after relief of chronic urinary tract obstruction.

In terminal renal failure the severe loss of filtering surface may lead to sodium retention. Observation of urinary sodium losses in patients with chronic renal failure and hyponatraemia is therefore important since the patient may change from a depletion of total body sodium to a preterminal phase of dilutional hyponatraemia.

Diagnosis of depletion of total body sodium. The signs and symptoms in depletion of total body sodium are described in Table 6. The clinical picture varies with the time taken to develop depletion and the magnitude of the sodium loss. Slight to moderate sodium depletion represents a total body sodium deficit of approximately 8 mmol/kg body weight, moderate to severe sodium depletion 8 mmol–11.5 mmol/kg body weight. Mild losses of total body sodium leads to loss of appetite and energy and postural fainting. These patients are susceptible to water loading and develop cramps more readily than normal subjects. Moderate to severe depletion produces symptoms and signs associated with a depleted intravascular volume. The sodium deficit under such circumstances is associated with a serum sodium of less than 135 mmol/l and provided the hyponatraemia has not been complicated by low perfusion, acute renal failure or hyponatraemia secondary to urinary sodium losses, the renal sodium concentration will be less than 30 mmol/l. The situation most commonly seen in the intensive therapy unit is that of non-renal losses of sodium.

Treatment. Treatment in moderate to severe depletion will require intravenous normal saline (150 mmol Na^+/litre) and in very severe depletion twice normal saline (300 mmol Na^+/litre) may be the initial replacement solution of choice. The rate of the infusion will depend upon the level of the serum sodium, the estimated sodium loss (see Table 10), the rapidity with which the patient has become sodium depleted,

Table 10. Guide to quantity of sodium lost in a patient with sodium depletion

Body weight in kg prior to illness = W
E.C.F. volume in litres   = F

E.C.F. Volume $(F) = W \times \dfrac{15}{100}$

Sodium deficit mmol/l = Normal serum sodium − calculated serum sodium
                         (mmol/l)   (mmol/l)

The total sodium deficit = $F \times$ sodium deficit (in mmol)

The sodium deficit may be replaced with normal saline or twice normal saline.

the acid base status and the state of the myocardium. In very severe depletion twice normal saline should be given at a rate of not greater than 2.0 mmol sodium ions per square metre body surface per minute (see Table 11 for calculation of body surface area from body weight) and should be limited to a total of 300 mmol. (Twice normal saline should only be used where there is severe hypotension, evidence of poor peripheral perfusion and oliguria). Sodium replacement can then be continued with normal saline (150 mmol Na^+/l). The rate of infusion should be slowed once the central venous pressure is 2 cm H_2O or above and the blood pressure systolic 100 mm Hg or above. An attempt should be made to replace $\frac{1}{3}$ to $\frac{1}{2}$ of the total estimated deficit over the first 12 hours plus replacing estimated sodium losses that are likely to occur during that period. Generally the kidneys can excrete the excess chloride ions given in the normal saline – but periodic estimations of acid-base status is advisable. A base deficit of greater than 10 should be corrected with sodium bicarbonate (see Table 3, p. 204). Sodium bicarbonate should not be given until the serum potassium is 3.5 mmol/l or greater.

Moderate to severe deficits can generally be treated with normal saline except where renal handling of water may be impaired when a small quantity of twice normal saline (up to 150 mmol) may be considered.

Table 11. Simplified body surface area chart*

Weight (kg)	Surface area (m²)
30	1.05
40	1.30
50	1.50
60	1.65
70	1.75
80	1.85
90	1.95
100	2.05

* From Crawford *et al.* (1950). Simplification of drug dosage calculation by application of surface area principle. (*Paediatrics* 5, 783, 1950.)

Excessive renal losses of sodium are most likely to occur following relief of urinary tract obstruction or during the diuretic phase of acute renal failure. Serious sodium depletion under such circumstances can be prevented by observation of the urinary sodium and replacing the excess loss. Sodium replacement in chronic renal failure should be performed with caution and rarely is sufficiently severe to warrant intravenous therapy. When intravenous sodium is required (generally because of vomiting) great care must be taken not to overload the patient.

2. *Dilutional hyponatraemia*

Water intoxication. The most common cause for water intoxication is the excessive administration of hypotonic solutions in the presence of an inadequate urine output. This may occur not only in association with renal failure but also following excess ADH excretion as a consequence of stress, and head injury and may be complicated by pulmonary oedema. Water intoxication may also follow colonic washouts with tap water and bladder washouts with distilled water. The condition is unlikely to occur in patients drinking spontaneously, for nausea and distaste for water occurs early in water intoxication. The symptoms of water intoxication depend upon the severity and the rapidity of onset. Acute intoxication is characterised by disorientation followed by convulsions which may proceed to fatal coma. There may be abnormal neurological findings such as assymmetrical pupils, altered reflexes and extensor plantar responses. When the onset is more gradual – the patient becomes lethargic, apathetic and disorientated. The serum sodium is generally less than 120 mmol.

Once diagnosed, intravenous fluids should be reduced to a minimum and sweating encouraged by placing the patient in a hot dry atmosphere. Acute severe intoxication should be treated with twice normal saline. 100 ml of twice normal saline should be infused hourly until convulsions have ceased or the serum sodium has reached 130 mmol/l. When water intoxication is associated with renal failure, the patient should be dialysed peritoneally with a hypertonic dialysate.

3. *Hyponatraemia secondary to a sodium shift* (see Tables 8 and 9)
Hyponatraemia may accompany potassium depletion when it is postulated that the sodium ions move into the potassium depleted cells.

Sick cell syndrome. This condition was discussed in detail by Flear and Singh (1973). They considered that in many diseases hyponatraemia arises not as a result of overproduction of ADH (the evidence for which in many hyponatraemic states is very limited) but because of widespread disturbance at the cellular level. This is undoubtedly one of the commonest causes for hyponatraemia in the critically ill and is becoming increasingly recognised as a bad prognostic sign. Flear and Singh (1973) believe that in severe illness sodium ions shift from the extracellular to the intracellular compartment. This concept is supported by various workers finding an increase in intracellular sodium in critically ill patients (Welt *et al.*, 1967; Smith, 1963).

Flear and Singh (1973) alternatively suggest that a widespread increase in the membrane permeability of sick cells allows intracellular solutes to leak out into the extracellular compartment together with potassium ions. By this mechanism the influx of sodium ions is balanced against the efflux of intracellular solutes, there being little net shift in water. Alternatively, the increased permeability may be secondary to inhibition of the membrane transport mechanism whereby sodium is transported out of the cell and potassium moved into the cell both against an electrochemical gradient. The energy required for this cation-exchange pump is supplied by ATP-ase from within the cell. The supply of ATP-ase may be reduced by any factors which impair cell metabolism, these commonly occur in the critically ill, and include anoxia, hypothermia and metabolic poisons. Cardiac glycosides are also known to inhibit part of the membrane ATP-ase system (Editorial, 1974).

Thus, in the critically ill patient a falling serum sodium concentration does not indicate a depletion of total body sodium and sodium ions should not be infused unless there is absolute evidence of excessive sodium losses. An attempt should be made to correct the underlying disease and measures should be taken to improve cell membrane transport. Tissue perfusion and oxygenation should be improved if at all possible and since insulin is known to stimulate ion exchange in cell membranes (independently of glucose uptake), its use should be considered. Allison and co-workers (1972) and Hinton *et al.* (1973) have used insulin glucose and potassium in patients suffering from severe burns. This regimen has been found to produce a sodium diuresis and to reduce the catabolic response after injury (Hinton *et al.*, 1971). The rate of glucose infusion should be no greater than 0.5 g/kg B.W./h and it is advisable to limit the quantity of glucose infused to not greater than 200 g during the first 24 hours. The quantity of glucose infused can be gradually increased over the subsequent 5 days – once the quantity of insulin required to maintain a blood glucose between 4 and 10 mmol/l has been estimated. It is rare to be able to give more than 500 g of glucose/24 h since it becomes difficult to control the blood glucose even with increasing insulin dosage. Insulin dosage is started at 1 unit per 4 g of glucose and may have to be increased to as high as 8 units per g. The insulin and dextrose can be placed in a 100 ml buretrol burette 100 ml 40% dextrose with insulin and potassium being infused over 2–4 hours (in an adult). The quantity of potassium required is variable – 40–180 mmol being required per 500 ml 40% dextrose infused (depending upon the potassium losses). This regimen is recommended in desperately ill catabolic patients once oxygenation acid base status and cellular perfusion has been improved by appropriate measures. The dangers of hyperglycaemia and hypokalaemia are high and the regimen should not be attempted without full monitoring facilities. Blood glucose should be checked initially 2–4 hourly especially if the renal threshold for glucose is suspected to be high or if the patient is in acute renal failure.

In any critically ill patient hyponatraemia is likely to develop if the patient is given excess fluid in relation to urine output. This is particularly likely to occur during and for the first 24 hours following a period of stress. Sequential weighing and central venous pressure monitoring are valuable guides to the total body fluid volume and the dynamic intravascular volume respectively.

Hypernatraemia. Aetiology, diagnosis and management, see the Hyperosmolar syndromes, Part 1, ch. VIII, p. 226.

ACUTE DISORDERS IN POTASSIUM BALANCE

Introduction

Potassium is the predominant cation of cells and thus its distribution is related to cell-mass. The total body potassium in a 70 kg male is approximately 3800 mmol and 70% of this is in the muscle cell. Energy is required to maintain potassium largely within and sodium predominantly outside the cell. A calculated negative balance of potassium ions does not necessarily mean a deficiency, this depending upon the capacity of the cells for potassium (being increased when the protein and glycogen content of the cells is increased).

The kidneys' ability (in contrast to sodium) to conserve potassium is limited; in severe depletion the urinary output of potassium (in the presence of normal renal function) should be less than 5.0 mmol/24 h. The kidneys also take 2–3 weeks to adapt to large increases in potassium load. Alterations in either intracellular or extracellular potassium concentrations affect membrane excitability by affecting the membrane potential. The membrane potential varies directly with the intracellular, extracellular potassium ratio. Generally, hypokalaemia is associated with an increased resting membrane potential – leading to weakness and paralysis and hyperkalaemia to a decreased potential and enhanced excitability. The serum potassium does not necessarily reflect the intracellular/extracellular potassium ratio (ki/ke ratio) and therefore slowly developing potassium depletion may lead to an equal quantitative fall in intracellular and extracellular potassium with resultant little change in membrane potential. Acute hyperkalaemia leads to a marked decrease in the ki/ke ratio (due to an increase in the extracellular potassium) and the resting membrane potential may be reduced to a point where depolarisation block occurs. The E.C.G. changes in hypokalaemia are helpful in making the initial diagnosis but the rate of improvement during potassium infusion may not correlate with the serum potassium changes, frequently lagging behind. During hypokalaemic states, the S–T segment on the E.C.G. becomes depressed, the U wave is exaggerated and the T wave amplitude is decreased without changing the actual duration of the Q − T interval. The P and QRS amplitude and duration may increase and the P–R interval may be prolonged (see Fig. 1). The combination of digitalis and

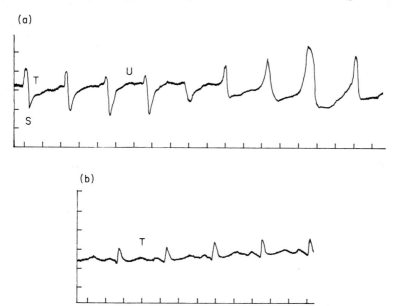

Fig. 1. E.C.G. changes – hypokalaemia.
(a) Lead III Se K 1.5 mmol/l. Low voltage flattening of waves. S-T segment depression. Prominent U wave. Last 4 complexes either a L.B.B.B. pattern due to defective conduction or a ventricular dysrhythmia.
(b) Lead III – same patient 48 h later after infusion of 300 mmol potassium ions. Se K 4.0 mmol/l.

quinidine may mimic the E.C.G. pattern of hypokalaemia. Low levels of Ke encourage ectopic pacemaker discharge and patients with a concentration of 3.2 mmol/l or less may develop supraventricular or ventricular ectopic beats. Arrhythmias may occur (in the absence of digoxin) such as junctional or atrial tachycardia with block.

Potassium is required for glucose uptake by the cell; impaired glucose tolerance has been found in patients who are potassium depleted. Potassium is also essential for protein synthesis enabling transfer of amino acids to polypeptides. The ion is also necessary for activation of certain enzyme systems essential for normal cell metabolism including the hydrolysis of adenosine triphosphate, acetylkinase and pyruvic phosphokinase.

At least four major factors are involved in the regulation of potassium excretion by the renal tubule, the cellular potassium concentration, the delivery of the sodium ions to the distal nephron, the acid base status and the level of the mineralocorticoids.

Good correlation exists between the level of cellular potassium and urinary excretion rate, whereas this correlation does not exist with the serum potassium. Clinical and experimental studies have shown that diminished sodium intake is associated with a decreased potassium excretion, whereas an increased sodium intake enhances excretion. There is an inverse correlation between the rate of hydrogen ion secretion and potassium secretion, for example in a metabolic acidosis

Table 12. Cation exchange across cells during acidosis and alkalosis

Intracellular compartment	Extracellular compartment	
	H^+ ←	Acidosis
Na^+	→	
K^+	→	
H^+	→	
	Na^+ ←	Alkalosis
	K^+ ←	

the hydrogen ion secretion is increased and that of potassium diminished. In a metabolic alkalosis there is excessive loss of potassium ions into the urine until the serum potassium falls to low levels when potassium ions are conserved and H ions are secreted instead. This leads to the paradoxical aciduria characteristic of a severe hypokalaemic metabolic alkalosis.

The metabolic status radically affects the serum potassium concentration. An acidosis is associated with hydrogen ion shift into the cell in exchange for potassium and sodium ions (see Table 12).

This relationship is such that for every rise or fall of 0.1 pH unit there is an average fall or rise of 0.63 mmol K^+/l. Factors which may affect the serum potassium and are likely to be encountered during the management of the critically ill are summarised in Table 13.

Hypokalaemia

Moderate potassium depletion, less than 10% of the total body potassium, produces no symptoms in healthy subjects (Black, 1967).

The urinary output over a period of several weeks falls to less than 10 mmol/day unless the cause for the potassium depletion is renal. When 10–30% of the total body potassium has been lost by feeding previously healthy subjects with a potassium exchange resin, symptoms included muscle weakness, apathy, anorexia, thirst and irritability. Tetany was also noted and the E.C.G. showed U waves (Fourman, 1954).

Table 13. Factors affecting potassium shifts between the intracellular and extracellular compartments

Changes in external balance

Alterations in K^+ intake	
Sodium excess	Loss of K^+ in urine. Se K $\downarrow$
Sodium deficiency	K comes out of the intracellular compartment Se K $\uparrow$
Severe sodium deficiency	Increased urinary K^+ loss Se K
Acidosis	K comes out of the cell in exchange for H^+ ions Se K $\uparrow$
Alkalosis	K enters the cell in exchange for H^+ ions Se K $\downarrow$

Changes in cell metabolism

Cellular uptake of glucose	Se K $\downarrow$
Depletion of glycogen stores	Se K $\downarrow$
Protein anabolism	Se K $\downarrow$
Protein catabolism	Se K $\uparrow$
Intravascular haemolysis	Se K $\uparrow$
Hyperpyrexia	Se K $\uparrow$

Miscellaneous factors

Insulin	Se K $\downarrow$
Adrenaline generally	Se K $\downarrow$
Succinylcholine	Se K $\uparrow$
Vasopressin	Se K $\uparrow$
Steroids	Se K $\downarrow$

Losses of greater than 30% of total body potassium is generally manifest as widespread damage to cell function and death. Potassium depletion may develop secondary to losses from the gastrointestinal tract, inadequate replacement therapy in patients unable to take food and fluids orally, and following prolonged periods of sweating or fluid loss from a damaged skin surface (e.g. burns). Intravenous feeding in the critically ill with inadequate potassium supplements may lead to a rapid fall in serum potassium. Drugs, in particular steroids and thiazide diuretics, commonly used in the intensive therapy unit, may be complicated by hypokalaemia. Potassium monitoring is essential during renal dialysis and during the institution of a forced alkaline diuresis for drug overdose.

Excessive renal losses of potassium may occur in conditions of sodium overload, protein catabolism, intravascular haemolysis and during periods of stress. Massive doses of corticosteroids as used in the treatment of septic shock, may in the presence of adequate renal function precipitate a heavy potassium diuresis. Patients suffering from cardiac failure or hepatocellular failure with oedema tend to lose large quantities of potassium in the urine secondary to high circulating aldosterone levels. This may be compounded by the use of thiazide diuretics. Renal disease, such as the diuretic phase following acute renal failure, high urine output following relief of urinary tract obstruction and chronic syndromes of renal tubular dysfunction, are commonly complicated by excessive potassium losses in the urine. Hypercalaemia may also be complicated by potassium depletion.

Since severe potassium depletion may lead to renal tubular dysfunction, the primary factor may be difficult to elicit. A metabolic alkalosis suggests a primarily non-renal cause for the potassium depletion, whereas osteomalacia and deficient formation of urinary ammonia suggests a renal cause.

Diagnosis and management of chronic potassium depletion

Patients suffering from *chronic potassium depletion* are rarely admitted to the unit except when complicated by another illness. In patients who are known to have been on thiazide diuretics and admitted with a supraventricular tachycardia, the serum potassium must be checked before administering a d.c. shock. Patients with a serum potassium of 3.5 mmol/l or less should have 30–60 mmol of potassium chloride infused in 100–200 ml $\frac{1}{5}$ N saline over a period of one hour before considering d.c. cardioversion. The serum potassium should be checked half an hour after finishing the infusion in order to give time for the potassium to enter the cells. The serum potassium should rise by at least 0.2 mmol/l with this regimen. Should the patient be in left ventricular failure secondary to a supraventricular tachycardia with a serum potassium of 3.5 mmol/l or less, the potassium can be infused over a period of 30 min and then cardioversion performed. Sodium bicarbonate should not be used to treat a metabolic acidosis if the serum potassium is 3.3 mmol/l or less. Under such circumstances when the pH is 7.2 or less or the B.D. greater than 10, the potassium should be infused rapidly (as above) followed by the administration of 50 mmol of bicarbonate ions over the subsequent 30 min. The serum potassium must then be rechecked. It is essential under such circumstances to monitor the E.C.G.

Generally, patients with chronic severe depletion (where the serum potassium is less than 2.8 mmol), can have the potassium replaced orally. In patients with ileus, the potassium can be given intravenously and provided potassium loss is not continuing, approximately $\frac{1}{3}$ to $\frac{1}{2}$ of the estimated total loss should be replaced over the first 24 h.

Diagnosis and management of acute moderate potassium depletion

In acute moderate potassium depletion (loss of approximately 10% of the total body potassium), the serum potassium is generally 3.2–3.5 mmol/l but occasionally the level may be above this figure when there is concurrent sodium depletion or a metabolic acidosis. Patients with moderate depletion receiving digitalis may manifest as a paroxysmal tachycardia with block (P.A.T.B.). Such a condition requires cancellation of the digoxin therapy and when complicated by heart failure, 40–60 mmol potassium chloride should be infused in 100 mls $\frac{1}{5}$ normal saline over a period of 1 hour. As a result of this therapy P.A.T.B. generally reverts spontaneously. Direct current shock should not be contemplated until the serum potassium is 3.5 mmol or above. It is essential during rapid intravenous potassium replacement to monitor the E.C.G. Rapid administration may occasionally produce ectopic junctional rhythms and very occasionally QRS or AV conduction prolongation. Such changes are an absolute indication to slow down the infusion rate. Particular care must be taken during rapid infusion of potassium in a digitalised patient.

In the absence of any serious cardiac dysrhythmia, $\frac{1}{3}$ to $\frac{1}{2}$ of the estimated potassium loss should be replaced over the first 24 h and to this must be added the continuing losses, e.g. from the gastrointestinal tract or in the urine.

Diagnosis and management of acute severe potassium depletion

Acute severe potassium depletion (greater than 10% loss of total body potassium) may occur rapidly in the presence of vomiting, fistula losses or diarrhoea. Muscle weakness is common and may be sufficiently severe to lead to paresis and inadequate ventilation. Muscle aching, abdominal distension and diarrhoea may also be noted. A metabolic alkalosis is common, frequently associated with albuminuria, a rising blood urea and inability to concentrate the urine. Potassium losses in the urine may be normal in spite of severe potassium depletion.

In acute severe depletion where potassium is still being lost and the serum potassium level is less than 2.8 mmol/l, large quantities of potassium may be required over the first 24 hours. Estimates should be made of the concentration of potassium being lost in the urine and other sites, e.g. fistulae – and this should be replaced 4 hourly. To this should be added approximately $\frac{1}{12}$ of the estimated loss of total body potassium. This may necessitate infusing up to 160 mmol of potassium chloride over the first 4 hours of treatment. This should be given in 1–2 litres of normal saline or $\frac{1}{5}$ normal saline, depending upon the fluid requirements. The patient should be monitored 2–4 hourly for serum potassium, electrolytes, acid base status, blood glucose and urinary output. The E.C.G. trace should be carefully assessed. Rapid potassium replacement may be complicated by tetany. Hypokalaemic tetany may be associated with hypocalcaemia or hypomagnesaemia and is more likely to arise when there is a severe metabolic alkalosis. Oliguria may also complicate rapid potassium replacement. Should the urine output fall fluid volume and potassium replacement must be estimated according to the central venous pressure and serum potassium levels – the serum potassium being only allowed to rise to approximately 4.0 mmol/l.

On rare occasions a hypokalaemic crisis manifested by a ventricular dysrhythmia and cardiac arrest or respiratory failure may necessitate more urgent therapy. A cardiac arrest complicated by a ventricular dysrhythmia should be treated with external cardiac massage, hand ventilation on oxygen, and infusion of 60 mmol of potassium chloride in $\frac{1}{5}$ normal saline over a period of 30 min. Cardioversion should be performed after approximately 30 mmol has been infused commencing at 20 J and repeating the shock with increasing increments of 50 J at 5 min intervals until cardioversion is successful. In hypokalaemic respiratory arrest, provided there is not a ventricular dysrhythmia, the patient should be intubated and ventilated on oxygen taking care not to hyperventilate the patient and maintaining the PaO_2 at 10.6–13.3 kPa (80–100 mm Hg). Potassium chloride 60 mmol should be infused intravenously (under E.C.G. control) in 100–500 ml of $\frac{1}{5}$ or normal saline over the first hour – subsequent dosage being estimated as for severe acute depletion of potassium.

Table 14. Causes of hyperkalaemia

Acute and chronic renal failure
Metabolic or respiratory acidosis
Adrenal insufficiency $\left\{\begin{array}{l}\text{Addison's disease} \\ \text{hypoaldosteronism}\end{array}\right.$
Hyperkalaemic periodic paralysis

Cell breakdown
    Hypercatabolic states
    Acute intravascular haemolysis
    Malignant hyperpyrexia

Iatrogenic
    Potassium sparing diuretics
    Exogenous potassium
    Massive transfusion of old blood
    Succinyl choline

Hyperkalaemia

Aetiology and diagnosis

The causes of hyperkalaemia are summarised in Table 14. The commonest and most rapid rise in serum potassium in the critically ill occurs when the onset of acute renal failure is missed. Other factors are frequently superimposed, e.g. red cell haemolysis, blood transfusion or potassium infusion which accelerates the rate of rise of serum potassium.

A mild hyperkalaemia is common in Addison's disease but in a crisis a flaccid quadriplegia associated with hyperkalaemia has been reported (Pollen and Williams, 1960).

Selective hypoaldosteronism is a rare condition characterised by relative or absolute deficiency of aldosterone secretion. The patient may manifest with hyponatraemia, dehydration, weakness and cramping of the muscles and Stokes–Adams attacks. Hyperkalaemia appears to be the cause for the cardiac dysrhythmias, muscular weakness and paresis. Hyperkalaemia may also occur shortly after removal of an aldosterone tumour.

The use of potassium retaining diuretics (triamterene or spironolactone) must be used with caution in any patient thought to be suffering from renal failure.

Cardiac arrest has been produced by massive transfusion of hyperkalaemic bank blood. On rare occasions plasma concentrations of potassium may reach five times as high in bank blood when stored for two weeks (Le Veen *et al.*, 1959). Cooling leads to an efflux of potassium from the cells into the plasma.

Hyperkalaemia leading to ventricular fibrillation has been reported in burned and traumatised patients after the administration of succinylcholine (Birch *et al.*, 1969). Succinylcholine is contraindicated in the management of patients who have sustained thermal trauma or direct muscle trauma and those who have neurologic motor deficits. Though succinylcholine induces a small release of K^+ in normal muscle, it produces a potentially lethal efflux in the presence of these disorders. This potassium releasing action begins about 5–15 days after injury and may persist for 2–3 months (Gronert and Theye, 1975). An elevation of serum potassium may occur in the test tube but not in the patient. The cause of the elevated level is release of potassium from

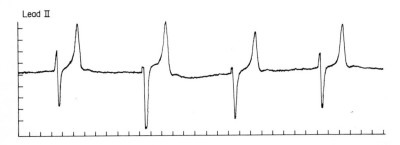

Fig. 2. E.C.G. charges – hyperkalaemia. Serum potassium 9.2 mmol/l. No definite evidence of atrial activity. Increase in the QRS interval. Tall peaked T waves.

platelets or white blood cells during clotting in samples containing high platelets or leucocytes (e.g. in polycythaemia, leukaemia). Apparent hyperkalaemia may also occur when the specimen is haemolysed. In all these conditions the plasma potassium will be normal and there will be no E.C.G. changes to suggest hyperkalaemia.

The toxic manifestations of hyperkalaemia are neuromuscular and cardiac. The neuromuscular effects rarely arise until the plasma potassium is greater than 8 mmol/l and include paraesthesia, tingling around the mouth, hands and feet, burning and numbness of the extremities, decreased or absent reflexes and a muscular paresis ranging from weakness to a flaccid quadriplegia. An ascending type of paralysis may occur and weakness may involve muscles of respiration or phonation. Fixed dilated pupils have been reported (Scherr *et al.*, 1962).

Electrocardiographic changes during hyperkalaemia generally closely correlate with the ke level. The T waves peaks when the plasma potassium reaches 5.5 mmol/l; the corrected Q-T interval is normal or shortens initially but may prolong as the QRS widens. The QRS widens when ke exceeds 6.5 mmol/l and above 7.0 mmol/l, the height of the P wave diminishes and the duration of this wave and the P–R interval becomes prolonged (Fig. 2). Surawicz and Gettes (1971) found that less than 25% of patients with hyperkalaemia developed the characteristic peaked T waves: it is therefore essential to estimate serial plasma potassium levels if a serious alteration in potassium is likely. The E.C.G. changes induced by hyperkalaemia can be reversed by increasing the concentration of plasma calcium and sodium, whereas a low sodium concentration or a metabolic acidosis enhances the changes. In the human, a plasma concentration of 8.5 mmol/l or more may be complicated by ventricular fibrillation and cardiac arrest.

Treatment of hyperkalaemia (for summary see Table 15)
The cause for the hyperkalaemia should be identified (see Table 14) and treated. Should the situation be readily reversible and renal function good, then drug therapy for the hyperkalaemia may be sufficient; in the presence of renal failure, drug therapy has frequently to be followed by dialysis. Blood glucose, B.U. electrolytes and acid base balance should be checked. Several drugs are available – glucose and insulin are preferable in the critically ill (see Table 15) which shifts extracellular potassium into the cells. The effect is noted within 15 min of stopping the infusion and lasts 2–4 h. This method is valuable where surgery is contemplated in a patient with a rising serum potassium and acute renal failure. The serum potassium can be further lowered by hyperventilating the patient during the operative procedure. Dialysis should be started immediately post-operatively. A continuous dextrose insulin infusion may enable dialysis to be postponed in acute hypercatabolic renal failure for up to 24 hours, when the original serum potassium was around 5.5 mmol/l. This regimen may be useful where the only indication for dialysis is a rising potassium and the circulation so unstable that deferment for 24 h is advisable. The usual dosage is 300–400 g dextrose plus the dosage of insulin required to maintain the blood glucose at 5–12 mmol/l infused continuously over 24 h. The insulin can be given intravenously as hourly bolus injections or infused continuously as 50% dextrose with the appropriate dosage of insulin, 100 ml being infused 4-hourly. The depolarising effect of a high extracellular potassium can be blocked by a high concentration of calcium. Although calcium does not alter the serum potassium it can rapidly reverse cardiotoxicity and should therefore be used as an extreme emergency where ventricular fibrillation has occurred. The

Table 15. Emergency management of acute hyperkalaemia

Drug	Dose	Onset of action	Duration	Comments
Calcium gluconate	10% 0.25 mmol Ca^{++}/ml 30 ml i.v. over 3 min	Min	Less than 1 h	Does not alter the serum potassium; rapidly eliminates cardiotoxicity; calcium chloride necrotic to veins
Calcium chloride	10% 0.45 mmol Ca^{++}/ml 15–20 ml i.v. over 5 min			
Sodium bicarbonate	8.4% 1 mmol HCO_3^-/ml Infuse 80–120 ml over 20 min	Min	Up to 2 h when given as a stat dose	Danger of sodium overload. May be infused continuously 80–120 mmol/h. Method of choice when there is hyponatraemia and hypovolaemia
Insulin and dextrose	40% dextrose 4 g CHO/ml Infuse 20–50 g with insulin 1 unit/4 g dextrose over 15–20 min	Min	Up to 4 h	Danger of hyperglycaemia. May be infused continuously 6-hourly with appropriate insulin dosage
Infusion mixture	Dextrose 40% 200 ml Sodium bicarbonate 8.4% 100 ml Infuse over 30 min Sol. insulin 20 units i.v. or i.m.	see above	see above	see above
Exchange resin in sodium or calcium phase	50–60 g in a sorbitol retention enema or via Ryles tube	approx. 30 min	4–6 h	Sodium overload with sodium phase resin. Diarrhoea. Has to be given via the gastrointestinal tract.

effect is almost immediate and generally only lasts about 30 min. The drug can be infused over 3–5 min; calcium chloride is more toxic on veins and therefore the gluconate is to be preferred. The gluconate is converted to bicarbonate which may also lead to a fall in serum potassium.

Sodium bicarbonate will counteract hyperkalaemia especially in patients with hyponatraemia or volume contraction. It should not be used where sodium overload is suspected since it may precipitate pulmonary oedema.

An infusion mixture using all the above methods may also be used but preparation may take time. Should a fall in serum potassium require to be maintained without dialysis, an exchange resin in the sodium or calcium phase can be given as a retention enema or via the Ryles tube. The effect lasts 4–6 h and may be repeated. This method is generally only used in patients receiving intermittent dialysis for acute renal failure where a rise in serum potassium is the only indication for dialysis. The resin in the sodium phase should not be used if there is any question of sodium overload.

ACUTE DISORDERS OF MAGNESIUM BALANCE

Introduction

The total body magnesium in an adult is approximately 15 mmol per kg body weight, half of which is in the bone. Only one per cent of the total body magnesium is extracellular, the remainder being intracellular where it is the second most abundant cation (the most abundant being potassium). The normal serum magnesium is 0.7–1.0 mmol/l about 35% of which is protein bound, the remainder being mostly ionised. Many of the basic energy processes of the cell are mediated by enzymes activated by magnesium. Most of the important features of magnesium depletion are directly related to its neuromuscular function. Parathyroid hormone as in calcium homeostasis is important for maintenance of the serum magnesium, the mechanism is uncertain. Experimental evidence suggests that elevation of plasma magnesium leads to inhibition of parathyroid secretion whereas hypomagnesaemia stimulates its release (MacIntyre et al., 1963). It is still unsettled whether the hormone affects magnesium directly or only through its action on calcium metabolism (Wacker and Parisi, 1968). Aldosterone has been found to cause an increased renal and faecal loss of magnesium whereas a deficiency of adrenal hormones produces hypermagnesaemia. Vitamin D can affect magnesium balance experimentally, physiologic doses increasing absorption whereas pharmacologic doses lead to hypomagnesaemia (George *et al.*, 1962). Patients with vitamin D intoxication may however have normal magnesium levels (Walser, 1962). The normal renal loss for magnesium is approximately 10 mmol a day which is reduced to less than 1 mmol in the presence of severe depletion.

The causes for magnesium depletion are numerous (see Table 16) and its lack is frequently associated with potassium and calcium depletion. Under conditions of depletion of potassium it is essential to estimate serum magnesium and calcium levels. The serum magnesium during the treatment of diabetic ketoacidosis with insulin follows a similar pattern to that of potassium. Hypomagnesaemic tetany has been reported, it has been recommended by Butler (1950) that replacement therapy should include 2.5 mmol of magnesium ions per litre of fluid infused. Hypocalcaemia is difficult to treat in the presence of hypomagnesaemia (Part 1, ch. VII, p. 191). Tetany caused by hypomagnesaemia does not respond to calcium.

Table 16. Causes of magnesium deficiency

Deficient intake
 Maintenance for prolonged periods on non-magnesium containing parenteral fluids
 Protein malnutrition

Decreased absorption
 Malabsorption syndromes
 Patients taking a high calcium diet

Excessive urinary loss
 Hyperaldosteronism primary or secondary
 Renal tubular defects
 Prolonged diuresis especially with thiazides

Excessive gastrointestinal loss
 Diarrhoea
 Aspiration of fistula losses

Transfer from extracellular fluid to other body compartments
 Insulin therapy in diabetic ketoacidosis (transfer of Mg^{++} into the cell)
 Following parathyroidectomy (transfer of Mg^{++} to bone)
 Acute pancreatitis (transfer of Mg^{++} to intraperitoneal fat deposits)

Diagnosis and treatment of magnesium deficiency

The manifestations of magnesium deficiency are similar to those of calcium depletion. Latent or overt tetany is the most distinctive feature and is frequently preceded by a period of vertigo, irritability and/or psychotic behaviour. Sleepiness, muscle weakness, tremor and purpose-less involuntary movements are often important features. The critical level for tetany is around 0.5 mmol/l but the percentage which is protein bound and the intracellular concentration are important factors. Hypocalcaemia and hypokalaemia are common. A metabolic alkalosis so commonly found in hypokalaemia will decrease the ionised fraction and hence increase the susceptibility to tetany. The symptoms of magnesium deficiency are exaggerated by a high calcium intake and even more so by a high phosphate intake. It should not be forgotten that intralipid contains phosphate as phospholipid – phosphate intake during intravenous nutrition may therefore be adequate in the presence of little or no magnesium intake – hence exaggerating the deficiency. Magnesium can be replaced orally, intramuscularly or intravenously (see Table 17) – oral absorption is good unless there is evidence of gastrointestinal dysfunction.

Table 17. Magnesium replacement solutions

Oral	
Magnesium hydroxide mixture B.P.C.	1 ml contains 4.5 mmol Mg^{++}
Magnesium chloride	1 g = 5.0 mmol Mg^{++}
Intramuscular	
Magnesium sulphate 50%	1 ml contains 2.0 mmol Mg^{++}
Intravenous	
Magnesium sulphate 50%	1 ml contains 2.0 mmol Mg^{++}

Dissolve 10 ml (20 mmol Mg^{++}) in 500 ml 5% dextrose solution.
Infuse at a rate not greater than 0.25 mmol/m² body surface per min (see Table 11).

The management of hypomagnesaemic tetany is with intravenous magnesium sulphate. Fifty mmol of magnesium should be infused in 500 ml to 1000 ml of 5% dextrose over a period of 2–4 h – the rate should not exceed 0.25 mmol/m² body surface per minute. (See Table 11 for estimation of body surface area in relation to weight). Subsequent dosage should be gauged according to the estimated losses and serial magnesium levels. Manifest hypomagnesaemia (serum magnesium 0.6 mmol or less) where losses have been heavy for several weeks and magnesium cannot be given orally, magnesium should be replaced intramuscularly daily as magnesium chloride 20–40 mmol daily for 2–3 days, then reducing to 6–12 mmol daily. The latter dosage can be given intramuscularly as magnesium sulphate. Maintenance dosage in patients on intravenous nutrition is discussed in Part 1, ch. IX, p. 252.

The treatment of hypomagnesaemia associated with hypocalcaemia is described in Part 1, ch. VII, p. 191.

In patients who are able to absorb magnesium orally and where the levels are not dangerously low (0.65–0.75 mmol/l), magnesium can be given orally as magnesium chloride or magnesium hydroxide, 50–100 mmol daily initially then decreasing to 12–20 mmol daily according to the serum magnesium level and the quantity of continued loss.

Magnesium excess

Symptomatic hypermagnesaemia most frequently occurs in patients with renal failure, it may also be induced by excessive and too rapid administration of magnesium intravenously. Cardiac conduction is affected at serum concentrations above 2.5 mmol/l resulting in increases of the PR and QRS duration and increased height of the T waves. Reflexes are lost at a concentration of around 5.0 mmol/l and respiratory paralysis occurs at 7.5 mmol/l. General anaesthesia occurs at these concentrations and cardiac arrest generally occurs at a level of approximately 12.5 mmol/l.

PHOSPHATE DEPLETION

Hypophosphataemia leads to a decrease in erythrocyte glucose-6-phosphate, fructose-6-phosphate, 2,3-diphosphoglycerate, adenosine triphosphate and other phosphate containing substances. The reduced amount of 2,3-diphosphoglycerate (2,3-D.P.G.) and adenosine triphosphate increases the affinity of haemoglobin for oxygen (Travis *et al.*, 1971). Phosphate depletion therefore decreases the oxygen availability to the cell and oxygen delivery has to be kept constant by a decrease in mixed venous tension.

In patients where cardiac output is already at an optimum (e.g. anaemia, hypoxia and increased energy demands), a further increase is not possible and the cells become deprived of oxygen. This results in a decrease in pH of the haemoglobin solution with resultant shift of the oxyhaemoglobin dissociation curve downwards and to the right, thereby decreasing the affinity of haemoglobin for oxygen and thus increasing the supply to the tissues. Thus the decrease in 2,3-D.P.G. may be offset by the presence of an acidosis. The development of a metabolic alkalosis in the presence of 2,3-D.P.G. deficiency can be dangerous since the tenacity of the red cell for haemoglobin will be increased and the stimulation of 2,3-D.P.G. synthesis, which normally occurs under such circumstances, is not possible because of phosphate depletion. It is therefore important, when phosphate depletion is suspected to maintain cardiac output and arterial oxygen pressure at an optimum and to prevent the onset of an alkalosis by the excessive use of sodium bicarbonate or through potassium depletion.

Hypophosphataemia is now being increasingly recognised in the critically ill and may be present whether or not hyperalimentation is used and in spite of phosphate supplementation (Watkins *et al.*, 1974). 2,3-D.P.G. deficiency is known to occur in A.C.D. stored blood and following massive transfusion. Phosphate should be infused daily at a rate of approximately 20 mmol/24 h until the phosphate levels have returned to normal. The normal daily requirement for phosphate in an adult on intravenous nutrition is 20–30 mmol, the higher dose being required in patients on high dextrose and/or protein regimens. This is generally readily supplied as Intralipid (2 g of fat/kg B.W. supplying 0.15 mmol of phosphorous/kg B.W., Aminosol 10% (18 mmol phosphate per litre) or Electrolyte Solution B (60 mmol phosphate per litre). When intravenous feeding is not being given, phosphate can be replaced with dipotassium hydrogen phosphate containing 1 mmol of inorganic phosphate per ml (see Table 2, p. 250) 10–20 mmol may be infused over a period of 6 h in 500 ml 5% dextrose, normal saline or $\frac{1}{5}$ normal saline. It must be remembered that this solution contains 2 mmol potassium ions per ml. Phosphate replacement should never be contemplated in patients who are oliguric or where renal functional impairment is suspected without careful monitoring of phosphate levels.

REFERENCES

Allison, S. P., Morley, C. J., Burns-Cox, C. J. (1972). Insulin, glucose and potassium in the treatment of congestive heart failure. *Brit. Med. J.* **3**, 675.

Bartter, F. C. (1958). The physiological control of aldosterone secretion. *Proc. roy. Soc. Med.* **51**, 201.

Birch, A. A. Jr., Mitchell, G. D., Playford, G. A. and Lang, C. A. (1969). Changes in serum potassium response to succinylcholine following trauma. *J.A.M.A.* **210**, 490.

Black, D. A. K. (1967). 'Essentials of Fluid Balance,' p. 2. Blackwell Scientific Publications, Oxford and Edinburgh.

Butler, A. M. (1950). Diabetic coma. *New Engl. J. Med.* **243**, 648.

Crawford, J. D. (1950). Simplification of drug dosage circulation by application of surface area principle. *Paediatrics* **5**, 783.

Danowski, T. S., Fergus, E. B. and Mateer, F. M. (1955). The low salt syndrome. *Ann. Intern. Med.* **43**, 643.

Editorial (1974). Sick cells and hyponatraemia. *Lancet* **I**, 342.

Elkington, J. R., Danowski, T. S. and Winkler, A. W. (1946). Haemodynamic changes in salt depletion and in dehydration. *J. Clin. Invest.* **25**, 120.

Flear, C. T. G. and Singh, C. M. (1973). Hyponatraemia and sick cells. *Brit. J. Anaesth.* **45**, 976.

Fourman, P. (1954). Depletion of potassium induced in man with an exchange resin. *Clin. Sci.* **13**, 93.

George, W. K., George, W. D. Jr., Haan, C. L. and Fisher, R. G. (1962). Vitamin D and magnesium. *Lancet* **I**, 1300.

Gronert, G. A. and Theye, R. A. (1975). Pathophysiology of hyperkalaemia induced by succinylcholine. *Anaesthesiology* **43**, 89.

Hayes, M. A., Williamson, R. J. and Heidenreich, W. F. (1957). Endocrine mechanisms involved in water and sodium metabolism during operation and convalescence. *Surgery* **41**, 353.

Hinton, P., Allison, S. P., Littlejohn, S. and Lloyd, J. (1971). Insulin and glucose to reduce catabolic response to injury in burned patients. *Lancet* **I**, 767.

Hinton, P., Allison, S. P., Littlejohn, S. and Lloyd, J. (1973). Electrolyte changes after burn injury and effect of treatment. *Lancet* **2**, 218.

Le Veen, H. H., Pasternack, H. S., Lustrin, I., Shapiro, P. B., Becker, E. and Helft, A. E. (1960). Haemorrhage and transfusion as the major cause of cardiac arrest. *J. Amer. Med. Ass.* **173**, 770.

MacIntyre, I., Boss, S. and Troughton, V. A. (1963). Parathyroid hormone and magnesium haemeostasis. *Nature* (Lond.) **198**, 1058.

Pollen, R. H. and Williams, R. H. (1960). Hyperkalaemic neuromyopathy in Addison's disease. *New Engl. J. Med.* **263**, 273.

Scherr, L., Lubash, G. D., Rubin, A. L. and Luckey, E. H. (1962). An unusual clinical sign; Mydriasis associated with hyperkalaemia and metabolic acidosis. *Ann. Intern. Med.* **56**, 508.

Smith, R. (1963). Hyponatraemia in infantile malnutrition. *Lancet* **I**, 771.

Surawicz, B. and Gettes, L. S. (1971). Effect of electrolyte abnormalities on the heart and circulation. *In* 'Cardiac and Vascular Diseases' (Ed. H. C. Conn, Jr. and O. Harowitz) Vol. 1, p. 539. Leo and Febiger, Philadelphia.

Taylor, W. H. (1965). 'Fluid Therapy and Disorders of Electrolyte Balance,' p. 143. Blackwell Scientific Publications, Oxford and Edinburgh.

Travis, S., Sugarman, H. J., Ruberg, R. L., Dadrick, S. J., Delivoria-Papadopoulos, M., Miller, L. D. and Oski, F. A. (1971). Alterations of red-cell glycolytic intermediates and oxygen transport as a consequence of hypophosphataemia in patients receiving hyperalimentation. *New Engl. J. Med.* **285**, 763.

Wacker, W. E. C. and Parisi, A. F. (1968). Magnesium metabolism. Medical progress: Magnesium metabolism. *New Engl. J. Med.* **278**, 712.

Walser, M. (1962). Separate effects of hyperparathyroidism, hypercalcaemia of malignancy, renal failure and acidosis on state of calcium, phosphate and other ions in plasma. *J. Clin. Invest.* **41**, 1454.

Watkins, G. M., Rabelo, A., Plzak, L. F. and Sheldon, G. F. (1974). The left shifted oxyhemoglobin curve in sepsis: a preventable defect. *Ann. Surg.* **180**, 213.

Welt, L. G., Smith, E. K. M., Dunn, M. J., Czerwinski, A., Proctor, H., Cole, C., Balfe, J. W. and Gitelman, H. J. (1967). Membrane transport defect: the sick cell. *Trans. Ass. Am. Physns.* **80**, 217.

Section 3: Acute Disorders of Calcium Metabolism

R. D. COHEN

INTRODUCTION

The body fluids contain only a minute fraction – approximately 0.1% of the total body calcium. The calcium content of the skeleton in an average man is about 1 kg. An ordinary diet contains about 1200 mg of calcium, of which the net absorption is only about 120–300 mg. Since losses through routes other than faeces and urine are very small, in a person in calcium balance the daily urinary calcium approximates that absorbed in the gut.

The level of calcium in the plasma is determined by three processes – gut absorption, renal excretion and bone excretion or resorption. About 55–60% of the plasma calcium is ionised, and most of the remainder is bound to protein, mainly to albumin. The ionised fraction is responsible for the physiological function of the ion. The homeostatic mechanisms summarised below which are responsible for regulating the plasma calcium are activated by changes in the ionised fraction. Since in clinical circumstances it is nearly always the plasma total calcium which is estimated, this measurement has to be interpreted in the knowledge of factors which may alter the proportion of ionised calcium; for example, in hypoalbuminaemic states, without any specific disturbance of calcium metabolism, the plasma ionised calcium is normal, although the plasma total calcium is low. Rules devised by Payne et al. (1973) enable the total plasma calcium to be interpreted given a value for plasma albumin; due account should be taken of the cautions and exceptions detailed by these authors.

Absorption of calcium is enhanced by vitamin D, and, indirectly by parathormone. The daily dietary requirement for vitamin D is about 100 international units (2.5 μg), and in the United Kingdom, where

189

skin synthesis of vitamin D under the influence of sunlight is often limited, vitamin D deficiency tends to be endemic in certain groups of the population (e.g. infants, adolescents, the aged and Asian immigrants). Vitamin D_3 (cholecalciferol) has to be converted by two successive hydroxylations, firstly to 25-hydroxycholecalciferol in the liver, and secondly to 1,25-dihydroxycholecalciferol in the kidney; the dihydroxy derivative is the active metabolite. Vitamin D_2 (ergocalciferol) is similarly handled. As well as being responsible for control of gut absorption of calcium, the final active metabolite also stimulates release of calcium from bone.

Urinary excretion of calcium is determined by the plasma level, and in a negative sense by parathormone, which stimulates tubular reabsorption of calcium. Parathormone also stimulates bone resorption and thus all three actions of parathormone – on bone, kidney and gut tend to raise the plasma calcium. Parathormone also has an important action in decreasing tubular reabsorption of phosphorus. Calcitonin secreted principally by the parafollicular cells of the thyroid, suppresses bone resorption and thus tends to lower both plasma and phosphorus; its precise physiological rɔle is, as yet, uncertain.

HYPOCALCAEMIA

The acute manifestations of low plasma ionised calcium are tetany (carpopedal spasm) and, less frequently, convulsions and laryngeal stridor. The level of plasma total calcium at which these occur is very variable, but symptoms are rare with plasma calcium greater than 1.88 mmol/l (7.5 mg/100 ml), and patients who have a sudden fall in plasma calcium appear to experience symptoms at a higher level than those with more chronic hypocalcaemia; paraesthesiae, particularly circumoral, are often premonitory manifestations of tetany. Causes of tetany other than hypocalcaemia should be remembered; these include alkalosis, commonly due to hysterical hyperventilation, potassium depletion (it also arises during the process of potassium repletion) and possibly in magnesium deficiency.

The most common causes of hypocalcaemia are malabsorption syndromes, particularly Crohn's disease and gluten-induced enteropathy, chronic renal failure, and acute postoperative situations after damage or removal of normal or hyperfunctioning parathyroid glands. Hypocalcaemia may also complicate acute pancreatitis. The hypocalcaemia of chronic renal failure seldom, however, gives rise to acute symptoms unless the metabolic acidosis which co-exists is corrected. In neonates and in the first few weeks of life, hypocalcaemic tetany is not uncommon and in many cases may be related to the high phosphate content of cows milk. Simple vitamin D deficiency, as in classical rickets, may produce sufficient hypocalcaemia to cause acute symptoms, but more usually plasma calcium is maintained at normal or near normal levels by secondary hyperparathyroidism.

The acute episode of tetany in the adult is readily treated by intravenous administration of 10–20 ml 10% calcium gluconate solution over about 10 min. If tetany recurs, 40–100 ml of 10% calcium gluconate may be added to isotonic sodium chloride solution and infused over 12–24 h. Plasma calcium should be monitored at intervals during the infusion. The further management of hypocalcaemic symptoms consists of (a) treatment of hypomagnesaemia, if present, (b) the administration of vitamin D in various forms and doses, and (c) giving oral or intravenous calcium supplements.

(a) *Treatment of hypomagnesaemia* (See Acute disorders of magnesium balance, Part 1, ch. VII, p. 183)

It is well established that hypocalcaemia is difficult to treat in the presence of hypomagnesaemia (Heaton and Fourman, 1965; Fourman and Royer, 1968). The latter often co-exists with hypocalcaemia in malabsorption states, particularly Crohn's disease and gluten-induced enteropathy. A rapid fall in plasma magnesium may occur after removal of a parathyroid adenoma, particularly in patients with marked osteitis fibrosa. Hypocalcaemia and hypomagnesaemia may also be found in chronic and acute alcoholism. In the presence of hypomagnesaemia there appears to be end organ resistance to parathyroid hormone, secreted in response to the low serum calcium (Estep *et al.*, 1969).

In these circumstances plasma calcium may often be restored to normal or nearly normal by magnesium supplements, and other forms of therapy for hypocalcaemia (e.g. vitamin D) become more effective. Oral therapy may suffice (Hanna *et al.*, 1960) and may be given as magnesium chloride or magnesium hydroxide 50–100 mmol daily initially. If this is ineffective or if a rapid response is desirable, magnesium salts may be given intravenously (Hanna *et al.*, 1960; Estep *et al.*, 1969). Magnesium sulphate 50 mmol daily in 1 litre 5% dextrose over 4–6 h for 1–3 days is a suitable regime. Caution is required in the presence of renal insufficiency and plasma magnesium should be measured daily during the initial phase of repletion.

(*b*) *Vitamin D therapy*

Vitamin D therapy of some sort is required in hypocalcaemia due to Vitamin D deficiency, malabsorption, surgical and idiopathic hypoparathyroidism and pseudohypoparathyroidism. It is only required in chronic renal failure if renal osteodystrophy is a problem; as indicated above, acute symptoms due to hypocalcaemia seldom arise in chronic renal failure. The dose required varies enormously, both with the type of Vitamin D congener employed and the condition under treatment.

In purely dietary Vitamin D deficiency, small oral doses of ergocalciferol (vitamin D_2) (e.g. 3000–6000 units (0.075–0.15 mg per day)) orally are all that is required. In malabsorption syndromes 50 000 units (1.25 mg) per day or more may be efficacious but it is often better to give ergocalciferol by intramuscular injection. There is a very wide range of dosage recommended (Fourman and Royer, 1968, p. 414; Nordin, 1973, p. 76); the writer's practice is to give a dose of 2.5 mg i.m. initially and then 1.25–2.5 mg fortnightly, adjusting the dose as required.

If ergocalciferol is used for the treatment of the various forms of hypoparathyroidism, very large doses may be required (1.25–10 mg per day) and stabilisation may be difficult but the recent introduction of 1α-hydroxycholecalciferol has put a new complexion on the treatment of these conditions (see below).

Other forms of vitamin D are also available. Cholecalciferol (vitamin D_3) is therapeutically approximately equivalent to ergocalciferol. Dihydrotachysterol (DHT) has an advantage over chole- and ergocalciferol in that the onset of its action in raising plasma calcium is more rapid, but, although some workers feel able to manipulate this drug satisfactorily, others feel that it is more unpredictable and less easy to control, giving rise to more episodes of hypercalcaemia (Hossain, 1970).

Though the more long-term management of patients requiring large doses of vitamin D congeners is outside the scope of this book, the physician dealing with the acute phase of the illness should, if he is not to follow the patient himself, transfer him to the care of someone well versed in the potential dangers of vitamin D therapy. Two important points are (*i*) the effect of daily oral high dose ergocalciferol therapy takes about 4–6 weeks to reach its maximum – the temptation to make increments in dosage at shorter intervals must, if possible, be resisted (Fourman and Royer, 1968, p. 337) and (*ii*) because of the occurrence of serious episodes of hypercalcaemia without apparent change in dose, no patient on long-term therapy should go for more than 3 months without having an estimation of plasma calcium. Patients should be warned of the common symptoms of hypercalcaemia (nausea, vomiting, thirst and polyuria) ; if they experience any of these they should stop taking the vitamin D preparation and report immediately to their doctor.

(c) Oral calcium supplements

It is usually desirable to give oral supplements of calcium in addition to the above measures. A suitable preparation is Sandocal, each tablet of which contains 400 mg of calcium as the lactate-gluconate (plus 4.5 mmol K^+ and 6.6 mmol Na^+). Two to 5 tablets per day are required.

Treatment of acute postoperative tetany

This may arise during surgery on the neck when the parathyroids are removed *in toto*, either by accident or design, or when a parathyroid tumour is removed, the other parathyroid glands being atrophic. Accidental removal (or damage to the blood supply) occurs occasionally during sub-total thyroidectomy for thyrotoxicosis; in these circumstances the onset of symptoms is very rapid – within 24–72 h of operation – since not only has circulating parathormone disappeared but, in addition, the bones in thyrotoxicosis are avid for calcium. A similar time scale is seen after removal of a parathyroid tumour. When, however, total parathyroidectomy is performed as a likely consequence of thyro-laryngectomy for carcinoma, symptoms may not be experienced for 6–9 days.

In most cases symptoms of hypocalcaemia after sub-total thyroidectomy for thyrotoxicosis resolve spontaneously or simply with oral or intravenous calcium supplements. A few patients, however, proceed to chronic hypoparathyroidism. Until recently, these patients have been treated as outlined above, but with the availability of 1α-hydroxycholecalciferol ($1\alpha(OH)D_3$) a synthetic congener of 1,25 dihydroxycholecalciferol, the final active metabolite of vitamin D_3, the situation appears to have become more satisfactory. The dose needed is 1–5 µg daily, i.e. about 1000 times less than that of vitamin D_2 or D_3 and the effect is very rapid, being apparent within 2 or 3 days (Russell *et al.*, 1974; Kooh *et al.*, 1975). It remains to be seen whether the acute hypercalcaemic episodes seen in chronic treatment with the other forms of vitamin D will be eliminated by this approach.

After total thyroidectomy for carcinoma of the thyroid or as part of operations for laryngeal or upper oesophageal carcinomas, all para-thyroid tissue is usually removed. This is, however, by no means certain and it is, therefore, wise to wait till the plasma calcium has fallen below 2.0 mmol/l (8.0 mg/100 ml). The writer has observed a rapid and satisfactory response to 2–3 µg 1α(OH)D$_3$ daily in these circumstances.

In the above account it has been implied that acute treatment for hypocalcaemia is only necessary when acute symptoms arise. Some patients have remarkably low serum calciums without any acute symptoms and it is not clear at what level of plasma calcium the hypocalcaemia itself becomes an indication for emergency treatment. However, it is well established that a low plasma calcium and a high plasma potassium is a particularly dangerous combination likely to produce cardiac arrest; it should be treated urgently. The injection of calcium gluconate is, of course, standard therapy in the severe hyperkalaemia of acute renal failure. Another circumstance where this combination occurs is after sub-total or total parathyroidectomy in the treatment of renal osteodystrophy, a rapid fall in plasma calcium often being associated with a rise in plasma potassium due to postoperative deterioration of renal function. Plasma calcium and potassium should, therefore, be monitored very frequently in the immediate post-operative period.

HYPERCALCAEMIA

The most common cause of hypercalcaemia is malignant disease, with or without bony involvement. Other conditions which may produce dangerously high levels of plasma calcium are primary hyper-parathyroidism, sarcoidosis, vitamin D intoxication and milk-alkali syndrome. Acute symptoms are seldom produced if the plasma calcium is below 3.0–3.25 mmol/l (12–13 mg/100 ml) but at higher levels nausea, vomiting, polyuria and thirst become increasingly common and the patient may become exceedingly ill because of dehydration and renal failure. The latter is due to a specific effect of calcium on the kidney, in addition to the dehydration caused by vomiting and polyuria, and is partly or, in many cases, wholly reversible.

The cause of hypercalcaemia in a particular patient may be obvious and will guide the choice of therapy. In those patients where the cause is not immediately obvious the object is to lower the plasma calcium to a safe level so that definitive investigations may proceed.

The first therapeutic measure is to rehydrate the patient; usually with isotonic sodium chloride but 5% dextrose may be needed in addition. Rehydration alone will usually lower plasma calcium by 0.25–0.75 mmol/l (1–3 mg/100 ml). If the plasma calcium is still above (12–13 mg/100 ml) a further non-specific but effective measure is the infusion of a neutral phosphate solution (Goldsmith and Ingbar, 1966). This contains 0.081 mol/l disodium hydrogen phosphate and 0.019 mol/l potassium dihydrogen phosphate (pH 7.4; 162 mmol/l Na$^+$; 19 mmol/l K$^+$). 500 ml are infused intravenously over about 6 h. The fall in plasma calcium starts during the infusion but continues after it has finished and may persist for several days. The infusion may be repeated if necessary, but more than 500 ml should only be given at a single session with great care since, if hypocalcaemia is induced, circulatory collapse may occur. Caution should be exercised in the presence of more than moderate renal failure (plasma urea 16.7 mmol/l (> 100 mg/100 ml)). Calcification of the vein at the site of infusion often occurs. Maintenance oral phosphate may be given in the form of phosphate Sandoz, 4–6 tablets per day (2–3 g elemental phosphorus/day).

The administration of calcitonin is also effective in hypercalcaemia (West et al., 1971). Although less dramatically effective than a phosphate infusion and much more expensive, it is perhaps somewhat freer of risk and has the advantage of not involving sodium, potassium and water administration, which may be undesirable in some circumstances. Porcine calcitonin ('Calcitare') 4–8 MRC units/kg/day intramuscularly in divided doses is a suitable dose; it may also be given intravenously. Salmon calcitonin ('Calsynar') is also effective in doses of 400 MRC units subcutaneously or intramuscularly; it may not be given intravenously. In subjects with a history of allergy, a skin test with diluted calcitonin should be performed before injection of the first dose.

Certain therapeutic measures are specific for a particular cause of hypercalcaemia. Thus oral cortisone acetate 50 mg t.d.s. (Anderson et al., 1954) or prednisone 10 mg t.d.s. is highly effective in sarcoidosis and vitamin D intoxication. Plasma calcium is usually restored to normal within 10 days. Steroids have no effect in primary hyperparathyroidism and are usually (but not always) disappointing in hypercalcaemia due to malignant disease. It has recently been shown that the hypercalcaemia of malignant disease associated with 'solid' tumours (rather than haematological malignancies) is induced by the osteolytic action of prostaglandins of the E series, possibly produced by the tumours themselves. Administration of inhibitors of prostaglandin synthesis such as indomethacin (75–150 mg/day) or aspirin (1.8–

4.8 g/day) often, but not always, produces striking falls in plasma calcium (Seyberth *et al.*, 1975). Primary hyperparathyroidism should, when the diagnosis has been established, be treated by removal of the parathyroid tumour, or, in the case of chief cell hyperplasia, removal of three glands and $\frac{1}{2}$–$\frac{2}{3}$ of the fourth. In vitamin D intoxication, the offending drug should be stopped temporarily whilst the above measures, including steroid administration in severe cases are instituted. In milk-alkali syndrome, the consumption of milk should be curtailed and the absorbable alkali replaced by a non-absorbable alternative. In haematological malignant disease, a remission induced by cytotoxic therapy will be accompanied by amelioration of co-existing hypercalcaemia. Mithramycin, an antibiotic which suppresses osteoclastic activity, may reduce hypercalcaemia in a wide range of circumstances, including myelomatosis (Stamp *et al.*, 1975); its toxicity is considerable and it should in general be reserved for when other measures have failed.

REFERENCES

Anderson, J., Dent, C. E., Harper, C. and Philpot, G. R. (1954). Effect of cortisone on calcium metabolism in sarcoidosis with hypercalcaemia. Possible antagonistic actions of cortisone and vitamin D. *Lancet* **2**, 720.

Estep, H., Shaw, W. A., Wallington, C., Hobe, R., Holland, W. and Tucker, St. G. (1969). Hypocalcaemia due to hypomagnesaemia and reversible parathyroid hormone unresponsiveness. *J. Clin. Endocr.* **29**, 842.

Fourman, P. and Royer, P. (1968). 'Calcium Metabolism and the Bone', Second Edition. Blackwell Scientific Publications, Oxford.

Goldsmith, R. S. and Ingbar, S. H. (1966). Inorganic phosphate treatment of hypercalcaemia of diverse etiologies.

Hanna, S., Harrison, M., MacIntyre, I. and Fraser, R. (1960). The syndrome of magnesium deficiency in man. *Lancet* **2**, 172.

Heaton, F. W. and Fourman, P. (1965). Magnesium deficiency and hypocalcaemia in intestinal malabsorption. *Lancet* **2**, 50.

Hossain, M. (1970). Vitamin D intoxication during treatment of hypoparathyroidism. *Lancet* **1**, 1149.

Kooh, S. W., Fraser, D., DeLuca, H. F., Holick, M. F., Belsey, R. E., Clark, M. B. and Murray, T. M. (1975). Treatment of hypoparathyroidism and pseudohypoparathyroidism with metabolites of Vitamin D: evidence for impaired conversion of 25-hydroxyvitamin D to 1α, 25-dihydroxyvitamin D. *New Engl. J. Med.* **293**, 840.

Payne, R. B., Little, A. J., Williams, R. B. and Milner, J. R. (1973). Interpretation of serum calcium in patients with abnormal serum proteins. *Brit. Med. J.* **4**, 643.

Nordin, B. E. C. (1973). 'Metabolic Bone and Stone disease'. Churchill Livingstone, Edinburgh and London.

Russell, R. G. G., Smith, R., Walton, R. J., Preston, C., Basson, R. and Henderson, R. G. (1974). 1,25-dihydroxycholecalciferol and 1α-hydroxycholecalciferol in hypoparathyroidism. *Lancet* **2**, 14.

Seyberth, H., Segre, G. V., Morgan, J. L., Sweetman, B. J., Potts, J. T. and Oates, J. A. (1975). Prostaglandins as mediators of hypercalcaemia associated with certain types of cancer. *New Engl. J. Med.* **293**, 1278.

Stamp, T. C. B., Child, J. A. and Walker, P. G. (1975). Treatment of osteolytic myelomatosis with mithramycin. *Lancet* **1**, 719.

West, T. E. T., Joffe, M., Sinclair, L. and O'Riordan, J. L. H. (1971). Treatment of hypercalcaemia with calcitonin. *Lancet* **1**, 675.

Section 4: Acute Disorders of Acid Base Balance

GILLIAN C. HANSON

INTRODUCTION

The body constantly attempts to maintain a pH between 7.38 and 7.42. pH is an inverse and logarithmic expression of hydrogen ion concentration ($[H^+]$). Any elevation of pH above 7.42 (i.e. a decline in ($[H^+]$) constitutes an alkalosis and any depression below 7.38 constitutes an acidosis. An *acid* is a substance which can donate a proton (hydrogen nucleus) and a *base* is a proton acceptor.

$$\text{Acid} \rightarrow \text{Proton} + \text{Conjugate Base}$$
$$\text{(proton donor)} \qquad \text{(proton acceptor)}$$
$$\text{Hx} \quad \rightarrow \quad \text{H}^+ \quad + \quad \text{X}^-$$

It is the effective concentration of 'activity' of the hydrogen ion in the blood that is assessed biochemically. Hydrogen ion is present in blood in minute amount and is heavily buffered. The relationship between pH, PCO_2 and the bicarbonate concentration is best seen in the Henderson–Hasselbalch equation:

$$pH = pK' + \log \frac{\text{bicarbonate}}{K \cdot PCO_2}$$

pK' is not a constant, but may be considered for practical purposes as 6.10, i.e.

$$7.4 = 6.10 + \log \frac{\text{bicarbonate}}{\text{'carbonic acid'}}$$

Thus the hydrogen ion concentration (degree of acidity) is directly proportional to the ratio of ventilatory function to metabolic function.

$$[H^+] \propto \frac{PCO_2}{[HCO_3]}$$

198

The units for hydrogen ions are nanomoles (mole $\times 10^{-9}$). Comparisons of nm/l and pH is shown in the following table.

pH	nm/l 10^{-9} m
6.80	158
7.00	100
7.10	79
7.20	63
7.40	40
7.70	20

Kassirer and Bleich (1965) noted that in the pH range 7.10–7.50 each change of one nm/l from 40 coincided with an approximate increase change of 0.01 pH unit from 7.40. The rate of production and excretion daily is similar to that of other cations, i.e. approximately 1 mmol/kg B.W. daily.

Hydrogen ion production is either respiratory or metabolic in origin. Respiratory acid is carbonic acid and is eliminated from the lungs as carbon dioxide. The arterial PCO_2 is a result of the relationship between production and excretion. Carbon dioxide is produced as a consequence of complete oxidation of fats and carbohydrate and provided ventilation is adequate excretion balances production. PCO_2 is thus a guide to respiratory function but is naturally affected by metabolism, the carbon dioxide production (and hence the level in the blood) and elimination being increased in hypercatabolic states. This should be remembered when artificially ventilating hypercatabolic patients – the minute volume having to be increased in order to eliminate the excess carbon dioxide produced. All hydrogen ions that are non-respiratory and depend upon kidney excretion for their elimination are considered metabolic. Production is affected by respiratory function as in hypoxia but it would appear that the PaO_2 supplying the cell has to fall to less than 4.8 kPa (36 mm Hg) before there is a rise in serum lactate (Carey, 1971). Failure of excretion of the 'metabolic' hydrogen ions via the kidneys, or an excess production, leads to a metabolic acidosis. The main sources of metabolic acid are 1. from the oxidation of sulphur-containing amino acids, and 2. from incomplete oxidation of fats and carbohydrates as in diabetic keto-acidosis, or in hypoxia where anaerobic glycolysis produces lactate plus hydrogen ions (lactic acid).

When hydrogen ion rises in the blood, the pH change is minimised by blood buffers. These buffers are chiefly haemoglobin and bicarbonate in whole blood, bicarbonate in the rest of the E.C.F. and proteins and organic phosphates in the I.C.F. It must be remembered that on rapid addition of H ions to the blood the H ion concentration will rapidly rise and reduce the blood buffering system – the hydrogen ion concentration if not increased (by further addition of H) will however steadily fall as the H^+ is buffered by extravascular buffers. The approximate contribution of individual buffers to total buffering in whole blood was described by Winters and co-workers (1967):

Buffers	Buffering in whole blood (%)
Haemoglobin and oxyhaemoglobin	35
Organic phosphates	3
Inorganic phosphate	2
Plasma proteins	7
Plasma bicarbonate	35
Erythrocyte bicarbonate	18

The two most reliable expressions of the metabolic component is standard bicarbonate and base excess or deficit (change in buffer base). Provided pH, $PaCO_2$ and base excess or deficit are estimated, standard bicarbonate gives no additional information. Buffer base is the sum of buffer anions and their relationship with electrolyte balance. This is best shown in the Gamble diagram (Fig. 1). It must be remembered that the sum of cations must equal anions in any body fluid and thus providing the sum of residual anions and residual cations remain equal, buffer base in mEq/l can be obtained by subtracting the chloride concentration from the sodium concentration. This calculation is only allowed if the protein concentration is normal as well as the residual anions or cations. Base excess or deficit is by definition the amount of acid or base respectively needed to bring a blood sample to pH 7.40 at PCO_2 40 mm Hg and 37°C. Thus:

Base Excess (B.E.) = Measured buffer base (M.B.B.) – Normal buffer base (N.B.B.)
Base Deficit (B.D.) = Normal buffer base (N.B.B.) – Measured buffer base (M.B.B.)

Therapeutically, changes in base deficit are used to calculate therapy making the assumption that only the extracellular fluid is involved. Since the H^+ ion produced becomes rapidly buffered by buffers within

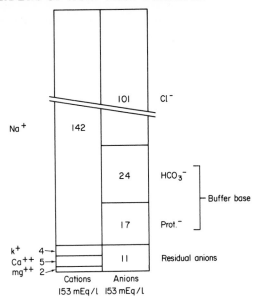

Fig. 1. The Gamble diagram. Anions and cations expressed as m/Eq/l in plasma.

the cell, this method of calculation invariably gives an overestimate of bicarbonate requirements. An overswing to a metabolic alkalosis in a critically ill patient should be avoided because:

1 A metabolic alkalosis will produce respiratory depression in a patient who is probably already hypoxic.

2 A metabolic alkalosis will increase the affinity of haemoglobin for oxygen thereby decreasing the availability to the cell.

3 For every ion of HCO_3^- infused, Na^+ is also administered which may be complicated by intravascular expansion and pulmonary oedema or a hypernatraemic hyperosmolar coma (see Part 1, ch. VIII, p. 226).

Certain acute situations associated with a metabolic acidosis tend to develop a metabolic alkalosis long-term – this may be increased even further after the over zealous use of bicarbonate. These include massive transfusion of A.C.D. stored blood, the citrate being ultimately metabolised to bicarbonate, and following the appropriate treatment of lactic acidosis, the lactate (in non-hepatic disorders) being ultimately metabolised to bicarbonate.

In acid base imbalance an attempt should be made to define the primary factor, commenting on the secondary compensatory mechanism should it be present.

Biochemical changes are often affected by the acid base balance of the blood. This in particular applies to the percentage of ionised calcium or magnesium, the level of potassium and inorganic phosphate. For example, in an acidosis there is a rise in plasma potassium, inorganic phosphate and the ionised fraction of calcium and magnesium.

Table 1. Factors, mechanism and treatment of primary metabolic acidosis likely to be encountered in the critically ill

1 *Hyperchloraemic acidosis*

Aetiology	Mechanism	Anion gap	Treatment
Diarrhoea	Loss of HCO_3^-	↑	Treatment of diarrhoea HCO_3^- B.D. >8
Small bowel losses	Loss of HCO_3^-		I.v. nutrition. Surgery to be considered HCO_3^- B.D. >8
Ureterosigmoid anastomosis	Cl^- reabsorbed in exchange for HCO_3^- from the urine draining into the colon	N O R	HCO_3^- Antibiotics Ileal loop
Proximal renal tubular acidosis	Inability to reabsorb HCO_3^-	M A	HCO_3^- and K^+ replacement
Distal renal tubular acidosis	Decreased acid secretion in the distal tubule	L	HCO_3^- and K^+ replacement
Excessive acid administration NH_4 Cl Arginine mono-hydrochloride	Excess H^+ ion load	↓	Discontinue

2 *High anion gap acidosis* (see p. 204)

Renal failure	Decreased excretion H^+ PO_4^{--} SO_4^{--}	↑	Treatment of renal failure (Pt 1, ch. IV)
Hepatic failure	Impaired removal and production of lactate Increased succinate fumarate	I N	Treatment of hepatic failure (Pt 1, ch. V)
Diabetic ketosis	Increased ketoacid production	C R	Treatment of diabetic ketoacidosis (Pt 1, ch. V
Lactic acidosis	See Table 4	E A S	HCO_3^-. Improvement of cellular perfusion and oxygenation
Toxic ingestion		E	
Methyl alcohol	↑Formic acid	decreased	D	HCO_3^- Dialysis
Ethylene glycol	↑Oxalic acid	cellular metabolism→		See treatment of
Paraldehyde	↑Acetic acid	lactic acid		overdose (Pt 2,
Salicylate	↑Salicylic acid	acidosis	↓	ch. VI, p. 620)

TREATMENT OF PRIMARY DISORDERS OF METABOLIC ACID BASE BALANCE

The factors, mechanism and treatment of primary disorders of metabolic balance which are likely to be encountered in the critically ill are tabulated in Tables 1 and 2.

Pure metabolic acidosis

A metabolic acidosis results from any process that tends to reduce bicarbonate, the exception being the metabolic compensation for a respiratory alkalosis. The diagnosis can be assisted by determining whether there is an increase in the serum unmeasured anions. The

Table 2. Factors, mechanism and treatment of primary metabolic alkalosis likely to be encountered in the critically ill

Chloride responsive alkalosis Aetiology	Mechanism	Urine chloride	Treatment
Gastric aspirate or vomiting	Cl^- depletion Severe potassium depletion	< 10–20 mmol/l	Sodium chloride Potassium chloride
Diuretic administration Villous adenoma of colon Residual alkalosis following correction of hypercapnoea			Sodium chloride
Chloride resistant Alkalosis Prolonged high dose administration of steroids	Increased distal tubular exchange of Na^+ for H^+ and K^+	> 10–20 mmol/l	Stop steroids Potassium chloride
Chronic potassium depletion	Shift of K^+ from the cell in exchange with H^+ →intracellular acidosis		Potassium re- placement
Rapid bicarbonate or lactate administration (in particular in renal failure) Citrate bladder irrigations	HCO_3^- load exceeding renal excretion		Discontinue admin- istration Consider arginine monohydrochloride

concentration of the serum anions (anion gap) is obtained by subtracting the sum of the bicarbonate and chloride concentrations from the serum sodium concentration. Normally the sum of un-measured ions (sulphates, phosphates, polyanionic plasma proteins and anions of organic acids) range from 5–12 mEq/l.

$$[Na^+] - [[HCO_3^-] + [Cl^-]] = 5\text{--}12 \text{ mEq/l}$$

In acidosis characterised by an excessive production of acid, e.g. lactic acid, the anion gap will be elevated, whereas the acidosis secondary to bicarbonate loss, e.g. diarrhoea, or failure to excrete an acid load, e.g. renal tubular acidosis, the anion gap will be normal.

Table 3. Calculation of bicarbonate ions required to correct a metabolic acidosis

---

Total body water (T.B.W.) $\simeq$60% of body weight (B.W.) in kg
Extracellular buffer base (B.B.) is accommodated in approximately 50% of T.B.W. i.e. 30% B.W. in kg
B.D. = deficit of HCO_3^- ions in mEq/l of whole blood
HCO_3^- mEq/l required to correct a calculated B.D.[1]
$$= 0.3 \times \text{kg B.W.} \times \text{B.D.}$$

---

[1] Invariably leads to overcorrection, not accounting for the buffer base accommodated in the extracellular nonvascular spaces and tending to overestimate T.B.W.

A rise in H^+ concentration of metabolic origin is associated with a compensatory rise in alveolar ventilation. Lennon and Lemann (1966) noted that the decline in $PaCO_2$ is highly proportional to the magnitude of HCO_3^- change, each 1 mEq/l fall in HCO_3^- resulting in an 0.15 kPa (1.1 mm Hg) change in $PaCO_2$. Subsequent to the initial respiratory compensation, the renal H^+ secretion may also increase. Should the relationship between the fall in $[HCO_3^-]$ and fall in $PaCO_2$ not exist – respiratory compensation should be considered inadequate and the patient be suffering from a mixed metabolic and respiratory acidosis.

The treatment of a metabolic acidosis is briefly summarised in Table 1. Sodium bicarbonate is the treatment of choice since it directly replaces lost bicarbonate. Lactate has no advantage over bicarbonate and because its effect depends upon oxidation of the lactate ion, may be ineffective in lactic acidosis. THAM (trihydroxymethyl-amino methane) has also been used but several serious side effects contra-indicate its clinical use (Bleich and Schwartz, 1966).

The dosage of bicarbonate ions required can be crudely estimated (Table 3). It is wise to correct the acidosis (according to this formula) to a B.D. of 10 since a swing to alkalosis should be avoided (p. 201). An initial dose of 50 mmol of bicarbonate ions should not be exceeded but in certain situations even this dosage should be queried. Since carbon dioxide tension generally remains low for several hours, small increments in plasma bicarbonate will have a striking effect on pH in the patient with severe acidosis. An attempt should be made to raise the standard bicarbonate to 4–6 mmol/l, the threat of a severe acidosis is then obviated and replacement should then be continued at a slower rate. Sudden and large increases in bicarbonate concentration has been held responsible for further acidification of the spinal fluid and deterioration in the level of consciousness (Posner and Plum, 1967). Because of the lack of predictability of alkali therapy, Astrup analyses should be performed 2–3 hourly.

Patients in cardiac or renal failure are predisposed to sodium overload when bicarbonate is used and peritoneal dialysis should be considered. The absorption of lactate across the peritoneal membrane is a source of bicarbonate and by decreasing the intravascular volume bicarbonate can be given intravenously. Such patients should have bicarbonate given intravenously under right atrial pressure monitoring control.

Bicarbonate should not be administered to a patient with a serum potassium of 3.0 mmol or less. Potassium replacement should proceed according to the recommendations on p. 177 and in a severe metabolic acidosis (pH 7.1 or less) 50 mmol bicarbonate should be infused after 40 mmol of potassium ions have been given intravenously. Continuous E.C.G. monitoring is essential.

Lactic acidosis. The principal sources of lactate entering the circulation under normal conditions are skeletal muscle, brain and erythrocytes. The increase in hydrogen ions is eliminated when the lactate ions are converted by the liver or kidney to glucose or oxidised. Either overproduction or failure of removal can result in a lactic acid acidosis. Two types have been defined – Type A and Type B (Editorial, 1973). The conditions which predispose to lactic acidosis are summarised in Table 4. Type A lactic acidosis is the commoner and results from inadequate cellular oxygenation, anaerobic glycolysis and the production of lactic acid. This is commonly seen in many forms of shock. It is probable that hepatic perfusion is reduced in shock states and thus removal of lactate is impaired. Moreover, severe acidosis itself completely inhibits hepatic removal of lactate in isolated perfused rat livers (Lloyd *et al.*, 1973).

Table 4. Conditions which predispose to lactic acidosis in the
critically ill

Underlying chronic renal or liver disease
Infection
Diabetes mellitus
Pancreatitis
Shock
Hypoventilation
Disseminated intravascular coagulation

Drugs: Phenformin Paraldehyde Fructose infusion
Ethyleneglycol Alcohol Methanol

The cause and treatment of Type B lactic acidosis is described by
Cohen in Section 5 (p. 208).

Pure metabolic alkalosis. The treatment of primary disorders of
metabolic alkalosis likely to be seen in the critically ill are summarised
in Table 2. The disorders causing a metabolic alkalosis can be defined
according to their response to sodium chloride administration and the
number of chloride ions in the urine. A severe alkalosis is relatively rare
but even with a moderate increase of standard bicarbonate pH rises
rapidly because there is little respiratory compensation. Sodium
chloride and potassium chloride correct an alkalosis by suppressing
renal acid excretion and increasing alkali excretion (Kassirer *et al.*,
1965). These methods are slow and where there is a severe alkalosis
BE > 20 and/or pH > 7.55, arginine monohydrochloride should be
considered. Arginine monohydrochloride should also be considered
in a patient with a chloride resistant alkalosis who is ventilating
inadequately spontaneously or where there is difficulty in maintaining a
PaO_2 above 9.3 kPa (70 mm Hg) in a ventilated patient, and in whom
the BE is 15 and/or pH > 7.5.

It is also important that the inorganic phosphate level is normal since
in depletion the red cell 2–3 D.P.G. is likely to be low. The administered
acid titrates excessive bicarbonate stores and effectively lowers pH. The
dose should be calculated according to the *following formula correcting to a
base excess of 10:*

Number of H ions required = kg B.W. × 0.3 (BE − 10) as arginine
monohydrochloride[1]

[1] Arginine monohydrochloride ($C_6H_{14}N_4O_2$ Hcl) 60% solution approximately 140 mmol H
per 50 ml.

Arginine monohydrochloride suspended in 500 ml $\frac{1}{5}$ normal saline should be infused over the subsequent 12 h. The effect should be assessed by serial Astrup analyses. Ammonium chloride or dilute hydrochloric acid (0.1–0.2 N) can also be given intravenously for severe alkalosis. Ammonium chloride may, however, produce central nervous system toxicity and dilute hydrochloric acid has the disadvantage that it has to be infused via a central vein because of the necrotic effect on peripheral veins.

Administration of arginine monohydrochloride should be accompanied by the appropriate infusion of sodium and/or potassium chloride. Patients with a severe metabolic alkalosis frequently suffer from impaired renal function and fluid balance should be observed carefully. The metabolic alkalosis is generally associated with potassium depletion and potassium should be used in treatment unless the serum potassium is 4.0 mmol or above.

The chloride composition of the urine is valuable in assessing whether the chloride stores have been replenished in those patients with an alkalosis responsive to sodium chloride. Excretion of greater than 60 mmol of chloride daily (in the presence of normal renal function) implies that the chloride stores have been adequately restored.

Patients with sodium chloride resistant alkalosis are generally severely potassium depleted – administration of large volumes of sodium chloride may exacerbate the hypokalaemia. Potassium chloride can be infused with $\frac{1}{5}$ normal saline or dextrose saline 4.3%/0.18% (see Part 1, ch. VII, p. 177).

REFERENCES

Bleich, H. L. and Schwartz, W. B. (1966). Tris buffer (THAM): an appraisal of its physiologic effects and clinical usefulness. *New Engl. J. Med.* **274**, 782.

Carey, L. C. (1971). Haemorrhagic shock. *In* 'Current Problems in Surgery' (Ed. M. M. Revitch). Year book, Medical publishers Inc., Chicago.

Editorial (1973). Lactic acidosis. *Lancet* **3**, 27.

Kassirer, J. P. and Bleich, H. L. (1965). Rapid estimation of plasma carbon dioxide tension from pH and total carbon dioxide content. *New Engl. J. Med.* **272**, 1067.

Lennon, E. J. and Lemann, J. Jr. (1966). Defences of hydrogen ion concentration in chronic metabolic acidosis. *Ann. Intern. Med.* **65**, 265.

Lloyd, M. H., Iles, R. A., Strunin, J. M., Layton, J., Simpson, B. R. and Cohen, R. D. (1973). The relation between intracellular pH and lactate metabolism in the isolated perfused rat liver in simulated metabolic acidosis. *Clin. Sci.* **44**, 27.

Posner, J. B. and Plum, F. (1967). Spinal fluid pH and neurologic symptoms in systemic acidosis. *New Engl. J. Med.* **277**, 605.

Winters, R. W., Engle, K., Dell, R. B., and Berkson, R. P. (1967). *In* 'Acid Base Physiology' Radiometer, Copenhagen.

Section 5: Treatment of Type B Lactic Acidosis

R. D. COHEN

INTRODUCTION

Lactic acidosis is a metabolic acidosis which is partly or entirely due to the accumulation of lactate and accompanying hydrogen ions. It is seen in two broad categories of situations. The first is in the presence of clinical evidence of poor tissue perfusion or oxygenation, as in shock; this variety may be referred to as Type A lactic acidosis. The second variety (Type B) (Editorial, 1973) occurs in the absence of such clinical signs. Both Type A and Type B lactic acidosis have poor prognoses but may respond to prompt and effective therapy. In Type A lactic acidosis the treatment of the acidosis is a part of the therapy of the shock syndrome which has been dealt with elsewhere in this book. This section will, therefore, be devoted to the management of the Type B variety.

CAUSES OF TYPE B LACTIC ACIDOSIS (Oliva, 1970; Cohen and Woods, 1976)

The most common single cause is the administration of the oral hypoglycaemic agent, phenformin, in patients whose renal or hepatic function is suspect. There are numerous other circumstances in which Type B lactic acidosis may arise, of which the more important are diabetic ketoacidosis, severe liver disease, intravenous infusion of fructose or sorbitol, ethanol ingestion, acute infections (especially septicaemia) and methanol poisoning. Renal failure is a frequent background to the development of lactic acidosis but is probably not a cause *per se*. There are many uncommon causes, e.g. the leukaemias, and a variety of inborn errors of metabolism, of which the best known is

Type I glycogen storage disease. The condition is due either to overproduction of lactic acid, impaired removal by the liver and kidneys, or a mixture of both.

PRESENTATION AND DIAGNOSIS

Severe hyperventilation, due to acidosis, is the most common presenting sign. Disturbances of consciousness, not infrequently proceeding to coma, abdominal pain and vomiting are also frequent accompaniments. The blood pressure is normal, there is no cyanosis and the periphery appears well perfused. Arterial pH (pH_a) is often below 7.0. Plasma electrolytes show a low bicarbonate level and an elevated anion gap (calculated as $([Na^+ + K^+]) - ([Cl^-] + [HCO_3^-])$ – normally 11–18 mEq/l). In the absence of ketoacidosis, salicylate poisoning or considerable uraemia, an acidosis associated with a high anion gap is almost certainly lactic acidosis. Blood lactate levels, normally about 0.5–1.2 mmol/l, lie between 5 and 35 mmol/l. Blood glucose is unremarkable. If moderate or severe lactic acidosis is untreated the patient eventually exhibits signs of shock and death is inevitable.

MANAGEMENT (Cohen and Woods, 1976)

The two main principles of treatment are:
1. The arterial pH should be restored to normal, or slightly above normal in 2–6 h, and subsequently held at that level.
2. The precipitating cause should, if possible, be eliminated.

1. Restoration of arterial pH

This should be achieved by the infusion of sodium bicarbonate. Review of the literature suggests that those patients in whom objective 1. is attained do much better than those in which restoration of pH_a is only partial, or is only temporary (there is a considerable tendency for relapse). Large quantities of bicarbonate may be required in severe cases (e.g. 1000 mmol); the situation is, therefore, quite different from that arising in the treatment of diabetic ketoacidosis, in which rehydration and insulin alone frequently suffice to deal with the acidosis, and if bicarbonate is given it is usually administered in amounts sufficient only to bring pH_a above 7.0–7.1. The bicarbonate should be administered as the approximately isotonic solution (1.4%– 163 mmol/l). Boluses of hypertonic bicarbonate (e.g. 8.4%–

1 mmol/ml) are in general contraindicated, since they may result in a rapid shift to the left of the oxygen dissociation curve due to the Bohr effect, and, if the patient is approaching the stage of shock this is particularly undesirable. However, after 2–3 litres of isotonic bicarbonate have been infused it is in the writer's experience safe to give a single dose of 100 ml 8.4% bicarbonate over about 30 min if restoration of pH_a is too slow.

Since large volumes of fluid may have to be administered a central venous pressure line should be set up for monitoring purposes, and a bladder catheter should be inserted. Otherwise fit patients will usually cope with the fluid volumes but difficulties may be experienced in patients with suspect myocardial function. Haemodialysis has been used as a method of fluid volume control during administration of sodium bicarbonate solution in Type B lactic acidosis. During the alkalinisation it will be found that the arterial pH will be restored to normal long before the arterial PCO_2 has risen to normal. This is a common feature of treatment of any acidosis and is due to the respiratory centre not having equilibrated to the new environment.

2. Elimination of the precipitating cause

All known precipitating drugs should be stopped – e.g. phenformin, fructose, sorbitol. Phenformin will be slowly excreted in the urine or hydroxylated to an inert metabolite in the liver. A number of lines of evidence suggest that two conditions have to be fulfilled before blood lactate levels fall, i.e. not only does the causal factor have to be dealt with, but the acidosis has to be eliminated. A situation may arise in treating phenformin-induced lactic acidosis where the pH problem has been resolved for some hours, but blood lactate is still not declining. In these circumstances the best course is to persist with sufficient bicarbonate to maintain pH_a normal or slightly greater than normal, and the blood lactate will eventually fall – presumably because body phenformin concentrations have fallen to a safe level. Infections should be dealt with in the usual way.

It will in general be found that the patient's condition will improve dramatically as the acidosis is corrected. It is preferable to have serial measurements of blood lactate to monitor therapy, but in any case the best manoeuvre after maintaining normal arterial pH for some hours is gradually to slow the rate of bicarbonate infusion, whilst carefully monitoring arterial pH. Any tendency for pH_a to fall should be immediately counteracted by raising the infusion rate. Eventually it will be possible to discontinue the infusion without a fall in pH_a occurring.

Other measures

Plasma potassium may fall during treatment and should be carefully monitored. It has been suggested that glucose and insulin, or intravenous methylene blue, are of value, but there is no sound evidence in support of these views. If the patient is diabetic, however, blood glucose should be monitored and hyperglycaemia dealt with as an independent problem. Diabetic ketoacidosis is accompanied in 8–10% of cases by minor to moderate elevations in blood lactate; in these circumstances the minor component of lactic acidosis usually responds to the ordinary treatment for diabetic ketosis. Rarely, more serious lactic acidosis arises after the ketoacidosis has been controlled; this requires the measures outlined above.

It is often helpful to have a radial artery cannula *in situ* to obviate the need for repeated arterial puncture.

Prognosis

A review of the literature approximately three years ago suggested that the overall mortality of phenformin-associated lactic acidosis was about 50% if treatment was started before shock had occurred, and about 65% if treatment was delayed. In lactic acidosis associated with infection, the mortality was even higher. It is the writer's impression that improved recognition of the syndrome and consequent speedier initiation of treatment are making a significant improvement in the outlook.

REFERENCES

Cohen, R. D. and Woods, H. F. (1976). 'Clinical and biochemical aspects of lactic acidosis.' Blackwell Scientific Publications, Oxford.
Editorial (1973). Lactic acidosis. *Lancet* **3**, 27.
Oliva, P. B. (1970). Lactic acidosis. *Am. J. Med.* **48**, 209.

Section 6: Acute Disorders of Uric Acid Metabolism

GILLIAN C. HANSON

INTRODUCTION

Plasma and urinary uric acid comes primarily from the regeneration of free nucleotides and of tissue nucleic acids and secondarily from ingested purine. The breakdown of nucleic acids involves multiple enzyme systems (Cartier and Hamet, 1974). Man can be maintained indefinitely on a purine-free diet (O'Sullivan, 1972), the purine being synthesised largely by the liver where it is transported by the blood to the tissues where nucleic acids are synthesised. The building of tissue nucleic acids liberates purines which are transported again to the liver where they undergo final oxidation into uric acid. Uric acid passes freely into the glomerular filtrate; it is completely reabsorbed from the proximal part of the tubule and then actively secreted back into the lumen. The existence of these two separate transport mechanisms accounts for the different effects of drugs on the net excretion of urate. The complex metabolic pathways involved in urate metabolism are described in detail by Cartier and Hamet (1974).

The plasma uric acid concentration depends upon sex, age and genetic constitution. Diet has little effect on the uric acid concentration. It is important to be aware of the normal uric acid concentration for your laboratory.

DIAGNOSIS AND MANAGEMENT

Hyperuricaemia may develop during the management of the critically ill under the following conditions:

Idiopathic gout

Myeloproliferative diseases and reticuloses, in particular during cytotoxic drug therapy

Haemolytic states

Drugs – Diuretics – in particular when the patient is suffering from idiopathic gout

Renal failure

Ketoacidosis associated with prolonged starvation or diabetes mellitus.

Hyperuricaemia may either precipitate acute gouty arthritis, or more seriously may affect renal function by producing acute obstruction to the collecting tubules of the kidney through precipitation of uric acid crystals. This is most likely to occur during the treatment of acute leukaemia, reticulosis and other widespread neoplasms in which large amounts of nucleic acids are degraded to uric acid in a short time. The stituation however may be compounded when diuretics are used during cytotoxic drug therapy and/or the patient has impaired renal function.

Under conditions where hyperuricaemia is likely to be precipitated, allopurinol should be used as a prophylactic so that the serum uric acid can be kept below the solubility limit of 0.4 mmol/l (7 mg/100 ml). Its activity is not influenced by associated renal disease.

Acute uric acid nephropathy has become more common as methods for treating these diseases have become more effective, thereby frequently causing severe and acute rises in uric acid (Pochedly, 1973). In the majority of cases treated by dialysis (either peritoneal or haemodialysis), recovery is quite rapid and is consistent with relief of tubular obstruction (Deger and Wagoner, 1972; Kjellstrand et al., 1974). Most reported patients treated by dialysis had a diuresis within 48 h after the uric acid level decreased below 1.5 mmol/l (25 mgm/100 ml) (Kjellstrand et al., 1974). The diuresis does not appear to correlate with the length of time oliguria persists, the total amount of uric acid removed, or the initial serum uric acid value. Delays in initiating dialysis may result in a more prolonged course (Steinberg et al., 1975). Steinberg and co-workers (1975) believe that acute uric acid nephropathy if treated vigorously has a good prognosis, the ultimate cause of the condition depending primarily on the initiating condition.

REFERENCES

Cartier, P. and Hamet, M. (1974). 'The Normal Metabolism of Uric Acid in Advances in Nephrology' (Ed. Hamburger, Crosnier and Maxwell) p. 3. Year Book, Medical Publ. Chicago.

Deger, G. E. and Wagoner, R. D. (1972). Peritoneal dialysis in acute uric acid nephropathy. *Mayo Clin. Proc.* **47**, 189.

Kjellstrand, C. M., Campbell, D. C. and Von Hartitzosch, B. (1974). Hyperuricaemic acute renal failure. *Arch. Intern. Med.* **133**, 349.

O'Sullivan, J. B. (1972). Gout in a New England town. *Ann. Rheum. Dis.* **31**, 166.

Pochedly, C. (1973). Hyperuricemia in leukemia and lymphoma. *N.Y. State J. Med.* **73**, 1085.

Steinberg, S. M., Galen, M. A., Lazarus, J. M., Lowrie, E. G., Hampers, C. L. and Jaffe, N. (1975). Haemodialysis for acute anuric uric acid nephropathy. *Am. J. Dis. Child.* **129**, 956.

Section 7: Acute Disorders of Porphyrin Metabolism

GILLIAN C. HANSON

INTRODUCTION

Porphyrins are intermediates produced during the synthesis of haem. Characteristic of the porphyrias is the excessive production of porphyrins or their precursors which can be measured in the faeces, blood or urine. Only certain of the porphyrias are likely to be encountered in the intensive care situation. The normal values and porphyrin level changes in the porphyrias likely to be encountered, are shown in Table 1.

Acute and severe manifestations are most likely to arise in acute intermittent porphyria – this condition is inherited as an autosomal dominant but in one third of cases there is no family history. Onset of symptoms is generally between 20 and 40 years and first attacks are unusual in people over 50 (Goldberg *et al.*, 1976). Porphyria variegata is also inherited as a Mendelian autosomal dominant and is particularly common in South Africans. Clinical features may be similar to acute intermittent porphyria and are associated with a bullous dermatosis. Hereditary coproporphyria is a less severe disease than acute intermittent porphyria, the neurological signs being absent. Photosensitive bullous lesions may be present on the face and hands.

Acute clinical manifestations may be precipitated by certain drugs in a patient unknown to be porphyric, and certain drugs and factors should be taken into account when treating a critically ill porphyric patient (Table 2).

CLINICAL MANIFESTATIONS

A porphyric may require intensive therapy because of neurological or

215

Table 1. Normal values and porphyrin level changes in the porphyrias likely to be encountered in intensive care. (Modified from Goldberg *et al.*, 1976)

	Urinary Aminolae-vulic acid	Urinary porphobilino-gen	Urinary uropor-phyrin	Urinary copropor-phyrin	Faecal protopor-phyrin	Faecal coropor-phyrin
Normal levels	0–40 umol/ 24 h	0–16 umol/ 24 h	0–49 nmol/ 24 h	1–432 nmol/ 24 h	0–200 nmol/g dry wt	0–76 nmol/g dry wt
Condition						
Acute intermit-tent porphyria	Raised – very high in attack	Raised – very high in attack	Usually raised	Sometimes raised	Sometimes raised	Sometimes raised
Porphyria variegata	Raised in attack	Raised in attack	Sometimes raised	Sometimes raised	Raised	Raised
Hereditary coproporphyria	Raised only in attack	Raised only in attack	Sometimes raised in attack	Usually raised – always raised in attack	Usually normal	Raised

Table 2. Drugs and factors which may aggravate or precipitate acute porphyria

DRUGS

Drugs unlikely to be used in the I.T.U.
Chlordiazepoxide
Sedormid
Chlorpropamide
Tolbutamide
Meprobamate
Glutethimide
Sex hormones including the contraceptive pill
Griseofulvin

Drugs which may be used in the I.T.U.
Sulphonamides
Barbiturates
Methyldopa
Anticonvulsants of the hydantoin and succinimide group

FACTORS
Menstruation
Decreased calorie intake
Infection
Alcohol excess

---

autonomic involvement or because of metabolic imbalance subsequent to vomiting. The symptoms and manifestations of acute intermittent porphyria (A.I.P.) are described in detail by Stein and Tschudy (1970).

The classic symptoms of an acute attack are abdominal pain, extremity pain, constipation and mental changes. Intermittent hypertension with postural hypotension, tachycardia and excessive sweating are common during the acute attack. Mental confusion, hallucinations and seizures are well recognised and paresis of the bulbar and peripheral musculature may occur. The paresis is generally asymmetrical and does not have an ascending pattern of development.

INVESTIGATIONS

Studies of glucose tolerance during attacks of A.I.P. have shown characteristically elevated blood sugars early and hypoglycaemia developing late after the administration of glucose (Stein and Tschudy, 1970). Hyponatraemia is common and is partly related to vomiting and the syndrome of inappropriate release of antidiuretic hormone (Ludwig and Goldberg, 1963). It is also possible that there is abnormal renal handling of sodium ions. Blood volume is characteristically low and may be one of the reasons why some of these patients exhibit postural hypotension.

MANAGEMENT

The management can be summarised under the following headings:

> Metabolic
> Cardiovascular
> Neurological
> Nutrition
> The skin

Metabolic management

Patients suffering from severe gastrointestinal fluid losses should have a central venous pressure line inserted and the metabolic abnormalities appropriately corrected. It is essential to observe fluid balance and sodium levels carefully, since should there be evidence of inappropriate release of antidiuretic hormone, water intoxication may develop (Part 1, ch. VII, p. 169). Promazine can be used quite safely to relieve vomiting remembering that in high dosage respiratory depression may develop.

Cardiovascular management

When there is severe hypertension, hypotensive agents may be used – keeping in mind that the blood pressure generally returns to normal after the acute attack. Should there be an associated tachycardia (greater than 100/min) it is wise to slow down the rate with intravenous propronolol given at a rate of 1 mg/min to a maximum dose of 10 mg stopping once the pulse rate is 80/min. This, in conjunction with intramuscular pethidine or morphine may in itself lower the blood pressure adequately. It is probable that intravenous or intramuscular hydrallazine will be safe in lowering the blood pressure in an acute hypertensive situation should the above methods fail. (20–40 mg being given by slow intravenous injection then subsequently intramuscularly.) Hydrallazine injection may be complicated by a tachycardia, it is therefore important to precede the injection with propranolol should the pulse rate be greater than 100/min. Methyl Dopa must not be used since it may precipitate or exacerbate an attack of A.I.P.

Neurological management

Evidence of weakening of the voice or inability to swallow are early signs of impending respiratory failure. Such patients should have their airway carefully observed in an intensive therapy unit. Respiration is a well recognised complication – a Ryles tube should be inserted into the stomach and magnesium trisilicate mixture should be instilled 4-hourly. A period of intermittent positive pressure ventilation may be indicated. Occasionally an ascending paresis may also require ventilation. Diazepam and phenoperidine are quite safe drugs to use in order to maintain the patient on the ventilator. Anticonvulsants of the hydantoin and succinimide groups are known to aggravate porphyria – a patient with seizures is best treated with intramuscular paraldehyde and/or diazepam given intramuscularly or intravenously. High doses of these drugs require careful observation of the airway.

Nutrition

It has been shown that withdrawal of protein and carbohydrate may precipitate an attack. The use of glucose has been shown to terminate the acute attack in a number of patients (Stein and Tschudy, 1970). Glucose generally has to be given intravenously – 200–300 g being infused daily as 10% or 40% dextrose. Should there be evidence of glucose intolerance, insulin may be necessary (Part 1, ch. IX, p. 263).

100–140 g of protein should be given daily either orally via the Ryles tube as albumaid, or intravenously as Vamin N or Vamin glucose.

The skin

The skin in porphyria variegata and hereditary coproporphyria may blister easily to produce vesicles or bullae. The skin should be protected against injury, the patient nursed on a smooth soft surface and turned gently at frequent intervals to avoid bed sores. The skin must not be exposed to sunlight and the face should be shielded from strong light. The usual U.V.R. sunscreens are of little value but dense visible sunscreens containing titanium dioxide are more effective. Blisters when they occur should be pinched and covered with paraffin gauze.

In the series of 46 patients with A.I.P. reported by Stein and Tschudy (1970), there were 4 fatalities. Two from prolonged respiratory failure with secondary infection and two from cerebral involvement possibly secondary to ventricular arrhythmias and inadequate cerebral perfusion. From this series it seems clear that the majority of patients should recover from the acute attack.

Acknowledgment

I am grateful to Dr J. S. Pegum, Senior Physician, Skin Department, London Hospital, London, E.1, for his advice on dermatological management.

REFERENCES

Goldberg, A., Beattie, A. D. and Campbell, B. C. (1976). The porphyrias and heavy metal intoxication. *Medicine* Second Series **13** (1), 600.

Ludwig, G. D. and Goldberg, M. (1963). Hyponatraemia in acute intermittent porphyria probably resulting from inappropriate secretion of antidiuretic hormone. *Ann. N.Y. Acad. Sci.* **104**, 710.

Stein, J. A. and Tschudy, D. P. (1970). Acute intermittent porphyria. A clinical and biochemical study of 46 patients. *Medicine* **49** (1), 1.

VIII

The Management of the Hyperosmolar Syndromes and Hyperglycaemia

Section 1: The Management of the Hyperosmolar Syndromes

GILLIAN C. HANSON

PATHOPHYSIOLOGY

Osmotic pressure is proportional to the molal concentration of particles. A molal concentration is expressed as moles solute per kilogram solvent on a solute to solvent weight basis. The units mosmol/kg vary linearly with freezing point depression. One mole of solute lowers the freezing point of water by 1.86°C. This observation is the basis for the most commonly used method of measuring osmolality. The normal serum osmolality falls in the range 275–295 mosmol/kg. Sodium and its salts and other electrolytes contribute approximately 275 mosmol/kg to the serum. Glucose and non-protein nitrogen contribute about 10 mosmol/kg. Protein is highly polyvalent and contributes little to the osmolality except when the concentration is very high, such as after the rapid infusion of amino acid solutions. Urea is included in the measurement of osmolality, but since it passes freely between the various body fluid compartments, it is unlikely to produce coma unless there are very large and rapid increases such as following therapeutic urea infusion for cerebral oedema. Dorwart and Chalmers (1975) compared methods for calculating serum osmolality from chemical concentrations and found that the following equation produced only ± 16 mosmol/kg difference.

$$\text{Osmolality} = 1.86\,\text{Na}\ (\text{mmol/l}) + \frac{\text{Glucose mg\%}}{18} + \frac{\text{B.U.N. mg\%}}{2.8} + 9$$

or

$$\text{Osmolality} = 1.86\,\text{Na}\ (\text{mmol/l}) + \text{Glucose mmol/l} + (\text{B.U.N. mmol/l} \times 2) + 9$$

The author of the letter following this reference stated that the formula should be simple and accurate and suggested the following to be of most benefit to the physician.

$$\text{Osmolality} = 2\,\text{Na}\ (\text{mmol/l}) + \text{Glucose (mmol/l)} + 2\ (\text{B.U.N. mmol/l})$$

When blood is taken for serumosmolality, the specimen should be immediately refrigerated since the level will rise after one hour in room temperature because of the formation of lactic acid.

A determined osmolality minus the calculated osmolality of more than 40 mosmol/kg is considered to reflect a grave prognosis. In the presence of gross hyperlipaemia or hyperproteinaemia, the difference may be greater than 40 mosmol/kg; the calculated osmolality being spuriously low, under such circumstances the determined osmolality will be accurate. Errors may arise when osmolality is calculated from blood taken during a lipid infusion.

The plasma osmolality will be raised in the presence of unusual solutes such as ethanol when cryoscopic osmometers are used (Glasser et al., 1973). Factors which may also cause an elevated osmolality include diabetic ketoacidosis and coma, nonketotic hyperglycaemia and hypernatraemia.

It is of considerable interest that Fulop and co-workers (1975) related stupor in ketotic diabetic coma (as in nonketotic diabetic coma), to serum osmolality and not to the severity of the acidaemia. They suggested that the absence of hyperosmolality (and the exclusion of hypoglycaemia) in a comatose diabetic patient would make one suspect that the stupor was not merely due to the diabetes.

Dorwart and Chalmers (1975) felt that the extra osmotically active

Table 1. Characteristics of major disturbances of intracellular and extracellular volume and solute concentration in the presence of *normal* renal function

Type of disturbance	Volume			Osmolality		Serum sodium
	Extracellular	Intracellular	Intravascular	Serum	Urine	
Predominant water depletion (other than diabetes insipidus)	D	D	D	I	I	I
Water intoxication (other than inappropriate ADH secretion)	I	I	I	D	D	D
Acute salt intake	I	D	I	D	I	I
Predominant salt loss	D	I	D	D	D	D
Acute sugar intake producing acute hyperglycaemia	I	D	I	I	I	N,D,I
Haemodilution e.g. C.R.F.				D	D generally	
Cardiac failure	I	I	N,D,I	D	N	D

D, deceased; I, increased; N, normal

Table 2. Aetological factors producing the hyperosmolar syndrome

PREDISPOSING FACTORS
Diabetes mellitus diagnosed or undiagnosed
Uraemia particularly acute
Pancreatitis acute or chronic
Stress, in particular associated with trauma and sepsis
Patients undergoing cardiopulmonary bypass
Patients undergoing peritoneal or haemodialysis

PRECIPITATING FACTORS
1 *Feeding preparations*
   Oral or intravenous glucose
   Oral and tube feeding elemental diets

2 *Drugs producing hyperglycaemia*
   Corticosteroids
   Adrenaline
   Glucagon
   Diazoxide

3 *Drugs producing hypernatraemia*
   Sodium bicarbonate
   Salt used as an emetic

4 *Irrigating solutions*
   Twice normal saline for stomach lavage or bowel washout
   Sodium citrate (6.3%) for bladder lavage
   Peritoneal dialysis solutions in particular when hypertonic

5 *Situations producing excessive water loss in excess of sodium*
   Diuretics – mannitol, thiazides, ethacrynic acid
   Burns
   Fistula losses, severe diarrhoea
   Starvation and dehydration

6 *Situations producing acute uraemia*
   Acute renal failure
   Intravenous urea

substances in the serum of dying shock patients would have to be nonionic. They suggested that a systematic search for these substances might give some insight into the mechanism of death from shock.

Certain characteristics of various pathological states of water and electrolyte metabolism are summarised in Table 1. The predisposing and aetiological factors producing the hyperosmolar syndrome are listed in Table 2.

The management of ketotic hyperglycaemia secondary to diabetes mellitus will be discussed on p. 232.

The patient in the intensive therapy unit is particularly predisposed to hyperglycaemia. In the acute phase of injury, insulin secretion is generally suppressed (Allison *et al.*, 1967). Following this acute phase, plasma insulin levels may be high in the presence of continuing glucose intolerance (Allison *et al.*, 1968). It is at this stage (which may continue for many days) that the critically ill stressed patients may become dangerously hyperglycaemic. Blood glucose monitoring and timely insulin therapy are essential during the management of the critically ill. Intravenous dextrose feeding in the absence of adequate blood glucose monitoring is one of the commonest precipitating factors. Urine glucose testing in the critically ill is totally unreliable, since in the presence of inadequate renal perfusion, glucose may be reabsorbed from the urine before it reaches the bladder. Stress may also alter the renal threshold for glucose. The use of massive doses of steroids for the treatment of shock may be followed by sodium retention, a potassium diuresis and hyperglycaemia. Glucagon may produce or increase the hyperglycaemia frequently seen in acute pancreatitis.

Several factors frequently are operating simultaneously, which in isolation would be unlikely to produce a hyperosmolar syndrome, for example the use of intravenous diazoxide (Charles and Danforth, 1971), intravenous glucose, corticosteroids, or thiazide diuretics in uraemia and the use of intravenous dextrose solutions in the presence of pancreatitis, undiagnosed diabetes mellitus, and burn injuries (Rosenberg *et al.*, 1957). The combination of a glucocorticoid and intravenous saline in a patient unable to take fluid orally may be dangerous, especially when sodium clearance is diminished or the patient is losing excess quantities of hypotonic fluid (e.g. diarrhoea). The elderly are particularly susceptible to hyperglycaemia following the use of oral elemental diets and tube feeds. Especially dangerous is the combination of a tube feed containing a high concentration of glucose and the simultaneous administration of glucose intravenously.

Hypernatraemia has been well documented following the use of saline as an emetic (Barer *et al.*, 1973), and sodium bicarbonate during resuscitation (Matter *et al.*, 1974). Hypernatraemia may develop in patients with diarrhoea where water replacement in relationship to sodium is inadequate and in relatively water depleted patients on dialysis.

Gastric bladder or bowel lavage should never be performed with hypertonic salt solutions. Death has been reported from the use of hypertonic saline for gastric lavage (Carter and Fotheringham, 1971).

DIAGNOSIS AND TREATMENT OF THE HYPEROSMOLAR SYNDROMES UNRELATED TO DIABETES MELLITUS

Clinical

Signs may be minimal in unconscious patients until the level of osmolality is dangerously high. The rate of deterioration may be a matter of hours in patients who have a rapid rise in serum osmolality due to the intravenous infusion, or irrigation with a hypertonic solution. In the hyperosmolar syndrome of slow onset, the patient may complain of severe thirst and this is followed by various changes in the sensorium, including meningeal signs, vestibular dysfunction, focal neurologic signs, tremors, generalised convulsions and hyperthermia.

In the hyperosmolar syndrome of acute onset, there is rapid onset of drowsiness, followed by twitching generalised convulsions, deepening coma and ultimately respiratory arrest. The most serious consequences of the hyperosmolar syndrome are severe brain shrinkage, distension of intracranial vessels and haemorrhage. In the acute syndrome where dehydration may not be present, there may be associated acute expansion of the intravascular space, left ventricular overload and pulmonary oedema. Renal failure occurring 6–12 hours after the acute precipitating event is also common.

Both experimental and clinical observations indicate that increases in plasma osmolality to levels exceeding 350 mosmol/kg are potentially fatal. When acute hyperosmolality is induced in animals with saline infusion, most of the animals die when the osmolality rises above 350 mosmol/kg (Sotos et al., 1960). Mortality from the acute severe syndrome with osmolalities above 350 mosmol is probably around 90% and in the syndromes of slower onset where the osmolality does not reach this level, is 30% or less. The mortality in patients where the syndrome has developed over a period of days and where the osmolality is allowed to rise above 350 mosmol/kg, is probably also extremely high. Such patients may recover but may be left with permanent brain damage.

Biochemical

The syndrome is characterised by a serum osmolality of 300 mosmol/kg or more, and the substance producing this rise will be obvious by biochemical analysis. Water depletion and evidence of extravascular dehydration is common in the case of slow onset. Urine osmolality will be increased in those patients who still have normal renal function. Experimental (Sotos et al., 1962) and clinical studies show that hypertonicity of the body fluids is associated with a severe degree of acidosis. This develops experimentally after the infusion of sodium chloride, sugar or urea, and develops irrespective of the plasma concentrations of sodium and chloride but is highly correlated with tonicity and can be reversed by infusion of hypotonic fluids (Sotos *et al.*, 1962). Sotos and co-workers (1962) surmised that hypertonicity of body fluids can cause disturbances in cellular metabolism, resulting in the formation and release of large quantities of hydrogen ion and the development of a severe extracellular metabolic acidosis. They found that restoration of osmolality towards normal by rehydration caused the acidosis to decrease. Death in hypertonicity is due to respiratory failure (Sotos *et al.*, 1960) (respiratory compensation for the severe metabolic acidosis rarely being evident), or from cerebral haemorrhage. Should the patient survive the first few hours the metabolic abnormalities may be complicated by the onset of acute renal failure. Metabolic acidosis is not always a feature of hypernatraemia developing after bladder irrigation with sodium citrate, most probably because the citrate ion is absorbed and, provided liver metabolism is adequate, is converted from lactate to bicarbonate.

Hypoxia is common, probably because of the catabolic state and absence of hypoxic drive; it may be complicated by the onset of acute pulmonary oedema through an acute hyperosmolar load, or because of excess fluid administration in the presence of acute renal failure.

Disseminated intravascular coagulation may be a complicating feature, which, if associated with a haemorrhagic diathesis may be an indication for intravenous heparin, replacement of clotting factors with F.F.P. and, on rare occasions, blood.

Treatment

Hyperosmolar syndrome of slow onset. Se osmolality < 350 mosmol/kg (see Table 3)

A history consistent with the slow development of the hyperosmolar syndrome does not necessitate dramatic treatment unless the calculated osmolality is > 350 mosmol/kg.

Predominant hyperglycaemia. Treatment consists of the administration of insulin for hyperglycaemia (Table 3) and fluid volume replacement either orally with water or intravenously with hypotonic saline (either half normal or $\frac{1}{5}$ N saline). Diuretics should not be used.

Predominant hypernatraemia. Here water should be given by mouth or via the Ryles tube. If oral absorption is not possible, fluid should be

Table 3. Summary of treatment of the chronic hyperosmolar syndrome serum osmolality <350 mosm/kg

---

Predominant hyperglycaemia
  Insulin soluble   20 units i.v. or i.m. stat then
                     4–8 units i.v. or i.m. hourly

  Check B.G. Reflomat[1] hourly. B.G. 4 hourly

  Stop insulin once B.G. 9 mmol/l or less
  Water via the Ryles tube and/or i.v. $\frac{1}{2}$ N or $\frac{1}{5}$ N saline
  Rate of fluid administration approximately 1 litre 4 hourly for 24 h – increase initial
     rate if there is evidence of severe dehydration

  Observe for hypokalaemia, onset of A.R.F. fluid overload or D.I.C.

Predominant hypernatraemia
  Fluids as above
  Observe for hyperglycaemia, hypokalaemia, onset of A.R.F. or C.C.F.

  DO NOT GIVE DIURETICS

  DIALYSE PERITONEALLY with a hypotonic dialysate should the B.D. be >10 or pH 7.1
     or less, or there is evidence of A.R.F.

  Dialysis solution – either HARTMANN'S SOLUTION if Se K$^+$ normal and B.G. 6 mmol/l or
     greater or 1 litre HARTMANN'S SOLUTION followed by 500 ml 1.3% DIALAFLEX
     solution

---

given intravenously as $\frac{1}{5}$ N saline. Should the patient be in renal failure and on dialysis – hypertonic dialysis should be stopped and the dialysate changed to either an isotonic or relatively hypotonic dialysing solution (Table 3). The blood glucose for patients on dialysis must be observed carefully and insulin given in a relatively low dosage (twice the blood glucose in mmol/l should the blood glucose be raised above 10 mmol/l). Insulin should be given subsequently i.m. or i.v. hourly in a dose of 4–8 units until the dextrostix or blood glucose checked hourly is 8 mmol or less (this may be estimated in the laboratory or by the Reflomat* system).

2. Hyperosmolar syndrome of acute onset or serum osmolality >350 mosmol/kg in a hyperosmolar syndrome of chronic onset (see Tables 4 and 5)

Predominant hypernatraemic. In situations where it is suspected that an excessive quantity of sodium ions has been given rapidly intravenously, the serum osmolality will reflect the gravity of the situation. With oral ingestion there may be delay in the rise in serum osmolality. Therapy should therefore not be guided by the initial biochemistry but by

---

* Boehringer Mannheim Lab. This system seems more reliable for ranges of high blood glucose than the Ames reflectance meter.

Table 4. Summary of treatment of the acute hyperosmolar syndrome or serum osmolality >350 mosm/kg in a hyperosmolar syndrome of chronic onset

Predominant hypernatraemia
  Oral ingestion. Remove gastric washings for analysis and washout with water.

$$\text{Expected rise in Na}^+ \text{ mmol/l} = \frac{\text{total vol. of initial gastric aspirate l} \times \text{Na}^+ \text{ conc. in the initial gastric aspirate mmol/l}}{\text{T.B.W. in litres (Part I, ch. VII, p. 159)}}$$

should the expected rise in the plasma Na be >30 mmol/l, commence

PERITONEAL DIALYSIS Solution – see Table 3
                     Rate – 500 ml every 20 min continuous recycling. Add potassium if necessary.

I.v. fluids. Set up C.V.P. and infuse up to a normal level with $\frac{1}{5}$ N saline. Maintain C.V.P. at a normal level. Infuse at a rate of approx. 1000 ml $\frac{1}{5}$ N saline/4 h. Slow down rate if C.V.P. >12 cm H_2O.

Do NOT give SODIUM BICARBONATE for a METABOLIC ACIDOSIS

CONVULSIONS treat with i.v. phenytoin if repeated, for I.P.P.V.
Should diazepam be used, observe ventilation.

I.P.P.V. Indications $\begin{cases} \text{Continuous twitching or convulsions} \\ \text{Inadequate airway maintenance} \\ \text{Inadequate ventilation} \\ \text{Increasing metabolic acidosis} \\ \text{Onset of pulmonary oedema} \\ \text{Rising PaCO}_2 \text{ or PaO}_2 \text{ 8.7 kPa (65 mm) or less} \end{cases}$

Use pancuronium to maintain on I.P.P.V. Maintain $PaCO_2$ 4.7–5.3 kPa (35–40 mm Hg) and PaO_2 10.6–13.3 kPa (80–100 mm Hg).

INTRAVASCULAR HAEMOLYSIS give whole blood if Hct 30% or less.

LUMBAR PUNCTURE
  Indications $\begin{cases} \text{deterioration in level of consciousness} \\ \text{localising neurological signs} \\ \text{neck stiffness} \end{cases}$

CATHETERISE if urine output <40 ml per hour in the presence of a normal C.V.P., suspect onset of A.R.F. *Check* u/p osmolality ratio – if ratio 1.2 or less, consider *peritoneal dialysis* (if not started).

Serial investigations On admission B.U. Electrolytes
                                       B.G. Serum osmolality
                                       C.S.F. osmolality (if taken) u/p osmolality ratio
                                       Blood gases acid-base status
                                       Hb P.C.V. Clotting indicies
  Check 2 – hourly as required.

INSULIN if B.G. 10 mmol/l or more (see Table 5 for dosage).
Observe for hypokalaemia, onset of A.R.F., fluid overload or D.I.C.

analysis of the total volume of the initial gastric aspirate, the stomach subsequently being washed out with water. A crude estimation of the possible effect on the intravascular concentration of sodium ions can then be made.

i.e.   expected rise in serum Na^+ mmol/l

$$= \frac{\text{total volume of} \atop \text{initial gastric aspriate l} \times \text{Na}^+ \text{ conc. in the} \atop \text{initial gastric aspirate mmol/l}}{\text{T.B.W. in litres (Part 1, ch. VII, p. 159).}}$$

Should the expected rise be greater than 30 mmol/l, then peritoneal dialysis with a hypotonic dialysate should be instituted on the basis that such a rise can be lethal. Insulin is invariably required to control a rise in blood glucose. A central venous pressure line should be inserted and intravenous $\frac{1}{5}$N saline administered until the C.V.P. is normal. Thiazide diuretics or mannitol *should not be given* since the loss of sodium ions in the urine is generally less than 145 mmol/l.

Table 5. Summary of treatment of the acute hyperosmolar syndrome or serum osmolality >350 mosm/kg in a hyperosmolar syndrome of chronic onset

---

Predominant hyperglycaemia

INSULIN   Soluble 2 × the B.G. in mmol/l i.v. or i.m., then 4–8 units i.v. or i.m. hourly.

Check B.G. Reflomat hourly and B.G. 4 hours after commencement. If B.G. not decreasing, increase i.v. or i.m. hourly insulin by 4 units.

I.V. FLUIDS   Set up C.V.P.
Give $\frac{1}{5}$ N saline or normal saline according to serum sodium.
Rate see Table 4.

DO NOT GIVE SODIUM BICARBONATE unless B.D. > 10 or pH 7.1 or less then *50 mmol* HCO_3^- *at the most.*

SODIUM BICARBONATE is *contraindicated* if Se osmolality 350 mosmol/kg or more.

CATHETERISE see Table 4.
Observe for fall in serum potassium, onset of fluid overload, A.R.F. or D.I.C.

Serial investigations see Table 4

The respiratory status must be carefully observed, inadequate ventilation, evidence of inadequate compensation for an increasing metabolic acidosis, the onset of left ventricular failure, increasing coma with a poorly maintained airway, or multiple convulsions are all indications for I.P.P.V. The patient requiring I.P.P.V. should be relaxed with intravenous pancuronium and phenytoin should be given to control convulsions. It is wise not to use opiates or diazepam since frequent assessment of the neurological status is indicated. Failure to breathe spontaneously after the electrolytes have been restored to normal for three days or more, is strongly suggestive of irreversible cerebral damage. An E.E.G. should be performed at this stage.

The younger patient who experiences a severe hyperosmolar syndrome may take many weeks to recover fully neurologically. During this period there is generally an initial phase of impaired level of consciousness followed by confusion and poor memory.

Lumbar puncture may be indicated to exclude a subarachnoid haemorrhage; blood may also be present if there has been an intracerebral bleed complicated by rupture into the subarachnoid space. The osmolality, sugar and sodium content of the C.S.F. should be estimated, since it would appear that severe neurological disturbances only occur when the C.S.F. osmolality is 8 mosmol/kg greater than the serum osmolality (Habel and Simpson, 1975).

The blood glucose must be carefully observed especially if the patient is on peritoneal dialysis. Insulin should be given if blood glucose is 10 mmol/l or more.

The metabolic acidosis should not be corrected with sodium bicarbonate – but will steadily subside with fluid volume replacement and dialysis. Acute oliguria invariably occurs when the serum osmolality due to hypernatraemia rises above 340 mosmol/kg and generally lasts 2–3 days. It is essential during this period to decrease the rate of rise of blood urea by giving adequate calories and continuing dialysis. Occasionally there is intravascular haemolysis during the acute phase of the illness – blood should not be given unless the Hct drops to 30% or less. Whole blood must be given. Treatment is summarised in Table 4.

Predominant hyperglycaemia. A rapid rise in blood glucose can generally be adequately controlled with insulin therapy coupled with intravenous isotonic or hypotonic saline. A metabolic acidosis is rare and renal failure unusual unless the patient is allowed to become severely dehydrated. Treatment is summarised in Table 5.

DIAGNOSIS AND TREATMENT OF THE HYPEROSMOLAR SYNDROMES ASSOCIATED WITH DIABETES MELLITUS

Introduction

Fulop and co-workers (1975) have shown that hyperosmolality exists in ketoacidotic hyperglycaemic coma and they suggested that it was the main metabolic factor producing stupor. It is well recognised that hyperosmolality is the major factor producing coma in the nonketotic hyperglycaemic patient. In the patient with diabetic ketoacidosis (D.K.A.) the hyperosmolality is largely due to glucose, whereas the nonketotic hyperglycaemic patients (N.K.H.) have a significantly higher serum sodium. This is probably because the nonketotic patients have a longer period of glucosuric diuresis during which they lose relatively more water than sodium (Smith, 1951) and also because these patients tend to be older and may have impaired renal tubular concentrating ability (Smith, 1951). Hyperosmolality seems necessary but not sufficient for the development of stupor in patients with D.K.A. and N.K.H., the additional factor probably being the rate at which it develops. These two factors presumably determine the severity of the blood brain osmotic disequilibrium and of brain cell hyperosmolality and dehydration. The close parallel between stupor and hyper-osmolality does not prove that hyperosmolality *per se* produces coma, it is known however that it can cause coma in other clinical settings.

Severe diabetic ketoacidosis (D.K.A.)

The essential cause of D.K.A. is insufficiency of insulin leading to hyperglycaemia, raised levels of fatty acids in the blood and consequently ketoacidosis. The osmotic properties of glucose and ketone bodies cause a diuresis and ultimate dehydration. The total electrolyte and water losses during ketosis are considerable; Maxwell and Kleeman (1962) give the average losses as:

Water   75–100 ml/kg
Na^+ 8 mmol/kg B.W.
Cl^- 5 mmol/kg B.W.
K^+ 6 mmol/kg B.W.

The load of ketoacids may overwhelm the body buffers so that the pH of the blood falls and there develops an increasing metabolic acidosis. The total loss of water may be as high as 10% of the total body weight, the plasma electrolytes are however diluted because of the high serum osmolality and the cells become extremely dehydrated. It is only in the final stages of D.K.A. that the serum sodium rises. A high serum sodium (> 150 mmol/l) is evidence of extreme dehydration and the patient is in imminent danger of circulatory collapse from hypovolaemia.

In diabetic ketosis the water loss is largely from the kidney but losses via the lungs (from compensatory hyperventilation up to 1500 ml daily) and in the vomit, are also considerable. The net loss of sodium ions from the body is generally in a concentration of $\frac{1}{5}-\frac{1}{2}$ N saline. This is important to remember when restoring fluid losses since hypernatraemia may develop if hypertonic sodium containing solutions are used (e.g. sodium bicarbonate) or even with the excessive use of N saline in the presence of inadequate renal tubular function. Magnesium, calcium, nitrogen and phosphate are also lost in the urine in excess.

The reported death rate from D.K.A. is 5–10% in good centres and up to 25% elsewhere (Alberti, 1975). Prevention and the early recognition and appropriate treatment of D.K.A. is therefore important.

Treatment

The treatment is summarised in Table 6. Controversy surrounds the dosage and route of insulin administration. Alberti *et al.* (1973) renewed the discussion about the optimal dosage of insulin suggesting an intramuscular stat dose of 10–20 units followed by 5 units i.m. hourly. He has subsequently suggested an alternative method of continuous infusion of insulin 2–6 units/h (Alberti, 1975). These results are in accord with previous studies that smaller doses of insulin are as effective as larger doses. From the data it would appear that none of the 14 ketoacidotic patients reported had a blood pressure systolic below 100 mm or a serum sodium above 145 mmol/l and the pH was less than 7.0 in only one patient. Keller *et al.* (1975) state that in clinical practice it is impossible to predict the response to a certain amount of insulin in a comatose patient and it may be that the doses of insulin recommended by Alberti (1975) would be too low to saturate the insulin receptors.

Table 6. Summary of treatment of severe diabetic ketoacidosis D.K.A.

ON ADMISSION   *Check*   B.G. serum osmolality
B.U. electrolytes
Blood gases. Acid-base status
Hb W.B.C. and diff. P.C.V.
Clotting factors

I.V. FLUIDS
Commence i.v. normal saline, give approximately 1000 ml in the first 30 min in a clinically dehydrated patient, otherwise 1000 ml in 1 h.
Set up C.V.P. and regulate subsequent infusion rate according to the C.V.P.

CATHETERISE
Subsequent fluids according to biochemistry

GENERAL
Maintain urine output at 40 ml/h or more.
Maintain C.V.P. at 6–10 cm H_2O. Slow down rate if C.V.P. > 12 cm.
Rate approximately 1 litre 2 hourly for 4 hours then 1 litre 4 hourly.
Type of fluid according to serial electrolytes, B.G. and osmolality.
P.P.F. as the first litre if patient shocked.   *(cont.)*

(*Table 6 cont.*)

Normal saline if Se Na < 145 mmol/l.

$\frac{1}{5}$ N saline or $\frac{1}{2}$ N saline if Se Na > 145 mmol/l

I.v. Potassium – approx. 10–20 mmol/h once Se K < 3.5 mmol/l *provided* urine output 40 ml/h or more.

Sodium bicarbonate – consider if pH 7.1 or less and BD 12 or more.

DO NOT give until Se K 3.2 or more and Se Na 150 mmol or less.

DO NOT give > 50 mmol HCO_3^- as the initial dose, then check acid base status $\frac{1}{2}$ h later.

INSULIN SOLUBLE

Intravenously   20–40 units stat

20 units B.G.–28 mmol/l or less

40 units B.G.–>28 mmol/l

continuous intravenous insulin infusion if there is evidence of poor perfusion.

Dose initially   4 units i.v. hourly–B.G. 28 mmol/l or less

8 units i.v. hourly–B.G. > 28 mmol/l

Check B.G.   3 h after commencing infusion if B.G. not fallen, double the dose.

Intramuscularly

No evidence of poor perfusion – pulse volume and B.P. good.

Dosage as above.

RYLES TUBE

Pass a Ryles tube – aspirate to dryness, then put down 15 ml sodium citrate 0.3 M.

INFECTION   Look for source of infection – treat appropriately.

EXCLUDE   Other factors precipitating D.K.A. e.g. pregnancy, overdose, vascular disorder.

VENTILATION   Consider if PaO_2 < 9.3 kPa   (70 mm Hg)   or $PaCO_2$ > 8.0 kPa (60 mm Hg) in a patient with no previous lung disease.

DIALYSE   Early if there is A.R.F. Observe Se sodium and B.G. carefully during dialysis.

Observe for cardiac failure, cardiac dysrhythmias, vomiting complicated by aspiration. Onset of A.R.F. Hypokalaemia. Hypernatraemia. Hypoglycaemia. Overcorrection of metabolic acidosis leading to respiratory depression.

Refractory shock, look for sepsis, onset of D.I.C.

Should level of consciousness not improve after 6 hours – reassess neurological status, consider lumbar puncture.

Subsequent management

B.G. check hourly – Reflomat system. B.G. lab. estimation 2–4 hourly.

Urea electrolytes – approx. 2–4 hourly.

Blood gases. Acid base status – 2–6 hourly.

STOP INSULIN once B.G. 12 mmol or less and set up a 5% dextrose drip with potassium supplements if required.

The route of insulin administration is also important. The plasma half-life of insulin given intravenously is only four to five minutes (Turner *et al.*, 1971) and therefore should preferably be administered as a continuous infusion. The absorption of currently used insulin to glass and plastic tubes should not be of major importance for the patient

(Page *et al.*, 1974). Preliminary observations suggest equal effectiveness with the use of a plastic paediatric infusion set rather than an infusion pump (Kidson *et al.*, 1974). This procedure is easy to perform in an intensive therapy unit.

Subcutaneous insulin is slowly absorbed and has a half-life of about 4 h so that there is delay in the onset of action and large depots of insulin may be created especially in the patient with poor skin perfusion. Subcutaneous insulin should therefore not be used for the initial management of D.K.A. Intramuscular insulin has a half-life of approximately two hours and can reasonably be used for the management of D.K.A. provided a rapid effect is not required and that there is no evidence of impaired tissue perfusion. Insulin sensitivity rapidly recovers in D.K.A. and therefore frequent glucose monitoring is imperative. A 5% glucose infusion should be started once the blood glucose has fallen to 12 mmol or less and the insulin stopped. Blood glucose monitoring, preferably using the Reflomat system (Boehringer Mannheim Lab.), should be continued hourly over the subsequent four hours since occasionally there is a delay in insulin activity if i.m. insulin has been used in the presence of preceding impaired peripheral perfusion.

Since hypotension and oliguria are a frequent complication, central venous pressure monitoring is essential in the management of severe D.K.A. Fluid volume replacement initially should be rapid, and in a hypotensive patient as much as 1000 ml of normal saline should be given within the first 30 min. Should the serum sodium be 145 mmol or above, this should be followed by $\frac{1}{2}$ N or $\frac{1}{5}$ N saline. In a septic patient or a patient suspected to be hypoalbuminaemic, plasma protein fraction should be the initial volume replacement solution of choice. Alkali therapy should not be used unless the pH is 7.10 or less, or the BD > 10, should be limited to 50 mmol, and should only be used once the central venous pressure has started to rise towards normal. Alkali is known to decrease venular tone and should therefore not be used if blood volume is grossly depleted (Harvey *et al.*, 1966). Severe acidaemia however is known to impair cardiac function (Ng *et al.*, 1967). Excessive use of bicarbonate may lead to hypernatraemia, augment the risk of hypokalaemia and if an alkalosis is allowed to develop, red cell diphosphoglycerate (2–3 D.P.G.) already markedly decreased (Alberti *et al.*, 1972) will further decrease P_{50} (Table 5, p. 345).

Potassium monitoring is essential and intravenous supplements are generally required within two hours of commencing therapy. Bicarbonate should not be given if there is a history of diarrhoea and/or vomiting until the serum potassium has been restored. The use of bicarbonate in a patient with an initial serum potassium of 3.2 mmol/l or less may precipitate fatal hypokalaemia. The onset of hypokalaemia is more gradual with the low dose insulin technique (Alberti *et al.*, 1973; Semple *et al.*, 1974).

Observation of urine output is essential since potassium supplements may be dangerous with the onset of acute renal failure. Since these patients are catabolic and acidotic, early peritoneal dialysis is indicated.

Associated conditions present should be treated appropriately. Infection is common and in these patients blood glucose tends to fall more slowly since anti-insulin hormones such as glucagon are higher (Rocha *et al.*, 1973). Pregnancy may be a factor precipitating D.K.A. – in such patients severe D.K.A. is associated with a high incidence of abortion. Drugs used under such circumstances must be carefully reviewed (Yaffe, 1975).

Intravascular coagulation associated with evidence of D.I.C. within the brain may well contribute to the mortality in D.K.A. (Timperley *et al.*, 1974). pH reduction and tissue hypoxia both cause cellular hypoxia and release of tissue thromboplastin. The cellular hypoxia in D.K.A. is accentuated by low concentrations of erythrocyte 2,3-D.P.G. A preliminary survey of the coagulation mechanism in ambulant diabetics has shown that this is often abnormal and that the right stimulus might rapidly cause D.I.C. (Timperley *et al.*, 1974). Prevention of D.I.C. includes rapid volume replacement in order to improve cellular oxygenation, maintenance of an adequate PaO_2 and careful correction (but not over-correction) of a severe metabolic acidosis. Heparin should be considered if D.I.C. is haematologically proven and the level of coma considered inappropriate for the severity of the metabolic abnormality. Prophylactic heparin is contraindicated because of the high incidence of erosive gastritis and gastrointestinal bleeding (Keller *et al.*, 1974).

A recent case study (Nobis *et al.*, 1972) suggests that in severe prolonged shock associated with D.I.C., should heparin fail to improve the clinical status, fibrinolytic therapy should be considered. In such patients peritoneal and/or haemodialysis also seems to be indicated (Chazan *et al.*, 1969).

Severe diabetic nonketotic hyperglycaemia (N.K.H.)

In common with all other hyperosmolar syndromes, N.K.H. causes stupor which progresses to coma. Since the disorder begins with an elevation in blood glucose without the subsequent development of severe ketosis and progresses towards the development of profound dehydration, it is possible to encounter the patient at any point of this clinical progression. It is proposed to discuss the management of patients who have developed severe N.K.H. There is a degree of overlap between D.K.A. and N.K.H. but it is important to elicit the dominant factors producing the coma. The pH occasionally may measure 7.35 or less (Arieff and Carroll, 1972) and is commonly associated with hypotension, hypoperfusion and a lactic acid acidosis. Serum lactate is generally only modestly elevated and not to the severe degree encountered in lactic acid acidosis (see Part 1, ch. VII, p. 205).

Patients with 2^+ acetonaemia (1:1 dilution) should be regarded as either mild ketosis or 'mixed' nonketotic coma. Flagrant diabetic ketoacidosis and 'pure' nonketotic coma appear to be two ends of a spectrum of lipid mobilisation. Several features other than serum ketones tend to distinguish ketoacidosis from nonketotic coma (Vinik *et al.*, 1970, Collins and Harris, 1971). Most frequently in N.K.A. blood glucose is above 44 mmol/l and very few cases have been reported with levels less than 33 mmol/l; serum osmolality is generally 340 mosm/kg or above and the average blood urea is higher, namely 13.3 mmol/l as opposed to 5 mmol/l in D.K.A. (Arieff and Carroll, 1972). The serum sodium concentration has a wide range in nonketotic coma but tends to be higher than the levels seen in D.K.A. Severe metabolic acidosis in N.K.H. is uncommon except terminally.

Treatment is summarised in Table 7.

Although there has been some suggestion that the amount of insulin required to treat the acute episode is smaller in N.K.H. than in D.K.H. other workers have found this not to be so (Arieff and Carroll, 1972). In cases of severe dehydration, the blood glucose may be raised through haemoconcentration – in such instances the blood glucose appears to fall rapidly once the intravascular volume has been expanded. Since the condition is insidious in onset, there is every reason to restore the blood glucose to normal values over a period of days as opposed to hours (Editorial, 1972). Hypoglycaemia is a danger and is another reason for lowering the blood glucose slowly. Fluid administration should be based on central venous pressure monitoring and should be as $\frac{1}{2}$ or $\frac{1}{5}$ normal saline. The average volume of fluid lost is 24% of the total body water – this should be replaced over 24–36 h. Should the patient be hypotensive with poor peripheral perfusion, the first litre of fluid should be given over 30–60 min. Sodium bicarbonate should be avoided unless the B.D. > 10 and/or the pH 7.1 or less. Fluid volume

Table 7. Summary of treatment of severe diabetic nonketotic hyperglycaemia

I.v. fluids   Set up C.V.P.
C.V.P. < 2 cm H_2O. Serum Na^+ > 150 mmol/l
$\frac{1}{5}$ N saline − 1 litre over 1 h then 1 litre 2-hourly until C.V.P. > 4.
C.V.P. < 2 cm H_2O. Serum Na^+ < 150 mmol/l
$\frac{1}{2}$ N saline − 1 litre over 1 h then $\frac{1}{5}$ N saline as above.
C.V.P. 4–12 cm H_2O
$\frac{1}{5}$ N saline approx 1 litre 4-hourly.
C.V.P. > 12 cm H_2O. No clinical or X-ray evidence of pulmonary oedema.
$\frac{1}{5}$ N saline as a fluid challange (Part 2, ch. II, p. 308) until C.V.P. > 12 cm then 1 litre
approx 8-hourly.
C.V.P. > 12 cm H_2O. L.V. overload present, proceed to—

Hypotonic peritoneal dialysis
Rate approx. 500 ml every 30 min. Observe serum K. B.G.
Maintain C.V.P. 4–10 cm H_2O with i.v. $\frac{1}{5}$ N saline.

Insulin soluble
B.G. < 25 mmol/l 16 units i.m. or i.v. stat. then 4 units i.v. or i.m. hourly.
B.G. > 25 mmol/l 20 units i.m. or i.v. stat. then 8 units i.v. or i.m. hourly.
Observe B.G. and Serum K. Stop insulin when B.G. 10 mmol or less.

Catheterise
Check u/p osmolality ratio. Urine output < 40 ml/h once C.V.P. normal and/or u/p
    osmolality rate 1.2 or less, start peritoneal dialysis.

Ryles tube
If gastric retention, aspirate and put down 15 ml 0.3 M sodium citrate.
Commence water 20 ml hourly – once able to absorb, slow down i.v. infusion.
Potassium
Once urine output > 40 ml/h give potassium at a rate of approx. 10–16 mmol/l
    (according to serum K^+)

Acidosis
Do *not* use sodium bicarbonate if serum Na > 150 mmol/l.
Do *not* give > 50 mmol i.v.
Dialyse if Se Na > 150 mmol pH < 7.1 or B.D. > 15.

Observe for vascular complications. Infection. Onset of renal failure. Deterioration of
    level of consciousness with respiratory depression. Hypokalaemia. Hypo-
    glycaemia.

Ventilation
Consider if gets respiratory depression, inadequate respiratory compensation for
    metabolic acidosis, convulsions uncontrolled with phenytoin sodium.

Check B.G. (Reflomat) hourly. B.G. Urea, electrolytes, Astrup 2–4 hourly.
Clotting factors – evidence of D.I.C. and clinical evidence of vascular occlusion,
    consider low doses of heparin.

replacement is commonly complicated by hypokalaemia and potassium replacement should be started as soon as the urine output is >40 ml/h. There must be frequent monitoring of the central venous pressure, blood pressure, urine output and plasma electrolytes. Renal failure may develop during metabolic correction and may necessitate peritoneal dialysis with a hypotonic solution (Table 3). It is important to assess clotting factors at the start of treatment and to look for any evidence of vascular occlusion. Arterial and venous thrombosis appears to be a particular hazard – mesenteric thrombosis (Whelton *et al.*, 1971) may require timely surgery. Tchertkoff and co-workers (1974) reported thrombosis of a cerebral artery and two patients with thrombosis of the mesenteric vessels. There was no record of clotting factors being performed. Clotting indices consistent with D.I.C. may be an indication for the use of low doses of heparin (see Part 2, ch. II, p. 366, Table 4).

REFERENCES

Alberti, K. G. M. M., Darley, J. H., Emerson, P. M., Hockaday, T. D. R. (1972). 2-3 diphosphoglycerate and tissue oxygenation in uncontrolled diabetes mellitus. *Lancet* **2**, 391.

Alberti, K. G. M. M., Hockaday, T. D. R. and Turner, R. C. (1973). Small doses of intramuscular insulin in the treatment of diabetic coma. *Lancet* **2**, 515.

Alberti, G. K. (1975). Comas in diabetes. *Medicine* **14**, Part 2, 640.

Allison, S. P., Prowse, K. and Chamberlain, M. J. (1967). Failure of insulin response to glucose load during operation and after myocardial infarction. *Lancet* **1**, 478.

Allison, S. P., Hinton, P. and Chamberlain, M. J. (1968). Intravenous glucose tolerance, insulin and free fatty acid levels in burned patients. *Lancet* **2**, 1113.

Arieff, A. I. and Carroll, H. J. (1972). Nonketotic hyperosmolar coma with hyperglycaemia; clinical factors, pathophysiology, renal function, acid base balance, plasma-cerebrospinal fluid equilibria and the effects of therapy in 37 cases. *Medicine* **51**, 73.

Barer, J., Hill, H., Hill, R. M. and Martinez, W. M. (1973). Fatal poisoning from salt used as an emetic. *Am. J. Dis. Child.* **125**, 889.

Carter, R. F. and Fotheringham, B. J. (1971). Fatal salt poisoning due to gastric lavage with hypertonic saline. *Med. J. Aust.* **1**, 539.

Charles, M. A. and Danforth, E. (1971). Nonketoacidotic hyperglycaemia and coma during intravenous diazoxide therapy in uraemia. *Diabetes* **20**, 501.

Chazan, B. L., Rees, S. B. and Balodinos, M. C. (1969). Dialysis in diabetics. *J. Amer. Med. Ass.* **209**, 2026.

Collins, J. V. and Harris, P. W. R. (1971). Non-keto-acidotic diabetic coma. *Post. Grad. Med. J.* (June Suppl.), 388.

Dorwart, W. V. and Chalmers, L. (1975). Comparison of methods for calculating serum osmolality from chemical concentrations and the prognostic value of such calculations. *Clin. Chem.* **21**, 190.

Editorial (1972). Hyperosmolal coma. *Lancet* **2**, 1071.

Fulop, M., Rosenblatt, A., Kreitzer, S. M. and Gerstenhaber, B. (1975). Hypersmolar nature of diabetic coma. *Diabetes* **24**, 594.

Glasser, L., Sternglanz, P. D., Combie, J. and Robinson, A. (1973). Serum osmolality and its applicability to drug overdose. *Am. J. Clin. Pathol.* **60**, 695.

Habel, A. H. and Simpson, A. H. (1975). Osmolar relation between C.S.F. and serum ion hyperosmolar hypernatraemic dehydration. *Arch. Dis. Child.* **80**, 331.

Harvey, R. M., Enson, Y. and Lewis, M. L. (1966). Haemodynamic effects of dehydration and metabolic acidosis in Asiatic cholera. *Trans. Ass. Amer. Physicians* **79**, 177.

Keller, V., Berger, W., Ritz, R. and Truog, P. (1975). Originals. Course and prognosis of 86 episodes of diabetic coma. *Diabetologica* **11**, 93.

Kidson, W., Carey, J., Kraegen, E. and Lazarus, L. (1974). Treatment of severe diabetes mellitus by insulin infusion. *Br. Med. J.* **2**, 691.

Matter, J. A., Weil, M. H., Shubin, H. and Stein, L. (1974). Cardiac arrest in the critically ill. II. Hyperosmolal states following cardiac arrest. *Amer. J. Med.* **56**, 162.

Maxwell, M. H. and Kleeman, C. R. (1972). *In* 'Diabetic Acidosis and Coma in Clinical Disorders of Fluid and Electrolyte Metabolism' p. 977. McGraw-Hill, New York.

Ng, M. L., Levy, M. N. and Zieske, H. A. (1967). Effects of changes of pH and of carbondioxide tension on left ventricular performance. *Amer. J. Physiol.* **213**, 115.

Nobis, H., Fischer, M., Fuchs, F. S. and Korp, W. (1972). Fibrinolysis and peritoneal dialysis in the treatment of diabetic coma, complicated by severe shock. *Diabetologia* **8**, 145.

Page, M. Mc.B., Alberti, K. G. M. M., Greenwood, R., Gumaa, K. A., Hockaday, T. D. R., Lowy, C., Nabarro, J. D. N., Pyke, D. A., Sönksen, P. H., Watkins, P. J. and West, T. E. T. (1974). Treatment of diabetic coma with continuous low-dose infusion of insulin. *Brit. Med. J.* **2**, 687.

Rocha, D. M., Sarteusario, F. and Faloona, G. R. (1973). Abnormal pancreatic-cell function in bacterial infections. *New Engl. J. Med.* **288**, 700.

Rosenberg, S. A., Brief, D. K., Kinney, J. M., Herresa, M. C., Wilson, R. F. and Moore, F. D. (1957). The syndrome of dehydration coma and severe hyperglycaemia without ketosis in patients convalescing from burns. *N. Engl. J. Med.* **272**, 931.

Semple, P. F., White, C. and Manderson, W. G. (1974). Continuous intravenous infusion of small doses of insulin in treatment of diabetic keto acidosis. *Brit. Med. J.* **2**, 694.

Sotos, J. F., Dodge, P. R., Meara, P. and Talbot, N. B. (1960). Studies in experimental hypertonicity: Pathogenesis of the clinical syndrome: Biochemical abnormalities and cause of death. *Paediatrics* **26**, 925.

Sotos, J. F., Dodge, P. R. and Talbot, N. B. (1962). Studies in experimental hypertonicity. II. Hypertonicity of body fluids as a cause of acidosis. *Paediatrics* **30**, 180.

Smith, H. W. (1951). *In* 'The Kidney: Structure and Function in Health and Disease' p. 308. Oxford University Press. New York.

Tchertkoff, V., Nayak, S. V., Kamath, C. and Solomon, M. I. (1974). Hyperosmolar nonketotic diabetic coma: vascular complications. *J. Amer. Ger. Soc.* **22**, 462.

Timperley, W. R., Preston, F. E. and Ward, J. D. (1974). Cerebral intravascular coagulation in diabetic ketoacidosis. *Lancet* **1**, 952.

Turner, R. C., Grayburn, J. A., Newman, G. B., Nabarro, J. D. N. (1971). Measurement of the insulin delivery rate in man. *J. Clin. Endocr. Metab.* **33**, 279.

Vinik, A., Seftel, H. and Joffe, B. I. (1970). Metabolic findings in hyperosmolar, non-ketotic diabetic stupor. *Lancet* **2**, 797.

Whelton, M. J., Walde, D. and Havard, C. W. H. (1971). Hyperosmolar nonketotic diabetic coma: with particular reference to vascular complications. *Brit. Med. J.* **1**, 85.

Yaffe, S. J. (1975). A clinical look at the problem of drugs in pregnancy and their effect on the foetus. *C.M.A.J.* **112**, 728.

Section 2: The Management of Hypoglycaemia

GILLIAN C. HANSON

PATHOPHYSIOLOGY

Hypoglycaemia exists when the blood glucose concentration is significantly below the lower limit of normal for the method used for analysis. It is important to know the lower limit of normality for your laboratory since they differ widely (see below). Plasma levels tend to be about 15% higher than whole blood values.

Method	Normal range (mmol/l)	Hypoglycaemia (mmol/l)
Somogyi–Nelson	3.3–5.6	2.5
Glucose-oxidase	3.0–5.3	2.5
Autoanalyser-ferricynide reduction		
Whole blood	3.6–6.0	2.8
Plasma	4.2–6.7	3.3

Hypoglycaemia is usually associated with symptoms of sweating, parasthesiae, visual disturbances, weakness and altered cerebral function – but these may be considerably modified in a patient sedated on a ventilator in an I.T.U. It has been postulated that the rate of fall of blood glucose may be more important than the absolute values. The blood glucose should be documented as being below the lower limit of normal and the patient's symptoms, clinical appearance (e.g. sweating), or level of consciousness, should improve with glucose administration. Diabetic patients with hypoglycaemia are rarely admitted to the I.T.U. unless there has been a prolonged period of hypoglycaemia complicated by cerebral oedema; prolonged hypoglycaemia is a well recognised complication of excessive oral hypoglycaemic therapy in a mild diabetic. One should be aware however that hypoglycaemia can be induced in the critically ill by excessive insulin administration, or by withdrawing a glucose source during insulin administration (e.g. stopping peritoneal dialysis). In certain circumstances the treatment of hypoglycaemia plays an essential part in the management of a medical condition.

Hypoglycaemic conditions which may be treated in the Intensive Therapy Unit are listed in Table 1. Patients with hypoglycaemia may

Table 1. Hypoglycaemic conditions which may be treated in the Intensive Therapy Unit

---

Hyperinsulinism due to islets cell neoplasm or hyperplasia

Hepatic disease:
    Generalised hypofunction
    Hereditary fructose intolerance
    Impaired gluconeogenesis and other factors
    Ethanol infusion
    Shock

Endocrine disturbance:
    Anterior pituitary insufficiency
    Adrenocortical insufficiency
    Hypothyroidism – myxoedema coma

Drug induced:
    Administration of insulin excess
    Oral hypoglycaemics

Tumours especially of mesodermal origin

Chronic renal failure

---

be admitted to the intensive therapy unit for management of convulsions or the suspected diagnosis of some form of cerebrovascular accident. Hypoglycaemia in hereditary fructose intolerance may be precipitated by using frucrose as an intravenous source of carbohydrate. Ethanol ingestion or infusion may be complicated by hypoglycaemia particularly in starving non-obese subjects. Glucose utilisation under such circumstances appears to be increased and this is associated (presumably through impaired gluconeogenesis) with an inhibition of supply (Searle *et al.*, 1974).

Alterations in carbohydrate metabolism have long been known to produce an important role in the host defence mechanism against shock induced by stresses such as endotoxin shock and gram negative sepsis.

The precise mechanism is unknown but is probably related to a defect in responsiveness to glucocorticoid permissive control of glucogenesis; a defect in induction or function of the gluconeogenic enzymes or some other impairment of liver cell metabolism (Filkins and Cornell, 1974). Hypoglycaemia is rarely encountered in humans in shock but occasionally the blood glucose is found to be close to the hypoglycaemic level, especially in patients suffering from severe sepsis.

Endocrine deficiency (see Table 1) may be associated with hypoglycaemia. Adrenal insufficiency may be associated with hypoglycaemia as a consequence of inadequate gluconeogenesis. Hypoglycaemia in patients with hypothyroidism is usually restricted to episodes of myxoedema coma.

Hypoglycaemia may complicate the presence of a sarcoma of fibrous nervous tissue origin (Field, 1963). Such tumours are commonly located in the retroperitoneal area but have also been found in the thorax or peritoneal cavity.

Chronic renal insufficiency may also be complicated by hypoglycaemia and it has been postulated that this is related to inadequate glycogenolysis (Brock and Rubenstein, 1970).

TREATMENT

Blood glucose should be routinely measured in all unconscious patients. The Dextrostix estimation (using the Ames reflectance meter) is reliable for estimation of blood glucose in the lower range. If there is any possibility that hypoglycaemia is the cause of the comatose state, then an intravenous bolus of 20–50 ml of 50% glucose should be given. Glucagon 1.0 mg i.m. may be given as an alternative but should not be used in an intensive care situation since it will not be effective if the glycogen stores are depleted.

The blood glucose level should be monitored closely after recovery since the patient may become hypoglycaemic again. Insulin should not be considered until the blood glucose is 12 mmol/l or more and should then only be given with careful glucose monitoring.

Hypoglycaemic coma secondary to oral hypoglycaemic drug therapy may be prolonged, the patient becoming rousable during glucose infusion. In this condition, and in those patients where a long acting insulin, or prolonged insulin-like effect is suspected, glucose should be given by continuous infusion, the dosage being titrated in order to maintain a blood glucose at 6 to 10 mmol/l.

REFERENCES

Brock, M. D. and Rubenstein, A. H. (1970). Spontaneous hypoglycaemia in diabetes with renal insufficiency. *J.A.M.A.* **213**, 1863.

Field, J. B. (1963). Differential diagnosis of hypoglycaemia. *Tex. Med.* **71**, 65.

Filkins, J. P. and Cornell, R. P. (1974). Depression of hepatic gluconeogenesis and the hypoglycaemia of endotoxic shock. *Amer. J. Physiol.* **227**, 778.

Searle, G. L., Sharnes, D., Cavaleri, R. R., Bagdade, J. D. and Porte, D. Jr. (1974). Evaluation of ethanol hypoglycaemia in Man: turnover studies with C–6^{14}C glucose. *Metabolism* **23**, 1023.

IX

The Long-term Metabolic and Nutritional Management of the Critically Ill Patient

GILLIAN C. HANSON

INTRODUCTION AND SEQUENTIAL OBSERVATIONS

In this category are included patients who require metabolic care after the acute metabolic phase of their illness is over. A certain number of these patients will be able to absorb food and fluid via the Ryles tube but the majority will require fluid, electrolytes, vitamins and nutrition intravenously.

The acute phase of a serious illness is generally over after 2–3 days and subsequently metabolic balance has to be maintained in order to allow the patient to recover. Patients most commonly coming into this category are those with extensive sepsis in particular intraperitoneal, intestinal fistuli associated with severe fluid and electrolyte losses, extensive trauma in particular associated with chest or head injuries and rarer causes such as tetanus and pneumonia requiring long-term ventilation.

The patient with a severe initial catabolic state is less likely to survive a prolonged illness or further complications arising from the original illness unless nutrition and metabolic status is maintained as close as possible to requirements.

Sequential observations

In order to maintain the nutrition and metabolic status as close as

247

possible to normal, certain sequential observations and investigations are essential (Table 1).

Table 1. Sequential observations and investigations in the long-term metabolic and nutritional management of the critically ill patient

Essential *Daily*	Fluid balance B.U. electrolytes Blood glucose Acid-base status Hb. P.C.V.

Advisable
    Daily
	Body weight
	Clinical nitrogen balance (Lee, 1975)
	Faecal and urinary nitrogen estimations in the presence of severe
	    diarrhoea.
	Urine and plasma osmolality
	Serum creatinine
	Electrolyte analysis of urine and gastrointestinal loss (if
	    excessive)

3 × Weekly or
    more frequently
    when indicated
	Serum calcium
	Serum magnesium
	Serum inorganic phosphate
	Serum proteins
	W.B.C. and differential. Platelet count and prothrombin time

Once a fortnight
    (i.v. nutrition
    for longer than
    3 weeks)
	Serum iron
	Serum B_{12}
	Serum folate

PATIENT MANAGEMENT

Fluid volume control

Following a period of stress the volume of water excreted by the kidney is decreased and the ability of the patient to handle a fluid load diminished. This generally persists for 3–5 days and during this period great care must be taken not to overload the patient. The volume of fluid required can be assessed by observations of fluid balance, assessment of the volume of fluid lost through temperature and sweat (Tables 1 and 2, Part 1, ch. VII, Section 2) and sequential weighing. In the presence of severe gastrointestinal losses, hyperventilation with inadequate humidification of the inspiratory gases and extensive fluid loss from the skin surface (e.g. following burns); daily weighing and monitoring of the central venous pressure is essential.

Table 2. Mineral content per litre of Aminosol 10%

		Approximate daily requirements per kg/B.W. in adults
Sodium	136 mmol	1.0–1.4 mmol
Chlorine	118 mmol	1.3–1.9 mmol
Calcium	0.68 mmol	0.11 mmol
Magnesium	0.4 mmol	0.1–0.25 mmol
Phosphorus	18 mmol	0.15 mmol
Copper	0.45 µmol	0.07 µmol
Zinc	18.4 µmol	0.3 µmol

Bed weighing is a difficult procedure to perform accurately and requires nursing skill. If at all possible the bed should be weighed before the patient is placed upon it – otherwise the patient plus the bed can be weighed daily to obtain a 'running weight'. Bedding must be noted and not changed between weighings, and all bottles and tubing must be taken off the bed for weighing.

Bed weighing beds are unsuitable for an intensive therapy unit because of poor access to the patient and limited versatility. Bed weighing can be performed mechanically (Avery bed scales) or electronically by placing transducer pads beneath the four feet of the bed (Datex bed weighing system).

It is essential when performing sequential daily weighing to note fluctuations in the light of treatment and other observations – in particular fluid balance, central venous pressure, serum electrolytes and serum osmolality. A low serum sodium in the absence of overt sodium losses during the first four days following stress is generally due to water overload and not to a depletion of total body sodium.

Patients suffering from severe stress (e.g. trauma) complicated by sepsis are those that are maximally catabolic. Water released from combustion of fat and protein may not be excreted by the kidneys during the oliguric phase, sodium excretion is also minimal. Such patients may therefore initially gain weight unless fluid balance is carefully controlled. Initially therefore the serum sodium may be noted to fall because of dilutional hyponatraemia. These patients are markedly predisposed to pulmonary oedema – a situation compounded by a rapidly falling serum albumin. With careful fluid balance control and avoidance of sodium overload, catabolic patients should lose approximately 500 g daily for the first 2–3 days which may increase to

1.0 kg daily over the subsequent 5–7 days. Patients should certainly not be allowed to gain weight during the first 3 or 4 days following stress. Intravenous feeding is generally started within the first 4 days and if well tolerated (so that adequate calories can be given) should prevent further slight loss after the initial 7–10 days depending upon the severity of the catabolic response.

The urine output should be maintained above 40 ml/h once the oliguric phase is over to enable the kidney to excrete the high osmolar load associated with a catabolic state. Water depletion must be avoided since patients who have developed a decreased creatinine clearance following a period of hypotension or sepsis are markedly predisposed to the development of acute renal failure.

Electrolyte and acid base control

Once the acute metabolic changes have been corrected, maintenance necessitates electrolyte estimations of the fluid lost (e.g. in the urine and gastrointestinal tract) and allowances for extra demands for particular ions (e.g. increased potassium requirements during feeding with intravenous dextrose or during steroid or thiazide diuretic therapy). Assessment of vital organ function in particular the heart, liver and kidneys should be made early in order to adjust the electrolyte requirements. The basal electrolyte requirements for a patient on long term nutrition either intravenously or via the gastrointestinal tract, is summarised in Table 2.

The average range of electrolyte concentrations in mmol/l of intestinal fluids in normal adults is shown in Table 7, Part 1, ch. VII, Section 2.

Stomach aspirate can generally be replaced with normal saline whilst watery diarrhoea can be replaced with $\frac{1}{5}$ or $\frac{1}{2}$ normal saline. Inadequate sodium maintenance is unusual unless inaccurate estimates are made of the volume lost in secretions which cannot be collected accurately e.g. sweat or bowel fistuli. Serum sodium must be observed carefully since the catabolic patient may gradually become hypernatraemic because of inappropriate use of sodium containing solutions to replace water losses. Hypernatraemia may also develop if the patient is hyperventilating in a dry environment and from evaporation through an area of skin loss (e.g. burns).

Potassium requirements may be extremely high in the presence of a small intestinal fistula or watery diarrhoea. These requirements have to be added to the average daily electrolyte requirements in the absence of excessive losses. It is essential that the ions are given in an adequate volume of fluid so that if an excess of an ion is given (e.g. sodium), there is sufficient water to enable it to be excreted by the kidney. Potassium and phosphate demands radically increase once glucose feeding is commenced. Glucose feeding should not be started until the serum potassium is above 3.5 mmol/l. A persistent metabolic alkalosis in the presence of a low/normal/serum potassium 3.2–3.5 mmol/l may be indicative of total body potassium depletion.

Large volumes of gastric aspirate if inadequately replaced with chloride may lead to an alkalosis.

Patients under stress are inclined to become acidotic – this may be related to inadequate peripheral perfusion and hence the production of excessive quantities of lactate, the use of fructose solutions or the use of amino acid solutions containing excess cationic amino acids. The patient with low gastrointestinal losses also tends to become acidotic. A mild metabolic acidosis can generally be corrected with small quantities (50–100 mmol) of sodium bicarbonate given daily. A persistent and increasingly severe metabolic acidosis associated with an anionic gap $(([Na^+] + [K^+]) - ([Cl^+] + [HCO_3^-]))$ of greater than 20 mmol/l, should make one look for a source of lactate (see Table 4, p. 206) or the insidious onset of renal failure (see Part 1, ch. IV). Should all these factors be excluded then the fluid electrolyte and nutritional regimen should be carefully reviewed.

Calcium supplements are not required if the patient is able to take food or calcium-containing fluids orally within one week of an acute illness. Exceptions include patients suffering from acute pancreatitis or severe losses of gastrointestinal fluid, and patients who were on calcium supplements or may have been calcium depleted before the onset of the acute illness. Apart from the latter, it is rare for the serum calcium levels to fall until late, in patients dependent upon intravenous fluids, because of the large calcium skeletal reserves. A continuous calcium supply is important in order to rebuild the skeleton and to maintain normal cell membrane permeability and nerve cell excitability. The daily calcium losses in an adult are approximately 8 mmol (320 mg) equivalent to 0.11 mmol/kg body weight. These losses may be increased through immobilisation or excessive gastrointestinal losses. Wretlind (1972) recommends 0.11 mmol daily per kg body weight for basal requirements – to this value should be added any losses above the normal (approximately 3 mmol) lost from the gastrointestinal tract. Calcium supplements should be started within 10 days in patients who are unable to take calcium orally and even earlier in patients with

Table 3. Additives which may be required during intravenous feeding in adults

	Dose and frequency	Route
Magnesium sulphate 50% 2.0 mmol Mg^{++}/ml	According to serum magnesium Maintenance requirement approx. 0.1–0.25 mmol/kg B.W. daily	i.m.
Calcium gluconate 10% 0.25 mmol Ca^{++}/ml or Calcium chloride 10% 0.45 mmol Ca^{++}/ml	According to serum calcium and maintenance requirement in the presence of a normal serum calcium	i.v. in carbohydrate solution
Sodium bicarbonate 8.4% 1 mmol HCO_3^-/ml 1 mmol Na^+/ml	According to acid base balance urine and plasma sodium levels	i.v.
DiPotassium hydrogen phosphate (K_2HPO_4) 2 mmol K^+/ml 1 mmol HPO_4^-/ml	According to serum phosphate and maintenance requirements. Allow for phosphate given in Intralipid and/or Aminosol	i.v. in carbohydrate solution
Potassium chloride 15% 2 mmol K^+/ml	According to serum potassium According to acid base status and potassium losses	i.v. in carbohydrate solution

excessive calcium losses. Calcium may be given intravenously as calcium chloride or gluconate (see Table 3) and may be added to the dextrose or saline infusion or given as Electrolyte Solution A (available on special request from Travenol Ltd. (see Table 11 for electrolyte content)).

Magnesium deficiency in patients on long-term intravenous therapy has been well documented (Paymaster, 1975) and should be prevented by supplementation within 10 days of commencing intravenous fluids. As with calcium therapy, magnesium supplements should be started earlier in patients with pancreatitis or severe gastrointestinal fluid losses. Wretlind (1972) recommends a basal supply of 0.1–0.25 mmol/kg of magnesium daily. The requirements for patients with severe gastrointestinal losses is higher and 12.5 mmol/day in an adult seems to be more realistic (Lee, 1974).

Magnesium is generally administered on a long-term basis as intramuscular magnesium sulphate (see Table 3), or as Electrolyte Solution A (see Table 11).

Phosphate supplements are rarely required during long-term intravenous therapy provided the protein hydrolysate Aminosol 10% is used as a source of nitrogen (approx. 18 mmol phosphorus per litre).

The phosphorus present in the Intralipid solution as phospholipid (15 mmol phosphorus per litre of 20% intralipid) may not be as freely available as once thought. Supplementation may therefore be needed with dipotassium hydrogen phosphate injection given in the carbohydrate infusion (Table 3), or as Electrolyte Solution B (see Table 11). This is particularly so when the dextrose insulin regime is being used or when pure crystalline amino acids without addition of phosphate are being used as a nitrogen source. Under conditions of severe catabolism when the insulin dextrose regime is being used together with a pure crystalline L-amino acid 15–30 mmol of phosphate may be required daily *in addition* to that present in Intralipid.

The requirements for trace metals for long-term intravenous therapy in adults is uncertain. It is probable that the trace metal supply is of particular importance during the intravenous feeding of infants and young children and may be also of importance when intravenous feeding or feeding via the Ryles tube is continued for more than two to four weeks. Wretlind (1972) uses the 'Addamel electrolyte solution' to replace trace metals (KabiVitrum Ltd) but other workers (Dudrick and Ruberg, 1971) have successfully used plasma for this purpose. 500 ml of dried plasma or fresh blood infused weekly should supply an adequate quantity of trace metals. Aminosol 10% also contains trace metals and phosphorus, which is absent from the crystalline amino acid preparation Vamin (see Table 2).

Table 4. Vitamin and haematinic requirements during nutritional management of the critically ill adult patient

Substance	Dose	Frequency	Route
Parenterovite	amps 1 and 2 h.p.	daily	i.v. as a bolus
Vit. K_1	5–10 mg	weekly	i.m.
Folinic acid	3–6 mg	daily	i.m.
Vit. B_{12}	500 μg	weekly	i.m.
Vit. D	1000 i.u.	weekly	i.m.
Iron (Imferon)	25–50 mg	weekly	i.m.

Zinc (Underwood, 1971) and copper deficiency (Mills, 1972) have been well documented in children. Zinc is involved in a wide range of cellular activities and is vitally concerned with the fundamental processes of R.N.A. and protein synthesis. Zinc may play a significant role in wound healing (Pories *et al.*, 1967), a deficiency should therefore be avoided. The daily zinc requirements are unknown, Wretlind (1972) suggesting that in adults 0.3 μmol per kg body weight should be supplied daily. This can be readily given as a litre of Aminosol 10% (Table 2) infused daily.

Vitamins

The water soluble and fat soluble vitamin requirements have been discussed in detail by Wretlind (1972, 1974). These are now available as Vitlipid and Solivito (KabiVitrum Ltd.). Their content is preferable to those recommended in Table 4 and is shown in Table 5. Ten ml of Vitlipid should be added to the Intralipid solution daily. The lypholised water soluble preparation Solivito should be dissolved in 10 ml of 5% dextrose solution and then added daily to the glucose solution being used for intravenous nutrition. At present vitamins in this country are

Table 5. Fat soluble and water soluble vitamin preparations to be used daily when intravenous feeding is being continued for more than two weeks

VITLIPID for adult		
Vitamin A (as retinol acetate)	0.75 mg retinol	
Vitamin D (as calciferol)	3 µg (120 i.u.)	
Vitamin K$_1$	0.15 mg	
Soybean oil	1000 mg	
Egg-yolk phosphatides	120 mg	
Glycerol	250 mg	
Aq. steril. ad	10 ml	
SOLIVITO (lyophilised)[1]		
Thiamine	1.2 mg as mononitrate	1.236 mg
Riboflavine	1.8 mg as Na-riboflavine phosphate	2.466 mg
Nicotinamide	10 mg as nicotinamide	10 mg
Pyridoxine	2 mg as pyridoxine chloride	2.431 mg
Folic acid	0.2 mg as folic acid	0.2 mg
Vitamin B$_{12}$	2 µg as cyanocobalamin	2 µg
Pantothenic acid	10 mg as sodium pantothenate	11.0 mg
Biotin	0.3 mg as biotin	0.3 mg
Ascorbic acid	30 mg as sodium ascorbate	34 mg
	amino-acetic acid (as body)	100 mg

[1] Some of the water soluble vitamins become inactivated on exposure to light. Solivito should be infused in the dextrose solution – the solution being shielded from light by the use of tinfoil over the container.

generally supplied as parenterovite 1 and 2 high potency ampoules – 1 of each being given intravenously daily. To this should be added vitamin D, approximately 2 i.u. per kg body weight intramuscularly and vitamin K$_1$ approximately 2 µg per kg body weight daily

(Wretlind, 1972). Both these vitamins are generally given weekly or twice weekly (Table 4). The dosage of vitamin K_1 administered is generally greater than the recommended requirement.

Haematinics (Table 4)

Vitamin B_{12} can be given as 500 µg i.m. weekly and folic acid is generally given intramuscularly as folinic acid 3–6 mg daily. Folate deficiency is becoming increasingly recognised. It may initially manifest as a pancytopenia, a megaloblastic marrow and/or a haemorrhagic diathesis secondary to thrombocytopenia. Patients particularly prone to this condition are patients receiving folate antagonists (e.g. trimethoprim in 'Bactrim' or 'Septrin' and phenytoin), patients losing excessive quantities of folate during renal dialysis, patients already depleted of folate prior to the onset of the acute illness, e.g. pregnancy malabsorption states, and patients receiving ethanol preparations during intravenous feeding (Wardrop *et al.*, 1975). Patients at risk who are unable to absorb an oral diet within three days of the onset of their acute illness should be commenced on intramuscular folinic acid and vitamin B_{12}. Thrombocytopenia with bleeding is a serious complication, the platelets rarely increasing for 3–7 days after starting therapy – during this period platelet infusions may be required in order to stop the bleeding. Leucopenia may also be present.

The quantity of folic acid available in Solivito (Table 5) is probably inadequate for patients already folate depleted or in patients who may be losing excessive quantities.

The administration of iron during prolonged intravenous nutrition is of particular importance since the iron reserves of the body are usually very small. The iron requirements are approximately 2.8 mg daily in menstruating women and approximately 1 mg daily for other adult patients. It is general to give approximately 2.8 mg daily during intravenous nutrition (Table 4), this being given as a weekly intramuscular injection.

NUTRITION

Introduction

A patient is unlikely to survive if they lose more than 30 per cent of their total body nitrogen during an acute illness. Following no food intake, a person may lose a third of their total body nitrogen in 15–25 days following major surgery and in 5–20 days following a major burn. The rapid onset of negative nitrogen balance leads to delayed wound healing, hypoproteinaemic oedema, and an increased susceptibility infection.

It is imperative therefore that nutrition should be started as soon as metabolic and fluid balance has been appropriately corrected. This can generally be started within 3 days of the onset of the acute illness. Feeding if at all possible should be via the gastrointestinal tract but generally in the critically ill, nutrition has to be commenced intravenously, intravenous feeding being steadily decreased as gastrointestinal absorption increases.

Intravenous nutrition

The aim of intravenous nutrition is to provide adequate calories and nutrients to maintain nitrogen balance in a specific patient. Its use is only indicated when oral or tube feeding (via the oesophagus, gastroenterostomy or jejeunostomy) is contraindicated or is inadequate.

Routes of administration

In the critically ill administration via a central vein is generally necessary, this also enables recording of the right atrial pressure. The use of a central venous catheter decreases the complications of venous thrombosis and thrombophlebitis but increases the risk of serious infection. The incidence of infection has been correlated with the duration the catheter remains in place (Schils, 1972). The catheter should be inserted by an experienced operator by a sterile non-touch technique. The catheter site should be cleaned with povidone-iodine before and after insertion – and sealed with a quickly drying plastic wound dressing such as Nobecutane or Op-site spray (antibiotic ointment may encourage the growth of fungi).

The site of insertion depends upon the availability of veins and the experience of the operator. The use of the subclavian vein should be avoided if at all possible in a patient on a volume cycled ventilator. A catheter inserted via the subclavian vein is found easier to manage, is more likely to enter the right atrium and because of the catheter length is less likely to become blocked. The method should not be used by an inexperienced operator since the incidence of complications is higher than that with antecubital vein catheterisation (pneumothorax, extravasation of fluid into the pleural cavity, arterial puncture, air embolism). The technique has been described by other workers (Dudrick and Wilmore, 1968; Yoffa, 1965).

In patients where intravenous feeding is unlikely to be prolonged for more than six weeks it is wise to change the catheter weekly. This is particularly important in septicaemic patients where the catheter tip may become secondarily infected thereby perpetuating the septicaemia. The catheter should also be changed whenever there is evidence of inflammation at the site of insertion, thrombophlebitis or fever where no other source of sepsis can be found. The catheter tip should always be cultured after removal – positive tip cultures may on occasions be difficult to interpret. Growth of *Candida*, *Staphylococcus alkus* or a bacteroides species in the absence of any constitutional upset may warrant careful observation without therapy. Where multiple intravenous injections are required it is preferable to give these via a peripheral vein drip keeping the central vein for feeding and monitoring of right atrial pressure.

Nutrient solutions

Calories should be sufficient to maintain weight for the adult patient under resting conditions, approximately 0.13 mJ/kg body weight (30 kcal/kg body weight) daily and to this should be added initially approximately 50 per cent more than the calculated value for resting metabolism. An additional number of calories should be added of approximately 0.013 mJ (3 kcal) daily per kg body weight per degree centigrade rise of body temperature above normal. The adequacy of calorie provision should be assessed according to daily or alternate day bed weighing and initially on estimated protein requirements (Table 8) with the knowledge that 0.65–0.87 mJ (150–200 kcal) should be provided per gram of nitrogen infused.

1 Carbohydrate solutions
Glucose is the carbohydrate solution of choice being the normal physiological substrate and essential for cerebral metabolism. Glucose tolerance is decreased following stress and glucose monitoring is essential in order to avoid serious complications such as hyperosmolar nonketotic hyperglycaemia coma (Wynick *et al.*, 1970), a metabolic acidosis (Winters *et al.*, 1964), convulsions secondary to acute osmotic changes and an osmotic diuresis with attendant sodium, potassium and water depletion.

Fructose offers no advantage, its use may be complicated by a lactic acid acidosis (Bergström *et al.*, 1968) and since the critically ill tends to have a metabolic acidosis, should not be initially used in patient management. Fructose infusions can decrease serum phosphate levels and raise lactate, bilirubin and urate levels (Schumer, 1970).

Sorbitol can only be utilised after its prior conversion to fructose in the liver and should therefore not be used in the management of the critically ill. It is also a powerful osmotic diuretic and has a greater tendency to produce dehydration than glucose in patients with liver disease, suggesting that the oxidation of sorbitol is impaired in hepatocellular failure (Lee *et al.*, 1972).

2 *Alcohol*

Ethanol is sometimes used as a source of calories, no more than 1.5 g/kg body weight should be given daily; even this dosage in the elderly may raise the blood alcohol level above 30 mg/100 ml when harmful pharmacological effects may be anticipated (Coats, 1972). Increasing evidence for a direct pharmacological effect on the liver cell makes its use questionable (Rubin and Lieber, 1971).

3 *Amino acids*

Amino acids are used in the body for protein synthesis and glyconeogenesis. Maximal utilisation requires a concomitant supply of energy, feeding should therefore not be commenced with amino acids. Kinney (1972) found that noncatabolic patients require 0.83 mJ (200 kcal) per gram of nitrogen, while 0.31 to 0.63 mJ (75 to 150 kcal) per gram of nitrogen appears sufficient in the catabolic patient in order to allow for optimal utilisation of amino acids for protein synthesis. Protein needs vary with age and the method of metabolism depends upon the route and rate of administration. Oral supply leads to absorption in the intestine and transport to the liver where they may be used for protein synthesis, but rapid absorption may lead to production of urea – making the amino acids unavailable for protein synthesis. Intravenous supply leads to a rapid distribution to all tissues where they may be transported to cells and directly used for protein synthesis. It has been found that the nitrogen requirements in different diseases is identical whether given orally or intravenously (Bergström *et al.*, 1972).

Adults require approximately 25% of the total nitrogen supply as essential amino acids (Furst *et al.*, 1970) exceeding this percentage in adults does not seem to be beneficial. It seems unlikely that this percentage will increase in catabolic states where the total nitrogen requirements are vastly increased. Studies are required to determine the proportions of essential amino acids yielding maximal utilisation for protein synthesis in different clinical situations. This may be of even greater importance in infants where the essential amino acid requirement is approximately 43% of the total nitrogen intake for maximal nutritional effect (Munro, 1972).

Efficient utilisation of essential amino acids for protein synthesis requires a supply of non-essential amino acids. The results of chromatographic studies on the urine suggest that the composition of the non-essential amino acids is as important as that of the essential amino acids (Tweedle, 1975). Excessive quantities of glycine in a solution may produce a rise in blood ammonia, it also tends to get excreted in the urine. Previous studies on oral feeding suggest that nitrogen balance can be improved by the addition of glutamic acid. Histidine and arginine should be considered semi-essential amino acids – histidine may not be synthesised in sufficient amounts during growth and regeneration (Synderman et al., 1959) and arginine has been found to reduce the blood ammonia rise produced by an infusion of essential amino acids (Fahey, 1957). Amino acid solutions containing an excess of cationic amino acids such as lysine, arginine and histidine may precipitate a metabolic acidosis whereas anionic amino acids such as glutamic and aspartic acids would tend to prevent this. It is therefore wise to find a solution providing a broad spectrum of non-essential amino acids when considering intravenous amino acid feeding.

For the synthesis of body proteins, only L-amino acids (except for D-methionine and D-phenylalanine) can be utilised. Intravenous amino acid can be provided as a casein hydrolysate Aminosol, or as pure crystalline laevorotatory amino acids. Tweedle (1973) compared post-operative nitrogen balance studies using various amino acid solutions. He concluded that Aminosol was as effective as the synthetic L-amino acid solutions Vamin and Aminoplex and better than Aminofusin in improving postoperative nitrogen balance. Aminosol has the disadvantage in containing a high ammonium content and peptides and therefore should not be used in patients with hepatic or renal insufficiency. Aminosol also contains a high concentration of sodium ions and should be avoided where renal handling of sodium is diminished. In adults requiring intravenous nutrition, Aminosol (which also contains many essential ions see Table 2) is the amino acid solution of choice except in the above situations when the pure crystalline laevorotatory amino acid preparation Vamin is probably the most convenient and best amino acid solution available at present.

A comparison of some of the amino acid solutions at present available is summarised in Table 6.

4 Fats

Fat emulsions have proven to be an excellent source of calories, the solutions are iso-osmolar and of neutral pH and are not lost in the urine or faeces. Phospholipids, cholesterol and fatty acids have an important structural function in maintaining membranes of all cells and sub-cellular units. Some dietary lipids have an important function in the regulation of body homeostasis, for example, the production of prostaglandins. Fat emulsions are probably a source of inorganic phosphate in the form of phospholipid (see p. 253). The fat emulsions available contain either cotton seed oil or soya bean oil and are nontoxic. The fat in the cotton seed oil preparations however accumulates in the reticulo endothelial cells and may reduce antibody formation (Lemperle *et al.*, 1970), whereas similar to natural chylomicrons, this was found not to be so with the soya bean oil preparation Intralipid. Huth *et al.* (1967) also found a decreased tolerance against *E. coli* endotoxin associated with hypercoagulation when Lipofundin (a cotton seed oil preparation) was used. After Intralipid infusion only insignificant effects were found. In view of these findings and the lack of toxicity experienced when a soya bean preparation is used for long-term nutrition, Intralipid appears to be the preparation of choice.

Hallberg (1965) found that adult subjects who had been fasting overnight cleared 3.8 g of fat as Intralipid per kg body weight in 24 h. This clearance rate appears to increase in subjects fasted for longer periods. The critically ill patient will generally tolerate 2–4 g of fat/kg as Intralipid infused over 24 h. The plasma should be viewed visually prior to giving a further infusion of Intralipid; should the plasma be clear the elimination capacity is not overloaded and a further infusion can be commenced. Until further experience is available, Intralipid should not be used in patients with hepatocellular failure, a haemorrhagic diathesis, a deficiency of lipoprotein lipase or hyperlipidaemia (Fredrikson type 1). The tolerance to fats appears to be diminished in patients with hepatic disease and in patients with extensive sepsis.

The practical aspects of intravenous nutrition and maintenance of metabolic balance

Intravenous feeding can be commenced once the initial metabolic disorder has been corrected, cellular and organ perfusion has been established as adequate and hepatic, renal, cardiac and pulmonary

Table 6. A comparison of some of the amino acid solutions at present available

Preparation	Constituents	N content per litre (g)	Remarks
Amigen 800	Casein hydrolysate 5% Ethanol 2.5% Fructose 12.5%	6.0	Ethanol and fructose contraindicated in the critically ill Contains peptides and ammonia ⎫ contra-indicated in renal or hepatic failure
Aminosol 10%	Casein hydrolysate 10%	12.8	High sodium content Contains peptides and ammonia High phosphate content (see Table 2) ⎭
Aminofusin forte	Synthetic L-amino acids	15.2	High glycine content. Therapeutic efficacy awaited
Aminoplex 14	Synthetic L-amino acids	13.4	Possible excess of lysine, arginine and glycine
Fre Amine	Synthetic L-amino acids	12.5	Has to be mixed with glucose – may develop glucose intolerance No glutamic acid
Synthamin 14	Synthetic L-amino acids	14.3	Contains phosphate Therapeutic efficacy awaited
Vamin N	Synthetic L-amino acids	9.4	Well utilised No phosphate or zinc (as in protein hydrolysates)

function has been assessed. Once fluid volume and metabolic deficiencies have been corrected subsequent electrolyte requirements can be added to the dextrose infusion or if large volumes of fluid are required above calorific requirements, may be added to normal saline or dextrose saline. The basal electrolyte requirements are summarised in Table 2 and to this must be added excess losses as sweat, fluid from the gastrointestinal tract (Tables 2 and 7, Part 1, ch. VII, section 2, respectively) and urine. It is important to give an adequate volume of fluid which should be 2500–3000 ml daily in a patient without excessive losses and in the absence of renal failure. Many of the feeding solutions are hypertonic (see Table 7) and therefore time must be given for them to be metabolised – urine glucose estimations may not reflect hyperglycaemia in the critically ill and serial blood glucose estimations are indicated when starting glucose feeding.

Table 7. Osmolalities of some intravenous solutions (plasma approximately 298 mosm/kg body water)

Solution	Water (mosm/kg)
Normal saline	308
10% Intralipid	280
20% Intralipid	330
10% glucose	523
50% glucose	3800
Aminosol 10%	925
Vamin glucose	1275

Observations should be conducted as suggested in Table 1. Provided these observations are taken the well recognised complications arising during intravenous feeding should not arise, these include –

> The hyperosmolar syndrome
> Metabolic acidosis
> Hypokalaemia, Hypomagnesaemia, Hypocalcaemia, Hypophosphataemia
> Water depletion or overload

Provided vitamins and haematinics are supplied according to Table 4 or Table 5, folate deficiency and vitamin deficiencies should not arise. Should the vitamin preparations mentioned in Table 5 be used – iron as Imferon should be given intramuscularly weekly in a dose of 25–50 mg. Serial folate estimations should be performed weekly in patients on renal dialysis and folate and iron estimations once a fortnight in patients on intravenous feeding for longer than three weeks. In critically ill septic patients fresh blood is often required in spite of these measures in order to maintain an adequate haemoglobin level. The haemoglobin level should be maintained between 7 and 10 g/100 ml. Mild anaemia may occur following prolonged administration of Intralipid (Jacobson, 1970). Intravenous feeding should commence with a 40 or 50% solution of dextrose. 40–50 g should be infused at a rate of not greater than 0.5 g/kg body weight per hour – a blood glucose should be performed before and one hour after the infusion has finished. Glucose should not be infused until the blood glucose is less than 12 mmol and should the level be between 8 and 12 mmol, 1 unit of soluble insulin should be added to the glucose solution in a ratio of 1 unit per 4 g of glucose. 20–40 mmol of potassium chloride is added per 40 g of dextrose infused – this has to be adjusted according to serial potassium levels, renal function and the potassium losses. In patients with severe glucose intolerance and blood glucose levels running at greater than 12 mmol, it is advisable to control the blood glucose with appropriate intra-muscular injections of soluble insulin at 2-hourly to 4-hourly levels and also to use insulin with the high glucose infusion. The ratio of insulin to glucose may have to be increased to as high as 4 units per 1 g of glucose infused. This situation particularly applies when continuous peritoneal dialysis is being performed where 200–300 g of glucose may be absorbed daily via the peritoneal membrane. It has been found that the insulin dextrose regime reduces the catabolic response in conditions of severe stress (Hinton et al., 1971), may limit the rise of urea and potassium in acute renal failure and produce a sodium diuresis in critically ill patients with sodium overload (Allison, 1976).

100–150 g of glucose is infused in 40–50 g alliquots in the first day – gradually increasing to 200–400 daily over the subsequent three days. In situations where calcium, magnesium and phosphate ions are required, glucose may be infused as Electrolyte Solution A or Electrolyte Solution B (see Table 11).

The protein requirements in diseases likely to be seen in the intensive therapy unit have been summarised by Munro (1974) see Table 8. Protein should follow the carbohydrate infusion and may be given as Aminosol 10%, Aminosol glucose, Vamin N or Vamin glucose depending upon calorific requirements, sodium and glucose tolerance and the condition being treated. The amino acid solution is generally infusion via a Y connector in conjunction with the Intralipid solution. Nitrogen balance studies should be conducted over the subsequent week in order to establish that sufficient protein is being provided.

Table 8. Protein requirements in diseases likely to be seen in surgical practice (1 g N_2 = 6.25 g protein) (modified from Munro, 1974)

Normal adult
(a) Normal equilibrium 0.55–0.7 g/kg
(b) Normal intake 1–2 g/kg

Following severe injury, major operation, sepsis or burning
(a) Acute phase – 2–4 g/kg
(b) Convalescence approximately – 2 g/kg

Gastrointestinal disease
(a) Ulcerative colitis 1–1.4 g/kg
(b) Ileocaecostomy 1–1.4 g/kg

Liver disease
Acute hepatic encephalopathy – nil to begin with increasing to level of tolerance

Renal disease
Renal failure no dialysis 0.5 g/kg
Catabolic acute renal failure 1.0–2.0 g/kg

Occasionally when nitrogen losses are high, Synthamin 14 or Aminofusin forte may have to be used as the nitrogen source. Studies assessing amino acid utilisation of these solutions are awaited.

Clinical nitrogen balance can be calculated according to Lee and Hartley (1975) see Table 9. Referring to Table 9, 6.25 is the conversion factor for conversion of nitrogen loss to protein catabolism. The figures 6/5 (for non-treated patients and those receiving crystalline amino acids) and 4/3 (for patients receiving protein hydrolysates) is the allowance for non-urea nitrogen. The conversion factor is 28/60 for urea into nitrogen, the gram molecular weight of urea being 60 which contains 28 g of nitrogen. This method however does not account for severe gastrointestinal losses, which if present should be calculated separately. In the non-dialysed acute renal failure patients, the formula can be used, the rate of rise of urea assuming greater importance (Lee and Hartley, 1975). Clearly the formula is not applicable to patients undergoing dialysis. In hypercatabolic renal failure dialysis should be commenced early and 400 g of carbohydrate should be administered daily (assuming 150 g will be absorbed from the peritoneum on continuous peritoneal dialysis) in order to reduce the rate of rise of blood urea. Fat as Intralipid is generally infused with the amino acid solution via a Y connector (Fig. 1). During the first day only 500 ml 10% Intralipid should be infused (unless there are contraindications to its use, see p. 260) gradually increasing the quantity infused to the level of tolerance – 2–4 g/kg body weight of Intralipid being given daily. Should the patient be losing a lot of water, this can be given as 10%

Table 9. Clinical nitrogen balance (Lee and Hartley, 1975)

Protein catabolism   = urea excretion (g/24 h) $\times$ 6.25 $\times \frac{6}{5} \times \frac{28}{60}$
                = urea excretion (g/24 h) $\times$ 3.5 = A $\Big\}$ For untreated patients and those receiving crystalline amino acids

Protein catabolism   = urea excretion (g/24 h) $\times$ 6.25 $\times \frac{4}{3} \times \frac{28}{60}$
                = urea excretion (g/24 h) $\times$ 3.9 = A $\Big\}$ For patients receiving protein hydrolysates

Blood urea correction = change in blood urea[1] (g/l) $\times$ total body water (60% body weight in kg) $\times \frac{28}{60} \times$ 6.25
                = change in blood urea (g/l) $\times$ body weight (kg) $\times$ 1.8 = B

Urinary protein correction
(usually negligible)   = g/24 h = C

Total protein catabolism/24 h = A + B + C

[1]Applies only to rise in blood urea.

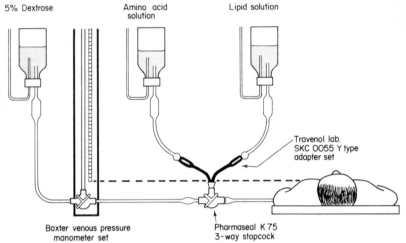

Fig. 1. Method of infusing amino acids and lipid solution via the central venous pressure line.

Intralipid instead of 20% Intralipid. No additives should be placed in the amino acid or Intralipid solutions. The rate of infusion of the amino acid Intralipid combination should be approximately 4 hours. Should the amino acid solution contain glucose – the level of blood glucose must be observed.

The energy requirements can be estimated according to p. 257, keeping in mind that approximately 0.63 mJ (150 kcal) are required per g of nitrogen infused and that 30% of the energy supplied should be

Table 10. Guide-lines for establishing an intravenous feeding regime in an adult

1 Provide protein according to Table 8.
2 Provide 0.65 mJ (150 calories)/g of nitrogen infused. (In an adult on a low protein diet provide at least 13 mJ (3000 calories)).
3 Provide 30% of calories as carbohydrate
4 Intralipid 2–4 g/kg body weight/24 h.
   (If Intralipid omitted because of contraindications to its use, ensure adequate replacement of phosphate.)
5 Provide approximately 5 mmol K^+/g nitrogen infused.
6 Ensure all electrolyte replacements are met.
7 Ensure fluid balance and acid base balance is correct.
8 Supply vitamins and haematinics.
9 Reassess requirements daily.
   (1 g N = 6.25 g protein)

as carbohydrate. The guide-lines for establishing an intravenous regime are summarised in Table 10; a suitable intravenous 24 hour regimen can be selected from Table 11.

Table 11. Five basic regimens for intravenous feeding in an adult (modified from Ellis et al., 1976)

Bottles		Contents/500 ml bottle	MJ	Water (ml)	Carbohydrate (g)	Nitrogen (g)	Fat	Na	K	Mg	Ca	PO$_4$
2		Vamin glucose[1]	1.36	460	50	4.7		25	10	0.8	1.3	
1		Aminosol 10%[1]	0.69	460		6.4		68	0.2			
1		Electrolyte Solution A with 20% w/v dextrose[2]	1.67	500	100					14	13	9
1		Electrolyte Solution B with 20% w/v dextrose[2]	1.67	500	100				30			30
1	1	Dextrose 50%	4.18	500	250							
1	1	Intralipid 20%[1,3]	4.18	400			100					
		Low sodium	10.24	2320	300	9.4	100	50	50	15.5	16	30
		Standard	9.57	2320	250	11.1	100	93	40	14.8	14	39
		Fat-free	9.57	2420	500	11.1		93	40	14.8	14	39
		Increased calories	13.75	2820	500	11.1	100	93	40	14.8	14	39
		Increased calories, low Na	14.42	2820	550	9.4	100	50	50	15.5	16	30

N.B. Electrolyte Solutions A and B should not be used in renal failure unless there is evidence of Ca^{++} Mg^{++} or PO_4^- depletion.

[1] KabiVitrum Ltd.
[2] Obtained by special request from Travenol Ltd.
[3] Contains phosphate as phospholpid (15 ml/l) which may not be freely available in the critically ill patient. Additives must not be added to this solution.

Energy 1 MJ = 239 Kcal.

Oral nutrition

Oral nutrition can rarely be started immediately in a critically ill patient but should be commenced as soon as is possible. The incidence of acute gastrointestinal haemorrhage from stress seems to have been reduced by the routine introduction of magnesium trisilicate mixture B.P. down the Ryles tube 4-hourly. Oral feeding should be commenced as soon as the gastric aspirate has decreased to less than 40 ml/h. Carbohydrate should be introduced initially in extremely low concentration. Caloreen* (an electrolyte free polyglucose polymer with weight for weight $\frac{1}{5}$ of the osmotic effect of glucose) should be initially introduced in a concentration of 20–50 g/l. One litre should be given (preferably by constant drip) over the first 24 h and gradually increased to 100 g/l. Once 100 g of Caloreen is tolerated Albumaid* (an hydrolysate of bovine serum proteins can be added) and progressively increased over the subsequent 7 days to the total estimated protein requirements, simultaneously increasing the oral fluid intake. At this stage the carbohydrate can be increased to total requirements and fat slowly added as medium triglyceride oil.* The following is an example of a feeding regime during the transition phase from intravenous to oral nutrition.

Via Ryles tube

100 g Albumaid
100 g Caloreen

Make up to 1000 ml with water given as a constant intragastric drip over 24 h.

Intravenous fluids
200 ml 40% dextrose, electrolytes and insulin if necessary
500 ml Aminosol 10%
500 ml Intralipid 20% } via Y connection
200 ml 40% dextrose + the above
500 ml Intralipid 20%

The final intravenous feeding solution to be stopped is generally Intralipid 20% – this can be given quite easily by peripheral vein.

Once on to feeding via the gastrointestinal tract, electrolytes and vitamins must be added. The same method can be applied to feeding via a gastrostomy or jejunostomy. It is essential not to increase the osmotic

* Scientific Hospital Supplies Limited.

load too rapidly otherwise the patient develops diarrhoea and losses of protein, fluid and potassium negate the effect of efficient gastro-intestinal feeding.

There seems to be little indication for the expensive elemental diets which arrive prepacked unless there are insufficient staff to make up a simple regime. On rare occasions the patient is able to take a liquid but not semi-solid diet orally – under these circumstances a liquid elemental diet may be more palatable than a liquid diet sent up from the diet kitchen.

REFERENCES

Allison, S. (1976). The metabolic response to injury. Metabolic disorders, No. 13, part 1. *Medicine*, second series, 608.

Bergström, J., Huttman, E. and Roch-Norlund, A. E. (1968). Lactic acid accumulation in connection with fructose infusion. *Acta Med. Scand.* **184**, 359.

Bergström, K., Blomstrand, R. and Jacobson, S. (1972). Long-term complete intravenous nutrition in man. *Nutr. Metab.* **14** (Suppl.) 118.

Coats, D. A. (1972). The place of ethanol in parenteral nutrition. *In* 'Parenteral Nutrition' (Ed. A. W. Wilkinson) p. 152. Churchill Livingstone, Edinburgh and London.

Dudrick, S. J. and Ruberg, R. L. (1971). Principles and practice of parenteral nutrition. *Medicine* **61** (6), 901.

Dudrick, S. J. and Wilmore, D. W. (1968). Long-term parenteral feeding. *Hosp. Practice* **3** (10), 65.

Ellis, B. W., Stanbridge, R. de L., Fielding, L. P. and Dudley, H. A. F. (1976). A rational approach to parenteral nutrition. *Brit. Med. J.* **1**, 1388.

Fahey, J. L. (1957). Toxicity and blood ammonia rise resulting from intravenous amino-acid administration in man. The protective effect of L-arginine. *J. of Clin. Invest.* **36**, 1647.

Furst, P., Jonsson, A., Josephson, B. and Vinnars, E. (1970). Distribution in muscle and liver vein protein of ^{15}N administered as ammonium acetate to man. *J. Appl. Physiol.* **29**, 307.

Hallberg, D. (1965). Studies on elimination of exogenous lipids from the blood stream. The effect of fasting and trauma in man on the elimination rate of a fat emulsion injected intravenously. *Acta. Physiol. Scand.* **65**, 153.

Hinton, P., Allison, S. P., Littlejohn, S. and Lloyd, J. (1971). Insulin and glucose to reduce catabolic response to injury in burned patients. *Lancet* **I**, 767.

Huth, K. W., Schoenborn, W. and Börner, J. (1967). Zur Pathogenese der Unverträglichkeitserscheinungen bei parenteraler Fettzufuhr. *Med. Ernahr* **8**, 146.

Jacobson, S. (1970). Complete parenteral nutrition in man for seven months. *In* 'Advances in Parenteral Nutrition from a Symposium Int. Soc. Parenteral Nutrition' (Ed. G. Berg) p. 6. Verlag, G.T., Stuttgart.

Kinney, J. M. (1972). Calories-nitrogen-disease and injury relationships. *In* 'Symposium on Total Parenteral Nutrition'. Sponsored by the Food Service Committee, Council on Foods and Nutrition of the American Medical Association, Nashville, Tennessee, Jan. 17–19.

Lemperle, G., Reichelt, M. and Deck, S. (1970). The evaluation of phagocytic activity in men by means of a lipid-clearing test. Abstract from 6th Int. Meeting of the Reticuloendothelial Society, p. 83.

Lee, H. A., Morgan, A. G., Waldram, R. and Bennett, J. (1972). Sorbitol: Some aspects of its metabolism and role as an intravenous nutrient. In 'Parenteral Nutrition' (Ed. A. W. Wilkinson) p. 121. Churchill Livingstone, Edinburgh and London.

Lee, H. A. (1974). Normal fluid and electrolyte requirements. In 'Parenteral Nutrition in Acute Metabolic Illness' (Ed. H. A. Lee) p. 108. Academic Press, London and New York.

Lee, H. A. and Hartley, T. F. (1975). A method of determining daily nitrogen requirements. Post. Grad. Med. J. 51, 441.

Mills, C. F. (1972). Some aspects of trace element nutrition in man. Nutrition 26, 357.

Munro, H. N. (1972). Basic concepts in the use of amino acids and protein hydrolysates for parenteral nutrition. In 'Symposium on Total Parenteral Nutrition'. Sponsored by the Food Service Committee, Council on Foods and Nutrition of the American Medical Association, Nashville, Tennessee, Jan. 17–19.

Munro, H. N. (1974). Protein metabolism in response to injury and other pathological conditions. Acta Anaesth. Scand. 55, (Suppl.) 81.

Passmore, R. (1969). Recommended intakes of nutrients from the United Kingdom reports on public health and medical subjects, No. 120, p. 34. Her Majesty's Stationery Office, London.

Paymaster, N. J. (1975). Post-operative Magnesium deficiency. Brit. J. Anaesth. 47, 85.

Pories, W. J., Henzel, J. H., Rob, C. G. and Strain, W. H. (1967). Acceleration of healing with zinc sulphate. Ann. Surg. 165, 432.

Rubin, E. and Lieber, C. S. (1971). Alcoholism, alcohol and drugs. Science 172, 1097.

Schils, M. E. (1972). Guidelines to total parenteral nutrition. J. Am. med. Ass. 220 (13), 1721.

Schumer, W. (1970). High caloric solutions in traumatised patients. In 'Body Fluid Replacement in the Surgical Patient' (Ed. G. G. Nahis and C. L. Fox, Jr.) p. 326. Grune and Stratton Inc., New York.

Synderman, S. E., Prose, P. H. and Holt, L. E. (1959). Histidine an essential amino acid for the infant. J. Dis. Child. 98, 459.

Tweedle, D. E. F. (1973). The effect of amino acid solutions of differing composition on the nitrogen balance of post-operative patients. J. Roy. Coll. Surg. Edinb. 18, 280.

Tweedle, D. (1975). Intravenous amino acid solutions. Brit. J. Hosp. Med. 13, 81.

Underwood, E. J. (1971). Zinc. In 'Trace Elements in Human and Animal Nutrition' (Ed. E. J. Underwood) p. 242. Academic Press, New York and London.

Wardrop, C. A. J., Heatley, R. V., Tennant, G. B. and Hughes, L. E. (1975). Acute folate deficiency in surgical patients on amino-acid/ethanol intravenous nutrition. Lancet 2, 640.

Winters, R. W., Scaglione, P. R., Nahas, G. G. and Verosky, M. (1964). The mechanism of acidosis produced by hyperosmotic infusions. J. Clin. Invest. 43, 647.

Wretlind, A. (1972). Complete intravenous nutrition. Nutr. Metabol. 14, (Suppl. 1).

Wretlind, A. (1974). Assessment of patient requirements. In 'Parenteral Nutrition in Acute Metabolic Illness' (Ed. H. A. Lee) p. 353. Academic Press, London and New York.

Wynick, W. J., Rea, W. J. and McClelland, R. N. (1970). Rare complications with intravenous hyperosmotic alimentation. J. Am. med. Ass. 211, 1697.

Yoffa, D. (1965). Supraclavicular venepuncture and catheterisation. Lancet 2, 614.

PART 2

Specific Management

1
Cardiac Arrest

GILLIAN C. HANSON

INTRODUCTION

Definition

Cardiac arrest can be defined as the sudden and often unexpected cessation of effective heart action with subsequent inadequate brain perfusion. This state is potentially curable for only four minutes in a previously healthy individual but the period is considerably lessened in patients with preceding hypoxia, impaired cardiac output, or brain perfusion.

Prevention of cardiac arrest

The prevention of cardiac arrest is an enormous subject and the discussion will therefore be limited to its prevention in patients who are already critically ill. Factors predisposing to cardiac arrest in the critically ill patient have been summarised by Camarata *et al.* (1971) and recognition and management of patients with depressed rhythmicity or conduction has been described in detail by Zoll (1971).

Heart disease

Factors predisposing to cardiac arrest
Cardiac arrest is most common in patients with heart disease; minor changes in blood volume, acid base status or blood oxygen tension in

273

such patients, is likely to precipitate a cardiac dysrhythmia. The blood pressure prior to the acute illness must be noted since a fall in the systolic pressure may lead to impairment of coronary artery perfusion. All patients, with a preceding history of heart disease should be monitored during surgery. Pain and anxiety is more likely to precipitate ventricular fibrillation in the patient with preceding cardiac disease.

Pulmonary embolism is a well recognised cause for cardiac arrest and is particularly likely to develop in patients who are on muscle relaxants for long-term ventilation. Heparin administration should be considered for all patients who are likely to be ventilated for more than one week.

Cardiac tamponade. Early recognition and appropriate treatment will prevent a cardiac arrest. Patients who are particularly predisposed to cardiac tamponade in the intensive therapy unit situation, include those who have had recent cardiac surgery, patients with chest injuries, and patients suffering from severe impact injuries, such as those due to high tension electricity, or bomb blast. Certain patients with extensive sepsis may develop cardiac tamponade, in particular following pneumococcal, staphylococcal and meningococcal infections. Various forms of pericarditis may also be complicated by tamponade.

Myocarditis. Patients with myocarditis are predisposed to serious dysrhythmias which may be precipitated by the introduction of catheters into the heart. Such cases include patients with meningococcal septicaemia (Korczyn *et al.*, 1971) and tetanus (Tsueda *et al.*, 1973).

Surgery. A third of all cases of arrest in the operating theatre happen during abdominal operations, and about a third during chest and/or heart operations (Nixon, 1965). Certain operative procedures are known to be particularly hazardous, e.g. operations where bone cement is used (Powell *et al.*, 1970) and orthopaedic procedures in patients known to have recently suffered from the fat embolism syndrome.

The incidence of arrest is increased in patients who are critically ill, and this is further magnified if a metabolic defect, hypoxia, blood volume changes or a cardiac dysrhythmia, is present or develops during an operation. All efforts should be made to correct these defects before surgery, and the patient should be monitored biochemically and electrocardiographically during surgery. Central venous pressure should be monitored throughout.

Drugs. Drugs can lead to arrest either through hypersensitivity (generally when the patient is ill or the heart is 'sick') or through direct depression on the heart muscle. The anaesthetic agents and drugs which may precipitate arrest have been summarised by Lorhan (1972). Drugs which cause particular concern when used in the very sick patient (particularly if hypertensive or in heart failure), include β-blockers, aminophylline (in particular when given into a central vein) (Camarata *et al.*, 1972), isoprenaline, adrenaline, lignocaine (Cheng and Wadhwa, 1973), edrophonium chloride (Gould *et al.*, 1971) and propanidid used for induction of anaesthesia (Jones, 1970). Certain drugs may produce metabolic changes which precipitate the arrest, such as the potassium rise induced by succinylcholine (Mazze *et al.*, 1969), or potassium penicillin G (Mercer and Logie, 1973) and potassium fall related to a thiazide diuretic, steroid therapy and the use of sodium bicarbonate.

Cardiac arrest may develop in a hypokalaemic patient on digoxin and patients on tricyclic antidepressants are markedly predisposed to arrhythmias (Williams, 1971). Ergometrine should be avoided in the obstetric patient with heart disease or hypertension (Browning, 1974).

Investigations. At least 5% of all arrests in hospital are the result of investigative procedures. The highest risk is in the X-ray department – all patients receiving intravascular contract media must have the heart monitored. Retroperitoneal insufflation with air may precipitate cardiac arrest as gas dissects up into the mediastinum. Errors may be made in the concentration of dextrose infusion used for intravenous cholangiogram – producing a hyperosmolar cardiac arrest. Intravenous administration of contrast media for pyelography may be followed by an anaphylactic reaction.

Visceral reflexes. Autonomic reflexes triggered through the vagus, e.g. anal dilatation, gall-bladder traction, urethral or tracheobronchial intubation, can precipitate a cardiac arrest. Under certain circumstances the bradyarrhythmia can be prevented by premedication with atropine. Provided the diagnosis is made quickly, the heart can generally be started easily by external cardiac massage and intravenous atropine.

Respiratory and metabolic disturbances. Hypoxia is one of the commonest causes for arrest – the critically ill patient is particularly predisposed to pulmonary aspiration during intubation or insertion of a Ryles tube. Hypoxia may develop acutely in a patient who sustains airway obstruction or a tension pneumothorax on a volume cycled ventilator. Critically ill patients may develop hypoxia secondary to pulmonary shunting or oedema, e.g. due to fluid volume overload during A.R.F. or in myocardial failure, in extensive sepsis and following severe trauma.

A gradually increasing arterial carbondioxide level may go undetected (especially in a patient being ventilated with a high oxygen percentage) generally terminating in ventricular fibrillation.

A metabolic acidosis may precipitate ventricular fibrillation. Hyperkalaemia may be undetected in a patient with polyuric renal failure and dangerous hyperkalaemia may be precipitated by inadequately ventilating a patient who is known to have hyperkalaemia; these patients commonly die in asystole or with a severe bradyarrhythmia. Dangerous hypokalaemia may develop by giving dextrose solutions, insulin or sodium bicarbonate in an already hypokalaemic patient.

Shock due to hypovolaemia, sepsis or inadequate cardiac output may precipitate cardiac arrest as a result of multiple factors.

Electrocution. Electrical or lightning injuries both cause death by inducing ventricular fibrillation.

DIAGNOSIS OF CARDIAC ARREST

Early diagnosis is essential. A conscious talking patient (unusual in an Intensive Therapy Unit) becomes progressively incoherent. Mental confusion and tachypnoea are early warning signs and in a series reported by Castagna *et al.* (1974) a respiratory arrest preceded cardiac arrest in 18% of patients. The skin is classically pale and becomes progressively more cyanosed, the pupils initially reacting, then dilate and become nonreactive. The only reliable sign that arrest has occurred is the absence of a pulse in a major artery, e.g. carotid or aorta (during thoracotomy or abdominal surgery): confirmation is by an electrocardiograph which shows asystole or ventricular fibrillation. It is probable, in patients who are not being monitored at the time, that ventricular fibrillation is the initial dysrhythmia proceeding to asystole as hypoxia increases. Occasionally the cardiograph shows some rhythm other than ventricular fibrillation or asystole but as there is inadequate cardiac output, cardiac arrest (in effect) has occurred.

TREATMENT

The efficient management of cardiac arrest requires a good plan based on five principles – determination to save the patient, speed of action, equipment availability, an efficient emergency call service, and finally, effective treatment (Nixon, 1965).

Immediate steps

Maintain the airway by elevating the jaw – clear out the mouth if there is evidence of obstruction or vomitus around the mouth. Leave the patient in the bed – if the bed has a firm base – otherwise place the patient supine on the floor and commence external cardiac massage. If the diagnosis is made early, the patient may breath spontaneously for several seconds before assisted ventilation is required. Two sharp blows

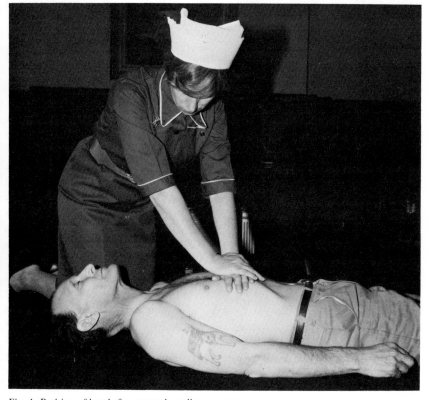

Fig. 1. Position of hands for external cardiac massage.

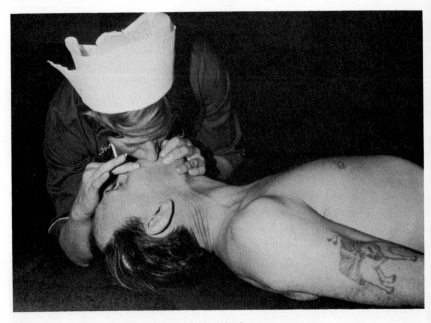

Fig. 2. Lung inflation by mouth to mouth resuscitation.

with the fist on the lower end of the sternum may restore the cardiac output. Should this be unsuccessful, external cardiac massage is performed by kneeling beside the patient and placing the base of the hand over the lower sternum, the second hand is placed over the first in order to maintain the correct position (Fig. 1). The lower part of the sternum is depressed firmly to a depth of 2–4 cm, and the sternum is allowed to rebound by release of the pressure. The rate should be approximately 60/min. (In a child one hand is used and in an infant two fingers will suffice.) A pause is made every 4–6 compressions to allow lung inflation. Lung inflation can be continued by mouth to nose, mouth to mouth (Fig. 2), or with the aid of a resuscitator such as an Ambu bag face mask and an oropharyngeal airway; a Brooke airway (Fig. 3), or a rebreathing bag with face mask and compressed oxygen (Fig. 4). The resuscitators have the advantage that oxygen can be entrained (Ambu system) or used alone but require some technical skill in their use. The cardiac arrest procedure using two operators is illustrated in Fig. 5. The chest must be seen to move with each gas inflation – should this not occur an obstructed airway must be excluded. Should the airway be obstructed and no anaesthetist be

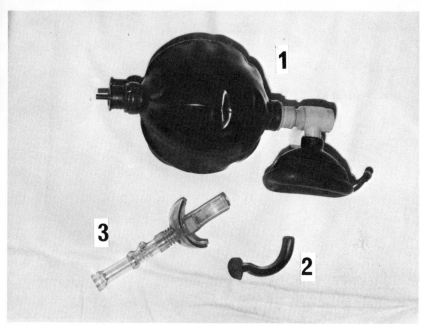

Fig. 3. *Resuscitators.* Ambu bag and face mask (1) and oropharyngeal airway (2). The Brooke airway (3).

available, an attempt should be made to intubate the patient. Laryngeal intubation can be confirmed by visible and auscultatory evidence of gas moving in and out of the lungs. Effective therapy will result in improvement in the patient's colour, a palpable pulse and a decrease in pupil size. Efficient external cardiac massage and mouth to mouth, or mouth to nose resuscitation may maintain adequate cerebral oxygenation for at least an hour. It is important to realise that stopping any of these procedures for even a few seconds may lead to cerebral damage – change over of resuscitators has to be planned beforehand so that change-over is efficient.

Definitive treatment

An intravenous infusion should be set up and 50 mmol of bicarbonate infused as sodium bicarbonate. Excess bicarbonate may precipitate the hyperosmolar syndrome (Máttar *et al.*, 1974) and subsequent dosage should be regulated according to sequential astrup analyses (see post-arrest management). Endotracheal intubation must be performed and the patient hand ventilated with oxygen.

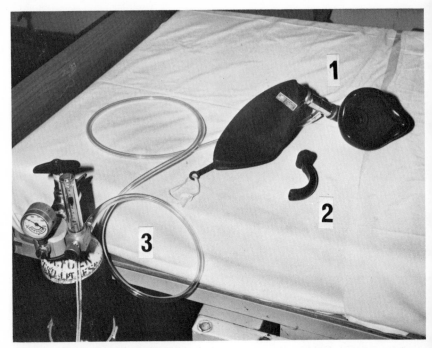

Fig. 4. *Resuscitation equipment*. Rebreathing bag and face mask (1), oropharyngeal airway (2) and source of compressed oxygen (3).

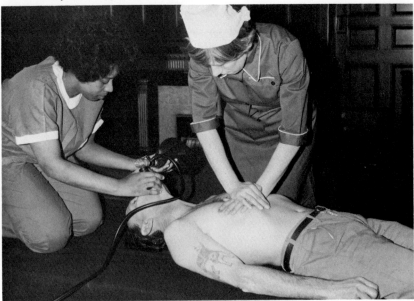

Fig. 5. Cardiac arrest procedure. Two operators. Respiratory resuscitation using an Ambu bag, face mask and entrained oxygen.

External cardiac massage is continued whilst the patient is connected to an E.C.G. oscilloscope using limb electrodes. The E.C.G. trace will show one of three abnormalities – ventricular fibrillation, asystole or occasionally an ectopic tachycardia sufficiently severe to produce an inadequate cardiac output. Direct current defibrillation can be performed without electrocardiographic verification and 100 J should be given if the trace is not easily obtainable. Grace *et al.* (1974) have improved the survival rate following cardiac arrest from 27 to 45% by performing blind defibrillation. Should fine ventricular fibrillation potentials be present electrocardiographically, 5 ml of adrenaline 1:10 000 should be injected into the ventricle with a fine long needle. Various sites are suggested for cardiac puncture, the one most commonly chosen being the fourth and fifth left intercostal space 2–3 inches from the sternum. Before the injection, it is important to withdraw blood to be sure that the needle tip is in a cardiac chamber. Injection of adrenaline into the heart muscle usually precipitates ventricular fibrillation which is resistant to therapy (Zoll, 1971). Intracardiac adrenaline generally coarsens the rhythm and increases the success rate with d.c. defibrillation. Shocks are administered

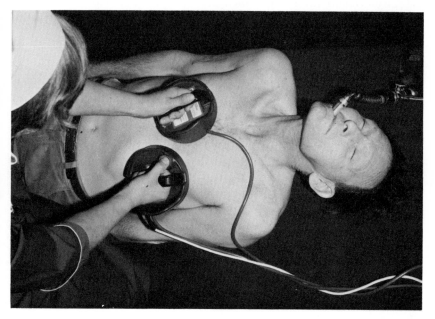

Fig. 6. Application of lubricated electrodes in preparation for d.c. shock. Patient intubated and lungs hand ventilated with oxygen.

starting at an energy level of 200 J and increasing by 100 at each shock to a level of 400 J. The lubricated electrodes should be placed as shown in Fig. 6 and hand ventilation should be continued until the shock is about to be given. The anaesthetist and all operators, apart from the individual administering the shock, should then stand well away from the bed. As soon as the shock has been given, hand ventilation and external massage should be recommenced. Even if the E.C.G. returns to sinus rhythm, external cardiac massage should be continued until a femoral pulse of good volume is palpable.

Treatment of particular problems

Refractory or recurrent ventricular fibrillation

Adrenaline is also valuable for ventricular fibrillation, refractory to d.c. shock – it should be given into one of the cardiac chambers as described previously. Calcium chloride should also be given in a dose of 5–10 ml of a 10% solution (2.25–4.5 mmol) added to 100 ml 1/5 normal saline and infused over 5 min or direct into a cardiac chamber – tonicity and cardiac contractility is thus frequently improved. Should counter shock be unsuccessful after these measures 100 mg lignocaine or 100 mg phenytoin should be given intravenously and the cardioversion repeated at 400 J.

Persistent ventricular arrhythmia

If ventricular fibrillation persists, or multifocal ventricular beats appear after cardioversion, procainamide or lignocaine should be given intravenously. Procainamide tends to depress myocardial contractility and lower blood pressure more than lignocaine. Lignocaine has a significant negative inotropic effect and should be given intravenously in graded doses of 60 mg repeating to a total dosage of 180 mg. The next dose of lignocaine should not be given if there is widening of the Q.R.S. and lengthening of the Q–T interval as shown on the E.C.G. Over-dosage of lignocaine may manifest as muscle twitching, followed by severe convulsive seizures – this may accentuate any hypoxia and metabolic acidosis that is already present. Once the ventricular extrasystoles have been stopped, lignocaine should be continued as a continuous infusion in a dose of 1–3 mg/min. Overdosage may lead to respiratory depression, muscle contractility or twitching. Continued ventricular arrhythmias, in spite of lignocaine, is an indication to add phenytoin to the present dosage of lignocaine. Other drugs which may be used are referred to on p. 46. It must be remembered that a refractory dysrhythmia may be related to hypoxia, a continuing metabolic acidosis, the onset of cardiac failure, or some other metabolic disorder such as the onset of the hyperosmolar syndrome, abnormalities in serum potassium, or more rarely serum calcium or magnesium. On rare occasions when ventricular fibrillation is recurrent in spite of myocardial depressants, these drugs may be given in conjunction with electrical stimulation.

In patients where there is evidence of A–V block and ectopic ventricular activity, an isoprenaline infusion should be commenced and arrangements made for intracardiac pacing. Four mg of isoprenaline is added to 500 ml 5% dextrose and the drip rate is steadily increased (starting at approximately 4 µg/min) until the ectopic activity is abolished (Zoll and Linenthal, 1963). Intravenous isoprenaline should be considered a temporary measure, an internal cardiac pacemaker being inserted as soon as possible (see Part 1, ch. III, p. 51). Should ectopic ventricular activity still be present, following insertion of a pacing catheter, a myocardial depressant such as lignocaine can be safely used without the danger of precipitating asystole or a serious bradyarrhythmia.

Asystole (see also Part 1, ch. III, p. 50)
The prognosis with asystole is extremely poor (Castagna *et al.*, 1974), except in cases where there is a rapidly correctable situation such as hypoxia, or an acute tension pneumothorax. Cardiac aystole is a well recognised complication of severe tetanus (Tsueda *et al.*, 1973), the heart can frequently be started by a sharp blow on the lower sternum. Attempts to achieve a co-ordinated rhythm or ventricular fibrillation are made with intracardiac adrenaline followed by an infusion of isoprenaline. Calcium chloride should be given if there is no evidence of digoxin toxicity. There is no indication for pacing these patients should the drugs fail, except in the case of a suspected digoxin toxicity where pacemaking should be considered (Citrin *et al.*, 1973).

Ectopic tachycardias sufficiently severe to produce an ineffective cardiac output
An ectopic tachycardia, whether supraventricular or ventricular, is treated by d.c. shock. In supraventricular dysrhythmias, the shock should be timed to occur just after the R-wave and avoiding the T-wave when a shock may cause ventricular fibrillation (Lown, 1967). It is wise to cardiovert before proceeding to a myocardial depressant which should be used in order to prevent recurrence. In refractory supraventricular dysrhythmias, intravenous verapamil has been found to be

particularly helpful (Krikler, 1974), given slowly in a dose of up to 5 mg since the injection may be complicated by transient asystole, bradycardia or hypotension (Benaim, 1972; Sacks and Kennelly, 1972). The drug should be given with extreme caution in patients who have recently received β-blockers. β-adrenergic blocking agents should be given with extreme caution in patients who are toxic, or are in congestive cardiac failure, since with even partial β-blockade serious bradycardia or asystole may arise. Other drugs used in supraventricular dysrhythmias are described in Part 1, ch. III, p. 43. A total β-blocker (propranolol) should be used in the rare supraventricular tachycardias that may complicate tetanus, a thyrotoxic crisis, or phaechromocytoma – the heart rate may be sufficiently rapid to produce a semblance of cardiac arrest – no peripheral pulses being palpable.

IMMEDIATE POST-ARREST MANAGEMENT

Cardiac management

Once the rhythm has been restored to normal – cardiac output generally steadily improves with associated manifestations of improved organ perfusion, e.g. increase in urine output and restoration of consciousness. Occasionally cardiac output does not improve and femoral pulses remain impalpable – in such circumstances cardiac massage should be continued until inotropic drug therapy has been tried. A sympathomimetic amine is the drug of choice under these circumstances such as isoprenaline, a pure β-adrenergic agent, having a strong chronotropic and inotropic effect with no vasoconstrictor activity. Adrenaline has a powerful α- and β-adrenergic stimulating effect and may produce a metabolic acidosis through peripheral vasoconstriction. Central venous pressure monitoring is essential when isoprenaline is used since peripheral vasodilatation may decrease the volume of blood returning to the heart, thereby decreasing cardiac output. The use of isoprenaline may be complicated by the onset of a supreventricular tachycardia or ventricular dysrhythmias – the dosage should therefore be titrated intravenously so that the heart rate does not increase above 140/min. Ventricular extrasystoles can be suppressed with the use of intravenous lignocaine, phenytoin or the cautious use of procaine amide (procaine amide tends to produce a greater decrease in myocardial contractility than lignocaine). A poor cardiac output may be related to a severe metabolic acidosis, hypokalaemia, or the insidious onset of cardiac failure. Intravenous digoxin should be considered in patients where the serum potassium and metabolic status is satisfactory provided there is nothing to suggest an overdose. The dose recommended is 0.5 mg titrated slowly intravenously whilst monitoring the E.C.G. The prognosis is extremely poor if cardiac output fails to improve by these measures.

Other drugs which may be considered in cardiogenic shock are discussed on p. 59. A combination of isoprenaline and dopamine may be particularly useful in patients where urine output remains poor and the pulse rate high (greater than 130/min) on an infusion of isoprenaline alone. On very rare occasions cardiac output may be improved by intra-aortic balloon counterpulsation (Part 1, ch. III, p. 62 and Part 4, ch. IV, p. 955).

Haemopericardium is a rare complication of cardiac massage. Should tamponade develop, the haematoma must be aspirated. Left ventricular failure should be treated along the usual lines.

Respiratory management

The patient should be sedated and hand ventilated with oxygen and *not* extubated should there be any factors complicating the arrest which may produce respiratory embarrassment. These factors include, the presence of left ventricular failure, rib fracture or pulmonary aspiration complicating resuscitation, or a period of prolonged arrest where cerebral oedema is likely. The patient should be sedated with diazepam and relaxation obtained with pancuronium. Ventilation has to be regulated so that there is adequate oxygenation and venous return. The $PaCO_2$ should be maintained at 3.7 kPa–4.0 kPa (28–30 mm Hg) in order to decrease any cerebral oedema which may be present. Pulmonary aspiration should be treated along the lines suggested in Part 2, ch. V, p. 573. The tolerance to P.E.E.P. is diminished following a cardiac arrest and should be instituted with extreme caution starting at levels of 1 cm H_2O and maintaining at the minimum level to achieve a $PaCO_2$ of 9.3 kPa (70 mm Hg) or above. Occasionally there is a fracture of the sternum and/or rib fractures so extensive that the patient requires prolonged ventilation as in a chest injury (Part 2, ch. III, p. 386). Under such circumstances the mortality is virtually 100%.

Cerebral management

Should the period of resuscitation before sinus rhythm and an adequate cardiac output be restored, last longer than 15 min, or the duration of arrest prior to the onset of resuscitation be longer than 2 min, then cerebral oedema should be presumed to have occurred. The patient should be hyperventilated – reducing the $PaCO_2$ to 3.7–4.0 kPa (28–30 mm Hg) and mannitol 200 ml 15% be infused over 30 min. Should there be evidence of left ventricular failure dexamethazone should be substituted for mannitol (4 mg intramuscularly 6 hourly for three days).

Metabolic and renal management

Blood should be taken for electrolytes, blood glucose, Astrup analysis and serum osmolality, as soon as sinus rhythm has been restored, or if the patient gets repeated attacks of ventricular dysrhythmia. A further dose of sodium bicarbonate should be given if the base deficit is eight, or greater, or the pH 7.2 or less. The dose given should not be above 50 mmol bicarbonate ions and be based on the formula:

$$0.3 \times \text{kg B.W.} \times (\text{B.D.} - 8) = \text{mmol } HCO_3^- \text{ required}$$

Bicarbonate should be infused over 15 min and the acid base status repeated 30 min after the infusion. Sodium bicarbonate must *not* be given if the serum potassium is 3.0 mmol or less – under such circumstances potassium must be infused first. A serum sodium level of greater than 150 mmol or a serum osmolality above 310 mosm/l is also a contraindication to the further use of sodium bicarbonate. A blood glucose of 15 mmol–30 mmol/l is an indication for hourly insulin administration (see Part 1, ch. IX, p. 263). A level above 30 mmol should be treated more aggressively because of the risk of a hyper-osmolar syndrome. Insulin in a dosage of two times the blood glucose in mmol, should be given intravenously followed by 12 units i.m. or i.v. hourly. Blood glucose monitoring is essential.

The patient should be catheterised as soon as is convenient and a urine plasma osmolality calculated (prior to diuretic therapy). A u/p osmolality ratio of 1.2 or less is indicative of renal failure – fluid volume control should therefore be judged on central venous pressure monitoring, and the serum potassium must be observed carefully. Most patients who develop acute renal failure following cardiac arrest, can be managed conservatively unless there are any complicating factors producing a catabolic state (see Part 1, ch. IV). In the absence of renal failure, the urine output should be maintained at 40 ml/h or more with the use of mannitol (0.2 g/kg B.W. i.v. over 15 min and repeated 4 hourly for 3 doses if urine output <40 ml/h), or frusemide. Hypokalaemia may complicate the repeated use of these agents should a diuretic response be obtained. Central venous pressure monitoring is essential in order to prevent the insidious onset of hypovolaemia.

SUBSEQUENT POST-ARREST MANAGEMENT

Should the patient require I.P.P.V. or C.P.P.V., ventilation should be continued until the PaO_2 (in a patient with normal lungs previously), is (9.3 kPa) 70 mm Hg or more on an F_IO_2 of 35% or less and P.E.E.P of 2.0 cm H_2O or less. Complicating factors such as pulmonary aspiration, multiple trauma to the chest wall, multiple arrests or previous chest disease, may require a planned tracheostomy 4–5 days following the initial arrest, in order to make weaning easier. A tracheostomy may also be required if the arrest was primarily respiratory in origin.

COMPLICATIONS AND PROGNOSIS

Complications of resuscitation

Injuries induced by resuscitation are rarely sufficiently serious to affect prognosis despite the numerous complications described. These include rib fractures in 47% (Himmelhock et al., 1964), haemothorax in 6% (Basinger et al., 1961), haemopericardium in 1–3% (Himmelhock and et al., 1964; Basinger et al., 1961). Himmelhock and co-workers (1964) noted a 40% incidence of fat embolism; this was described as marked in 15%. Late rupture of the liver and spleen has also been reported.

Prognosis

A well organised resuscitation team effectively increases survival following unexpected cardiac arrest (Lemire and Johnson, 1972; Hollingsworth 1971), between 12 and 20% of patients leave hospital alive (Sandoval, 1965; Stiles et al., 1971). In a follow up of 230 patients who left hospital alive Lemire and Johnson (1972) found that 74% were alive at the end of one year and 51% alive after three years. The effectiveness of resuscitation in patients who are already critically ill is very much less, the incidence of recurrence is greater as is also the incidence of asystole. Permanent cerebral damage following successful resuscitation is unusual (Norris and Shrandasekar, 1971 and Castagna et al., 1974).

Conclusion

The outline of cardiac arrest management circularised to the wards in

Whipps Cross Hospital is shown in Table 1 and the post-cardiac arrest management is summarised in Table 2.

Table 1. Treatment of cardiac arrest

Phase I
(*a*) If patient connected to drips or suction, place board on bed and roll patient on to it. The floor is preferable.
(*b*) Lower the head and clear the airway.
(*c*) Raise the legs.
(*d*) Thump middle of sternum once.

Phase II
(*a*) Begin closed chest massage.
(*b*) Mouth to mouth respiration – an Ambu bag, rebreathing bag connected to air or oxygen or a Brooke airway should be used if possible.
(*c*) Send for assistance *once instituted*.

Phase III
(*a*) Intubate the trachea.
(*b*) Erect an intravenous drip.
(*c*) Record an E.C.G.

Phase IV – Definitive treatment
(*a*) 50 mmol sodium bicarbonate i.v.
(*b*) 10 ml 10% calcium gluconate via drip tubing.
(*c*) 1 ml 1/1000 adrenaline hydrochloride via drip tubing if small magnitude ventricular fibrillation is present.
(*d*) Defibrillate externally or apply the pacemaker as necessary.

Phase V – Supportive treatment
(*a*) If consciousness does not quickly return, use I.P.P.V. with 100% oxygen.
(*b*) Elevate head of bed if B.P. adequate.
(*c*) Catheterise the bladder.
(*d*) Give i.v. mannitol 0.2 g/kg B.W. over 2–3 min.
(*e*) Measure urine output over the next 3 h.
(*f*) Check acid-base; correct if necessary.
(*g*) Cool the patient to 32–33°C rectal if necessary.

Table 2. Immediate post-arrest management

I. CARDIAC
  Poor cardiac output
  Isoprenaline infusion (1–6 µg/min) maintain heart rate <140/min. Should cardiac output remain poor and pulse rate >130/min consider dopamine.
  Should ventricular extrasystoles arise, use intravenous lignocaine, phenytoin or procaine amide.
  In refractory cases consider other antidysrhythmics (see Part 1, ch. III).
  Exclude a metabolic abnormality: cardiac failure, haemopericardium.
  Consider i.v. digoxin.
  Consider intra-aortic balloon counterpulsation (see Part 4, ch. IV, p. 955).

II. RESPIRATORY

Do not extubate should factors be present which may produce respiratory difficulty.
Should I.P.P.V. or C.P.P.V. be indicated:

Maintain on diazepam and pancuronium.

Maintain PaO_2 9.3–13.3 kPa (70–100 mm Hg) $PaCO_2$ at 3.7–4.0 kPa (28–30 mm Hg).

Treat pulmonary aspiration (Part 2, ch. V, p. 573).

Treat extensive chest trauma (Part 2, ch. III, p. 386).

III. CEREBRAL

Period of arrest prior to resuscitation >2 min, or period or resuscitation >15 min, give:

Mannitol 200 ml 15% i.v. over 30 min followed by dexamethasone 4 mg i.m. 6 hourly for 3 doses.

Hyperventilate [$PaCO_2$ 3.7–4.0 kPa (28–30 mm Hg)].

IV. METABOLIC AND RENAL

Metabolic

Check Astrup B.G. B.U., Electrolytes, Se Osmolality.

B.D. >8 and/or pH <7.2, give sodium bicarbonate not >50 mmol over 15 min. (0.3 × kg B.W. × (B.D. − 8) = mmol HCO_3^- ions required.)

Do not give bicarbonate if Se K^+ <3.0 mmol/l, Se Na^+ >150 mmol/l, Se Osmolality >310 mosmol/kg body water.

Blood glucose 15–30 mmol/l – hourly insulin, >30 mmol/l – i.v. insulin 2 × B.G. them i.m. or i.v. hourly

(B.G. monitoring essential)

Renal

Catheterise – u/p osmolality ratio 1.2 or less in A.R.F. u/p osmolality ratio >1.2 maintain urine output >40 ml/h with mannitol (0.2 G/kg B.W. i.v. over 15 min 4 hourly as required for 3 doses), or frusemide.

Monitor C.V.P. and serum potassium

ACKNOWLEDGEMENTS

I wish to thank the operating theatre technicians and nursing staff for their co-operation in producing the figures for this chapter.

REFERENCES

Basinger, J. R., Saleman, E. W., Jones, W. A. and Friedlich, A. L. (1961). External cardiac massage. *New Engl. J. Med.* **265**, 62.

Benaim, M. E. (1972). Asystole after verapamil. *Brit. Med. J.* **2**, 169.

Browning, D. J. (1974). Serious side effects of ergometrine and its use in routine obstetric practice. *Med. J. Aust.* **1**, 957.

Camarata, S. J., Weil, M. H., Harashiro, P. K. and Shubin, H. (1971). Cardiac arrest in the critically ill. 1. A study of predisposing causes in 132 patients. *Circulation* **44**, 688.

Castagna, J., Weil, M. H. and Shubin, H. (1974). Factors determining survival in patients with cardiac arrest. *Chest* **65**, 527.

Cheng, T. O. and Wadhwa (1973). Sinus standstill following intravenous lidocaine administration. *J.A.M.A.* **223**, 790.

Citrin, D. L., O'Malley, K. and Hillis, W. S. (1973). Standstill due to digoxin poisoning treated with atrial pacing. *Brit. Med. J.* **2**, 526.

Gould, L., Zahir, M. and Gomprecht, R. F. (1971). Cardiac arrest during edrophonium administration. *Am. Heart J.* **81**, 437.

Grace, W. J., Kennedy, R. J. and Nolte, C. T. (1974). Blind defibrillation. *Am. J. Cardiol.* **34**, 115.

Himmelhock, S. R., Dekker, A., Gazzaniga, A. B. and Like, A. A. (1964). Closed-chest cardiac resuscitation: A prospective clinical and pathological study. *New Engl. J. Med.* **270**, 118.

Hollingsworth, J. H. (1969). The results of cardiopulmonary resuscitation. *Ann. Intern. Med.* **71**, 459.

Jones, G. (1970). Cardiac arrest following induction with propanidid. *Brit. J. Anaesth.* **42**, 74.

Korczyn, A. D., Kessler, E. and Bornstein, B. (1971). Meningococcal disease with cardiac death. *Confin. Neurol.* **33**, 271.

Krikler, D. (1974). Verapamil in cardiology. *Europ. J. Cardiol.* **2**, 3.

Lemire, G. and Johnson, A. L. (1972). Is cardiac resuscitation worthwhile? A decade of experience. *New. Engl. J. Med.* **286**, 970.

Lorhan, P. H. (1972). Diagnosis, management and treatment of cardiac arrest in acute anaesthetic emergencies. *In* 'International Anaesthesiology Clinics' (Ed. Lorhan), p. 81. Little Brown & Co., Boston.

Lown, B. (1967). Electrical reversion of cardiac arrhythmias. *Brit. Heart J.* **29**, 469.

Máttar, J. A., Weil, M. H., Shubin, H. and Stein, L. (1974). Cardiac arrest in the critically ill. II. Hyperosmolal states following cardiac arrest. *Amer. J. Med.* **56**, 162.

Mazze, R. I., Escue, H. M. and Houston, J. B. (1969). Hyperkalaemia and cardiovascular collapse following administration of succinylcholine to the traumatised patient. *Anaesthesiology* **31**, 540.

Mercer, C. W. and Logie, J. R. (1973). Cardiac arrest due to hyperkalaemia following intravenous penicillin administration. *Chest* **64**, 358.

Nixon, G. F. (1965). 'The Treatment of Cardiac Arrest in Intensive Care and Resuscitation in Heart Disease' (Ed. K. S. Smith), p. 15, Waterlow and Sons, London.

Norris, J. R. and Shrandrasekar, S. (1971). Anoxic brain damage after cardiac arrest. *J. Chronic. Dis.* **24**, 585.

Powell, J. N., McGrath, P. J., Lahiri, S. K. and Hill, P. (1970). Cardiac arrest associated with bone cement. *Brit. Med. J.* **3**, 326.

Sacks, H. and Kennelly, B. M. (1972). Verapamil in cardiac arrhythmias. *Brit. Med. J.* **2**, 716.

Sandoval, R. G. (1965). Survival rate after cardiac arrest in a community hospital. *J.A.M.A.* **194**, 675.

Stiles, Q. R., Tucker, B. L., Meyer, B. W., Lindesmith, G. G. and Jones, J. C. (1971). Cardiopulmonary arrest, evaluation of an active resuscitation program. *Am. J. Surg.* **122**, 282.

Tsueda, K., Jean Francois, J., and Richter, R. W. (1973). Cardiac standstill in tetanus: review of seven consecutive cases. *Internat. Surgery* **58**, 599.

Williams, R. B. (1971). Cardiac complications of tricyclic antidepressant therapy. *Ann. Intern. Med.* **74**, 395.

Zoll, P. M. (1971). Rational use of drugs for cardiac arrest and after cardiac resuscitation. *Amer. J. Cardiol.* **27**, 645.

Zoll, P. N. and Linenthal, A. J. (1963). Prevention of ventricular tachycardia and fibrillation by intravenous isoprotenerol and epinephrine. *Circulation* **27**, 5.

II

Shock

Section 1: Introduction and Pathophysiology

GILLIAN C. HANSON

INTRODUCTION

Shock is a term used by the clinician to describe a condition characterised by inadequate cellular perfusion and consequent failure of function of various tissues and organs.

PATHOPHYSIOLOGY

Various mechanisms can result in shock, the most obvious being pump failure, obstruction to the main channel of flow (e.g. constrictive pericarditis, massive pulmonary embolism) and depletion of the circulating blood volume. The latter is discussed in greater detail in Section 3, p. 333.

Shock associated with sepsis is complex and is discussed in more detail in Section 4, p. 355.

Certain areas of the body and factors closely associated with these areas are commonly affected to a greater or lesser extent in all forms of shock. These will be discussed under the following headings: *Microcirculation, Blood – rheological properties, Blood – coagulation, The heart, Affect of shock on function of other organs.*

Microcirculation

Pump failure, obstruction to flow, and circulating blood volume depletion if not quickly treated will affect function of the capillary bed.

293

MODEL OF THE MICROCIRCULATORY UNIT

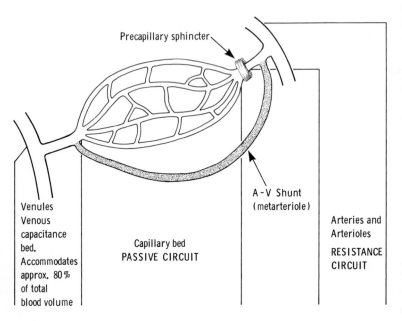

Fig. 1. Diagram of a microcirculatory unit.

The microcirculation appears to be affected earlier and to a greater degree in shock associated with sepsis. The microvascular unit is illustrated in Fig. 1. Blood enters from an arterial conduit via a muscular arteriole which breaks up into smaller units, the metarterioles. At the origin of the arterial capillary from the metarteriole, there is often a condensation of vascular smooth muscle, the precapillary sphincter. The muscular arterial components form the resistance part of the circuit. The capillaries downstream from the precapillary sphincters also undergo caliber changes but these effects are probably the passive result of caliber changes in the resistance vessels. The capillary bed then forms the passive component of the circuit. Blood flow through the capillary bed and fluid filtration between the intravascular and interstitial fluid compartments are largely regulated by humoral and neurogenic controls on the precapillary arterial circuit and the post-capillary venules. The venules are the return channels from the microvascular unit and serve as a capacitance bed. The capacitance bed acts as a storage reservoir for blood and changes in capacitance largely regulate the volume of blood circulating at any one time and hence the volume of blood returning to the heart. The metarterioles bridge the arterioles with the venules – blood under certain conditions can therefore be shunted from the resistance to the capacitance circuit thus bypassing the capillary unit.

It must be recalled that the degree of organ or tissue perfusion in relation to a falling systemic arterial pressure is variable. Sometimes the skin and to a lesser extent skeletal muscle react passively, perfusion falling as the systemic blood pressure falls, whereas perfusion in the renal, coronary and cerebral vascular bed remains almost the same until a pressure of about 50 mm Hg is reached, when flow falls precipitously. Vascular autoregulation has the effect of conserving vital organ function until the blood pressure has fallen to seriously low levels; the critical level where autoregulation is lost however depends upon the state of the vessels – autoregulation being lost earlier in patients with vascular atheroma.

As the blood pressure falls various compensatory mechanisms come into play which initially have a valuable part to play in maintaining adequate oxygenation to vital organs – if allowed to continue however, the release of cellular metabolites may either perpetuate or increase the severity of shock. The initial compensatory mechanism is vasoconstriction principally affecting vessels supplied with alpha-adrenergic receptors. These are stimulated by the catecholamines secreted by the adrenal medulla and sympathetic endings (Hokfelt et al., 1962). The initial affect of catecholamines on the microcirculatory unit is marked constriction of the arterioles, precapillary sphincters and moderate constriction of the venules. Perfusion therefore continues but at a considerably reduced rate and volume, the mean capillary pressure is not increased and thus fluid is still taken up from the interstitial spaces. Should perfusion fail to improve, transcapillary exchange of essential substrates and especially oxygen is impaired. Tissue hypoxia is initially compensated for by anaerobic metabolism with accumulation of lactic acid (Broder and Weil, 1964; Weil and Afifi, 1970). In spite of the continued high circulation of catecholamines, it is thought that different components of the capillary circulation have an altered reactivity to the accumulation of tissue metabolites – in particular lactate. The precapillary resistance vessels (arterioles) tend to relax as does the precapillary sphincter; the tone of the venules also decreases but to a lesser degree. Owing to this new microcirculatory pattern, blood begins to pool in the capillary bed, capillary hydrostatic pressure rises to values which exceed colloid osmotic pressure and fluid enters the interstitial space. The precarious blood volume which could previously support an adequate systolic pressure in central vessels is thus suddenly decreased, first by blood sequestration in the capacitance bed and then by plasma leakage into the interstitial space. This results in a generalised circulatory collapse which may lead to irreversible shock and death.

Blood – rheological properties

As a consequence of plasma loss from the intravascular space, haemoconcentration occurs. Haemoconcentration and vasoconstriction radically affect the rheological properties of blood. The rheology of blood or its flow properties include the intrinsic properties of blood and the influence on these properties by the behaviour of the vasculature. The viscosity of blood is one of several rheologic properties and denotes the ratio of sheer stress (force imposed per unit area of fluid plane) to sheer rate (difference in the velocity of two planes divided by the distance between them – velocity gradient). The main factors which affect blood viscosity are flow rate, the haematocrit, plasma protein and fibrinogen concentrations, erythrocyte flexibility and vessel bore. Poiseuille's Law (see below) states that flow is directly related to the driving pressure and to the fourth power of the radius of the lumen and is inversely related to the viscosity and length of the tube. Flow rates are a linear function of the driving force or pressure when the velocity of flow is constant. Suspensions, such as blood, have a constant viscosity value at high flow rates and at low flow rates the viscosity rises sharply and there is no longer a linear relationship between pressure and flow.

Poiseuille's Law

$$\text{Rate of flow} = \frac{P_1 - P_2}{8L} \times \frac{\pi r^4}{\eta}$$

Where, $P_1 P_2$ = pressures at either end of the vessel, L = length of the vessel, r = radius of the vessel, η = viscosity of the fluid

One of the major reasons for the rapid rise in viscosity as flow falls is that during fast flow rates the blood cells tend to course in the stream's axis, leaving an outer rim of clear plasma which produces minimal resistance, since the highest rate of shear is near the vessel wall. However if the flow slows the cells aggregate adjacent to the vessel wall further limiting flow and encouraging stagnation. As haematocrit rises (due to loss of fluid into the interstitial space), viscosity rises exponentially. A linear relationship has been found between erythrocyte flexibility and fibrinogen concentration (Editorial, 1975). Any factor which promotes fibrin formation such as stasis, high blood viscosity or excessive platelet stickiness, will make the red cells less flexible. Inflexibility of the red cells prevents them being squeezed through the smaller vessels and under these conditions the relative viscosity is largely independent of haematocrit up to values of 80%. Thus, a combination of factors leads to stasis in the microcirculation during shock, a fall in flow rate, a rising haematocrit, decreased erythrocyte flexibility (due to stasis and an increasing viscosity) and a decrease in the vessel bore secondary to vasoconstriction.

It can therefore be seen that during treatment of severe shock, therapy must be directed towards decreasing the shearing forces within the microcirculation and towards modification of the colloid environment. Attempts to manipulate blood viscosity by such agents as dextran are often counterproductive in that, while they lower the haematocrit and reduce aggregation, they make the red cells inflexible (Editorial, 1975). Even haemodilution tends to lower the fibrinogen level and hence decreases erythrocyte flexibility. In spite of these findings Hint (1968) found that oxygen transport capacity is highest at a haematocrit level of 30%. Hopkins and co-workers (1974) have shown however that profound anaemia may contribute to continued haemorrhage in patients with gastrointestinal haemorrhage. They found that the flow of blood from a glass capillary tube doubled when the haematocrit was reduced from 45 to 15% and was inversely proportional to the viscosity. It seems reasonable therefore that haematocrit should not be allowed to fall too low especially where there is likelihood of small vessel bleeding. An haematocrit of around 30% therefore seems a reasonable level to aim for during volume replacement of a patient with severe shock where there is evidence of diminished tissue and organ perfusion.

Blood – coagulation

Prolonged hypotension, hypoxia and acidosis with or without septicaemia are known to cause disseminated intravascular coagulation. This is probably related to the lactic acidosis which develops during severe shock and is known to cause endothelial damage (Colman *et al.*, 1972). Microthrombosis will obviously stop flow through certain capillaries thereby perpetuating the cellular hypoxia. Microthrombosis has been found to develop in many organs during shock and is probably the ultimate factor producing respiratory failure and/or renal failure.

Microthrombosis may not necessarily be associated with signs of hypocoagulation, this depending upon the extent of thrombus formation and the rate of production of coagulation factors. Should shock progress however, an initial hypercoagulability may progress to hypocoagulability because the consumption of coagulation factors exceeds their production (Simmons *et al.*, 1969).

The heart

It is becoming increasingly recognised that the heart can be adversely affected in septic and hypovolaemic shock. Many of these factors are fairly obvious, the elderly patient being more susceptible. The onset of cardiac dysrhythmias frequently secondary to hypoxia and/or metabolic acidosis and overload of the circulation with overenthusiastic volume replacement may lead to biventricular failure. Other factors producing a deterioration in cardiac function have been less easy to define. During prolonged and severe hypotension patchy necrosis of myocardial cells has been demonstrated (Hackel *et al.*, 1974). Lee and Downing (1974) studied ventricular function in cats subjected to sustained haemorrhagic shock. They suggested that the progressive reduction of ventricular contractility was consequent upon the interplay of three key factors – metabolic acidosis, reduced coronary perfusion pressure (and presumably reduced coronary flow), loss of sympathetic support in the presence of myocardial ischaemia and increasing metabolic acidosis.

The circulatory response to extensive infection is characterised by a high cardiac output and low systemic vascular resistance (Clowes *et al.*, 1966; MacLean *et al.*, 1967). Failure of the cardiovascular system to supply the increased circulatory requirement is associated with a low cardiac output, high systemic vascular resistance, falling blood pressure, and progressive acidosis leading to death (Gunnar *et al.*, 1973; MacLean *et al.*, 1967). Factors producing the fall in cardiac output include fluid translocation leading to a fall in the dynamic blood volume, increasing pulmonary vascular resistance accompanied by right heart failure (Clowes *et al.*, 1970), direct damage to myocardial cells by endotoxin (Hinshaw *et al.*, 1972) and possibly the presence of a myocardial suppressor factor (M.D.F.). This substance is thought to originate in the ischaemic pancreas and may reach the systemic circulation via the lymphatic system (Lefer, 1973). No evidence was found of a myocardial suppressor factor in sustained haemorrhagic shock (Lee and Downing, 1974).

Affect of shock on function of other organs

Mention has already been made of the autoregulatory mechanisms for controlling blood flow in the heart and kidneys. The effect of shock on lung function is described in Part 2, ch. V, p. 545. Acute intrinsic renal failure may follow a period of shock, many factors have been implicated but decreased renal blood flow appears to be the most important (Tristani and Cohn, 1970). It is frequently a combination of factors which leads to renal failure, these include, intravascular haemolysis, circulating endotoxins, intravascular coagulation obstruction of the tubules by casts and ischaemic tubular necrosis. Blood volume depletion leads to the production of renin which when converted to argiotensin II, stimulates the adrenal cortex to release aldosterone. Aldosterone conserves body sodium and thus maintains blood volume.

Smart and Rowlands (1972) in experiments on rats showed that liver damage was produced during haemorrhage when liver perfusion was impaired. Filkins and Cornell (1974) found that endotoxin administration to rats depressed hepatic gluconeogenesis. They suggest that the development of hepatic gluconeogenic capability is a critical event in survival during endotoxin shock and that the depression of gluconeogenesis may induce hypoglycaemia and contribute to circulatory decompensation. Jaundice is considered to be a grave prognostic sign in patients recovering from shock (Nunes et al., 1970).

Drucker et al. (1972) observed pancreatic function during experimentally induced hypovolaemic shock. The pancreatic output of insulin appears to be a two phase system – the initial output represents release from pancreatic stores in response to acute reduction in blood volume. The second phase of insulin output depends upon insulinogenesis which can occur during hypovolaemia in response to hyperglycaemia but may be inhibited by a reduction in pancreatic blood flow and increased levels of catecholamines in the blood.

It is possible that the ischaemic pancreas may have an important part to play in the perpetuation of shock by releasing a myocardial suppressant factor.

REFERENCES

Broder, G. and Weil, M. H. (1964). Excess lactate: An index of reversibility of shock in human patients. *Science* **143**, 1457.

Clowes, G. H. A. Jr., Vucinic, M., and Weidner, M. G. (1966). Circulatory and Metabolic alteration associated with survival or death in peritonitis. *Ann. Surg.* **163**, 866.

Clowes, G. H. A. Jr., Farrington, G. H., Zuschneid, W., Cossette, G. R. and Saravis, C. (1970). Circulating factors in the etiology of pulmonary insufficiency and right heart failure accompanying severe sepsis (peritonitis). *Ann. Surg.* **171**, 663.

Colman, R. W., Robboy, S. J. and Minna, J. D. (1972). Disseminated intravascular coagulation (D.I.C.). An approach. *Am. J. Med.* **52**, 679.

Drucker, W. R., Gallie, B. L., Lau, T. S., Farago, G., Levene, R. A. and Haist, R. E. (1973). The effect of persisting hypovolaemic shock in pancreatic output of insulin. *Advances in Exper. Med. and Biol.* **33**, 187.

Editorial (1975). Haemotheology, blood flow and venous thrombosis. *Lancet* **2**, 113.

Filkins, J. P. and Cornell, R. P. (1974). Depression of hepatic gluconeogenesis and the hypoglycaemia of endotoxin shock. *Amer. J. Physiol.* **227**, 778.

Gunnar, R. M., Loeb, H. S., Winslow, E. J., Blain, C. and Robinson, J. (1973). Haemodynamic measurements in bacteremia and septic shock in man. *J. Infect. Dis.* **S.295**, 128.

Hackel, D. B., Ratliff, N. B. and Mikat, E. (1974). The heart in shock. *Circulat. Res.* **35**, 805.

Hinshaw, L. B., Greenfield, L. J., Owen, S. E., Black, M. R. and Guenter, C. A. (1972). Precipitation of cardiac failure in endotoxin shock. *Surg. Gynec. Obstet.* **135**, 39.

Hint, A. (1968). The pharmacology of dextran and the physiological background for the clinical use of Rheomacrodex and Macrodex. *Acta anaesth. Belg.* **19**, 119.

Hokfelt, B., Bygdeman, S. and Sekkenes, J. (1962). The participation of the adrenal glands in endotoxin shock. *In* 'Shock: Pathogenesis and Therapy' (Ed. K. D. Bock), p. 106. Springer Verlag.

Hopkins, R. W., Fratianne, R. B., Rao, K. V. and Damewood, C. A. (1974). Effects of haematocrit and viscosity on continuing haemorrhage. *J. Trauma* **14**, 482.

Lee, J. C. and Downing, S. E. (1974). Critical oxygen tension and left ventricular performance during shock. *Amer. J. of Physiol.* **226**, 9.

Lefer, A. M. (1973). Blood-borne humoral factors in the pathophysiology of circulatory shock. *Circulat. Res.* **32**, 129.

MacLean, L. D., Mulligan, W. G., McLean, A. P. H. and Duff, J. M. (1967). Patterns of septic shock in man – A detailed study of 56 patients. *Ann. Surg.* **166**, 543.

Nunes, G., Blaisdell, F. W. and Margaretten, W. (1970). Prognosis of jaundice following shock. *Archs. Surg.* **100**, 546.

Simmons, R. L., Heisterkamp, C. A., Moseley, R. V. and Doty, D. B. (1969). Postresuscitative blood volumes in combat casualties. *Surg. Gynec. Obstet.* **128**, 1193.

Smart, C. J. and Rowlands, S. D. (1972). Oxygen consumption and hepatic metabolism in experimental posthaemorrhagic shock. *J. Trauma* **12**, 327.

Tristani, F. E. and Cohn, J. N. (1970). Studies in clinical shock and hypotension. VII Renal haemodynamics before and during treatment. *Circulation* **42**, 839.

Weil, W. H. and Afifi, A. A. (1970). Experimental and clinical studies on lactate and pyruvate as indicators of the severity of acute circulatory failure (shock). *Circulation* **41**, 989.

Section 2: Monitoring in Shock

E. D. Bennett and Gillian C. Hanson

INTRODUCTION

Much research work continues to be carried out to elucidate the multiple factors producing shock refractory to conventional forms of therapy in order to find a more rational mode of therapy. Those reading these articles may get the impression that the shocked patient cannot be resuscitated without elaborate monitoring systems – this is entirely untrue. The majority of severely shocked patients can be appropriately treated with a select and limited amount of monitoring providing the staff are well trained in the progressive steps to be taken in management. It is also essential that the staff have a thorough understanding of the physiological principles on which the monitoring is based. It is proposed, therefore, to describe these principles and then the monitoring that is considered essential for the proper clinical management of the shocked patient.

PHYSIOLOGICAL PRINCIPLES

The ability of both ventricles to pump blood depends on a number of factors, including the filling pressures, the intrinsic 'contractility' of the ventricular muscle, the venous capacity and the peripheral resistance.

The relationship between filling pressure and ventricular output is shown in Fig. 1 by a series of Frank–Starling curves. These show that there is a curvilinear relationship between output and filling pressure so that at low filling pressures the output is small. As filling pressure

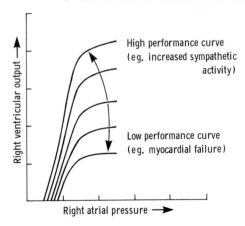

Fig. 1. Diagram showing the relationship of right ventricular output to right atrial pressure (Frank–Starling curves). The right ventricular output increases as the right atrial pressure increases but above a certain level of right atrial pressure, right ventricular overload leads to a fall in cardiac output.

increases a concomitant rise in output occurs, until a plateau is reached. Any further increase in filling pressure will not further increase output and may in fact lead to a decrease.

Each curve describes cardiac function for a particular state of intrinsic contractility which in turn is related to the balance between sympathetic and parasympathetic activity. Thus an increase in sympathetic activity improves ventricular performance from the same filling pressure, whereas increased parasympathetic activity has the opposite effect.

The resistance offered by the peripheral circulation also plays a part in the control of ventricular output. For a given level of filling pressure and contractility an increase in peripheral resistance will reduce ventricular output and vice versa. Furthermore any sudden increase in peripheral resistance may in itself lead to a rise in filling pressure as the heart empties less completely with each beat. The normal heart compensates for this and filling pressure rapidly returns to the initial level. There is therefore subtle interaction between filling pressure, contractility and peripheral resistance. However, increases in cardiac output which is the product of stroke volume and heart rate, are probably to a large extent governed by the heart rate; although increased emptying of the ventricle due to a higher level of contractility also plays a role. Thus for a given level of ventricular performance a slow heart rate will lead to a low cardiac output and an increase in heart rate will result in a higher cardiac output.

The physiological principles described above apply to both the right and left ventricles. However, there are differences in behaviour which are of clinical significance. The right ventricle is more sensitive than the left ventricle in terms of output, to changes in filling pressure. For a given increase in filling pressure, therefore, particularly in an abnormal heart, the right ventricular output may increase more than that of the left. If this difference is considerable the pulmonary circulation becomes overfilled and pulmonary oedema may result.

Right ventricular filling pressure is largely determined by the volume of blood returning to it. This is governed by the amount of blood within the circulation and the state of the venous tone. If the circulation is depleted because of acute blood loss or plasma loss as in burns or vomiting, the right ventricular filling and therefore the right atrial pressure (central venous pressure) will be low resulting in a low right ventricular stroke output. The heart will attempt to maintain cardiac output by an increase in heart rate.

As blood is incompressible an increase in venous tone will shift blood towards the right ventricle and elevate right ventricular filling pressure. A normal ventricle will rapidly deal with this increased volume and eject it into the pulmonary circulation. However, if the pulmonary circulation is already overloaded as a result of perhaps left ventricular failure, the right sided filling pressure (central venous) will remain elevated. A similar situation occurs if the circulation is overfilled for example by too rapid infusion of blood or other fluid. On the other hand the output of the left ventricle is rather more sensitive to changes in peripheral arterial resistance. As already mentioned, the normal left ventricle can readily adjust to changes in peripheral resistance, when, however, left ventricular function is depressed, a sudden increase in arterial resistance may rapidly lead to the onset of left ventricular failure with elevation of filling pressure and fall in cardiac output.

This brief description of the physiological principles indicates some of the variables which should be considered during management of the critically ill.

These variables include pulse rate, blood pressure, central venous (right atrial pressure), left atrial pressure and cardiac output. The monitoring of these variables will now be considered.

Pulse rate, pulse volume and blood pressure

The pulse rate may be detected by palpation, by detecting the R-wave on the E.C.G. monitor or with the use of a peripheral pulse sensor (see also Part 4, ch. I, p. 899). The E.C.G. is susceptible to electrical artefacts which are less likely to occur when sensing the peripheral pulse by photoplethysmography. Where the blood pressure is low and there is peripheral vasoconstriction, the peripheral pulse signal may not be detectable. Pulse rate is an extremely delicate reflector of cardio-vascular status but may be radically affected by drugs, e.g. digitalis, β-blockers, atropine, neostigmine and by alterations in the level of certain hormones – in particular adrenaline and noradrenaline. A rising pulse rate is one of the earlier warning signs of loss in circulating blood volume and may precede or occur simultaneously with a fall in central venous pressure. A steadily rising pulse rate in the absence of fluid loss and in the presence of a falling blood pressure should make one consider sepsis, acid base, electrolyte or blood gas imbalance, fluid overload, or myocardial damage, as the underlying cause.

Pulse volume has been underrated as a valuable sign in the management of the shocked patient. It is a far more reliable indicator of haemodynamic status than the blood pressure. A crude assessment of femoral pulse volume by palpation in the presence of an impalpable radial artery pulse is an excellent guide to volume replacement, whilst awaiting insertion of a central venous line. The presence of a barely palpable femoral pulse of low volume and rapid rate in the absence of evidence of a diminished dynamic blood volume indicates a poor prognosis and warrants appropriate and immediate action.

Blood pressure

The blood pressure is commonly measured with a mercury manometer, using an inflatable cuff and a stethoscope. Systemic blood pressure is rarely recordable by this system below a level of 60 mm Hg. In the management of the shocked patient it is therefore recommended that an intra-arterial line should be inserted and a pressure transducer used to record blood pressure and to demonstrate minor changes in pressure not detectable by the cuff technique. Direct measurement of arterial pressure is described in Part 4, ch. I, p. 901. Insertion of an intra-arterial line in a severely shocked patient is not without its dangers. Radial artery cannulation results in a significant incidence of radial artery thrombosis and some of these patients have an inadequate collateral circulation with resultant ischaemic loss of tissue in the hand.

Femoral artery catheterisation using the Seldinger technique is probably the method of first choice. There are now commercially available kits which are pre-sterilised and contain a needle, guide wire and teflon catheter with connecting tube and tap with luer lock fitting. With care, these catheters can be left *in situ* for up to three days with virtually no morbidity. A further advantage of using the femoral artery is that it seems less affected by arterial constriction than the radial artery. This is important in the presence of severe hypotension, when radial artery pressure may not accurately reflect arterial pressure.

The small volume displacement achieved by modern pressure transducers makes it possible to work with small lumen catheters which have an external diameter of only 0.8 mm. These catheters can be connected to a variety of transducers via a three way tap. The catheters can be continuously flushed with heparinised 5% dextrose or 1/5 N saline, at a rate of 4 ml/h. This low rate of flushing does not interfere with the pressure measurements. Blood should never be allowed to run back into the cuvette of the transducer and it is important not to apply a dangerously high pressure to the transducer when flushing. Arterial samples may be taken from the side arm of the three way tap. Blood pressure should be quoted in reference to a particular plane – (commonly the midaxillary line) – the transducer should be so mounted that the reference level can be maintained when the patient's position is altered. Conventionally blood pressure is referred to atmospheric pressure at the height of the heart. Should the site of measurement not be at the heart level, a correction of -7.8 mm Hg must be made for every 100 mm below this level. Sterilisation is of extreme importance – the transducer must not be autoclaved but sterilised with a cold chemical such as activated glutaraldehyde (Cidex) or ethylene oxide. A description of the various transducers available, their calibration and the effect of various hydraulic systems on the frequency response is described by Hill and Dolan (1976). No air should be allowed to enter the system since the damping effect is considerable.

Indirect automatic monitoring of blood pressure is described in Part 4, ch. I, p. 900. Indirect automatic measurement of the brachial artery pressure based on the ultrasonic Doppler principle is becoming increasingly popular (Kontron Instruments). The method involves application of the transducer (using coupling gel) on to the brachial artery and securing the transducer with an inflatable cuff. Two mercury manometers are used to measure the cuff pressure, one recording systolic and the other diastolic pressure (see Fig. 2). Readings can be made on demand or at requested intervals and can be recorded on a pen

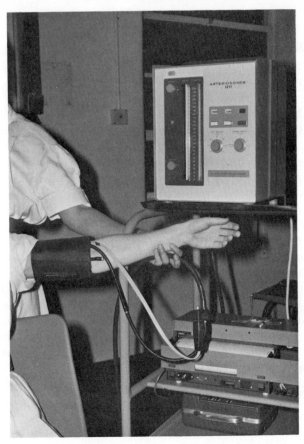

Fig. 2. Indirect Blood Pressure Monitoring System based on the ultrasound principle (Kontron Instruments) showing cuff (with transducer placed over the brachial artery) display panel and write-out system.

write-out. We have found this method convenient and accurate, pressures can be recorded as low as 40 mm S.P., the mercury levels are easy to see at a distance and are maintained at the last recorded pressure making ready assessment of progress. Good reports on the accuracy of this method have been given by Kazamias *et al.* (1971). Buggs *et al.* (1973) have investigated the method in hypotensive patients and found that the Doppler technique recorded systolic blood pressure when this was not detectable by auscultation or palpation.

Central venous pressure

The monitoring of central venous pressure is an excellent dynamic guide of haemodynamic status. The relationship between central venous pressure and cardiovascular functions have already briefly been described. An excellent description of the role of the central venous pressure in cardiovascular dynamics has been given by Russell, 1974.

As indicated, right atrial pressure monitoring gives a reliable measure of the balance between systemic venous return and right ventricular performance. Thus it is a valuable indicator of the level of the circulating blood volume.

Sequential changes are more important than the initial value, the absolute value depending upon the zero reference point being used. In general, a high right atrial pressure indicates true overload of the circulation, whether secondary to excess volume replacement or to acute left ventricular failure. However, in certain circumstances, a high right atrial pressure does not reflect these conditions; this is seen most commonly in patients with chronic or acute pulmonary hypertension. A high pulmonary vascular resistance is associated with an increased resistance to right ventricular emptying and right ventricular pressure must rise so that blood can flow into the pulmonary artery. Right atrial pressures in consequence must also rise and will be measured as a high central venous pressure. Should blood loss occur in such a patient the central venous pressure may only fall to a level which would otherwise be considered normal. The patient may, therefore, not have the volume replacement that is needed. On the other hand a high right atrial pressure in patients with chronic pulmonary hypertension must not be interpreted as indicating an elevated left ventricular filling pressure, which may, in fact be low. Diuretics may be entirely inappropriate and have a markedly deleterious effect.

Another situation where care is needed in the interpretation of central venous pressure is in patients where mechanical ventilation has been instituted. In this situation, particularly if positive end expiratory pressure has been added, a decrease in central venous pressure may occur, resulting in a fall in right ventricular output. With higher levels of pulmonary end expiratory pressure, the right atrial pressure may be normal or elevated but inadequate to maintain right ventricular filling pressure. During mechanical ventilation it is the transmural pressure which accurately reflects the haemodynamic state. Under these circumstances right atrial filling pressure measured relative to atmospheric pressure are unreliable (Qvist et al. 1975). The situation may be

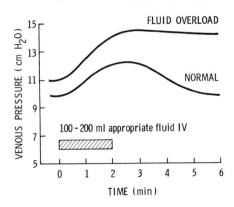

Fig. 3. Diagram showing the effect of a 'fluid challenge' on a patient with a high normal central venous pressure where diminished venous return is suspected.

clarified by the method of fluid challenge, or measurement of cardiac output: Sykes (1963) and Weil (1969) have advocated a fluid load to test cardiac performance. In an adult 100–200 ml of an appropriate fluid is infused over 2 min and the central venous pressure monitored subsequently (Fig. 3). A rise in central venous pressure of more than 3 cm H_2O indicates that the right ventricle cannot handle any more volume. Should there be a rise and fall to the preceding level in a patient on P.E.E.P. with decreased urine output, fall in pulse volume and/or blood pressure, the fluid challenges should be repeated until the central venous pressure no longer returns to the initial level. Should the aetiology of the shock state be obscure, or there are problems in obtaining a reliable response with monitoring of right atrial pressure, facilities permitting, the fluid challenge should be conducted in conjunction with measurement of right ventricular output (see p. 322) and monitoring of mixed venous oxygen tension from the pulmonary artery (see p. 319).

Because the right ventricle is more compliant than the left, in situations where rapid haemodynamic changes are occurring, right atrial pressure will not necessarily reflect left atrial pressure. An increased fluid load therefore may increase left atrial pressure more than right atrial pressure. When left atrial pressure exceeds 22 mm Hg pulmonary oedema occurs because the hydrostatic pressure now exceeds the osmotic pressure. In certain circumstances, however, pulmonary oedema may be secondary to an increase in capillary permeability. It is wise, therefore, to maintain the central venous pressure (right atrial pressure) at a low normal level (4–8 cm H_2O)

unless there is evidence of a decrease in cellular perfusion (decreased urine output, poor skin perfusion, tachycardia or decreased pulse pressure) when it is reasonable to conduct a fluid challenge. It should be stressed that pulmonary oedema as a result of fluid overload can occur in severely ill patients who otherwise have normal hearts, this is probably related to poor renal perfusion, high levels of circulating catecholamines, ADH and corticosteroids. It is essential, therefore, in the critically ill shocked patient to establish a good baseline for central venous pressure and to avoid an upward trend. A sudden rise in right atrial pressure may be related to pulmonary vasoconstriction or an increase in intrathoracic pressure such as following the institution of P.E.E.P., the development of tension pneumothorax or cardiac tamponade.

MONITORING SYSTEMS USED IN CLINICAL PRACTICE

Indications for right atrial pressure (central venous pressure) monitoring

Right atrial pressure monitoring should be instituted in any shocked patient, the possible exception being in the young patient where a brief period of shock is rapidly and permanently corrected by blood volume replacement.

Technique of measurement

There are several techniques in current use for the insertion of central venous catheters.

Ante-cubital vein

A 60 cm catheter should be inserted by a strictly sterile non-touch technique – the operator being gowned, gloved and masked. In patients over 176 cm (6 ft) high, a 90 cm catheter should be used especially if insertion into the left antecubital fossa is proposed. The most medial vein should be selected in the antecubital fossa and once the catheter has been inserted to the level of the axilla, the arms should be abducted at right angles from the chest and the patient's head turned towards the side of insertion. By this method, the catheter is less likely to enter the internal jugular vein. The catheter should be inserted to the hilt and the position adjusted so that the tip is in the right atrium. This can be confirmed by chest X-ray.

The disadvantage of this technique is that it is somewhat time consuming and difficulties can sometimes be encountered in locating a suitable ante-cubital vein. On some occasions even when a suitable vein has been located there may be considerable difficulty due to anatomical variations in actually passing the catheter into the right atrium.

Subclavian vein

The supra-clavicular approach is preferable to the infra-clavicular approach. The technique has been described in detail by Yoffa (1965), Ashbangh and Thomson (1963), Davidson *et al.* (1963) and Rushman *et al.* (1970). Both approaches expose the patient to the risk of pneumothorax and this is particularly so when patients are being respired with positive pressure ventilation. Under these circumstances, therefore, the subclavian approach should not be used.

Internal jugular vein

This technique has been described by English *et al.* (1969). It exposes the patient to very little risk, and with practice is relatively easy to perform. Its main disadvantage is that the patient has to be lying flat, and this may be impossible with a breathless patient. Using a Seldinger kit (i.e. needle, spring guide wire and teflon catheter) the right carotid artery is located at the mid point of the neck with the finger tips. The internal jugular vein lies just lateral to the artery. The needle with fluid filled syringe attached is firmly inserted at an angle of 45°. The plunger of the syringe is withdrawn and when the vein is entered dark blood will enter the syringe. The needle is held firmly, the syringe detached, and the guide wire gently passed down the needle. The needle is then removed and the teflon catheter then passed over the guide wire, which is then withdrawn. The catheter is then connected via a three way tap to the manometer.

Once in position, whichever technique is used the entry site of the catheter should be sealed with a clear plaster spray (not antibiotic ointment because of the danger of fungal infection) and the dressing taken down daily. Any evidence of infection around the insertion site, or a pyrexia for which no cause can be found, is an indication for removal of the catheter and culture of the catheter tip. The catheter should be preferably removed after 5 days and replaced in another site if necessary because of the increasing incidence of infection the longer the catheter is *in situ*.

It is probable that those in charge of critically ill patients should be familiar with all the techniques of insertion, and should develop their own preference. The central venous catheter is connected to a column filled with 5% dextrose, normal saline or 1/5 normal saline. The

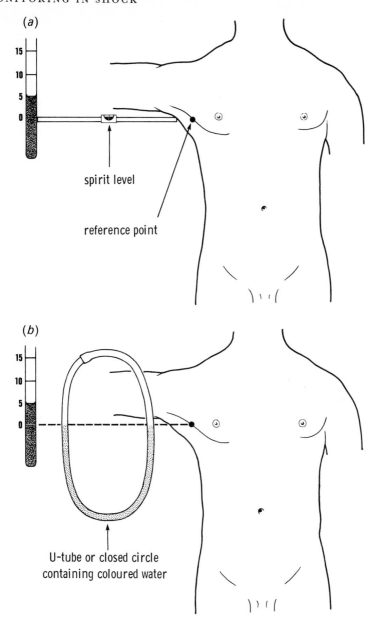

(a)

spirit level

reference point

(b)

U-tube or closed circle
containing coloured water

Fig. 4. Two methods for determining the reference level for measurement of central venous pressure. (*a*) Using a spirit level. (*b*) Using a U-tube or a closed circle (thereby avoiding spillage) containing coloured water.

catheter and column are connected via a three way tap to an infusion bottle containing one of the above fluids. The zero pressure reference point should be reproducible and meaningful. Many levels have been used (De Brunner and Bühler, 1969), the most simple being the midpoint between the arteroposterior diameter of the thorax at the level of the fourth intercostal space. The reference level should be marked on the patient's chest and readings should be taken using a fluid level or a U-tube (Snow and Dobnik, 1975) from the reference point to the zero level on the manometer scale – the patient being positioned in the horizontal plane (Fig. 4).

The method of measurement is relatively simple, reliable and does not need sophisticated technology. It should once again be stressed, that although the initial level of central venous pressure offers useful information it is the trend over the subsequent hours related to other appropriate clinical findings which is of greater significance.

Central venous pressure does not under certain circumstances accurately reflect left atrial pressure – this may be particularly important if left ventricular function is at all impaired. When such circumstances are thought to exist it may be necessary to measure pulmonary artery and pulmonary capillary wedge pressure and cardiac output. These measurements assess left ventricular function more accurately, a description is given later in this chapter. The measurements are time consuming and are not, therefore, applicable to most critically ill patients where time cannot be wasted in instituting treatment. The development of more rapid non-invasive techniques for assessing left ventricular function (see later section) may therefore have a further significant effect on the clinical management of such patients.

Apart from the monitoring of pulse, blood pressure and right and left atrial pressure there are other physiological variables which can give valuable information. These will now be considered.

Skin and core temperature differential

When nursing the critically ill shocked patient, an electrical method for monitoring skin and core temperature is essential. Two main principles of operation are used in these probes, either the change in electrical resistance of the probe element with its temperature or the generation of a thermal electromotive force by two dissimilar metals whose junctions are at different temperatures. The details of different probes available are described by Hill and Dolan (1976).

The measurement of core temperature is essential in order to prevent

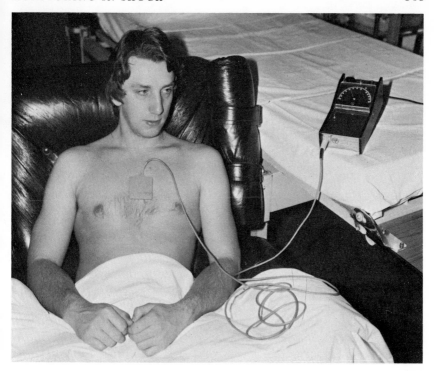

Fig. 5. Monitoring system for measuring core temperature.

dangerous fluctuations (which may affect cardiac rhythm) and as a comparison with the skin temperature. The temperature measured in the oesophagus at heart level is very close to that in the aorta (Cooper and Kenyon, 1957) and is considered an accurate indication of cardiac temperature. Rectal temperature should not be relied upon as an indicator of core temperature when the rectum is loaded; the probe should be strapped in position since movement of the patient may cause displacement. Rectal probes are uncomfortable for the patient and are impossible to retain when the patient is restless or has diarrhoea – a far more suitable and reliable method of core temperature monitoring has been developed by the Bioengineering Division of the M.R.C. England (Fox *et al.*, 1973: Solman and Datton, 1973) and is shown in Fig. 5. The measuring pad is attached to the patient by double-sided adhesive tape and is generally placed over the centre of the sternum. Fifteen to twenty minutes have to be allowed for the pad to heat to skin temperature, once this has occurred a direct recording is made of core temperature. The newer versions have upper and lower temperature alarms. The only disadvantages of this method is the time taken for the initial recording (which can be obviated by taking an oesphageal or rectal temperature if this is considered urgent). The pad (because of its size) tends to become displaced in patients with a small anterior chest wall and the cable from the pad may snap if unduly angulated.

Skin temperature (as measured from the medial aspect of the big toe) has been found to be a reliable indicator of cardiac output and indirectly an indicator of systemic blood flow (Joly and Weil, 1969; Eberhart and Trezek, 1974). Joly and Weil (1969) studied the temperature of the medial aspect of the big toe in patients with shock and found that if the temperature of the toe 3 hours after admission was less than 27°C, or the difference between toe and ambient temperature was less than 2°C, the likelihood of death was high (67%).

Continuous and simultaneous measurement of toe and core temperature has been found to be a valuable indicator of adequacy of skin perfusion – the difference between the two decreasing as skin perfusion improves. It is of interest to note that skin measurements may be extremely low (less than 30°C) during the initial phase of severe shock and may suddenly rise over a period of 30–45 min to levels within 4°C of core temperature once peripheral perfusion improves. In elderly patients it is important to check that peripheral arterial pulses are present once the systolic pressure rises above 80 mm Hg since a failure to improve skin temperature may be related to arterial thrombosis.

A persistently low skin temperature (less than 32°C) in the presence of a metabolic acidosis, adequate volume replacement and a low systolic pressure, should make one consider the use of peripheral vasodilators.

Urine volume per hour, U/P osmolality ratio

The hourly measurement of urine output is valuable in the assessment of renal perfusion in the shocked patient. An output of less than 40 ml/h is generally noted with a urine plasma osmolality ratio (U/P ratio) of 1.4 or less; an increase in urine output is one of the earliest reflectors of improvement in organ perfusion. It is important to check the U/P osmolality ratio prior to diuretic therapy.

The use of diuretics or the insidious development of high output renal failure may invalidate these measurements. A U/P osmolality ratio around 1.0 in the presence of polyuria and the absence of diuretic therapy is generally related to the onset of renal failure. The measurement of free water clearance has been suggested as an early predictor of renal failure and recovery (Baek *et al.*, 1973).

The diagnosis of acute renal failure is described in greater detail in Part 1, ch. IV, p. 76.

Respiratory rate and blood gas analysis

An early and ill appreciated sign of shock associated with sepsis is an increase in the respiratory rate. This is generally related to ventilation perfusion inequality and consequent hypoxia. The respiratory rate in the patient with hypovolaemic shock (unrelated to chest or head injury) generally remains normal until more than 30% of the blood volume has been lost. When more than 40% of the blood volume has been lost the patient characteristically develops air hunger because of depletion of oxygen carrying capacity. Various methods are available for monitoring respiratory rate in adults (Hill and Dolan, 1976) but generally reliance is made on nursing observations. A failure to increase the respiratory rate in a patient known to be hypoxic would suggest a depression in respiratory drive due to drugs, inadequate cerebral perfusion or brain trauma. Blackburn (Part 4, ch. I, p. 903) describes various systems for monitoring respiratory rate and tidal volume and methods for detecting gas concentrations in the inspired and expired air. Details are also given regarding apnoea detection systems used in units responsible for the management of the critically ill neonate.

All shocked patients should have arterial blood taken for blood gas estimation, preferably before giving oxygen or during the administration of a known inspiratory oxygen percentage. Intravascular polarographic electrodes for the continuous monitoring of PO_2 are now available and a monitoring system for the future may be continuous monitoring of the PaO_2 through the skin (Part 4, ch. I, p. 909). Maintenance of an adequate PaO_2 is one of the most important factors in the management of the shocked patient. It is generally found that all patients with sepsis with a systolic blood pressure below 100 mm Hg have a PaO_2 of 8.6 kPa (65 mm Hg) or less when breathing air; this may be particularly profound in cases of intra-abdominal sepsis.

Early onset of severe hypoxia following trauma with mild to moderate hypovolaemic shock should make one suspect pulmonary aspiration, pulmonary oedema due to fluid overload, or the early onset of the fat embolism syndrome. A reliable assessment of the alveolar-arterial oxygen gradient is not possible in a shocked patient breathing spontaneously.

Acid base status

The importance of the acid base state and treatment of disorders in acid base balance has been discussed on p. 108. The extent of cellular hypoxia subsequent to inadequate peripheral perfusion is reflected in the blood pH and serum lactate. Both initial levels and the directional changes in serum lactate may be used as prognostic indicators. Carey *et al.* (1971) found that in haemorrhagic shock the magnitude of lactate elevation was not a reliable indicator of survival but there was a relationship between the severity of shock and the degree of lactic acidaemia. A persistently raised blood lactate following resuscitation generally indicated a bad prognosis. Serial lactate levels may be valuable in indicating the adequacy of resuscitation but the estimation is time consuming and is rarely indicated during treatment of shock, measurement of pH and base deficit giving adequate information for appropriate therapy.

Haemoglobin, haematocrit and clotting factors

The quality of haemoglobin is essential for adequate oxygen uptake and delivery to the cell and the level of the haematocrit can radically effect blood viscosity (p. 296). In shock multiple estimations of Hct are essential in order to maintain the level at an optimum for oxygen transport. Optimal oxygen transport capacity has been found at an Hct of around 30% (Hint, 1968) and will not fall below normal values (provided normovolaemia is maintained) until the Hct is less than 25% (Messmer *et al.*, 1972).

Early base line assessment of clotting factors is essential in the management of the shocked patient. Prolongation may indicate the early onset of disseminated intravascular coagulation or deficiency of labile factors due to replacement with old blood (see p. 365, Table 3). A fall in the platelet count, in the absence of haemorrhage, may suggest shock related to sepsis. Severe haemorrhage followed by replacement with old blood is commonly associated with thrombocytopenia. Thrombocytopenia in the absence of any clotting factor abnormality is not indicative of disseminated intravascular coagulation.

MONITORING SYSTEMS USED IN THE EVALUATION OF THE CRITICALLY ILL SHOCKED PATIENT WHO FAILS TO RESPOND TO TRADITIONAL THERAPY

In this section an attempt will be made to rationalise investigations so that appropriate therapy can be started. It is tempting to obtain far too

Table 1. Monitoring methods considered essential in the management of the majority of shocked patients

Analysis	Method	Function assessed
Pulse Rate	Manual or from E.C.G.	Overall haemodynamic state
Pulse volume ⎫ Blood pressure ⎭	Manual or mechanical cuff technique Intra-arterial line and pressure transducer	
Central venous pressure (C.V.P.)	Right atrial line. Water manometer or pressure transducer	Right ventricular function Pulmonary artery pressure Venous return
Skin and core temperature	Skin probe Rectal or central body probe	Skin perfusion in relation to central body perfusion
Urine volume/h Urine plasma osmolality ratio (U/P ratio) before diuretics	Urinary catheter – burette Semiautomated system Osmometry	Renal function and perfusion
Respiratory rate Blood gas analysis	Generally visual Arterial sample rapid analysis Intravascular polarographic electrode	Pulmonary function
Acid base status	Arterial or arterialised capillary sample	Reflection of pulmonary and metabolic function and cellular perfusion
Hb Haematocrit	Venous blood in appropriate sampling bottles	Rough estimation of oxygen carrying capacity related to blood viscosity
Clotting factors		Prolongation may reflect inadequate capillary perfusion, loss of clotting factors due to haemorrhage, or the presence of factors which depress coagulation

many indices which when inaccurate or interpreted incorrectly may lead to greater errors in management than would exist if therapy was based on simpler tests (Table 1). The more complex the test the greater the likelihood of error and this is particularly true in the severely shocked patients where appropriate catheter placement may be difficult. On occasions it is wise to start therapy before more elaborate investigations are started since delay may result in death. Some of these investigations are still being evaluated by units experienced in their use and it is hoped that the procedures will become fewer and simpler.

A non-invasive technique for assessment of left ventricular function is urgently needed and it is hoped that transcutaneous aortovelography may meet this requirement (see p. 323).

Alveolar arterial oxygen gradient – respiratory index – percentage saturation of blood in the right atrium – difference between arterial and mixed venous oxygen content

The indications for ventilation in the critically ill shocked patient are generally based on the respiratory rate and the blood gases. Ventilation is generally indicated when the respiratory rate is greater than 35 (in an adult) and the PaO_2 on oxygen via a mask is less than 9.3 kPa (70 mm Hg). The $PaCO_2$ generally rises terminally in the shocked patient unless there has been preceding respiratory failure.

Once the patient is ventilated, the alveolar arterial oxygen gradient can be readily calculated (Part 1, ch. II, p. 21) and not only gives a guide to the oxygen required in order to maintain an adequate PaO_2 but also can be used sequentially to assess patient progress (Woo and Hedley-Whyte, 1973). Goldfarb *et al.* (1975) have evolved a respiratory index based on the alveolar arterial oxygen gradient divided by the PaO_2. An index of 6.1 or greater was associated with a mortality of 41% (see also Part 2, ch. V, p. 555).

It is preferable to make the calculation on the inspired oxygen percentage the patient is already receiving since (1) with prolonged ventilation, exposure to 100% oxygen should be avoided, and (2) exposure to 100% oxygen even for a short period may alter the pulmonary shunt (see Part 2, ch. V, p. 553).

The measurement of percentage oxygen saturation in the right atrium has been found to correlate with right ventricular output in shock (Lee *et al.* 1972). This (though less reliable) may be used as a guide to the right ventricular response on the institution of P.E.E.P. if pulmonary artery sampling is not possible. Lee and co-workers (1972) found that a percentage oxygen saturation in the right atrium of less than 65% was related to a cardiac index of less than 2.0 l/m²/min and greater than 70% was related to a cardiac index of 2.7 l/m²/min or above. As with most indices, sequential changes are more helpful as a therapeutic guide than isolated recordings. A fibre optic catheter for continuous monitoring of oxygen saturation is now available. A calculation of the difference in oxygen content between blood taken simultaneously from the right atrium (via the central venous catheter) and an artery appears to provide prognostic data (Wilson *et al.*, 1974). A low A–V O$_2$ difference (especially less than 1.0 vol/100 ml) or a high venous oxygen saturation, is a bad prognostic sign indicating poor peripheral oxygen utilisation or peripheral systemic shunting.

Pulmonary artery pressure (P.A.P.) – Pulmonary capillary wedge pressure (P.C.W.P.) – Arterial and mixed venous oxygen content difference

The pulmonary artery pressure can be monitored by the introduction of a flow directed balloon tipped catheter. This may be either of double lumen (for measuring P.A.P., P.C.W.P. and mixed venous oxygen content as described by Swan *et al.* (1970) or of triple lumen (Ganz *et al.* 1971). The triple lumen catheter permits measurement of the P.A.P., P.C.W.P., mixed venous oxygen content and central venous pressure.

The technique of balloon flotation catheterisation is described in detail by Swan and Ganz (1975). When using the triple lumen catheter, the lumens for monitoring P.A.P. and C.V.P. should be filled with sterile saline and the lumen measuring P.A.P. attached to a pressure transducer and the trace displayed on an oscilloscope. The E.C.G. should be monitored continuously during insertion because of the danger of dysrhythmia. The catheter is inserted as for monitoring of the central venous pressure (see p. 309), the catheter reaching the right atrium after 45–55 cm insertion from the left, and 35–40 cm from the right antecubital fossa and approximately 10 cm from the subclavian vein (supraclavicular technique) and 8 cm from the subclavian vein (infraclavicular technique). Entry into the thorax is shown by pressure oscillations on the oscilloscope, the balloon is then inflated with 0.8 ml of air and the catheter advanced gently under monitoring control. Entry into the pulmonary artery is confirmed by a trace showing the same systolic pressure as the right ventricle but a higher diastolic pressure. The catheter may then be advanced a little further if P.C.W.P. is required. The balloon should then be deflated. Should the catheter fail to record pulmonary capillary wedge pressure after advancement of more than 16 cm from the ventricle, the catheter should be withdrawn to the right ventricular position and reinsertion commenced.

With the increasing use of flow directed balloon tipped catheters, more dangers are being reported. These include damage to the pulmonary capillaries which is generally small but may lead to pulmonary infarction if solutions are injected at relatively high pressure through the catheter lumen. Pulmonary damage should be avoided in the critically ill patient whose pulmonary functional reserve is very limited. Pulmonary infarction may follow prolonged wedging and therefore the balloon should be deflated after each recording. Other complications include cardiac dysrhythmias, balloon rupture, catheter knotting, thromboembolism and infection. Greene and Cummings (1973) reported an incidence of 9.3% of autopsy cases with aseptic right-sided endocarditis who had received monitoring with a pulmonary artery catheter during their terminal hospital course. The incidence of sepsis is probably similar to that for any central line (Schils, 1972).

In the management of the critically ill pulmonary artery catheters have been left in place for 7 days or more. Swan and Ganz (1975) however now recommend that 48 h of continuous use in a single patient should be the upper limit of safe utilisation. This they state is because the latex of the balloon tends to take up lipoproteins from the blood with consequent deterioration in elastic property and a tendency towards disintegration. P.C.W.P. recordings may not reflect left atrial pressure when the patient is receiving P.E.E.P. or in the patient with high airways pressure. Lozman et al. (1974) found that in 5 postoperative open-heart surgery patients receiving P.E.E.P., P.C.W.P. did not reflect changes in directly measured left atrial pressure in 9 of 32 data sets. These failures occurred at levels of P.E.E.P. 10 cm H_2O or above. The measurement of P.C.W.P. appears to be a reliable index of left atrial pressure in patients during spontaneous respiration or during administration of intermittent positive pressure ventilation (Lappas et al., 1973). P.C.W.P. monitoring will generally be considered in the critically ill shocked patient when the central venous pressure is running high and the question is raised whether this is related to an increase in pulmonary artery pressure or reflecting a rise in left atrial pressure. Many of these patients are receiving P.E.E.P. (in order to maintain an adequate PaO_2) and under these conditions measurement of P.C.W.P. does not always accurately reflect left atrial pressure (see above). Another significant error is the phenomenon called 'over-wedging'. Here a spuriously high P.C.W.P. is recorded probably because the balloon is overinflated and partially seals over the open end of the catheter.

The monitoring of P.A.P. is less difficult, less subject to error and is unlikey to be complicated by pulmonary damage unless the catheter is forced too far distally during placement (Cerra *et al.*, 1972). Unfortunately the results obtained do not reflect left atrial pressure in the critically ill, being affected by an increase in pulmonary vascular resistance or a raised intrathoracic pressure. Many authors claim that the measurement of the central venous pressure is an unreliable estimation on which to base fluid balance and therapeutic management of the critically ill. These claims are correct – if readings are taken in isolation, without relating to preceding records and placing sequential recordings into context with other findings. Sequential accurate readings and careful observation of a trend however can be vital in the management of the critically ill. We do not consider that the monitoring of P.C.W.P. is essential in the management of the critically ill shocked patient and should be used in a situation where the central venous pressure recordings are steadily rising (without the sudden rise which generally occurs on commencing P.E.E.P.) and where no other index of left ventricular function is available.

During the institution of P.E.E.P. a comparison of right atrial pressure, P.A.P. and right ventricular cardiac output before and after introduction of P.E.E.P., are probably far more reliable indices on which to base subsequent management (see p. 327). The monitoring of the difference between arterial and mixed venous oxygen content taking the mixed venous sample from the pulmonary artery, is obviously a better prognostic indicator than sampling from the right atrium and is also more reliable as an index of right ventricular output. Four volumes per cent suggests a normal cardiac output, greater than 6 volumes per cent a low cardiac output and less than 3 volumes per cent a high cardiac output (Berk, 1975).

Accurate estimation of oxygen content can only be made with the technique of Van Slyke and Neil (1924). This is particularly time consuming and not applicable to the clinical situation. It is now possible to measure blood oxygen content directly using the Lex O_2 Con equipment. This gives a direct digital read out of oxygen content and is now coming into more general use in the management of critically ill patients.

Accurate estimation of haemoglobin saturation can also now be made using a transmission oximeter (IL Co-oximeter). This measures the optical density of haemoglobin at three different wavelengths and presents the value of haemoglobin and haemoglobin saturation in digital form.

Cardiac output, systemic vascular resistance – Assessment of left ventricular function

The most suitable method of measuring cardiac output at the bedside is the thermodilution technique (Part 4, ch. I, p. 905). Using the Swan–Ganz triple lumen catheter, which also has a temperature sensitive thermistor embedded on its outer surface near the distal tip, it is possible to make the following measurements: right atrial pressure, pulmonary artery pressure and pulmonary capillary wedge pressure (P.C.W.P.). Assessment of P.C.W.P. requires that the balloon on the pulmonary artery catheter is inflated and the catheter allowed to float into and wedge in a pulmonary capillary. Cardiac output is determined by injecting 10 ml of either ice cold or room temperature 5% dextrose into the lumen that opens in the right atrium. This bolus is mixed in the right atrium and right ventricle and the change in temperature of the blood is detected by the thermistor lying in the pulmonary artery. Several thermo-dilution computers are commercially available and these integrate the area under the thermo-dilution curve presenting the value for cardiac output in analogue or digital form.

With the introduction of these more automated systems of cardiac output measurement the monitoring of right ventricular output will become more readily available. This will be of particular importance in the management of the shocked patient where volume, blood gas and metabolic imbalance has been corrected, together with any cardiac dysrhythmia or left ventricular failure; but where organ perfusion remains poor (as measured by urine output, skin core temperature difference and acid base status). Severe hypoxia may necessitate the use of P.E.E.P. which may be lethal if instituted in the presence of inadequate right ventricular output. It will also enable (in conjunction with other indices) a more scientific approach to drug therapy for improvement of organ perfusion.

Once central venous pressure, mean arterial pressure and cardiac output has been measured, an indicator of peripheral perfusion can be calculated – total systemic vascular resistance (Berk, 1975)

$$T.S.R. = \frac{M.A.P. - C.V.P.}{C.O.} \; 79.8$$

Where T.S.R. = total systemic vascular resistance (dyne-s-cm^{-5}), M.A.P. = mean arterial pressure (mm Hg), C.V.P. = central venous pressure (mm Hg), C.O. = cardiac output l/min.

Berk (1975) has found that the T.S.R. is usually elevated in cardiogenic shock (greater than 1500 dyne-s-cm^{-5}), whereas a normal or low resistance (1000 dyne-s-cm^{-5}) or less suggests an associated hyperdynamic state and sepsis. A normal or elevated T.S.R. in shock associated with sepsis may suggest inadequate blood volume replacement (Berk, 1975).

Assessment of left ventricular function
With the data for P.C.W.P. and cardiac output obtained from the Swan–Ganz thermodilution catheter, and with a satisfactory measurement of mean systemic blood pressure it is possible to calculate stroke work using the following formula:

$$S.W. = \frac{S.V. \times (M.S.P. - P.C.W.P.) \times 1.36}{100}$$

Where S.W. = stroke work gm m, S.V. = stroke volume (cardiac output/heart rate) ml, M.S.P. = mean systemic blood pressure mm Hg, P.C.W.P. = mean pulmonary capillary wedge pressure mm Hg.

The value for stroke work can then be plotted against the P.C.W.P. which is taken to represent left heart filling pressure. If the left heart filling pressure can be varied then a classic Frank–Sterling curve can be obtained. This is a particularly time consuming operation and is, therefore, not generally applicable to critically ill patients; it may be useful however in the management of patients with severe acute myocardial infarction or following cardiac surgery.

There is, however, a new non-invasive technique (Transcutaneous Aortovelography) which may ultimately prove to be of value in the sequential assessment of transaortic flow in the shocked patient. The measurement is based on the Doppler principle and uses an ultrasonic beam with a transmission frequency of 2 mHz. The emitted energy is back-scattered by red cells moving round the aortic arch with a frequency shift proportional to the aortic blood velocity. The system has recently been evaluated (Light, 1976; Sequira *et al.*, 1976) and preliminary investigation has found it to be of great value in the therapeutic assessment of the shocked patient (Buchtal *et al.*, 1976). The characteristic wave form appearances in different types of shock are illustrated in Fig. 6. Sequential changes following various therapeutic

Cardiogenic shock following myocardial infarction

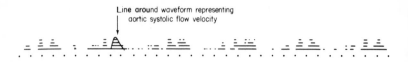

Septic shock (central venous pressure normal)

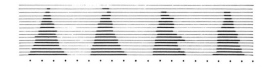

Hypovolaemic shock

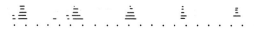

Fig. 6. Transcutaneous aortovelography (T.A.V.) traces obtained from patients admitted with various forms of shock.

manipulations are of particular value in assessing patient progress. Quantitation of the wave form is useful in evaluation of less obvious wave form changes and the initial systolic acceleration may prove to be an index of left ventricular function. The following references are of value for those readers interested in the initial clinical evaluation (Buchtal *et al.*, 1976; Hanson, 1976; Bilton *et al.*, 1978).

Pulmonary compliance

Suter and co-workers (1975) found that when cardiac output or true mixed venous blood is not available, compliance may be used to indicate the end-expiratory pressure likely to result in optimum cardio-pulmonary function.

A decrease in pulmonary compliance may also prove to be an early indicator of the onset of the 'shock lung syndrome' (Part 2, ch. V, p. 539). Sequential analysis of total pulmonary compliance is now possible with some of the more modern ventilators and the sequential evaluation should be considered in patients who have recovered from a period of shock, in patients with extensive sepsis and before and after the institution of P.E.E.P.

Table 2. Monitoring methods used in the evaluation of the critically ill shocked patient who fails to respond to traditional therapy, such as volume, blood gas and metabolic correction and correction of left ventricular failure and cardiac dysrhythmia

Analysis	Method	Function Assessed
Alveolar-arterial oxygen gradient	Measurement of PaO_2 on a known inspiratory oxygen percentage	Pulmonary function
Respiratory index (see text)		
Right atrial percentage oxygen saturation	Blood sample from right atrial C.V.P. catheter Continuous monitoring fibre optic catheter (Part 4, ch. I, p. 909)	Right ventricular output Oxygen uptake
Pulmonary artery pressure (P.A.P.)	Catheterisation of the pulmonary artery. Pressure transducer and display	Right ventricular output Pulmonary vascular resistance
Pulmonary capillary wedge pressure (P.C.W.P.)	Catheter sited correctly in wedge position. Pressure transducer and display	Left atrial pressure
Difference between arterial and mixed venous oxygen content	Measurement of oxygen content in the pulmonary artery and peripheral artery	Right ventricular output
Cardiac output	Dye dilution technique Thermo dilution technique Transcutaneous aortovelography (T.A.V.)	Right ventricular output Index of left ventricular function
Total systemic vascular resistance	Calculated (p. 322)	Peripheral perfusion
Pulmonary compliance	Calculated from pressure and flow traces during ventilation Method for assessment using the Servo ventilator-Elma-Schönander. (Ingelstedt *et al.*, 1972) (Sequential recordings more valuable than one isolated reading)	Pulmonary 'elasticity' May predict onset of pulmonary failure Of value for assessment of effect of P.E.E.P. on haemodynamic state and pulmonary function

Table 3. Normal range of values of some indices referred to in Tables 1 and 2

Index measured	Normal value	Comments
Central venous pressure (C.V.P.)	2–8 cm H_2O (1.5–6 mm Hg)	Affected by venous return, R.V. function, P.A.P., I.T.P.* and L.V. function
Right atrial percentage oxygen saturation	70–80%	Possible index of R.V. function and oxygen uptake
Difference between arterial and mixed venous oxygen content	3–6 vol %	>6 vol % suggests low and <3 vol % a high R.V. output
Pulmonary artery diastolic pressure (P.A.D.P.)	6–12 cm H_2O (4.4–9 mm Hg)	Affected by R.V. function, P.A.P., I.T.P.* and L.V. function
Pulmonary capillary wedge Pressure (P.C.W.P.)	8–14 cm H_2O (6–10.4 mm Hg)	Reflects L.V. function except when I.T.P.* or pulmonary capillary pressure high
		>24 cm H_2O suggests early pulmonary oedema in the absence of the above.
Cardiac output (C.O.)	>4.0 l/min	Average at rest 5.0–13.0 l/min
Cardiac index	2.5–3.0 l/min/m²	Cardiac minute output per m² of body surface
Total systemic vascular resistance	1000–1500 dyne/s/cm^{-5}	For calculation see p. 322
		May be valuable in conjunction with C.O. for deciding upon appropriate drug therapy for shock
Alveolar arterial oxygen gradient	4.0–9.3 kPa (30–70 mm Hg)	Valuable for assessment of progress in pulmonary function and appropriate oxygen therapy
Skin core temperature difference	<2°C	Index of skin perfusion in relation to central body perfusion

* I.T.P. = Intrathoracic pressure

With the development of electronically controlled servo-ventilators it is possible to obtain on-line measurements of airway resistance and total pulmonary compliance. This can be calculated from analogue outputs of pressure and flow. The relevance of these measurements in the clinical management of critically ill patients remains to be determined.

Conclusion

The monitoring methods considered essential in the management of the majority of shocked patients are tabulated in Table 1. Should the patient fail to improve with 'traditional' methods of treatment (blood volume replacement, acid base and electrolyte correction, correction of blood gases and correction of cardiac dysrhythmias or overt left ventricular failure), more sophisticated methods of monitoring may be indicated in order to decide upon appropriate drug therapy. The institution of P.E.E.P. for severe hypoxia in a shocked patient poses a special problem and is discussed below.

The monitoring methods enumerated in Table 2 are more elaborate and are not readily available to the average clinician. Monitoring of the alveolar-arterial oxygen gradient may be sufficient to decide upon the severity of pulmonary failure and sequential determination of the right atrial percentage oxygen saturation is helpful in indicating right ventricular function. It is probable that future monitoring of the shocked patient unresponsive to traditional methods of treatment will be narrowed down to monitoring of right atrial pressure, right ventricular cardiac output (and hence T.S.R.), the alveolar-arterial oxygen gradient, pulmonary compliance and T.A.V. as an indicator of left ventricular function. Initial recordings of these indices will evaluate right and left ventricular function, pulmonary function and the state of the peripheral circulation. Sequential evaluation will indicate response to various therapeutic manoeuvres and also may predict the onset of pulmonary failure.

A summary of the normal values for some of the less well-known indices referred to in Tables 1 and 2 are shown in Table 3.

THE MONITORING OF A PATIENT BEFORE AND AFTER THE INTRODUCTION OF P.E.E.P.

The haemodynamic responses to mechanical ventilation with P.E.E.P. are now becoming increasingly recognised (Qvist et al., 1975; Suter et *al.*, 1975). These responses are more pronounced in the critically ill and cardiac output may fall sufficiently to decrease organ perfusion. The patients particularly at risk are those with poor right ventricular function (due to myocardial suppression or cardiac disease) or those with hypovolaemia or diminished blood volume reserve.

The indications for the use of P.E.E.P. are detailed elsewhere but may be summarised as those patients (with presumed preceding normal pulmonary function) whose PaO_2 on mechanical ventilation is 9.3 kPa (70 mm Hg) or less on an inspiratory oxygen percentage of 50, and those patients where, because of lung pathology, P.E.E.P. is considered beneficial (aspiration syndrome, pulmonary atelectasis). Cardiac output is unlikely to decrease at levels of P.E.E.P. below 5 cm H_2O, and may even increase (Hobelman *et al.*, 1975) but once it is proposed to use P.E.E.P. at higher levels – a degree of monitoring is essential. There is considerable evidence that the maximal PaO_2 is often achieved by levels of P.E.E.P. above 10 cm H_2O (Downs *et al.*, 1973; Falke *et al.*, 1972) and that patients with the greatest degree of pulmonary dysfunction have the largest increases in PaO_2 following P.E.E.P. (Ashbaugh and Petty, 1973; McMahon *et al.*, 1973). Suter and co-workers (1975) found that the end expiratory pressure resulting in maximum oxygen transport (cardiac output times arterial oxygen content) was achieved when the maximal venous oxygen tension, cardiac output and pulmonary compliance were obtained with sequential increases of P.E.E.P. Hobelman and co-workers (1975) found a fall in cardiac output at levels of P.E.E.P. higher than 10 cm H_2O but it is probable that a fall did not occur before then since all their patients had baseline cardiac indices of 3 l/min/m² or greater. At levels of P.E.E.P. as high as 20 cm H_2O the cardiac index was found to fall as much as 2.26 l/min/m². Attempts should be made therefore to correct a low right ventricular output before introducing P.E.E.P. Arterial blood pressure may not change in spite of major alteration in right ventricular output and the steady increase in C.V.P. with increases of P.E.E.P. may not correlate with the decrease in right ventricular output (Hobelman *et al.*, 1975). When intrathoracic pressure (I.T.P.) rises, the effective right ventricular filling pressure (C.V.P. minus I.T.P.) can only be maintained if the C.V.P. also rises. It is possible that the rise in C.V.P. may protect against a change in cardiac output by maintaining an effective right ventricular filling pressure. Qvist and co-workers (1975) have found experimentally that the fall in right ventricular output can be reversed by blood volume augmentation; it is preferable however to reduce the level of P.E.E.P. to levels below which right ventricular output falls

Table 4. Monitoring systems which may be required during the use of P.E.E.P.

A–aO$_2$ difference
Mixed venous oxygen tension (measured from the pulmonary artery)
Central venous pressure
Right ventricular cardiac output
Pulmonary compliance
Possibly T.A.V. (in the future)

unless an adequate PaO$_2$ cannot be maintained. Volume augmentation may be followed by pulmonary oedema on withdrawal of P.E.E.P. (Qvist *et al.*, 1975).

Hobelman and co-workers (1975) found that the use of P.E.E.P. up to 10 cm H$_2$O is quite safe provided the patient had an initial cardiac index of 3 l/min/m^2 or more. P.C.W.P. was found to increase above these levels and was generally a sign that a fall in cardiac output had occurred. Since most of these patients have severe pulmonary dysfunction and monitoring has frequently to be continued for many days – the sequential analysis of mixed venous oxygen tension, and/or pulmonary compliance and if possible right ventricular output seem to be a safer method of forecasting a deterioration in right ventricular function in patients being ventilated on levels of P.E.E.P. of 8 cm H$_2$O or more.

Table 5. Guidelines for management of the critically ill patient on mechanical ventilation with P.E.E.P.

Prior to starting P.E.E.P.

Measure right atrial pressure – and 'top up' with fluid if measuring 10 cm of water or
  less, to a level of 10 cm H$_2$O

Measure percentage oxygen saturation from the right atrium (1)

If facilities permit – Measure pulmonary compliance (2) or Mixed venous oxygen
  tension (from the pulmonary artery) (3) or Right ventricular cardiac output (4)

DO NOT commence P.E.E.P. if there is suspected hypovolaemia

Start P.E.E.P. at 2 cm H$_2$O and increase at 30 min intervals with 2 cm H$_2$O increments.
  (Sequential monitoring may not be possible if the patient is desperately ill)

Measure after 20 minutes at the set level of P.E.E.P. the indices above

A suitable level of P.E.E.P. is reached once the PaO$_2$ is 9.3 kPa (70 mm Hg) or greater
  on 50% inspiratory oxygen

DO NOT increase P.E.E.P. above a level at which the indices (1) (2) (3) or (4) start
  to fall. It may be necessary to have to accept a PaO$_2$ of 8.0–9.3 kPa (60–70 mm Hg).

The monitoring systems which may be required in order to ensure optimum right ventricular output, pulmonary perfusion and oxygen transport before and during the institution of P.E.E.P. are summarised in Table 4. Future work may show that the monitoring of transaortic flow by the method of T.A.V. in conjunction with sequential analysis of mixed venous oxygen tension, may be equally as rewarding. Guidelines for monitoring patients on P.E.E.P. are summarised in Table 5.

REFERENCES

Ashbaugh, D. and Thomson, J. W. W. (1963). Subclavian-vein infusion. *Lancet* **2**, 1138.

Ashbaugh, D. G. and Petty, T. L. (1973). Positive end-expiratory pressure; physiology, indications and contraindications. *J. Thorac. Cardiovasc. Surg.* **65**, 165.

Baek, S. M., Brown, R. S. and Shoemaker, W. C. (1973). Early prediction of renal failure and recovery: sequential measurement of free water clearance. *Ann. Surg.* **177**, 253.

Berk, J. L. (1975). Monitoring the patient in shock. *Surg. Clin. N. Amer.* **55**, 713.

Bilton, A. H., Brotherhood, J., Cross, G., Hanson, G. C., Light, L. H. and Sequeira, R. F. (1978). Transcutaneous aortovelography as a measure of central blood flow. *J. Physiology*. Proceedings of the Physiological Society. (In press).

Buchtal, Anna., Hanson, Gillian C. and Peisach, A. R. (1976). Transcutaneous aortovelography. Potentially useful technique in management of critically ill patients. *Brit. Heart J.* **38**, 451.

Buggs, H., Johnson, Jr. P. E., Gordon, L. S., Balguma, F. B. and Wettach, G. E. (1973). Comparison of systolic arterial blood pressure by transcutaneous doppler probe and conventional methods in hypotensive patients. *Anaesth. Analg. Curr. Res.* **52**, 776.

Carey, L. C., Lowery, B. D. and Cloutier, C. T. (1971). Haemorrhagic Shock. *In* 'Current Problems in Surgery' (Ed. M. M. Ravitch), p. 11. Year Book Medical Publishers Inc., Chicago.

Cerra, F., Milch, R. and Lajos, T. Z. (1972). Pulmonary artery catheterisation in critically ill surgical patients. *Ann. Surg.* **1**, 37.

Cooper, K. E. and Kenyon, J. R. (1957). A comparison of temperatures measured in the rectum, oesophagus and on the surface of the aorta in hypothermia in man. *Brit. J. Surg.* **44**, 616.

Davidson, J. T., Ben-Hur, N. and Nathan, H. H. (1963). Subclavian venepuncture. *Lancet* **2**, 1139.

De Brunner, F. and Buhler, F. (1969). Normal C.V.P., the significance of the reference point and normal range. *Brit. Med. J.* **3**, 148.

Downs, J. B., Klein, E. F. and Modell, J. H. (1973). The effect of incremental P.E.E.P. on PaO_2 in patients with respiratory failure. *Anaesthesiol. Analg.* (Cleve) **52**, 210.

Eberhart, R. C. and Trezek, G. J. (1974). Central and peripheral rewarming patterns in post-operative cardiac patients. *Critical Care Med.* **1**, 239.

English, I. C. W., Frew, R. M., Pigott, J. F. and Zaki, M. (1969). Percutaneous catheterisation of the internal jugular vein. *Anaesthesia* **24**, 521.

Falke, K. J., Pontoppidan, H. and Kumar, A. (1972). Ventilation with end-expiratory pressure in acute lung disease. *J. Clin. Invest.* **51**, 2315.

Fox, R. H., Solman, A. J., Isaacs, R., Fry, A. J. and McDonald, I. C. (1973). A new method for monitoring deep body temperature from the skin surface. *Clin. Sci.* **44**, 81.

Ganz, W., Donoso, R. and Marcus, H. S. (1971). A new technique for measurement of cardiac output by thermodilution in man. *Amer. J. Cardiol.* **27**, 392.

Goldfarb, M. A., Clurij, T. F., McAslan, T. C., Sacco, W. J., Weinstein, M. A. and Cowley, R. A. (1975). Tracking respiratory therapy in the trauma patient. *Amer. J. Surg.* **129**, 255.

Greene, J. F. and Cummings, K. C. (1973). Aseptic thrombotic endocardial vegetations. A complication of indwelling pulmonary artery catheters. *J.A.M.A.* **225**, 1525.

Hanson, Gillian C. and Buchtal, Anna. (1976). Clinical experience with transcutaneous aortovelography. *In* 'Application of Electronics in Medicine.' Inst. of Electronic & Radio Engineers, London.

Hill, D. W. and Dolan, A. M. (1976). The measurement of blood pressure. *In* 'Intensive Care Instrumentation.' p. 4. Academic Press, London and New York.

Hill, D. W. and Dolan, A. M. (1976). The monitoring of body temperature. *In* 'Intensive Care Instrumentation.' p. 159. Academic Press, London and New York.

Hill, D. W. and Dolan, A. M. (1976). Respiratory measurements. *In* 'Intensive Care Instrumentation.' p. 76. Academic Press, London and New York.

Hint, H. (1968). The pharmacology of dextran and the pathophysiological background for the clinical use of Rheomacrodex and Macrodex. *Acta. Anaesth. Belg.* **19**, 119.

Hobelman, C. F. Jr., Smith, D. E., Virgilio, R. W., Shapiro, A. R. and Peters, R. M. (1975). Haemodynamic alterations with positive end-expiratory pressure: the contribution of the pulmonary vasculature. *J. Trauma* **15**, 951.

Ingelstedt, S., Jonson, B., Nordström, L. and Olsson, S. G. (1972). A servo-controlled ventilator measuring expired minute volume, airway flow and pressure. *Acta. Anaesthesiol. Scand.* (Suppl. 47) 7.

Joly, H. R. and Weil, M. H. (1969). Temperature of the great toe as an indication of the severity of shock. *Circulation* **39**, 131.

Kazamias, T. M., Gander, M. P., Franklin, D. L. and Ross, Jr. J. (1971). Blood pressure measurement with doppler ultrasonic flow meter. *J. Appl. Physiol.* **30**, 585.

Lappas, D., Lell, W. A., Gabel, J. C., Curetta, J. M. and Lowenstein, E. (1973). Indirect measurement of left-atrial pressure in surgical patients – pulmonary-capillary wedge and pulmonary-artery diastolic pressures compared with left-atrial pressure. *Anaesthesiology* **38**, 394.

Lee, J., Wright, F., Barker, R. and Stanley, L. (1972). Central venous oxygen saturation in shock: a study in Man. *Anaesthesiology* **36**, 472.

Light, H. (1976). Transcutaneous aortovelography. A new window on the circulation? *Brit. Heart J.* **38**, 433.

Lozman, J., Powers, C. R., Older, T., Dutton, R. E., Roy, R. J., English, M., Marco, D. and Eckert, C. (1974). Correlation of pulmonary wedge and left atrial pressures. *Archs. Surg.* **109**, 270.

McMahon, S. M., Halprin, G. M., Sieker, H. O. (1973). Positive end-expiratory airway pressure in severe arterial hypoxemia. *Am. Rev. Resp. Dis.* **108**, 526.

Messmer, K., Sunder-Plassmann, L., Klövekorn, W. P. and Holper, K. (1972). Circulatory significance of haemodilution: rheological changes and limitations. *Adv. Microcirculat.* **4**, 1.

Qvist, J., Pontoppidan, H., Wilson, R. S., Lowenstein, E. and Laver, M. B. (1975). Haemodynamic responses to mechanical ventilation with P.E.E.P. *Anaesthesiology* **42**, 45.

Rushman, G. B., Ferguson, A. and Boulton, T. B. (1970). Catheterisation of the superior vena cava. *St. Bart's Hosp. J.* **74**, 363.

Russell, W. J. (1974). 'Central Venous Pressure. Its Clinical Use and Role in Cardiovascular Dynamics.' Butterworths, London.

Schils, M. E. (1972). Guidelines to total parenteral nutrition. *J. Am. med. Ass.* **220** (13), 1721.

Sequeira, R. H., Light, L. H., Cross, G. and Raftery, E. B. (1976). Transcutaneous aortovelography. *Brit. Heart J.* **38**, 443.

Snow, J. C. and Dobnik, D. B. (1975). Central venous pressure monitoring – a simple device to determine zero level. *Anaesthesiology* **43**, 678.

Solman, A. J. and Datton, J. C. P. (1973). New thermometers for deep tissue temperature. *Bio-Med. Engineering* **8**, 432.

Suter, P. M., Fairley, H. B. and Isenberg, M. D. (1975). Optimum end-expiratory airway pressure in patients with acute pulmonary failure. *New Engl. J. Med.* **292**, 284.

Swan, H. J. C., Ganz, W., Forrester, J., Nerais, H., Biamond, G. and Chonette, D. (1970). Catheterisation of the heart in man using a flow-directed balloon tipped catheter. *New Engl. J. Med.* **283**, 447.

Swan, H. J. C. (1975). Commentary. Balloon flotation catheters. *J.A.M.A.* **233**, 865.

Swan, H. J. C. and Ganz, W. (1975). Use of balloon flotation catheters in critically ill patients. *Surg. Clin. N. Amer.* **55**, 501.

Sykes, M. K. (1963). Venous pressure as a clinical indication of adequacy of transfusion. *Ann. R. Coll. Surg.* **33**, 185.

Van Slyke, D. D. and Neill, J. M. (1924). Determination of gases in blood and other solutions by vacuum extraction and manometric measurement. *J. Biol. Chem.* **61**, 523.

Weil, M. H. (1969). Progress in the bedside management of shock. *J. Trauma* **9**, 154.

Wilson, R. F., Wilson, Jaqueline A., Gibson, D. B. and Lucas, C. E. (1974). Arterial-central venous differences in critically ill and injured patients. *J. Trauma* **14**, 924.

Woo, S. W. and Prof. Hedley-Whyte, J. (1973). Oxygen therapy. *Brit. J. Hosp. Med.* **487**.

Yoffa, D. (1965). Supraclavicular subclavian venepuncture and catheterisation. *Lancet* **2**, 614.

Section 3: The Management of the Patient Suffering from Severe Trauma

GILLIAN C. HANSON

INTRODUCTION

The metabolic consequences of trauma and some of the effects on organ function have already been discussed.

The assessment of the severity of damage to various organs as a consequence of shock is discussed elsewhere (Part 1, chs IV and V). Initial assessment is of extreme importance since subsequent therapy (e.g. artificial ventilation) may mask the site or extent of organ damage. A history should be obtained if at all possible from a witness at the site of the accident. Examination should be conducted by a clinician experienced in the management of patients suffering from severe trauma who should preferably be accompanied by an anaesthetist. The order of assessment may be altered if one organ is so severely damaged that treatment is required urgently – but systematic examination is vitally important and should be followed by a decisive course of action.

ASSESSMENT OF RESPIRATORY FUNCTION AND INITIAL EMERGENCY MANAGEMENT

The respiratory rate, signs of upper airway obstruction, and the colour of the lips should be noted. The chest wall should be examined (anteriorly and posteriorly) for any external evidence of trauma, the configuration of the chest wall and its movement should be assessed.

333

Evidence of upper airway obstruction is an indication for immediate clearance and probably endotracheal intubation. Emergency tracheostomy is rarely required unless there is actual severance of the trachea.

The position of the trachea and cardiac apex is important – deviation to one side may suggest a tension pneumothorax on the opposite side, or massive collapse on the ipsilateral side.

An inflated poorly moving hemithorax associated with a hyper-resonant percussion note and diminished breath sounds in a cyanosed patient is consistent with an acute tension pneumothorax. A needle with trochar should be inserted on the affected side, should air drain out and the patient improve, the diagnosis is confirmed. Leaving the trochar in position the patient should now be X-rayed – but if the chest injury is extensive, intubation and hand ventilation should be started after inserting a chest drain and the chest X-ray performed later. Chest X-rays should include an erect film in order to detect accumulation of fluid in the thoracic cavity. The assessment of chest injuries in relation to subsequent management is summarised in Table 1. Initial careful

Table 1. Initial assessment of a patient suffering from a chest injury and guidelines for subsequent treatment

Classification		Clinical features	Treatment
Grade	Descriptive		
1	Mild	Fractured ribs – few Cough adequate No ventilatory impairment $PaCO_2 \downarrow PaO_2$ normal or slightly $\downarrow$	Humidified oxygen Percentage appropriate to lung condition Pain relief by local or regional blockade
2	Moderate	May have floating segment Cough inadequate Ventilatory impairment $PaCO_2 \downarrow PaO_2$ generally $\downarrow$ Other injuries fairly common	Consider regional blockade Consider tracheostomy (mandatory in chronic lung disease) Humidified oxygen percentage appropriate to lung condition I.P.P.V. probably necessary
3	Severe	Floating segment or segments As in 2 $PaCO_2 \uparrow PaO_2 \downarrow$ Other injuries common	Tracheostomy I.P.P.V. Oxygen percentage administered appropriate to lung condition

evaluation is important, since once the patient is artificially ventilated many of the physical signs are lost.

Should intubation be considered necessary, initial hand ventilation by the anaesthetist should be preferably performed in the presence of another clinician. An acute tension pneumothorax may develop necessitating urgent insertion of a chest drain.

Hypotension in the presence of a chest injury and in the absence of overt blood loss would suggest, bleeding into the thorax, acute tension pneumothorax, acute mediastinal emphysema or cardiac tamponade.

A patient with a chest injury should be connected to an E.C.G. monitor since cardiac dysrhythmias are common.

Blood gases must always be taken. Severe hypoxia – where the PaO_2 on 100 per cent oxygen fails to rise above 9.3 kPa (70 mm Hg) may be due to many factors including extensive pulmonary oedema (from many causes), bilateral tension pneumothorax, a ruptured main bronchus, and a grossly impaired cardiac output either due to outflow obstruction, hypovolaemia or myocardial failure.

Further details on initial assessment and subsequent management of chest injuries are discussed in Part 2, ch. III, p. 386.

ASSESSMENT OF THE SHOCKED PATIENT

A shocked patient with extensive trauma should be presumed to be hypovolaemic until proven otherwise – two intravenous lines should therefore be inserted immediately and volume replacement commenced. A quick examination should make it possible to assess the extent of blood loss. Replacement of the estimated volume of blood lost without clinical improvement would suggest:

1   Incorrect assessment of the initial volume of blood lost.
2   Haemorrhage from a hidden source.
3   Continued bleeding.
4   Shock from some other cause.

Assessment of the initial volume of blood lost

An assessment of the fluid loss from burns is described on p. 450.

The volume of blood loss in relation to clinical criteria and percentage of total blood volume is shown in Table 2. Young patients may lose more blood before clinical decompensation occurs – a raised pulse rate and decreased pulse pressure being a much more delicate guide than systolic blood pressure. The range of volumes of blood lost

Table 2. Haemorrhagic shock. Classification in relation to clinical criteria and percentage of total blood volume lost

Classification	Blood loss as a percentage of total blood volume	Blood pressure (mm Hg)	Symptoms and signs
Compensated preshock	10–15	Normal	Palpitations Dizziness Tachycardia
Mild	15–30	Slight fall	Palpitations Thirst Tachycardia Weakness Sweating
Moderate	30–35	70–80	Restlessness Pallor Oliguria
Severe	35–40	50–70	Pallor Cyanosis Collapse
Profound	40–50	50	Collapse Air hunger Anuria

Table 3. Approximate volume of blood lost from various sites of injury in a 70 kg male (blood volume 5.0 litres). (Modified from London, 1968)

Site of injury	Extent of injury and approximate volume of blood required (ml) and expressed as a percentage of blood volume (5.0 l)			
	Moderate	Percentage of total blood vol.	Severe	Percentage of total blood vol.
Arm and forearm	400	8	1200	24
Foot and ankle	400	8	800	16
Leg	800	16	1800	36
Thigh	1200	24	2500	50
Pelvis	1200	24	5000	100
Abdomen	1200	24	5000	100
Chest	1200	24	5000	100

Table 4. Estimated blood volume in health as a percentage of body weight. (Abstracted from Moore, F. D., 1959, Publ. Documenta Geigy Scientific Tables, 7th Edition)

Body build	Blood volume as percentage of body weight	
	Men	Women
Normal	7.0	6.5
Obese	6.0	5.5
Thin	6.5	6.0
Muscular	7.5	7.0

from various sites is shown in Table 3. These approximate volumes refer to a normal 70 kg male with a blood volume of 7% of body weight (5.0 litres) and should be increased or decreased according to the estimated blood volume of the patient shown in Table 4.

A central venous pressure line should be inserted as soon as possible; this is of particular importance in the presence of chest injury, in patients where cardiac function may be impaired, in the presence of severe shock or where the volume of blood lost is uncertain.

In severe or profound traumatic shock, adequate oxygenation (often requiring intubation and hand ventilation) and rapid volume replacement, is essential. Time must not be wasted with percutaneous insertion – if no veins are obvious a cut down onto an antecubital vein should be performed immediately. An infusion should not be set up in the lower limbs if there is any question of blood loss from the abdomen or pelvis, even percutaneous insertion into the subclavian vein by an experienced operator may be difficult in profound shock. The infusion fluid must be warmed if replacement is rapid, otherwise there may be a rapid fall in core temperature.

Once volume replacement is underway a decision has to be made as to whether the patient requires an urgent operation to stop further blood loss or whether the patient should be transferred to the Intensive Therapy Unit.

The metabolic consequences of sustained haemorrhage, its management, and the type of fluid to be used, are discussed on pp. 346 and 361.

1. *Incorrect assessment of the initial volume of blood lost*
By referring to Tables 3 and 4 it should be possible to assess the volume of blood loss. This should correlate with the clinical findings of Table 2. Lack of correlation would suggest continued bleeding, haemorrhage

from a hidden source, or shock from another cause. Failure to correct shock in a traumatised patient is most commonly related to inadequate blood volume replacement. Oozing from a scalp wound can add up to a large volume of blood – this may be marked by the inappropriate and incorrect placement of a pressure bandage when suturing is indicated.

2. *Haemorrhage from a hidden source*

The most common 'hidden' sites for haemorrhage are intraperitoneal, retroperitoneal, into the thoracic cavity, or into the thigh following a pelvic fracture.

Increasing abdominal distension with continued shock is an indication for peritoneal tap or diagnostic peritoneal lavage; fractures of the lower rib cage may be additional features consistent with rupture of the liver or spleen.

Back pain, in particular in a patient with a back or pelvic injury would suggest a retroperitoneal bleed – bruising often takes 24 h to appear. An X-ray of the lumbar spine may show a fractured vertebral transverse process which may sever one of the lumbar venules and produce profound haemorrhage. Increasing abdominal distension, in the absence of blood in the peritoneum from diagnostic tap, ileus and/or oliguria with no known cause to precipitate acute renal failure, are all features suggestive of a retroperitoneal bleed. Multiple rib fractures are frequently complicated by an intrathoracic bleed. A considerable amount of blood may be lost following a pelvic fracture – clinical manifestations may include a palpable mass in the iliac fossa, and/or distension, and pain in the upper thigh.

3. *Continued bleeding*

Persistent shock following replacement of the assessed volume lost may be due to continued bleeding or shock from another cause. A continuously falling central venous pressure, after volume 'top-up', oliguria and a high pulse rate are all signs consistent with this diagnosis. Continued bleeding is generally associated with clinical evidence of intra-abdominal haemorrhage – where after initial resuscitation an emergency laparotomy is indicated. On occasions bleeding is so severe that an emergency operation is required in the presence of inadequate blood volume replacement. Under such circumstances at least two good intravenous lines must be running and a central venous pressure line should be inserted as soon as possible. A muscle relaxant should not be used during the initial anaesthetic management of a severe intra-abdominal bleed – its use relaxing the anterior abdominal wall and

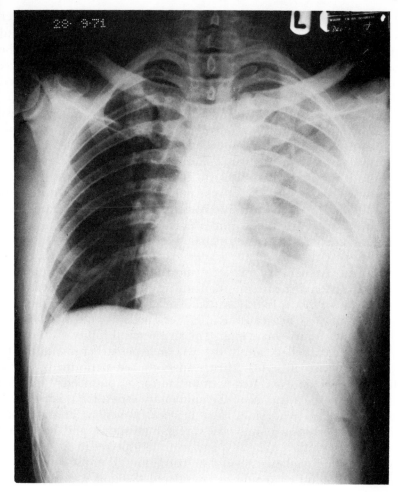

Fig. 1. Chest X-ray showing ruptured left hemidiaphragm. At laparotomy the spleen had ruptured and was bleeding into the left thoracic cavity.

increasing the capacity of the peritoneal cavity for blood. It may be given as soon as the peritoneum has been incised. Haemorrhage into the thoracic cavity generally stops spontaneously – but continued fresh blood draining via the chest drain would indicate bleeding from a major vessel, a ruptured lung, a torn pericardium or a ruptured diaphragm associated with bleeding from the abdominal cavity (Fig. 1). These are indications for emergency thoracic or thoracoabdominal surgery.

4. *Shock from some other cause*

Continued shock is an absolute indication for insertion of a central venous pressure line. A steadily rising central venous pressure in the absence of any bleeding source, or where the calculated volume of blood lost has been replaced, would suggest some other cause for the low blood pressure.

In the absence of central venous pressure monitoring, it is very easy especially in the elderly, or the patient in acute renal failure, to move insiduously from a period of hypovolaemic shock to fluid overload. The central venous pressure is a very delicate reflector of this transition and therefore it is wise to be satisfied with a low normal central venous pressure $(2-6$ cm $H_2O)$ provided the pulse volume is good, the rate less than $110/min$, the blood pressure systolic 100 mm Hg or greater, and skin core temperature differential $3°C$ or less.

Other causes for hypotension include a cardiac dysrhythmia tamponade, or outflow obstruction due to acute mediastinal emphysema. Sepsis complicating primary traumatic haemorrhage is unusual. A ruptured gall bladder, stomach, intestine, or acute traumatic pancreatitis may be associated with shock. Extravasation of urine due to a ruptured ureter or bladder may also be a cause. Rupture of a hollow viscus may follow a direct contact injury, blast injury, or an electrical injury.

A severe metabolic acidosis, hypoxia or hypercarbia should not be allowed to arise if serial Astrup analyses are performed. Severe refractory hypoxia associated with an increasing pulmonary vascular resistance may be a feature of the pulmonary aspiration syndrome, or the fat embolism syndrome. Here the central venous pressure may reflect the increasing pulmonary vascular resistance and be a poor guide to venous return. When hypovolaemia is suspected in these circumstances – a fluid challenge should be tried (Fig. 3, p. 308) and other systems of monitoring should be considered (Section 2, p. 301). The institution of P.E.E.P. in a patient with poor right ventricular function or borderline hypovolaemia may produce hypotension, but under such circumstances preceding monitoring, and the onset of hypotension within 15 min of starting P.E.E.P., makes the diagnosis relatively easy.

Rarer causes of shock following trauma unrelated to hypovolaemia include the sudden onset of acute bronchospasm complicated by a decreasing venous return and hence left ventricular output, anaphylactic shock, severe head injury or acute bowel ischaemia secondary to volvulus or embolism. Severe acute bronchospasm associated with tachycardia, hypertension and commonly histamine wheals, may follow the use of dextran 70 or Haemaccel. An awareness of this rare complication is important since during resuscitation the onset of acute bronchospasm may be missed. The use of dextrans during resuscitation of patients subject to bronchospasm should be questioned. Lorenz and co-workers (1976) found that histamine release was always found with allergy related to Haemaccel but there was no significant release with reactions to dextran.

CHOICE OF FLUIDS TO BE USED DURING THE MANAGEMENT OF HAEMORRHAGIC SHOCK

Restoration of the circulating blood volume to normal is one of the most important aspects of treatment in many forms of shock. In acute hypovolaemic shock the rate and volume of replacement is probably more important than the type of fluid infused. This concept probably applies to all patients with mild to moderate hypovolaemic shock, provided volume does not continue to be lost and the volume of fluid given is therefore unlikely to be more than one third of the total blood volume. In severe shock however, in patients who suffer from repeated depletion of blood volume, or patients where serum albumin is low before the onset of blood volume loss, the type of fluid infused should be carefully considered. It is probable that in such patients the ultimate prognosis may be affected by the type and volume of fluid infused.

The aim of fluid replacement in hypovolaemic shock is to ensure adequate oxygenation of the peripheral cell. Blood volume is maintained with an equilibrium established between the plasma and the interstitial fluid. Fluid tends to leave the vascular bed under the influence of the capillary hydrostatic pressure and to a lesser extent by the osmotic effect of the proteins in the interstitial fluid. This filtration force is opposed by the osmotic pressure of the plasma proteins and to a minimal extent by the hydrostatic pressure within the interstitium. When plasma is lost there is an initial transcapillary movement of water and salt, and because plasma proteins cannot be replaced immediately the body replaces fluid by decreasing the capillary hydrostatic pressure and thus increasing trans-capillary movement of salt and water. Skillman and co-workers (1968) have shown that when 10–15% of the blood volume is lost acutely in haemorrhage, plasma albumin is replenished at a rate of 40 g/h with initial fluid refill of approximately 1 ml/min. When fluid is not given within 24 h the vascular volume returns to prehaemorrhagic levels. In volunteers bled 10–20% of their total blood volume, no alteration in serum albumin is found (Pruitt *et al.*, 1967) but when patients are bled large amounts, serum albumin becomes severely depressed (Carey *et al.*, 1971). A decrease in serum albumin below 25 g/l requires that the interstitial hydrostatic pressure becomes elevated in order to maintain plasma volume. This is the reason why very much more crystalloid is required in severe haemorrhage to replace the volume of blood lost. De Palma and co-workers (1970) found that three times the calculated volume of blood lost was required to resuscitate rats bled 47% of their blood volume, than when crystalloids were used. In humans a ratio of 3:1 lactated Ringer's Solution for lost blood has been recommended by Shires *et al.* (1964). Cervera and Moss (1974) however calculated the volume of crystalloid to be replaced for lost undiluted blood, and found it to be approximately 7:1. It is probable that the use of crystalloids for blood volume replacement, in particular in patients with impaired cardiac pulmonary or renal function, may lead to pulmonary oedema.

During replacement of blood volume following haemorrhage the rheological properties of blood should be taken into account. Optimal transport capacity coincides with an haematocrit of around 30% provided normovolaemia is maintained and the haemotocrit is not allowed to fall below 25% (Hint, 1968). Should the blood volume fall, the oxygen transport capacity will immediately decrease. Thus, in hypovolaemic shock blood volume should be replaced as quickly as possible and an haematocrit of around 30% should be aimed for. This means that blood volume should be replaced with a solution other than blood until approximately one third of the blood volume has been lost when whole blood should be used. The choice of solutions to be used include plasma protein fraction, salt-free albumin, dextran 70 and Haemaccel.

Plasma protein fraction and salt-free albumin

Plasma protein fraction is the plasma expander of choice when the serum albumin is suspected to be below 25 g/l, where the patient is septic, and in patients with severe or profound shock where there is an increased likelihood of pulmonary oedema. The solution is hepatitis antigen free, is isotonic, has the same sodium content as plasma, a potassium content of 2.2–2.4 mmol/l and a protein content of 46 g/l. The plasma half-life in healthy individuals is 15–17 days whereas the half-life of salt-free albumin is 17–21 days (Swain, 1976). Salt-free albumin should be used in preference to plasma protein fraction if there is any possibility of sodium overload as in renal failure or in patients with a low serum sodium suspected to be due to the sick cell syndrome

(p. 170). Plasma protein fraction may also have to be used in profound haemorrhagic shock where the maximum volume of dextran 70 (1.5 g/kg B.W./24 h) has been given, or where there has been an allergic reaction to the dextran solution. In both these circumstances Haemaccel should not be used as an alternative since firstly, in profound shock the serum albumin will fall below 25 g/l and secondly Haemaccel may also be complicated by allergic reactions. In severe shock, increased capillary permeability may lead to loss of the infused protein into the extracellular fluid producing oedema which subsequently slowly resolves. Swain (1976) wonders therefore whether a larger molecule (M. W. albumin 67 000) should be used in profound shock since even albumin under such circumstances may lead to pulmonary oedema. At present, however, there does not appear to be a better plasma expander in shock where the maximum volume of dextran 70 has been given and large volumes of fluid have been lost.

In our experience the use of plasma protein fraction has not been complicated by any allergic reactions, occasionally the use of salt-free albumin may be followed by a low grade erythematous rash.

Dextran 70 and Haemaccel

Dextran 70 has been advocated as the volume expander of choice in haemorrhagic shock (Gruber, 1969; Gruber et al., 1976). This is a polymolecular polysaccharide with an average molecular weight of 70 000, 6 g of dextran being present per 100 ml of solution, normal saline or 5 per cent dextrose being used as the vehicle. The solution is slightly hyperoncotic and approximately 1 g of dextran binds 25 ml of water. Dextran 70 is excreted in the urine and approximately 40% appears in the urine after 24 h. It is therefore an excellent volume expander, the only disadvantages being that the dosage should be limited to 1.5 g dextran/kg body weight and that allergic reactions have been reported (Lorenz et al., 1976). Reissigl (1969) reported a decrease in platelets, a prolongation of bleeding time and decreases in Factor V, A.H.F. and fibrinogen when doses above this are given. Gruber (1969) states that doses up to 1.5 g dextran/kg body weight do not produce measurable changes in clotting mechanisms and this has certainly been the author's experience.

Dextran 70 should not be used if there is evidence of a bleeding diathesis. It is wise to avoid the use of dextrans in severely shocked patients who are known asthmatics or have bronchospasm at the time of the infusion. Gelatin solutions may cause histamine release (Messmer et *al.*, 1970), the manifestations being similar to that with dextran; their use should be similarly restricted.

Dextran 40 should not be used for volume expansion, firstly because it decreases platelet adhesion, and secondly because there have been reports of renal functional impairment following its use (Morgan *et al.*, 1966).

Haemaccel is a 3.5% gelatin solution in a balanced electrolyte vehicle. The gelatin has an average molecular weight of 35 000 and has a colloid osmotic pressure which is comparable to that of normal plasma. Haemaccel being iso-osmotic does not take up fluid from the interstitial space and 100% is recovered from the circulation 10 min after the infusion, the volume expanding effect begins to fall after 1 h and only 50% of the volume expanding effect is present after 4 h, whereas with dextran 70, 50% is still present after approximately 8 h (Giebel and Horatz, 1969).

The volume of Haemaccel that may be given appears to be unlimited, no coagulation defects have been found and large volumes (as with dextran 70) do not affect renal function (Lutz and Hallwacks, 1969). The disadvantage of Haemaccel is the transient plasma expanding effect and like dextran 70, the occasional reported case of allergy.

Indications for the use of blood during haemorrhagic shock

Blood is indicated once one third of the calculated blood volume has been lost or the haematocrit has fallen to 30% or less. The primary purpose of giving whole blood to a patient is to increase the oxygen delivery to the tissues. At the present time blood drawn routinely for transfusion is stored either in acid citrate dextrose (A.C.D.) or citrate phosphate dextrose (C.P.D.). The pH of freshly drawn blood in A.C.D. is 7.0 and that of C.P.D. is 7.2. The pH of both falls progressively during storage to 6.1 after 21 days, and 6.8 after 28 days of A.C.D. and C.P.D. preserved blood respectively (McConn, 1975). As a result of the fall in pH there is a progressive fall in P_{50} (PaO_2 at 50% saturation under standard conditions) and red cells 2,3-D.P.G. this being greater in A.C.D. preserved blood. Thus, transfusing the patient with stored blood can result in a lowering of the patient's 2,3-D.P.G. and a shift of the dissociation curve to the left, the magnitude of these changes depending upon the age and the amount of blood transfused. The use of sodium bicarbonate for correction of a metabolic acidosis may also produce a left shift of the oxyhaemoglobin dissociation curve. The

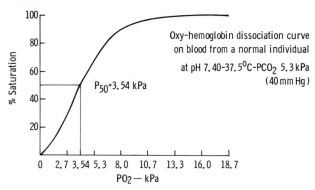

Fig. 2. The dissociation curve for a normal individual (P_{50} 3.54 kPa).

oxyhaemoglobin dissociation curve in whole blood is shown in Fig. 2.

For normal man with a body temperature of 37.5°C, the P_{50} is 3.54 kPa (26.52 mm Hg). During resuscitation of a patient with haemorrhagic shock it is important to be aware of the factors which may influence the position of the dissociation curve – a tendency towards a left shift as a result of blood transfusion should not be compounded by other factors which may do the same (Table 5).

Hypoxia is known to increase red cell 2,3-D.P.G. and may be an important factor in the metabolic response to hypoxia. It is important to be aware that 2,3-D.P.G. may be depleted in phosphate deficiency (commonly seen in long-term critical illness). Maintenance of an adequate phosphate level is therefore essential during the management of the critically ill.

In view of these changes in preserved blood, blood used during the treatment of severe or profound shock should be less than 3 days old and should more than 10 units be required over a period of 24 h, fresh blood, or blood collected within the previous 24 h, is advisable. These

Table 5. Factors influencing the position of the dissociation curve of whole blood

Factor	Relationship
Temperature	$P_{50} \downarrow$ temp $\downarrow$
	$P_{50} \uparrow$ temp $\uparrow$
Bohr effect (lowering red cell pH)	$P_{50} \uparrow$ pH $\downarrow$
2,3-D.P.G.	$P_{50} \downarrow$ 2,3-D.P.G. $\downarrow$

recommendations are of even greater importance in the alkalotic patient or in the patient where phosphate depletion is suspected. It is hoped that washed deep frozen red cells (which retain 2,3-D.P.G. and are hepatitis antigen free) will shortly be available for treatment of profound haemorrhagic shock.

Stroma-free haemoglobin may ultimately become available as an oxygen-carrying blood substitute (Palani et al., 1975).

Consideration has been given towards the therapeutic manipulation of the oxyhaemoglobin dissociation curve. There is at the moment little support for the usefulness of increased 2,3-D.P.G. levels as a therapeutic modality to increase oxygen delivery in the acutely ill (McConn, 1975). It is of interest to note however that methylprednisolone sodium succinate (Solu-medrone) which may be used in septic shock, has been found to increase the P_{50} in the acutely ill (Bryan-Brown et al., 1973). This increase in P_{50} was not always accompanied by an increase in 2,3-D.P.G., furthermore it was associated with an improvement in oxygen consumption, a fall in mixed venous oxygen saturation, and a transient increase in cardiac index (Bryan-Brown et al., 1974). Should these findings be confirmed by other authors, its use might be seriously considered as a bolus dose in the management of profound haemorrhagic shock. Improvement in cellular oxygenation may well be one of the methods whereby massive doses of steroids are claimed by various workers to improve the prognosis in septic shock (Christy, 1971).

CARDIOVASCULAR, RESPIRATORY AND METABOLIC CHANGES RELATED TO ACUTE HAEMORRHAGIC SHOCK

Increased peripheral resistance which begins shortly after the onset of haemorrhage is one of the first observable haemodynamic changes (Shoemaker, 1970). With continued blood loss the cardiac output progressively decreases and arterial pressure is maintained initially by constriction of capillary beds. Increasing blood loss leads to the onset of a metabolic acidosis, accumulation of lactic acid and relaxation of the arteriolar sphincter leading to the capillary bed. This is followed by a fall in peripheral vascular resistance and a further fall in the circulating blood volume. A low cardiac output is unlikely to be seen after blood volume replacement unless there is concomitant cardiac insufficiency (Shoemaker, 1970). Almost immediately after the onset of haemorrhage and trauma there develops an increased pulmonary artery pressure and pulmonary vascular resistance, the degree of increase is related to the severity of trauma or blood loss and the magnitude and duration correlates with morbidity and mortality (Shoemaker, 1970). Subsequently pulmonary shunting develops and increases with the severity of shock. Ventilatory perfusion imbalance leads to severe hypoxia which may be accentuated by the accumulation of water in the interstitium (Moss et al., 1973). Thus, in severe haemorrhagic shock hypoxia and hypocarbia is common, frequently associated with a falling pH due to the accumulation of lactic acid. pH in haemorrhagic shock is a poor reflector of the severity of acidosis, largely because of the extent of respiratory compensation (Cloutier et al., 1969); a base deficit is invariably present in severe haemorrhagic shock.

Biochemical and respiratory monitoring has proven to be a valuable guide to prognosis, the biochemical changes returning to normal levels 15 min before the central venous pressure and pulse rate, and almost 70 min before the blood pressure (Schumer et al., 1975). Schumer and co-workers (1975) based their findings on a 'gas index' pH + $PaCO_2$ + PaO_2 and a 'biochemical' index serum lactate + inorganic phosphate + serum alpha-amino acids. They found a direct relationship between the 'biochemical index' and number of deaths and an indirect relationship between the number of deaths and 'gas index'. It is evident that a falling pH and PaO_2 and an increasing base deficit and/or serum lactate in the face of good volume replacement and attempts at adequate oxygenation (with intubation and C.P.P.V.) portray a bad prognosis.

The electrolyte changes which result from severe trauma and haemorrhage are not well understood. The classic findings of a low serum sodium and chloride and elevated potassium levels may not be present and clearly several factors have to be considered when evaluating blood electrolytes in the shocked patient. The serum sodium level frequently falls to 128–130 mmol/l and does not necessarily reflect total body sodium depletion, this is probably due to shift of sodium ions into the interstitial space and into the cells (Fox and Keston, 1945). A persistently low serum sodium (more than 48 hours after resuscitation) associated with a high urinary sodium loss and oliguria should make one suspect the early development of a traumatic I.A.D.H. syndrome (Part 2, ch. III, p. 409).

One of the most feared electrolyte changes in resuscitation for severe haemorrhagic shock is that of hyperkalaemia. A high incidence of hyperkalaemia might be anticipated because of the high potassium content of stored blood, the rapid potassium loss from damaged and anoxic tissues and the reduced potassium excretion from oliguria. After massive transfusion Wilson *et al.* (1971) found that patients are normally normokalaemic, 10.1% becoming hypokalaemic and 12.1% hyperkalaemic. Hyperkalaemia may be related to the onset of acute renal failure in a catabolic patient, the presence of a metabolic acidosis, the use of succinylcholine, and rarely to intravascular haemolysis.

The blood glucose commonly rises before resuscitation from haemorrhagic shock (Carey *et al.*, 1971) and is generally associated with low levels of circulating insulin (Cerchio *et al.*, 1973). It has been postulated that the inhibition of insulin release to a glycaemic stimulus may play an important role in the immediate survival during acute circulatory impairment, allowing more glucose to be diverted to the non-insulin dependent organ, the brain and ensuring an adequate energy supply during the acute phase of stress. Blood glucose levels should be monitored and insulin used if the blood glucose rises above 12 mmol/l, thereby eliminating the danger of hyperosmolar coma (p. 226).

The incidence of complications following massive transfusion are remarkably few (Wilson *et al.*, 1971). Massive transfusion for profound shock using uncrossmatched O negative blood is rarely followed by intravascular haemolysis or a severe reaction, mild jaundice commonly develops 24 to 72 h later and is probably related to the period of impaired hepatocellular perfusion or the absorption of haemoglobin from a site of loculated blood. Hypothermia is a complication of massive blood transfusion – the blood should always be warmed prior to infusion. Blood that has been stored for more than 48 h has no effective platelets and grossly reduced amounts of Factors V and VIII. Thrombocytopenia is largely dilutional and adequate clotting may take place at levels as low as 30–40 000/mm³. Factors V and VIII should be replaced with fresh frozen plasma.

Following the use of large volumes of blood, a metabolic alkalosis commonly develops on the first postoperative day. Since this will seriously affect the oxyhaemoglobin dissociation curve (p. 344) it is wise not to overcorrect a metabolic acidosis during transfusion. There is no justification in the routine use of bicarbonate according to the volume of blood given; sodium bicarbonate should be given according to sequential analysis of acid base status in conjunction with assessment of the rate of improvement and adequacy of peripheral perfusion.

Data derived from haemorrhagic experiments in dogs have shown that disseminated intravascular coagulation is often observed. In humans, it is important to differentiate between haemorrhage from a bleeding source, bleeding secondary to the use of old blood and the lack of labile factors, and true disseminated intravascular coagulation

(D.I.C.). D.I.C. is exceptionally rare in severe haemorrhagic shock unless there is associated sepsis, and if it is present, rarely requires treatment. D.I.C. is most commonly recognised in patients with extensive lung trauma, and postoperatively following obstetric, gynaecological procedures or operations on the bladder or prostate. Postoperative oozing from an extensive raw or infected area may also be complicated by D.I.C. D.I.C. is discussed in detail on p. 654.

A.C.D. stored blood contains debris when stored for more than 24 h, the amount of debris generally increases with storage time. Definite indications for microfiltration of blood have not yet emerged, the occurrence of the shock lung syndrome following massive transfusion of unfiltrated blood is controversial and the author has been surprised by the remarkable lack of pulmonary complications provided adequate perfusion, oxygenation, metabolic balance and cardiac function is maintained. Clearly multiple factors contribute towards the development of the shock lung syndrome (p. 542) but in the light of recent evidence, it seems reasonable to filter blood more than 48 h old. The blood filters available and the justification for their use, are discussed in greater detail in Part 4, ch. III, p. 940.

SUMMARY OF TREATMENT OF HAEMORRHAGIC SHOCK

In the light of the preceding discussion, the treatment of haemorrhagic shock can be summarised as follows:

Treatment should be based on the estimated volume of blood lost (Table 3) and the severity of the shocked state (Table 2). Should these two estimates fail to correlate, another cause for the shocked condition must be looked for (p. 335). The ratio of blood to other fluids to be used is as follows:

Estimated total volume of blood loss as a percentage of total blood volume	Therapeutic regime
<30	Blood not required
30–80	Ratio of blood to other fluid 1:1
>80	*Idem* 2:1 50% should preferably be as blood stored for less than 3 days

The type of other fluid used depends upon various factors, the most important being the severity of shock, preceding organ function (renal, pulmonary and cardiac) and the preceding level of serum albumin.

In previously healthy patients aged 40 or less and a total blood loss less than 30% of the total blood volume, fluid may be replaced with dextran 70 or Haemaccel – should there be a history of allergy or asthma, it is probably wise to use normal saline instead of dextran 70 or Haemaccel. Haemaccel has a shorter intravascular life than dextran 70, so that should there be a possibility of a further bleed, it is wiser to use dextran 70.

With blood loss of 30 to 80% of the total blood volume, initial volume is replaced with dextran 70 (maximum dose 1.5 g/kg B.W.) or Haemaccel and blood is introduced in a ratio of 1 : 1. Should bleeding continue and more than 50% of the estimated blood volume has been given as dextran 70, Haemaccel or normal saline singly or in combination; plasma protein fraction or salt free albumin should be substituted in a 1 : 1 ratio with blood (because of the inevitable fall in serum albumin).

When more than 80% of the estimated blood volume has been lost, blood should be replaced in a ratio of 2 : 1, the other solution of choice being similar to the preceding recommendations. In patients where the serum albumin is suspected to be less than 25 g/l, where there is associated sepsis or where there is a known allergic susceptibility, or bronchial asthma, plasma protein fraction (P.P.F.) is the fluid of choice when more than 50% of the blood volume has been lost. Because of the shortage of P.P.F. it is reasonable to restrict its use to patients 65 years or less.

The routine adopted in the management of haemorrhagic shock at Whipps Cross Hospital is as follows:

Table 6. Summary of treatment of haemorrhagic shock

I   FLUIDS

Compensated preshock (10–15% of blood volume lost)	Set up drip. Crossmatch.
Mild shock (15–30% of blood volume lost)	Replace blood volume with dextran 70, Haemaccel or normal saline.
Moderate shock (30–35% of blood volume lost)	Replace initially with dextran 70 (Max. 1.5 g/kg B.W./24 h), Haemaccel or normal saline. Give blood after full crossmatch, ratio of blood to other fluid 1 : 2. Warm the blood. Filter if more than 48 h old.

Severe shock (35–40% of blood volume lost)	At least 2 drips running. Insert a C.V.P. line. Restore blood volume as quickly as possible; blood can generally be partially crossmatched (see Part 3, ch. 1, p. 814). Ratio of blood to other fluid 1 : 1. Warm the blood. Filter if blood more than 48 h old.
Profound shock (greater than 40% of blood volume lost)	Observe the airway, give oxygen. Consider intubation. Ratio of blood to other fluid 1 : 1 until 80% or more of the blood volume lost. Under such circumstances give emergency A.B.O. and rhesus specific blood (see Part 3, ch. 1, p. 814). Ratio blood to other fluid 2 : 1. Give 50% of blood requirement as blood stored less than 2 days. Packed cells should not be used. Maintain Hct around 30%. Use P.P.F. as non-haemoglobin containing fluid of choice. Insert C.V.P. line. Catheterise. Monitor E.C.G., electrolyte, acid-base status and coagulation profile. Give 3 packets of F.F.P. for every 4000 ml of blood infused.

II   DRUGS

1. *Sodium bicarbonate* to be given if base deficit > 10 and/or pH 7.2 or less. (Aliquots of 50 mmol HCO_3^- or less).
2. *Calcium chloride* 10 ml 10% (4.5 mmol calcium ions) i.v. every 3000 ml blood infused.
3. *Mannitol* give 0.2 g/kg B.W. over 2–3 min if C.V.P.* > 4 cm H_2O, B.P. S.P. > 90 mm Hg and urine output < 40ml/h.
Check u/p osmolality ratio before giving mannitol.
4. *Potassium chloride* if SeK 3.5 mmol or less, give cautiously in patients with suspected renal failure.
5. *Digitalis* consider in elderly patients and in patients with a preceding history of heart failure.
6. *Insulin* consider if B.G. > 12 mmol/l.
7. *Oxygen* if PaO_2 < 9.3 kPa (70 mm Hg) on oxygen via a face mask, intubate and ventilate.   8. Do not use vasoconstrictors.
9. Do not use muscle relaxants in patients with severe haemorrhagic shock due to an intra-abdominal bleed until blood volume replacement is adequate and the peritoneum has been incised.

III   Should the patient's condition remain serious, in spite of the above measures:
1. Re-evaluate the respiratory status.   2. Search for obscure sources of bleeding.
3. Consider haemorrhage complicated by sepsis.   4. Assess cardiac function.
5. Exclude a bleeding diathesis.

---

* May be higher than this level in patients with preceding high airway pressures or pulmonary hypertension and may be raised acutely because of pulmonary oedema. Under such circumstances this level would not reflect an adequate right ventricular filling pressure.

Certain factors may perpetuate a condition of shock in spite of adequate volume replacement.

Hypoxia and/or hypercarbia with an increasing respiratory acidosis may induce a tachycardia or cardiac dysrhythmia and a falling blood pressure. A sudden increase in intrathoracic pressure (e.g. acute pneumothorax pulmonary collapse) may decrease venous return and hence cardiac output. This may also occur with the acute onset of a pneumomediastinum or haemorrhage into the pericardial sac.

Sepsis on occasions may be complicated by haemorrhage in particular from an acute gastric erosion related to stress. Hypotension may be related to a combination of hypovolaemia and septicaemia.

A bleeding diathesis is most commonly secondary to the use of old blood with inadequate replacement of labile factors. There may be a preceding coagulation abnormality (Part 2, ch. VIII, p. 653), or on rare occasions profound sustained haemorrhagic shock may be complicated by disseminated intravascular coagulation (Part 2, ch. VIII, p. 654).

REFERENCES

Bryan-Brown, C. W., Back, S., Makabali, G. and Shoemaker, W. (1973). Consumable oxygen: availability of oxygen in relation to oxyhaemoglobin dissociation. *Crit. Care Med.* **1**, 17.

Bryan-Brown, C. W., Back, S., Makabali, G. and Shoemaker, W. (1973). Consumable haemodynamic responses and oxygen delivery after methyl prednisolone sodium succinate. *In* 'Steroids and Shock' (Ed. Glen, T.) p. 361. Baltimore Univ. Park Press.

Carey, L. C., Lowery, B. D. and Cloutier, C. T. (1971). 'Haemorrhagic Shock in Current Problems in Surgery' (Ed. Ravitch, M. M.). Yearbook, Medical Publishers Inc., Chicago.

Cerchio, G. M., Persico, P. A. and Jeffay, H. (1973). Inhibition of insulin release during hypovolaemic shock. *Metabolism* **22**, 1449.

Cervera, A. L. and Moss, G. (1974). Crystalloid distribution following haemorrhage and haemodilation. *J. Trauma* **14**, 506.

Christy, J. H. (1971). Treatment of gram-negative shock. *Am. J. Med.* **50**, 77.

Cloutier, C. T., Lowery, B. D. and Carey, L. C. (1969). Acid-base disturbances in haemorrhagic shock in 66 severely wounded patients prior to treatment. *Archs. Surg.* **98**, 551.

De Palma, R. G., Robinson, B. A. and Holden, W. D. (1970). Fluid therapy in hypovolaemic shock: experimental evaluation. *J. Surg. Onc.* **2**, 349.

Fox, C. L. Jr. and Keston, A. S. (1945). The mechanism of shock from burns and trauma traced with radio sodium. *Surg. Gynec. Obstet.* **80**, 561.

Giebel, O. and Horatz, K. (1969). Behaviour of blood volume and its components after replacement with Dextran and gelatin plasma substitutes following bleeding in the healthy young male. Bibl. haemat. No. 33, p. 171. Karger, Basel and New York.

Gruber, U. F. (1969). 'Blood Replacement'. Springer, Heidelberg.

Gruber, U. F. (1970). Recent developments in the investigation and treatment of hypovolaemic shock. *Brit. J. Hosp. Med.* **4**, 631.

Gruber, U. F., Sturm. Verena and Messmer, K. (1976). Fluid replacement in shock. *In* 'Shock. Clinical and experimental aspects' (Ed. Ledingham, I. McA.) p. 231. Ex Cerpta Medica – Amsterdam, Oxford and New York.

Hint, H. (1968). The pharmacology of dextran and the pathophysiological background for the clinical use of Rheomacrodex and Macrodex. *Acta Anaesth. Belg.* **19**, 119.

London, P. S. (1968). Traumatic shock. *Brit. J. Hosp. Med.* **I** (3), 312.

Lorenz, W., Doenicke, A., Messmer, K., Reimann, H.-J., Thermann, M., Lahn, W., Berr, J., Schmal, A., Dormann, P., Regenfuss, P. and Hamelmann, H. (1976). Histamine release in human subjects by modified gelatin (Haemaccel) and Dextran: an explanation for anaphylactoid reactions observed under clinical conditions? *Br. J. Anaesth.* **48**, 151.

Lutz, H. and Hallwacks, O. (1969). Changes in Renal Function after Shock and Volume Replacement with Various Plasma Substitutes. *In* 'Modified Gelatins as Plasma Substitutes'. Bibl. haemat. No. 33 (Ed. Lundsgaard-Hansen, P., Hässig, A. and Nitschmann, Hs.) p. 398. Karger, Basel and New York.

McConn, R. (1975). The oxyhaemoglobin dissociation curve in acute disease. *Surg. Clin. N. Amer.* **55** (3), 627.

Messmer, K., Lorenz, W., Sunder-Plassman, L., Klöuekorn, W. P. and Hutzel, M. (1970). Histamine release as cause of acute hypotension following rapid colloid infusion. *Naunym-Schmiedeberg's Arch. exp. Path. Pharmak.* **267,** 433.

Morgan, T. O., Littler, J. M. and Evans, W. A. (1966). Renal failure associated with low-molecular-weight dextran solution. *Brit. Med. J.* **2**, 737.

Moore, F. D. (1939). 'The Metabolic Care of the Surgical Patient'. Saunders, Philadelphia.

Moss, G. S., Des Gupta, T. K., Newson, B. and Nyhus, L. M. (1973). Effect of haemorrhagic shock on pulmonary interstitial sodium distribution in the primate lung. *Ann. Surg.* **177**, 211.

Moss, G. S. and Saletta, J. D. (1974). Traumatic Shock in Man. *New Engl. J. Med.* **290**, 724.

Palani, C. K., De Woskin, R. and Moss, G. S. (1975). Scope and limitations of stroma-free haemoglobin solutions as an oxygen-carrying blood substitute. *Surg. Clin. N. Amer.* **55**, 3.

Pruitt, B. A., Moncrief, J. A. and Mason, A. D. (1967). Efficacy of buffered saline as the sole replacement fluid following acute measured haemorrhage in man. *J. Trauma* **7**, 767.

Reissigl, H. (1969). Scope and limitations of therapy with plasma substitutes. Differential indications for substitutes, blood preparations and electrolyte solutions. *In* 'Modified Gelatins as Plasma Substitutes.' Bibl. haematol. No. 33, p. 32 (Ed. Lundsgaard-Hansen, Haussig, A. and Nitschmann, Hs.). Karger, Basel and New York.

Schumer, W., Erve, P. R. and Miller, B. (1975). Biochemical monitoring of the surgical patient. *Surg. Clin. N. Amer.* **55**, 11.

Shires, G. T., Coln, D., Carrico, J. and Lightfoot, S. (1964). Fluid therapy in haemorrhagic shock. *Archs. Surg.* **88**, 688.

Schoemaker, W. C. (1970). Systemic and Pulmonary Hemodynamic Patterns in Hemorrhagic and Traumatic Shock. *In* 'Body Fluid Replacement in the Surgical Patient' (Ed. Fox, C. L. and Nahas, G. C.) p. 32. Grune and Stratton, New York and London.

Skillman, J. J., Eltringham, W. K., Goldensen, R. H. and Moore, F. D. (1968). Transcapillary refilling after haemorrhage in the splenectomised dog. *J. Surg. Res.* **8**, 57.

Swain, P. (1976). Personal communication.

Wilson, R. F., Mammen, E. and Walt, A. J. (1971). Eight years of experience with massive blood transfusions. *J. Trauma* **2** (4), 275.

Section 4: Shock and Infection

GILLIAN C. HANSON

INTRODUCTION

The pathophysiology of shock has been discussed on p. 293. In this discussion certain aspects of shock associated with sepsis are mentioned.

Only approximately 50% of patients in shock associated with sepsis have positive blood cultures. Reasons for this include antibiotic therapy prior to taking the blood cultures, poor culturing technique, or the presence in the blood stream of factors either released from the bacteria or released from other sites because of the presence of sepsis, which contribute to the development of shock. The clinical presentation of gram negative shock in man resembles shock produced by endotoxin in animals and it has been suggested by Glynn and Howard (1973) that the two are the same. Patients suffering from gram negative shock may however have no evidence of circulating endotoxin demonstrable by the limulus test (Levin *et al.*, 1970) and patients suffering from gram positive shock (where endotoxin is absent) may manifest in a similar manner. The limulus test is considered by some workers, however, to be of little clinical usefulness in the detection of endotoxaemia or gram negative septicaemia (Ellin *et al.*, 1975). It is probable that either endotoxin or exotoxin have an important part to play in the production of shock associated with sepsis.

The haemodynamic changes found in septic shock appear to be extremely variable, but with the use of more sophisticated monitoring techniques it has become apparent that the majority of the patients with shock associated with sepsis initially manifest (once dynamic volume has been restored) with a normal or increased cardiac output and a

355

decreased or normal peripheral vascular resistance (Wilson *et al.*, 1967; Siegal *et al.*, 1967). The high peripheral vascular flow with reduced oxygen extraction may be due to three mechanisms, pathological shunting which by-pass the capillary beds, defective oxygen transfer from the capillary to the cell, and finally the oxidative metabolic pathway of the cell may be primarily damaged. The first mechanism is supported by many workers, defective oxygen transfer may exist in patients with 2,3-D.P.G. deficiency (commonly seen in patients with inadequate phosphate replacement, malnutrition or chronic sepsis) and Wright *et al.* (1971) have sufficient experimental evidence to support the theory that in septic shock (unlike pure hypovolaemic or cardiogenic shock) a primary cellular defect occurs and that the hyperdynamic circulation seen in this situation may be a compensatory mechanism. The cellular defect may be the direct effect of toxin on cells or the presence of circulating vasoactive polypeptides (Thal and Sardesai, 1965). It is clear that during the treatment of septic shock, restoration of an adequate circulating blood volume is one of the most important objectives.

It is probable, that patients who manifest with a low cardiac output have either an inadequate circulating blood volume, preceding myocardial dysfunction, or have developed cardiac failure as a consequence of the inability of the heart to keep up with the circulatory demands, the onset of a cardiac dysrhythmia, or a failure of the right heart because of increasing pulmonary hypertension.

It is of interest to note that few patients who present with shock associated with sepsis when efficiently and appropriately treated, die within the first 48 h of admission (Ledingham, 1975). Those with severe prolonged shock and extensive sepsis (especially abdominal) tend to die, however, several days later from continuing uncontrolled sepsis, secondary infection, or most commonly multiple organ failure – presumably a consequence of inadequate cellular oxygenation during the period of shock. Right heart failure as a consequence of pulmonary failure, secondary to shock and sepsis, is one of the commonest causes of death and is often terminally associated with renal and hepatic failure. Ledingham (1975) has reported gastrointestinal bleeding (generally due to an erosive gastritis) as a late cause of death – the early regular use of magnesium trisilicate mixture seems to reduce the incidence. Patients may present with acute erosive gastritis and extensive sepsis – here Cimetidine (given intravenously or orally) is extremely valuable.

Disseminated intravascular coagulation is a well recognised complication of sepsis and may be one of the major factors producing multiple organ failure. The mechanism by which endotoxin may stimulate intravascular coagulation is a problem of much interest. Endotoxin may initiate the intrinsic clotting system by activating the Hageman factor. Once local hypoxia secondary to shock develops – vessel wall and endothelial cell damage occurs thereby initiating the extrinsic clotting system.

THE SOURCE OF INFECTION AND THE BACTERIA INVOLVED IN SHOCK ASSOCIATED WITH SEPSIS

The incidence of staphylococcal septicaemia has decreased from 27% in 1961 to 15% in 1965 and the incidence of gram negative and enterococcal septicaemia has increased from 40 to 50% over the same period (Finland, 1970). In children the portal of entry of the organism is frequently obscure (Kaufman, 1976) and children are more predisposed to the development of shock in association with the pneumococcus, streptococcus and meningococcus. Newborn infants are particularly prone to develop gram negative bacteraemia.

In adults the portal of entry is most commonly the genitourinary tract but other sources include the gastrointestinal tract, wounds, the respiratory tract and the biliary tract. Certain situations are known to predispose the patient to septicaemia. In surgical practice operations on the biliary and urinary tract in the presence of infection, and laparotomy for peritonitis without adequate or appropriate antibiotic cover, are particularly hazardous. Infection may be introduced at operation, in particular during cardiac surgery, or during the introduction of catheters for investigative procedures, or for prolonged intravenous infusion.

Septicaemia associated with shock is most likely to develop in certain patients particularly at risk, the diabetic, the patient with leucopenia or hypoproteinaemia, the patient in renal failure, or the patient on steroids. There is a higher incidence and higher mortality from shock associated with sepsis in the very young and in the patient over 60 years.

The organisms most commonly involved in the gram negative series producing death from septic shock are the *E. coli*, *P. aeruginosa*, *K. pneumoniae*, Proteus, Enterobacter, Bacteroides species and fungi. In the gram positive series the commonest cause of death is associated with the *Staphylococcus aureus*, Enterococcus, Clostridium species, the Streptococcus, Pneumococcus and Meningococcus. The incidence of Pseudomonas, Proteus and fungal septicaemia is high in patients on broad spectrum antibiotics or receiving immunosuppressives.

DIAGNOSIS OF SHOCK ASSOCIATED WITH SEPSIS

Many patients with septicaemia can be saved provided the diagnosis is made early and management is correct. The signs of septic shock can be subdivided into early and late (Table 1). Many of these signs may be thought to be due to other factors and consequently the diagnosis is made too late.

Septicaemia from whatever cause is frequently preceded by a period of pyrexia or rigors. In the early stages, the patient is frequently alert, restless and tachypnoeic and this progresses to a state of coma. Dyspnoea is invariably present unless the patient has developed central nervous depression secondary to drug therapy, hypotension, or carbon dioxide narcosis in a patient receiving oxygen with preceding chronic respiratory failure. Central cyanosis may be absent in spite of a low PaO_2. The presence of hypoxia in association with a low $PaCO_2$ and inability to raise the PaO_2 to adequate levels with oxygen via a face

Table 1. Differential diagnosis of septic shock

Early signs	Alternative diagnosis
Pyrexia (occasionally absent)	Myocardial failure
Sweating	Pulmonary embolism
Restlessness	Amniotic fluid embolism
Some confusion	Adverse drug reaction
Tachypnoea	Incompatible blood transfusion
Tachycardia 90–110/min	Transfusion of old blood
Slight fall in B.P. 80–100 mm Hg systolic pressure	Blood volume loss in the absence of septicaemia
Mild jaundice	
Deterioration during anaesthesia or failure to regain consciousness after an anaesthetic	

Late signs	Alternative diagnosis
Coma	Cerebral catastrophe
Tachypnoea often associated with central cyanosis	Myocardinal failure
Cold pale extremities with peripheral cyanosis	Pulmonary ⎰ aspiration ⎱ thrombotic embolism ⎰ amniotic fluid embolism
Skin cold and clammy	
Tachycardia >110/min	Hepatocellular failure
Hypotension <80 mm Hg	Blood volume loss in the absence of septicaemia
Moderate jaundice	
Oliguria	
Coagulation abnormalities	

mask, is characteristic. Chest X-ray at this stage may show early pulmonary oedema (in the absence of hilar engorgement), the Stage 1 of the shock lung syndrome (p. 540), or may be passed as normal.

Coma generally occurs relatively late and is a bad prognostic sign. On rare occasions tachypnoea due to myocardial failure may be noted: this generally arises in cases seen late where hypotension has been assumed to be due to hypovolaemia and the patients have been over infused in the presence of oliguria.

Tachycardia is always present and in the presence of a normal central venous pressure and the absence of overt fluid loss, should raise the suspicion of early septic shock. On rare occasions the pulse rate rise is not significant ($<100/\text{min}$) because of the preceding use of β-blockers, the use of opiates for pain, digoxin toxicity, or heart block.

Drugs may on occasions produce similar clinical signs. A patient (who had recently undergone surgery for perforated diverticulitis) was on an aminophylline infusion for his bronchial asthma. The tachycardia and restlessness was attributed to this drug. It was not until the infusion had been stopped for 2 h and the symptoms persisted, that the diagnosis of *E. coli* septicaemia was made.

Haemolysis secondary to an incompatible blood transfusion is rare and mild jaundice, in the presence of sepsis, should be considered infective until proven otherwise. The clostridial organism has a particular reputation for producing severe and rapid haemolysis. Rapidly increasing jaundice, in the presence of a fall in blood haptoglobin concentration and frank haemoglobinuria, should make one suspect clostridial myonecrosis. Jaundice may develop in the absence of intravascular haemolysis, this may be secondary to hepatocellular necrosis subsequent to hypoxia and hypotension, or portal thrombophlebitis.

Many of these potentially septicaemic patients are subjected to a general anaesthetic for removal or drainage of the infected source. Manipulation of the infected organ may provoke a bacteraemia. The anaesthetist may notice the patient develop central cyanosis, a tachycardia, a fall in blood pressure, or a failure to regain consciousness following the anaesthetic. These signs may be misinterpreted and the diagnosis made too late.

Certain bacteria are known to produce characteristic skin rashes – in particular the Meningococcus (Fig. 1) and the typhoid and paratyphoid organisms. Patients with meningococcal septicaemia and skin rash may have haematological evidence of disseminated intravascular coagulation. Skin haemorrhages associated with a coagulation disorder

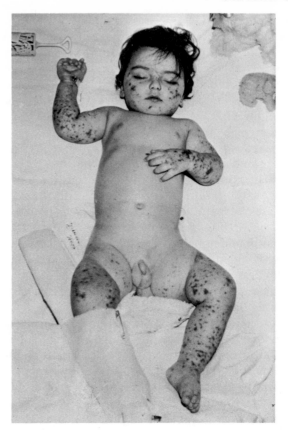

Fig. 1. Appearances of the meningococcal skin rash.

are commonly seen in septicaemias due to the Meningococcus, Pneumococcus, Pseudomonas, Proteus and Bacteroides species. Cold cyanosed extremities may be indicative of severe impairment of peripheral blood flow associated with disseminated intravascular coagulation; this is commonly associated with the late stages of septic shock and evidence of multiple organ failure, in particular pulmonary, hepatic and renal.

It is important to realise that, after the administration of an antibiotic endotoxin may be released from lysed organisms and trigger the haemodynamic crisis of septic shock (Weil *et al.*, 1964). The onset of late signs (Table 1) is associated with a bad prognosis, these patients commonly dying several days after the shocked condition has been corrected from organ failure, continued sepsis, or rarely, acute haemorrhage from stress.

EVALUATION OF THE PATIENT WITH SEPTIC SHOCK

A thorough history should be obtained, if necessary from a relative. The surgeon should be consulted if there has been a recent operative procedure. An assessment of the volume of fluid or blood lost over the preceding few days should be made, and a history obtained of any recent drug therapy. Past history of drug allergies, renal, hepatic or cardiovascular disease is of importance.

Physical examination provides information regarding the source of infection, organ function and the severity of the shocked state. The mental state, the femoral pulse volume and the state of skin perfusion are valuable signs. Cold cyanosed extremities in a comatose patient with an impalpable or rapid low volume femoral pulse indicates a bad prognosis.

The monitoring methods considered essential in the management of the patient in shock associated with sepsis, is enumerated in Table 1,

Table 2. Summary of treatment of septic shock

1. Assess adequacy of ventilation. Give oxygen and, if necessary, use mechanical ventilation.
2. Assess electrolyte and acid-base status. Insert a C.V.P. line. Restore the circulating blood volume and if possible, correct metabolic imbalance.
3. Take blood and other cultures and start appropriate antibiotic therapy. Give antibiotics intravenously. Consider hyperbaric oxygen therapy.
4. Should there be a poor response to (2) and (3), give massive doses of methylprednisolone intravenously.
5. Should the C.V.P. be raised consider digitalis.
6. Should the condition remain critical consider monitoring cardiac output and the use of drugs affecting cardiovascular function. (See Table 5).
7. Measure the urine/plasma osmolality ratio (U/P ratio).
8. If the U/P ratio is less then 2:1, insert a bladder catheter and measure urine output. If less than 50 h have elapsed from the onset of oliguria and the U/P ratio is less than 1:2, give up to three doses of mannitol (0.2 g/kg body weight) i.v. over 2–3 min at 2-hourly intervals until the urine is at least 50 ml/h.
9. If there is no response to mannitol, consider massive doses of frusemide.
10. Should there be no increase in urine volume, establish the conservative regime for acute renal failure. Assess the appropriate time for dialysis. Reassess the drug dosage in the light of impaired renal function.
11. Assess the haematological status, including evidence of intravascular haemolysis, hypercoagulation or hypocoagulation.
12. Consider surgery.

p. 317. It is rare for more sophisticated methods to be required in initial management but should be considered in patients who fail to improve with restoration of blood volume, correction of blood gas, acid base and electrolyte imbalance and antibiotics, and where drug therapy is being considered for treatment of the shocked state (Table 2, p. 325). More sophisticated monitoring methods may also be required when deterioration in cardiac function is suspected or where respiratory failure is sufficiently severe to warrant P.E.E.P. and there is concern about the haemodynamic response to its use (p. 327).

TREATMENT OF SHOCK ASSOCIATED WITH SEPSIS

The aims of treatment are to restore an effective circulating blood volume, to attempt to correct the metabolic, respiratory, haematological and microcirculatory disturbances, and to eradicate the source of infection. A summary of treatment is shown in Table 2.

Volume replacement. Correction of abnormalities in metabolic balance

Our experience suggests that a high percentage of shocked patients have a depletion of the circulating blood volume. Institution of right atrial pressure monitoring as soon as is feasible is therefore essential. A low level (less than 4 cm H_2O at the mid-thoracic level) warrants rapid volume replacement. Approximately 500 ml of fluid should be infused over 20 min and the right atrial pressure recorded. Should the value be the same and yet the femoral pulse volume and blood pressure remain low, more fluid should be infused at a rate of approximately 200 ml every 15 min until either the blood pressure reaches 100 mm Hg systolic pressure, or above, or the central venous pressure has risen to 10 cm H_2O or more. A normal central venous pressure (pp. 307–309) in the presence of hypotension is an indication for a series of fluid challenges (p. 308). By this method an 'optimum' dynamic blood volume can be restored and is frequently associated with an improvement in pulse pressure and a systolic pressure above 80 mm Hg. When the right atrial pressure is above 15 cm H_2O, either cardiac failure has occurred or there is suggestive evidence of an increase in pulmonary artery pressure due to pulmonary failure, or there has been a rise in intrathoracic pressure due to the institution of P.E.E.P., bronchospasm, acute pneumothorax, or cardiac tamponade. A severe acidosis may also produce an increase in pulmonary artery pressure which resolves once the acidosis is corrected. When the right atrial pressure is thought to be raised because of an increase in pulmonary artery pressure, a fluid challenge of 200 ml over 5 – 15 min may be tried. A sudden rise of the right atrial pressure by 2 cm H_2O or more is an indication to stop, but occasionally the right atrial pressure remains static and a series of fluid challenges can be given until the right atrial pressure shifts. Clearly, under such circumstances the right ventricle is under considerable stress, and the introduction of a triple lumen catheter should be considered in order to monitor right ventricular output (p. 322). Fluid loading can be clearly continued if the right ventricular output steadily rises but should be stopped once the systolic pressure is 80 mm Hg or more and urine output has increased. Under these circumstances of pulmonary failure in association with sepsis, the monitoring of P.C.W.P. as an indicator of left ventricular function may be misleading. It is hoped that transcutaneous aortovelography may ultimately prove valuable as an indicator of left ventricular function (p. 323). The type of fluid to be used during volume replacement should be considered. Clearly if there is a base deficit of 10 or more, sodium bicarbonate should be used in order to restore the base deficit to 10. A pH of 7.2 or less in an adult in the absence of a correctable respiratory deficit is also an indication for the use of bicarbonate. Sodium depletion should be replaced with normal saline or twice normal saline, keeping in mind that a low serum sodium may represent the 'sick cell syndrome' (p. 170). Potassium, calcium, magnesium and phosphate deficits should be replaced as quickly as possible. Hypokalaemia is a serious complication of septic shock and warrants appropriate and immediate replacement (p. 177). Phosphate, magnesium and calcium depletion is common in patients who have been suffering from malnutrition in association with chronic sepsis and inadequate electrolyte replacement. It is important to assess renal function before ionic replacement since dangerous hyper-kalaemia may develop in patients with renal failure.

Fluid therapy should never be instituted 'blind' in a patient with shock associated with sepsis, since on rare occasions the shock is secondary to fluid overload in the presence of oliguric renal failure or the onset of frank left ventricular or right ventricular failure. Under such circumstances volume depletion by diuretics, venesection and/or dialysis may correct the shock state.

In the absence of any metabolic deficit, dextran 70 is a suitable volume expander in patients with normal serum albumin levels. In patients with suspected hypoalbuminaemia, either P.P.F. or salt-free albumin should be used, salt-free albumin being the solution of choice in patients with renal failure.

Management of respiratory failure

One of the most important aspects of treatment is maintenance of the airway and restoration of normal blood gases. The majority of patients in shock associated with sepsis have PaO_2 levels of 9.3 kPa (70 mm Hg) or less, even on oxygen via a face mask. Early intubation and the introduction of I.P.P.V. or C.P.P.V. is imperative, firstly because hypoxia may perpetuate the shocked state, secondly because the onset of pulmonary oedema in association with sepsis may be prevented by early C.P.P.V., thirdly because severe shock is generally associated with an impaired cough reflex – aspiration being a common complication, fourthly because miliary atelectasis is common and may be one of the factors producing the 'shock lung' and finally the work of breathing increases oxygen demands and is frequently complicated by exhaustion.

The management of the patient with pulmonary failure associated with sepsis is described in Part 2, ch. V, p. 552.

Haematological abnormalities and their management

Patients in septic shock will usually show an initial granulocytopenia followed by granulocytosis and thrombocytopenia. The granulocytosis is particularly prominent in patients suffering from meningococcal or pneumococcal septic shock. Granulocytopenia is frequently associated with metamyelocytes and myelocytes in the blood stream and may on occasions be sufficiently severe to suggest a hypoplastic marrow. On rare occasions a megaloblastosis may be present, together with a megaloblastic marrow. Our limited experience suggests this is related to folic acid deficiency and is seen in patients on folate inhibitors before the onset of septic shock (e.g. phenytoin sodium), or in patients who may be folate depleted because of inadequate replacement therapy (patients on dialysis or on intravenous fluids only). The use of trimethoprim (in septrin or bactrim) may lead to folate depletion, thrombocytopenia and leucopenia.

Thrombocytopenia may be due to peripheral platelet destruction, disseminated intravascular coagulation or suppression of the bone marrow due to sepsis and shock. Thrombocytopenia in isolation rarely causes bleeding even when the platelet count falls to 40 000/mm³ or less. Sequential platelet counts should however be performed, since patients with platelet counts of 40 000/mm³ or less should have platelets restored before any operative procedure, a steady rise in the platelet count is generally a good prognostic sign.

In septic shock there is generally an oscillatory pattern of early hyper-coagulability followed by hypocoagulability (Attar *et al.*, 1966a; Attar *et al.*, 1966b). Analysis of large series of patients with gram negative septicaemia and shock reveals changes in coagulation parameters consistent with intravascular coagulation (Corrigan *et al.*, 1968; Wilson *et al.*, 1967). The condition disseminated intravascular coagulation (D.I.C.) has been reviewed in some detail by Colman and workers (1972) and is also described in Part 2, ch. VIII, p. 654. The baseline clotting indices estimated in the patient with shock varies in different centres – but indices serving an adequate baseline and reflecting coagulation changes are listed in Table 3.

Table 3. Baseline coagulation studies. Changes following massive transfusion and D.I.C.

Coagulation test	Normal levels	Aetiology	
		Massive transfusion	D.I.C.
Platelet count (per mm³)	250 000 ± 50 000	Generally < 150 000	< 150 000
Prothrombin time (s)	12.0 ± 1.0	> 15.0	> 15.0
Thrombin time (s)	20.0 ± 1.6	Normal	> 25
Fibrinogen level (mg/100 ml) or	230 ± 35	Normal	< 160
Fibrinogen titre	$\frac{1}{128}$ or greater	Normal	$\frac{1}{32}$ or less

An early diagnosis of D.I.C. can best be made on the regular frequent analysis of these indices. Results must be interpreted in the light of massive transfusion with old blood, or replacement of labile clotting factors with fresh frozen plasma. The diagnosis of D.I.C. requires that three out of four of these indices should be abnormal. The presence of fibrin degradation products may be an early indicator of D.I.C. but may not take place if there is endogenous inhibition of fibrinolysis or if the patient has been treated with fibrinolytic inhibitors. (*Inhibitors of fibrinolysis are contraindicated in the treatment* of coagulation problems in association with septic shock.)

The time when D.I.C. should be treated is controversial. Treatment is summarised in Table 4.

Frequently the diagnosis is made in the absence of overt bleeding.

Table 4. Treatment of disseminated intravascular coagulation associated with severe sepsis

Diagnosis based on 3 out of the 4 coagulation indices shown in Table 3 being positive. Exclude any deficiency of vitamin K, folic acid, or the presence of any drug anticoagulant.

In the absence of overt bleeding
1. Treat the sepsis with appropriate antibiotics and surgical drainage if necessary.
2. Treat the shock, thereby improving cellular perfusion.
3. Replace labile clotting factors with F.F.P. (1 packet of F.F.P. raises the fibrinogen titre by approximately 25 mg/100 ml in a 70 kg man). *Do not* give platelets unless the platelet count is 40 000/mm³ or less.
4. Check the fibrinogen level (or titre) 1 hour after giving F.F.P. and record the result. Should the level (or titre) have not risen or have fallen, consider heparin. Should the level have risen repeat the fibrinogen titre another hour later, should it have fallen, consider heparin.

In the presence of overt bleeding
1. As above. *Do not* operate until at least 4 packets of F.F.P. have been given and should the platelet count be 40 000/mm³ or less, cover the operation with fresh blood, platelet enriched plasma, or platelets. Give 4 packets of platelets or platelet enriched plasma before and during the operation.
2. As above.
3. As above.
4. Consider the use of heparin in cases where bleeding is severe (e.g. oozing from operation sites, extensive purpura, bleeding from the mouth or gums).
5. Use heparin in all cases where the clotting factors deteriorate in spite of repeated replacement of clotting factors.

Heparin therapy

50–100 units per kg B.W. i.v. as a bolus then 10–15 units per kg B.W. hourly as a continuous infusion.
Use lower dosage if platelets < 100 000/mm³.
Monitor coagulation indices (Table 3), reduce the dosage of heparin if thrombin time becomes prolonged longer than 40 s after starting therapy.
E.A.C.A. or tranexamic acid should *not* be used.

Generally, treatment with heparin is not commenced until overt bleeding occurs – replacement of clotting factors with F.F.P. being used first. This clearly may perpetuate the situation, more clotting factors being provided to enable further microcoagulation to take place. However, D.I.C. in the presence of septic shock is generally self-limiting and spontaneously resolves once the source of infection and/or the organism involved is treated. Further work may suggest that heparin should be used earlier in order to prevent microcoagulation which is thought to be one of the major factors in producing multiple organ ailure. At the present moment a compromise is struck between the early use of heparin as soon as D.I.C. is detected and heparin used too late when bleeding has become uncontrollable and there is existence of multiple organ failure. The management of D.I.C. is summarised in Table 4. In the majority of patients clotting factors spontaneously improve after correction of shock, appropriate treatment of the sepsis and initial replacement with F.F.P.

In pregnancy associated with sepsis it has been recommended that heparin should be used early, but generally the condition resolves as with other sources of sepsis (see Part 2, ch. XI, p. 723).

Heparin has to be used most frequently in conditions where rapid elimination of the source of infection is impossible – this in particular applies to patients with chronic intra-abdominal sepsis where total surgical drainage is not feasible.

The heparin dosage should be regulated according to the thrombin time, the dosage may have to be increased above that recommended because of heparin resistance. Heparin may take several hours to take effect and during this time in patients with severe bleeding, blood volume should be maintained as recommended on p. 349. Blood when required should be as fresh as possible. The initial effect of heparin is clinical, i.e. major bleeding stops and no new purpura develops. The prothrombin time generally falls within hours and falls by at least 5 seconds or returns to normal within one day (Colman *et al.*, 1972). The platelet count may take several days to rise or may even fall and is therefore not a reliable therapeutic indicator. The fibrinogen level or titre may take several days to rise but in conditions of sepsis is generally artificially increased by the use of F.F.P.

Heparin therapy is often stopped too soon, and once commenced should be continued for at least 3 days following return of the prothrombin time to normal. In situations where sepsis is difficult to eradicate, or is likely to recur, heparin therapy should be continued for at least 10 days.

Drug therapy

Drug therapy is rarely required in the treatment of shock associated with sepsis and should generally only be considered under the following circumstances:

1. Blood pressure less than 70 mm S.P. for >30 min after adequate volume, electrolyte, acid base and blood gas control.

2. Evidence of deterioration or continued poor function in two of the following systems – kidneys, lungs or skin.
3. Evidence of a poor cardiac output.

The drugs available are enumerated in Table 5 and the choice can now be more scientifically selected according to the basic disorder.

High doses of methylprednisolone sodium succinate (30 mg/kg B.W.) given as a bolus is probably the initial drug of choice in septic shock. Experimental work suggests that steroids get at the basic cause of shock in sepsis, namely the effect of toxin on cells. A specific vasodilator action has been proposed for pharmacologic doses of corticosteroids (Lillehei et al., 1964) but this effect has not been subsequently confirmed (Altura and Altura, 1974). They do however exert modifying effects on the action of vasoactive agents on the peripheral vasculature. All these agents (catecholamines, vasopressin angiotensin and serotonin) are known to be released into the blood in shock and produce peripheral vasoconstriction. Their effect is inhibited or attenuated by massive doses of methylprednisolone. Methylprednisolone has been found to be more effective than hydrocortisone (Altura and Altura, 1974).

Weil and co-workers (1974) reviewed the effect of pharmacological doses of glucocorticoids on normal human volunteers and on patients and animals suffering from shock associated with sepsis. They concluded that routine treatment of bacterial shock states (especially shock associated with bacteraemia due to gram negative bacteria), with pharmacological doses of glucocorticoid constituted rational treatment. They found that the survival rate of patients receiving cortisone or its equivalent in doses greater than 300 mg/day, increased from 17% in those not receiving the drug to 43%. Their conclusions make a double blind trial in such critically ill patients difficult to justify. The timing of steroid therapy is difficult, but since in limited doses there seems to be no harmful effect, it is preferable to give it early rather than too late.

The indications for its use include:

1. The septic patient requiring emergency surgery whose systolic blood pressure is 100 mm Hg or less. Methyl prednisolone (30 mg/kg B.W.) should be given as a bolus approximately 30 min before operation.
2. Evidence of impaired cellular perfusion. A urine output of less than 40 ml/h in the presence of a normal circulating blood volume (as assessed by the C.V.P.), a low skin temperature which fails to rise after volume, acid base and blood gas correction, and/or a steadily increasing B.D. or pH of 7.2 or less following the use of bicarbonate.

One has the impression that the drug takes approximately 30 to 60 minutes to improve skin perfusion and/or acid base state or blood pressure, during this period additional support may be necessary using one of the drugs listed in Table 5.

Methyl prednisolone may have to be repeated on 2 or 3 more occasions in the same dosage (30 mg/kg B.W.) at 4 hourly intervals until impaired cellular perfusion has resolved.

A very high percentage of these patients develop renal failure but if renal function is still present, a potassium diuresis may develop within 45 min of steroid usage. A diuretic response frequently requires volume replacement and potassium supplementation.

The next drug of choice is probably digitalis. Digitalis is of particular value in the elderly where the onset of atrial fibrillation is common and may be fatal. Intravenous digoxin may increase cardiac output even in the presence of a sinus tachycardia (Ledingham, 1975) and should therefore be used in conjunction with steroids in any patient 40 years or over, or in younger patients where the pulse rate is 120/min or above. It is imperative to exclude digoxin toxicity or hypokalaemia prior to its use; frequently a dose of 0.5 mg titrated slowly intravenously under E.C.G. monitoring control may be adequate to tide the patient over the critical phase. Patients in atrial fibrillation should be fully digitalised, the dosage being estimated according to blood levels because of the high incidence of digoxin toxicity.

There is experimental evidence to suggest that early digitalisation maintains integrity of the myocardial cell (Coalson *et al.*, 1972). The use of steroids and digitalis generally tide the patient over the critical phase of shock and it is rare that other drugs have to be used. The mortality in patients requiring other drugs (approximately 5% of patients presenting with blood pressure systolic of 100 mm or less) is extremely high and since inappropriate drug therapy is dangerous selection should be based (if possible) on reliable physiological data. These data are referred to in Tables 1 and 2, pp. 317 and 325 respectively and should include monitoring of right atrial pressure, right atrial percentage oxygen saturation, right ventricular cardiac output and skin core temperature difference. An indicator of left ventricular function is also of value (e.g. Transcutaneous Aortovelography) but is at present clinically rarely possible.

Should steroids and digoxin be indicated and the patient sufficiently ill to suspect other drugs may have to be used, a triple lumen catheter should be inserted in order to measure mixed pulmonary oxygen tension and cardiac output (by thermodilution). Should the systolic blood

Table 5. Drugs used in the treatment of septic shock

Name of drug	Activity	Possible indications for its use	Disadvantages
Isoprenaline	β-adrenergic stimulator. Inotropic and chronotropic. Arterial vasodilation largely skeletal and mesenteric. Volume of capacitance bed $\downarrow$ $\therefore$ inc. in venous return.	Poor cardiac output in conjunction with a high arterial resistance. May be used in conjunction with dopamine hydrochloride (see text).	Increase in ventricular rate may increase oxygen demand. Ventricular dysrhythmias. Increased A–V shunting with decreased cellular oxygenation. May require volume replacement.
Noradrenaline	Small doses β-adrenergic stimulator. Larger amounts α-adrenergic effect (venous and arterial constriction).	None.	Loss of blood volume due to rise in capillary hydrostatic pressure. $\downarrow$ renal corticol flow. Local tissue necrosis.
Dopamine hydrochloride (precursor of noradrenaline)	Predominant β-adrenergic effect on the heart. Direct specific vasodilatory effect on the mesenteric and renal vessels. α-adrenergic effect on the skeletal muscle vascular bed producing vasoconstriction. Effect on the peripheral vascular resistance – small doses tend to produce a decrease, larger doses an increase. Oxygen consumption less than isoprenaline.	Poor cardiac output especially when associated with a high pulse rate i.e. instead of isoprenaline. Poor urine output.	Do not use until central venous pressure above the lower limits considered normal for that patient. May require volume 'top-up', may produce peripheral vasoconstriction when used in a dose high enough to achieve an adequate cardiac output.

Phenoxybenzamine	α- and β-receptor-blocker. Reduces arteriolar and vascular resistance, increase in capillary flow. Mobilisation of volume pooled in venous capacitance vessels.	Cardiac output normal or high. Severe vasoconstriction with high arteriolar and vascular resistance (because of length of activity and difficulty in control, preferable to use phentolamine).	Greater volume of blood accommodated in the circulation, relative fall in blood volume. Volume replacement invariably required. Adrenergic blockade may last for several days.
Phentolamine mesylate	As above.	As above. Preferable to phenoxybenzamine – reversed rapidly once infusion is stopped.	Greater volume of blood accommodated in the circulation, relative fall in blood volume. Volume replacement invariably required. Large doses needed.
Corticosteroids (synthetic)	Various claims – action uncertain. Prevention of the effect of vasoconstrictors released subsequent to the onset of shock in sepsis. Restoration of R.E.S. function. Reduction of release of lysoenzymes following shock.	Possibly drug of first choice in the management of severe shock associated with sepsis when volume acid base, electrolyte and blood gas control fails to produce improvement.	No increase in susceptibility to infection or reduced wound healing provided only used in limited doses.

pressure fail to rise above 80 mm S.P. after 45 min following the use of methylprednisolone and digoxin (should this be indicated) or there is evidence of further deterioration in cardiac output or skin, renal or pulmonary function, the use of one or two of the following drugs should be considered – dopamine hydrochloride, isoprenaline hydrochloride or phentolamine mesylate (Table 5).

Much more experience is required in additional drug therapy in shock associated with sepsis. It is extremely rare for patients to recover once these drugs are used. The subsequent advice is based on very limited experience and the impression that the few initial recoveries obtained might well have survived without their use. The majority of these patients die subsequently of disordered cellular function following upon inadequate tissue perfusion. Terminal pulmonary failure is common (see Part 2, ch. V, p. 539).

Vasoconstrictors are contraindicated in any patient with a low cardiac output (C.I. 2.5 l/min/m²), the mortality being increased five times above those patients in shock not receiving vasoconstrictors (Wilson et al., 1971). Noradrenaline is therefore contraindicated in patients suffering from shock primarily related to sepsis (Table 5).

Wilson and co-workers (1971) found that vasodilators (which are theoretically ideally suited) used for treating patients with sepsis and severe peripheral vasoconstriction seem to be detrimental. Their use should therefore be restricted to patients with a skin core temperature difference of more than 5°C (the core temperature being 33°C or more) and a cardiac index of 3.0 l/min/m² or above. Vasodilators are contraindicated in patients with a core temperature of less than 33°C because of the resultant heat loss. Phentolamine mesylate is the drug of choice and should be given as 5 mg intravenously over 1 min followed by 0.1 mgm per min (see Table 5). Cardiac output should be checked every 15 minutes and a fall associated with a fall in central venous pressure is an indication for fluid top-up. Should the systolic pressure and cardiac output fall, in spite of adequate fluid top-up, either dopamine should be added to the regime, or phentolamine stopped and isoprenaline with or without dopamine used. A brief summary of the pharmacological activity of isoprenaline and dopamine hydrochloride is described in Table 5. The most significant difference between isoprenaline and dopamine is the effect on lowering peripheral vascular resistance, isoprenaline producing a considerably greater effect. The action of isoprenaline may be valuable in patients with severe peripheral vasoconstriction, but when combined with a low cardiac output may be sufficiently intense to lower vital organ perfusion (Talley *et al.*, 1969). Under such circumstances a lower dose of each drug infused simultaneously may produce the necessary benefit. The combination of drugs should also be used where there is severe peripheral vasoconstriction associated with a low cardiac output and a pulse rate of greater than 140/min, or the presence of multiple ventricular extrasystoles.

Dopamine hydrochloride has been recently reviewed in a symposium held at the Royal Society of Medicine (Proceedings of the R.S.M., 1976). It appears to be of maximum value where the cardiac output is low (less than 3.0 l/min/m²) and there is evidence of impaired renal perfusion in the absence of a lowered circulating blood volume. In general, small doses of dopamine tend to decrease peripheral vascular resistance, while larger doses tend to produce an increase. Talley *et al.* (1969) when treating a series of patients with shock of varied aetiology, found that the infusion concentration of dopamine required to produce optimal clinical and haemodynamic data was usually associated with an increase in peripheral vascular resistance. Where the skin core temperature is greater than 5°C and there is an associated metabolic acidosis, dopamine hydrochloride should only be considered when isoprenaline fails to produce haemodynamic improvement or where isoprenaline is contraindicated (increasing hypoxia, tachycardia). Under such circumstances the drug should be started in the lowest concentration and any evidence of deterioration in peripheral perfusion without achieving the required haemodynamic effect, would be an indication to combine the drug with low doses of isoprenaline or phentolamine.

The dosage of dopamine hydrochloride recommended is 2–30 µg/kg/min. The infusion should be started at the lowest concentration and steadily increased until the systolic blood pressure had reached approximately 30 mm Hg below the estimated 'normal' level. The dosage should not be increased if the pulse rate is 130/min or greater.

Antibiotic therapy

The appropriate choice of antibiotic forms a vital role in the treatment of septic shock. Prior to treatment both anaerobic and aerobic blood cultures should be taken. In most forms of blood stream infection, the numbers of bacteria in the blood are small and only cultivation reveals them. On rare occasions direct staining of the blood film may reveal bacteria, this in particular applies to the anthrax bacillus and *Cl. welchii*. In order to get immediate confirmation of the bacteria involved, any source of suspected sepsis should be drained, directly stained and cultured anaerobically and aerobically. This in particular applies to fluid from the pleural cavity, joints, urine, spinal fluid, skin abscesses, stools, bile, wound sites and vaginal discharge.

The bacteriologist should be consulted prior to taking the blood cultures since special media may be suggested for certain bacteria. There is an increasing incidence of septicaemias due to Bacteroides, anaerobic Streptococco, Klebsiella and fungi, and this should be taken into account when antibiotic therapy is instituted. There has also been an increased incidence of septicaemia due to two bacterial species, which makes therapy particularly difficult. This situation is particularly likely to arise following septic abortion (where Clostridia and a gram negative organism may be involved) in chronic intra-abdominal and urinary tract infections and in patients on immunosuppressives where a fungal infection may also be present.

Chemotherapy for septic shock is reviewed by Seneca and Grant (1976) and Kirby (1976). The drugs to use prior to the exact organism being known is based on gram stain of any infected source, the suspected source of infection, previous antibiotic therapy and the clinical presentation. There is still controversy about the best drug combination in patients suffering from suspected gram negative sepsis. In patients recently hospitalised, with no preceding operation or antibiotic therapy (e.g. perforation and shock), it is reasonable to commence with a combination of cephalothin and clindamycin (clindamycin for the possible presence of Bacteroides). Should shock be severe, and fails to respond to volume replacement, and a resistant Klebsiella or coliform be suspected, treatment should also include gentamicin. Preliminary bacterial sensitivities can generally be obtained within 24 h when it may be possible to stop gentamicin therapy. The combination of a cephalosporin and gentamicin may produce nephrotoxicity – but this has not been our experience if the combination is used for 24 h or less and cephalothin is used. Gentamicin is a difficult antibiotic to use, the dosage varying from one patient to another, even when renal function appears normal. In critically ill patients overdosage is wiser than underdosage and the initial loading dose should be 2.5 mg/kg followed by 1.5 mg/kg every 8 h. The initial dose should be given intravenously and subsequent doses intramuscularly. Subsequent dosage must be adjusted according to peak and trough blood levels. Cephalothin should be given as a 2.0 g intravenous bolus, followed by 1.0–2.0 g 4 hourly. Clindamycin is preferable to lincomycin in the treatment of suspected Bacteroides infection, since the organism may take several days to culture, it is wise to continue therapy for three to four days until a negative culture is obtained.

In suspected Proteus or Pseudomonas infections, a combination of carbenicillin and gentamicin should be used. A synergistic action occurs against most bacteria and the combination appears to depress the incidence of gentamicin-resistant bacilli* (Kirby, 1976). Carbenicillin should be given in doses of 24–30 g daily in patients with normal renal function, the dosage should be reduced according to blood levels in patients with impaired renal function. Staphylococcal septicaemia should be treated with a combination of Fucidin and methicillin (methicillin being less protein bound than oxacillin or cloxacillin) until the sensitivity of the staphylococcus is established.

Pneumococcal, meningococcal, and most septicaemias due to the Streptococcus, are most appropriately treated with a combination of benzyl penicillin and sulphonamide. Because of possible bacterial resistance, cephalothin should be added to this regime until sensitivities are obtained. Septicaemia in association with meningitis warrants intrathecal benzyl penicillin.

Once Bacteroides septicaemia is diagnosed intravenous metronidazole should be combined with clindamycin, other antibiotics being stopped. Metronidazole is now available for intravenous use (May and Baker Ltd.), the dosage being 500 mg in 100 ml of buffered isotonic aqueous solution – this being infused over 30 min 8-hourly. Oral therapy should be resumed as soon as possible. Side effects are remarkably rare – there has been no evidence of nephrotoxicity in one patient with severe renal failure treated with long-term oral metronidazole. Haemodialysis may however produce two to three fold reduction in blood levels (Ingham et al., 1975). Blood levels should therefore be estimated in patients on dialysis.

The specific management of gas forming infections and chronic intra-abdominal sepsis are described in Part 2, ch. IV, pp. 499 and 511.

Many patients sufficiently ill to warrant intensive therapy are susceptible to secondary infection. Lackner and co-workers (1974) found that the incidence of bacteraemia increased in the second and third weeks – a pyrexia during the first week of admission being commonly abacteraemic. They found that most of the organisms isolated were resistant to the drugs of the penicillin and cephalosporin type. Aminoglycoside therapy is therefore generally indicated in patients developing septic shock whilst being treated in the intensive therapy unit.

* In hospitals known to harbour gentamicin-resistant bacilli tobramycin should be substituted. The dosage being adjusted according to peak and trough blood levels.

During the last few years a striking increase in the incidence of clinically significant and sometimes fatal systemic fungal disease in hospitalised patients has been reported (Bernhardt *et al.*, 1972). The natural virulence of most fungi is low and certain predisposing factors are generally present. These include, extreme youth or age, debilitation and malnutrition, drug addiction, neoplasm including leukaemia, diabetes mellitus, renal failure, transplantation, treatment with certain drugs (immunosuppressives, steroids, broad spectrum antibiotics) and prolonged indwelling catheters. The diagnosis must depend on a combination of clinical and laboratory findings and careful consideration of the multiplicity of factors comprising the clinical setting (Rodrigues and Wolff, 1974). Potent fungal toxins have been isolated (Salvin, 1952) and fungaemia may present with a shock state similar to gram negative sepsis. D.I.C. may be present (Philippidis *et al.*, 1972). Initial blood cultures may fail to yield the organism or isolation may be too late for effective institution of therapy. The presence of any of the above factors, a leukaemoid reaction in the peripheral blood film and budding fungi in the urine is strong evidence in favour of a disseminated fungal infection. Such evidence in a shocked patient may warrant the use of antifungal therapy.

The chemotherapy for the systemic mycoses has been excellently reviewed by Utz (1976). The most common septicaemia encountered is that due to the Candida species. The septicaemia is frequently either promptly fatal or self-limited, and when associated with endocarditis, chemotherapy is generally ineffective (Utz, 1976). The drug of choice is flucytosine (which is now available intravenously) since it is less toxic than amphotericin B. In desperately ill patients flucytosine should be combined with amphotericin B. Flucytosine toxicity has been most frequently reported in uraemic patients and the dosage should be regulated according to the creatinine clearance. Flucytosine was found effective in patients who relapsed following amphotericin B therapy.

Amphotericin B, combined with deoxycholate and buffer, forms a colloidal state in glucose solutions and can be infused intravenously. Renal insufficiency does not appear to affect the serum levels or urinary excretion and the drug (because of possible lipoprotein binding) is excreted for periods of up to 3 weeks after stopping treatment. There is no universal agreement about the optimal daily dose. The initial dose, 1 mg, is added to 100 ml 5% glucose and infused over 4 h. The dose is then increased on alternate days by 5 mg – increments to a maximum of 50 mg or 1 mg/kg B.W. (depending upon the patient's weight). A more rapid increase in the critically ill is frequently complicated by tachycardia, sweating and vomiting. The total dose generally given is 1.5–2.5 g given over a period of 4–6 weeks. Creatinine clearance should be monitored on alternate days and the rate of dose increase should be decreased should there be deterioration. Hypokalaemia and a metabolic acidosis are the complications which should be treated as soon as they arise. Maintenance of a high urine output is essential.

The use of Miconazole (an imidazole derivative) in the treatment of systemic mycoses has been recently reported (Symoens, 1977). Symoens (1977) found that intravenous treatment with Miconazole brought about recovery of 90% of patients with gastrointestinal or systemic candidiasis. Meningitis requires intrathecal administration. Side effects of the drug are few and it can be used quite safely in seriously ill patients – it is possibly less effective than amphotericin B in the treatment of C. albicans. Preliminary work suggests that Miconazole and amphotericin B when given in combination is less effective than either alone – the combination should therefore be avoided until more data is available (Schacter et al., 1976).

In the critically ill patient with renal failure, the combination of intravenous flucytosine and intravenous Miconazole* may prove to be the drugs of choice in fungal septicaemia.

For the management of other rarer fungal infections, reference should be made to the papers by Bennett (1974), Cartwright (1975) and Utz (1976).

Surgery

It is imperative, at the initial clinical assessment, to consider whether there is any septic focus that can be removed surgically. 'Medical' resuscitation may improve the patient initially but should there be an extensive nidus of infection, medical treatment alone will not save the patient.

Intraperitoneal leakage of bile, urine, blood or gastrointestinal contents may necessitate an emergency laparotomy. An obstructive uropathy associated with a pyonephrosis and septicaemia, or a perinephric abscess, may require urgent drainage. Pelvic examination by an experienced clinician is mandatory whenever septic shock develops from an unknown source, or when pelvic sepsis is suspected.

Laparotomy may be indicated when an intraperitoneal or pelvic infection is suspected and where drainage could prove to be lifesaving.

* Not immediately available but may be available on application to Janssen Pharmaceutical Ltd.

These patients are desperately ill and the time taken for resuscitation prior to laparotomy is critical. Once blood volume, acid base electrolyte and blood gases have been corrected and the systolic pressure 100 mm Hg or more, laparotomy should be performed within the subsequent hour. When there is a loculated infection, initial resuscitation is often successful but rapid deterioration may occur several hours later unless the infection is drained. Death is unlikely during the operation provided the timing is correct and the laparotomy and subsequent appropriate surgical procedure is performed by an experienced surgeon. It is imperative that during laparotomy, should no obvious source of infection be found, that the examination be thorough, since should the patient deteriorate again at least an intraperitoneal, retroperitoneal or pelvic infection is unlikely and another source of infection must be searched for.

Preparation for operation includes the resuscitative procedures indicated in Table 2. Digoxin (unless there is a contraindication) 0.5 mg should be titrated slowly intravenously and 30 mg/kg B.W. of methylprednisolone hemisuccinate given intravenously approximately 30 minutes pre-operatively. Arterial oxygen on oxygen via a face mask is invariably less than 9.3 kPa (70 mm Hg); intubation and ventilation should preferably be performed prior to transfer of the patient to theatre. Central venous pressure and E.C.G. monitoring during the operation is essential. Adequate anaesthesia in the critically ill can be obtained with nitrous oxide, oxygen, phenoperidine, diazepam and a muscle relaxant such as pancuronium.

The U/P osmolality ratio should be checked pre-operatively and if 1.2 or less, renal failure should be suspected. Should serum potassium be 5.0 mmol or more, the operation should be covered with insulin and glucose intravenously and the anaesthetist ensure that the patient does not develop a respiratory acidosis. Surgery should not be considered until the B.D. is less than 10, the pH 7.3 or greater and the serum potassium at least 3.5 mmol/l. Clotting factors must be checked pre-operatively and if the fibrinogen level or titre be low, 3 packets of F.F.P. should be infused pre-operatively and a further 3 packets be available if oozing develops per or postoperatively. A platelet count of 40 000/mm³ or less is an indication for a platelet or platelet enriched plasma infusion pre-operatively and during operation; 4 packets pre-operatively and 4 packets during the operation (platelet enriched plasma eliminates the need for F.F.P.).

Blood as fresh as possible should be available for all patients if the Hct pre-operatively is 35% or less.

Should the patient be in renal failure, a peritoneal dialysing catheter or arteriovenous shunt can be inserted in theatre in preparation for renal dialysis. It is wise, if the peritoneum is opened, for the peritoneal dialysing catheter to be inserted under direct vision away from the operating site (generally in the iliac fossa). It is important that the catheter is inserted correctly, simple peritoneal drains are not satisfactory for dialysis. Peritoneal 'lavage' should be considered in patients with severe nonlocalised peritonitis in the absence of renal failure. Isotonic dialysing fluid at a rate of 500 ml every 30–45 min until the fluid is clear (i.e. generally 2 days) may be valuable – this in particular applies to patients with biliary peritonitis, sepsis associated with pancreatitis and severe faeculent peritonitis. Peritoneal lavage may be interrupted twice daily for the instillation of noxythiolin – 5 g of noxythiolin is dissolved in 500 ml of normal saline, the solution is run into the peritoneal cavity and drained out after 2 h. This is repeated 12 hourly for a period of 24–72 h.

Postoperatively, clotting factors, electrolytes (including blood glucose), blood gases and chest X-ray should be rechecked. The patient should not be allowed to breathe spontaneously for at least 12 h postoperatively (even if the blood gases are normal on an F_IO_2 of 35% or less).

D.I.C. may develop postoperatively especially if extensive pelvic sepsis or oozing at the operative site occurs, clotting factors may therefore have to be replaced. Surgical drainage of the infective source may be followed by a potassium diuresis, potassium monitoring is therefore important. The blood glucose, even in the nondiabetic may rise to levels sufficiently high (> 12 mmol/l) to warrant insulin therapy. Soluble insulin is preferably given as a stat dose of 20 units or less, followed by 4–8 units hourly either intramuscularly or intravenously until the blood glucose has fallen to 8 mmol/l or less.

Since the haemodynamic disturbance is profound in these patients, it is preferable (in patients with renal failure) to defer dialysis for at least 24 h postoperatively. The rate of rise of urea and potassium can be reduced by the insulin dextrose regime – 200–300 g of dextrose being infused over the subsequent 24 h with appropriate glucose monitoring and insulin supplementation (Part 1, ch. IX, p. 263).

REFERENCES

Altura, B. M. and Altura, B. T. (1974). Peripheral vascular actions of glucocorticoids and their relationship to protection in circulatory shock. *J. of Pharm and Exper. Ther.* **190**, 300.

Attar, S. M. A., McLaughlin, J., Mansberger, A. R. and Cowley, R. A. (1966a). Prognostic significance of coagulation studies in clinical shock. *Surg. Forum* **17**, 8.

Attar, S., Mansberger, A. R., Irani, B., Kirby, W., Masaitis, C. and Cowley, R. A. (1966b). Coagulation changes in clinical shock: II Effects of septic shock on clotting times and fibrinogen in humans. *Ann. Surg.* **164**, 41.

Bennett, J. E. (1974). Drug therapy: Chemotherapy of systemic mycoses. *New Engl. J. Med.* **290**, 30.

Bernhardt, H. E., Orlando, J. C., Benfield, J. B., Hirose, F. M. and Foos, R. Y. (1972). Disseminated candidiasis in surgical patients. *Surg. Gynecol. Obst.* **134**, 819.

Cartwright, R. Y. (1975). Antifungal drugs. *J. Antimicrob. Chemother.* **1**, 141.

Coalson, J. L., Woodruff, H. K., Greenfield, L. J., Guenter, C. A. and Hinshaw, L. B. (1972). Effects of digoxin on myocardial ultrastructure in endotoxin shock. *Surg. Gynec. Obstet.* **135**, 908.

Colman, R. W., Robboy, S. J. and Minna, J. D. (1972). Disseminated intravascular coagulation (D.I.C.): an approach. *Am. J. Med.* **52**, 679.

Corrigan, J. J. Jr., Ray, L. and May, N. (1968). Changes in the blood coagulation system associated with septicaemia. *New Eng. J. Med.* **279**, 851.

Ellin, R. J., Robinson, R. A., Levine, A. S. and Wolff, S. M. (1975). Lack of clinical usefulness of the limulus test in the diagnosis of endotoxemia. *New Engl. J. Med.* **293**, 521.

Finland, M. (1970). Changing ecology of bacterial infections as related to antibacterial therapy. *J. Infect. Dis.* **122** (5), 419.

Glynn, A. A. and Howard, C. J. (1973). *In* 'Recent Advances in Clin. Path. (Ed. Dyke, S. C.). Churchill-Livingstone, Edinburgh.

Ingham, H. R., Rich, G. E., Selkon, J. B., Hale, J. H., Roxhy, C. M., Betty, M. J., Johnson, R. W. C. and Uldall, P. R. (1975). Treatment with metronidazole of three patients with serious infections due to Bacteroides fragilis. *J. Antimicrob. Chemother.* **1**, 235.

Kaufman, J. J. (1976). Septicemia: Pathogenesis and frequency. *J. Antibiotic Chemother.* **21**, 62.

Kirby, M. M. (1976). Antimicrobial therapy. *In* 'Antibiotics and Chemotherapy' (Ed. Garrod, L. P., Seneca, H., Jawetz, E. and Fereres, J.) Vol. 21, 191. Karger, Basel.

Lackner, F., Haider, W., Orbes, S., Pichler, H., Rotter, M. and Werner, H. P. (1974). Septicaemia in critical care patients treated with high doses of antibiotics. *Resuscitation* **3**, 205.

Ledingham, I. McA. (1975). Septic shock. *Brit. J. Surg.* **62**, 777.

Levin, J., Poore, T. E., Neil, P., Zauber, B. A. and Oser, R. S. (1970). Detection of endotoxin in the blood of patients with sepsis due to gram-negative bacteria. *New Engl. J. Med.* **283**, 1313.

Lillehei, R. C., Longerbeam, J. K., Bloch, J. and Marax, W. G. (1964). Nature of irreversible shock: experimental and clinical observations. *Ann. Surg.* **160**, 682.

Philippidis, P., Namar, J. I., Sibinga, M. S. and Valdes-Dapnea, M. A. (1972). Disseminated intravascular coagulation in *Candida albicans* septicaemia. *J. Pediatr.* **80**, 78.

Proceedings of an International Symposium held by Arnar-Stone Laboratories. Royal Society of Medicine, June 1976. Dopamine Hydrochloride. *Proc. Roy. Soc. Med.* **70**, (Suppl. 2) 1977.

Rodrigues, R. J. and Wolff, W. I. (1974). Fungal septicaemia in surgical patients. *Ann. Surg.* **180**, 741.

Salvin, S. R. (1952). Endotoxin in pathogenic fungi. *J. Immunol.* **69**, 89.

Schacter, L. P., Owellen, R. J., Rathbun, H. K. and Buchanan, B. (1976). Antagonism between Miconazole and Amphotericin B. *Lancet* **2**, 318.

Seneca, H. and Grant, J. P. Jr. (1976). 'Chemotherapy in Antibiotics and Chemotherapy' (Ed. Garrod, L. P., Seneca, H., Jawetz, E. and Fereres, J.) Vol. 21, 77. Karger, Basel.

Siegel, J. H., Greenspan, M. and Delguercio, L. R. (1967). Abnormal vascular tone, defective oxygen transport and myocardial failure in human septic shock. *Ann. Surg.* **165**, 504.

Symoens, J. (1977). Clinical and experimental evidence on Miconazole for the treatment of systemic micoses: a review. *Proc. Roy. Soc. Med.* **70** (Suppl. 1), 4.

Talley, R. C., Goldberg, L. I., Johnson, C. E. and McNay, J. L. (1969). A haemodynamic comparison of dopamine and isoproterenol in patients in shock. *Circulation* **39**, 361.

Thal, A. P. and Sardesai, V. M. (1965). Shock and the circulating polypeptides. *Amer. J. Surg.* **110**, 308.

Utz, J. P. (1976). Chemotherapy for the systemic mycores. *Brit. J. Hosp. Med.* **15**, 112.

Weil, M. H., Shubin, H. and Biddle, M. (1964). Shock caused by gram-negative micro-organisms. Analysis of 169 cases. *Ann. Intern. Med.* **60**, 384.

Weil, M. H., Shubin, H. and Nishijima, H. (1974). Corticosteroid therapy in circulatory shock. *Internat. Surg.* **59**, 589.

Wilson, R. F., Chiscano, A. D., Quadros, E. and Tarver, M. (1967). Some observations on 132 patients with septic shock. *Anesth. Analg.* **46**, 751.

Wilson, R. F., Sarver, E. J. and Rizzo, J. (1971). Haemodynamic changes, treatment and prognosis in clinical shock. *Archs. Surg.* **102**, 21.

Wright, C. J., McLean, A. P. H., MacLean, L. D. (1971). Regional capillary blood flow and oxygen uptake in severe sepsis. *Surg. Gynec. and Obstet.* **132**, 637.

III

The Management of Specific Injuries

Section 1: Introduction to Trauma

G. W. ODLING-SMEE

INTRODUCTION

Trauma is dynamic transfer of energy to living tissue, which is in a lower energy state, either directly or through a secondary medium. This results in disruption of morphological structure, with a corresponding alteration in function of the cells and eventually of the whole body. The host system responds to this by the classical inflammatory reaction. So that when trauma has occurred there is a zone of tissue disruption, surrounded by a zone of intact cells which are not functioning (cellular shock) and surrounded by a third zone of reactive hyperaemia with outpouring of extracellular fluid and blood. As a result, cellular and humoral mechanisms bring to the site of injury agents for removing cell debris, rendering innocuous toxic metabolites liberated from the cells and dealing with bacteria introduced. Radiation injury is slightly different, in that no gross injury pattern is observable, but the effect may be on the chromosomes, and may be detected in the descendants of the cells injured. Snakebite is an example of localised injury spreading to adjoining areas until the whole body is affected.

383

Trauma and healing should be thought of as one continuous dynamic process. Following the transfer of energy there is a propagation of the energy wave over adjacent tissue. As the cells in the zone of cellular shock recover, dead cells in the central zone act as the stimulus for the inflammatory reaction. The contraction and retraction of the blood vessels may be thought of as the first stage in healing.

INJURIES CAUSED BY DIRECT CONTACT

These injuries are the type commonly seen in accident departments in hospitals. They include road traffic injuries, industrial injuries, and gunshot and bomb blast wounds. Wounds inflicted by the surgeon incising the skin should also be included in this category. The following factors are important:

(a) Time scale of contact. Wounds may be caused by a single contact, by repetitive contact or by sustained contact.

(b) Angle of contact. The damage sustained will depend on whether the blow is struck, end-on, angular, tangential or oblique, or whether the injury is an avulsion injury.

(c) The direction of the wound on the skin. This is related to (a) and (b) but is clearly important, as collagen deposition is exactly perpendicular to the direction of muscle pull (Narasimhan and Day, 1975).

BLAST INJURIES

Following an explosion, a wave of compression hits the body and may penetrate its orifices. The various constituent anatomical parts are compressed to differing degrees, depending on the elasticity, resilience, compliance and tensile strength. These compression injuries are often first manifest on the brain, because it is suspended by the falciform ligament in a fluid medium, and shear forces will act upon it. Also the neurones and brain cell bodies have different physical properties and these will result in a differential sliding of one on another, producing a temporary state of unconsciousness (concussion). Other injuries are rupture of the tympanum, rupture of hollow viscera caused by first compressing the viscera containing air, and then decompressing, causing the high pressure areas to perforate; and injuries to the lungs. There is a differential acceleration between the lungs and the thoracic wall and this will cause an 'explosion' of the alveoli, and extensive interstitial haemorrhage. Blast injury may also cause air and fat emboli.

SOUND AND ULTRASOUND INJURY

Pain is felt at 140 decibels, and noise above this level has a blocking effect on neuronal transmission in the auditory nerve. Ultrasound has the same effect, and has been used to cause a general neuronal blockage similar to general anaesthesia. Epiphyseal plate cells can be disrupted.

THERMAL INJURY

(a) *Heat*. Following a burn there is local denaturing of proteins and varying degrees of wider involvement; neuronal and hormonal systems, especially the hypothalamic and adrenal systems, may be involved. Vasodilatory and circulating amines (the kinins etc.) contribute to the overall picture. Burn injuries are described in greater detail in Section 7, p. 443.

(b) *Cold*. There is widespread necrosis of cells, and concomitant vasoconstriction resulting in ischaemia and tissue anoxia. Crystals of ice may form in the cells and alter the osmotic relationships. This may be the cause of cell death.

(c) *Electrical*. The damage sustained may be related to the direction of the current, a current passing from head to toe causing much more damage than that passing from one arm to another, because the medulla is not involved. Electrical and lightning injuries are described in greater detail in Section 8, p. 467.

RADIATION INJURY

Ionising radiation produces slow damage to tissue. The injury is the same whether caused by X-rays or beta or gamma rays. The first week sees an erythema followed by a vasoconstriction, and in the sixth week necrosis begins to occur. There is a release of metabolites, and an increase in capillary permeability. There is an early loss of D.N.A. and lipid from cardiac cells, and later a decrease in actinomyosin and potassium concentrations.

REFERENCES

Narasimhan, M. J. and Day, S. B. (1975). Biological perspectives of some trauma injuries. *In* Trauma (Ed. S. B. Day). Plenum, London and New York.

Section 2: The Management of Chest Injuries

D. L. Coppel

The majority of chest injuries occur as a result of road traffic accidents but in some communities injuries from bullets, knife stabbings or bomb explosions may be just as common. Other causes include industrial, domestic and agricultural accidents.

Major injury to the chest may produce instability of the thoracic cage and contusion of the lungs. This reduces pulmonary ventilation leading to hypoxia and hypercarbia, with resulting acidosis, atelectasis, pulmonary oedema and pneumonia. All these factors inter-relate and can lead to death if treatment is not prompt and effective.

TREATMENT

Emergency treatment

The initial management of patients with chest injuries differs very little from general principles described by Jones (1966) and Ballinger *et al.* (1968) and now universally adopted for any severely injured patient. The immediate priority is to establish a clear unobstructed airway. Respiratory obstruction may have resulted from direct injury, bleeding or aspiration of vomit.

An intravenous catheter is inserted for the administration of colloid or crystalloid fluids, blood and drugs. A catheter should be placed into the superior vena cava to measure central venous pressure (C.V.P.) and act as a guide to fluid replacement and enable cardiac tamponade to be detected rapidly. Arterial blood should be drawn for gas analysis, electrolyte, haemoglobin and urea estimations, as well as for grouping and cross matching. Serum amylase estimations may be indicated in the presence of seat belt injuries to detect damage to the pancreas.

Inspection of the chest wall, front and back, will reveal an open or sucking wound. If present, this can be temporarily occluded with a large gauze dressing, as exposure of a previously normal lung to the atmosphere will result in collapse and shift of the mediastinum to the uninvolved side. The patient may have clinical signs of a pneumothorax or a haemothorax and, provided the patient is not unduly distressed, chest X-rays should be taken to confirm this. In crushing injuries, lateral views of the spine should also be taken to exclude fractures.

Chest drains can be inserted under local or general anaesthesia by placing the catheters on the affected side or sides, one just above the diaphragm in the mid-axillary line and the second anteriorly in the 2nd intercostal space (Cohn, 1972). The amount of blood or air which escapes into the underwater seal must be measured accurately using a graduated bottle and a Wrights Spirometer, since excessive loss may be an indication for thoracotomy. If the lung fails to expand, even with the free escape of air, low pressure suction (3 to 5 cm water) should be used. Massive leakage of air usually indicates injury to the trachea, large bronchi or massive lung lacerations. Persistent haemorrhage from an intercostal or internal mammary artery may continue but bleeding from the lung itself, although initially profuse, usually stops within a few minutes.

The presence of shock in patients with thoracic injury indicates haemorrhage or cardiac tamponade or may be secondary to respiratory distress, pain or other factors.

Further treatment of the patient with chest injuries depends not only on other associated injuries including head, abdominal, spine or fractures of long bones but also on any pre-existing disease (chronic bronchitis, emphysema and asthma), or a history of heavy smoking, particularly in obese or elderly patients.

Abdominal injuries are often difficult to diagnose accurately because of guarding and tenderness associated with fractures of the lower ribs. The absence of haemorrhage from the intercostal drains with hypotension, tachycardia, oliguria and a low central venous pressure (C.V.P.) should make one suspicious. Four quadrant peritoneal tap and lavage is helpful if the diagnosis is uncertain.

Many believe that prophylactic measures are important in preventing patients with injuries of the chest from developing frank respiratory failure (Roscher et al., 1974). These include adequate analgesia without inducing respiratory depression or obtunding the cough reflex, provision of effective humidification and chest physiotherapy, and treatment and maintenance of acid base balance blood gases, electrolyte and nutritional status. Indeed, if these measures are unduly delayed treatment becomes extremely difficult and prolonged and the outcome unsuccessful (Sankaran and Wilson, 1970).

Patients usually fall into two groups – those who can be treated without artificial ventilation (conservative treatment) and those for whom ventilation is essential.

Conservative treatment (Treatment without artificial ventilation)

Despite its terminology this requires skilled nursing and frequent reviews of progress and is often more demanding on staff and patients than more aggressive treatment. The principles involved are listed in Table 1; some of these will be discussed in detail.

Table 1. Conservative treatment

1. Analgesia
2. Warm humidified oxygen
3. Tracheo-bronchial suction
4. Chest drains
5. Rehydration
6. Blood gas analysis, electrolyte and acid base estimations
7. Antibiotic therapy

Conservative treatment is suitable when the injuries are of a minor nature but, because of severe pain, the patient is unable to cough and clear the secretions from the tracheobronchial tree. This may result in atelectasis and infection, producing hypoxia and hypercarbia. It must be remembered that there is reflex increase in bronchial secretions (mediated through the vagus nerve) secondary to trauma, and this may overwhelm the patient.

Conservative treatment is usually only required for 3 to 4 days and can really only be successful in patients without extensive injuries. The nature of the injuries and the form of treatment should be explained to the patient in order to obtain maximum co-operation. Progress can be monitored by blood gas, electrolyte and acid base analyses. Antibiotics (such as ampicillin) are given initially to all patients and then modified according to culture and sensitivity. This procedure seems to modify an infection which is almost impossible to prevent.

Franz *et al.* (1974) suggests that artificial ventilation can be avoided in severe lung contusion by the use of pharmacological doses of methylprednisolone in association with fluid restriction, diuretics, albumin, tracheobronchial suction and intercostal nerve blocks. The mechanism of protection is thought to be lysosome preservation, decreasing capillary permeability and acute inflammatory response.

Analgesia

It may not be possible to achieve adequate analgesia with conventional dosages of parenteral narcotics (e.g. 10 mg morphine 4 hourly) without causing respiratory insufficiency. Intravenous lignocaine is often effective in providing pain relief without depression of consciousness, respiration or cough reflex. Close observation is required to detect the onset of convulsions, should infusion be too rapid, and the adult dosage should be restricted to a maximum of 100 mg in 1 h. It can be used successfully in association with low doses of narcotics (5 mg morphine or 50 mg pethidine intravenously 4 hourly) and regulated to provide optimum pain relief to coincide with physiotherapy.

Inhalational analgesia using premixed nitrous oxide in oxygen (Entonox) or low concentrations of methoxyflurane or trichlorethylene can often relieve pain and at the same time retain the patient's co-operation. Unfortunately their prolonged inhalation is not without danger.

Regional analgesia is valuable when the chest wall is stable and pulmonary damage is small. Intercostal nerve blocks provide adequate pain relief in ribs fractured from 1st to 5th ribs. Bupivacaine (0.25%) with 1:400 000 adrenaline will often be effective for up to 8 hours. Thoracic extradural analgesia has its advocates, because consciousness is retained, pain relief is consistent and coughing is not troublesome. It can be employed with fractures below the fifth ribs. The tip of the catheter is placed in the mid zone of the affected segment.

This form of analgesia is seldom required after 7 days (Gibbons et al., 1973b). If there are multiple fractures or suspected hypovolaemia extradural thoracic analgesia is probably unsuitable as severe hypotension may result (Collie and Lloyd, 1967).

Oxygenation

Oxygen is delivered to the patient from a cascade type humidifier (e.g. Puritan) in amounts sufficient to maintain the PaO_2 within the normal range. The mist should be warmed, since cold reflexly increases airway resistance. In addition to maintaining an airway, tracheal intubation may be required to facilitate removal of tenacious secretions, to perform bronchial lavage or re-expand atelectatic areas. If required more than twice in 24 hours tracheostomy should be considered (Gibbons et al., 1973a).

Artificial ventilation

This is indicated in patients with extensive lung damage, some pre-existing disease or associated injury, or in those that deteriorate with conservative treatment.

The technique for controlling the open chest during thoracotomy was extended to patients with severe chest injuries by Jensen in 1952. This concept of 'internal pneumatic stabilisation' (Avery et al., 1956) now known as intermittent positive pressure ventilation (I.P.P.V.) has now largely replaced all other methods of controlling paradoxical respiration and ensuring adequate ventilation and oxygenation in patients with severe chest trauma (Grimes, 1972). It is well documented by Bendexin et al., 1965 and Sykes et al., 1969.

Some idea of the frequency of its application is shown by the fact that 70% of 164 patients with severe chest injuries who were admitted to the author's intensive care unit required I.P.P.V. for an average of 13 days. One half of these had associated injuries and the mortality was 23%. This is similar to the experience of Lloyd et al. (1965), James et al. (1974), Lewis et al. (1975).

Our indications for ventilation are summarised in Table 2. I.P.P.V. should be undertaken when the $PaCO_2$ is greater than 8 kPa or PaO_2 is less than 8 kPa when breathing 70% oxygen.

There is renewed support for operative stabilisation of the chest wall in the presence of paradoxical respiration (Moore, 1975) (Powers, 1975), in the belief that this will avoid I.P.P.V. and tracheostomy and reduce the number of days spent in hospital. This philosophy not only ignores the underlying lung pathology but also the fact that the vast proportion of patients also have associated head, abdominal or bony injuries. A few patients, however, with fractures of the sternum and ribs with minimal lung contusions are suitable for external fixation. Traction, however, often does not adequately control paradox and may lead to necrosis of bone and soft tissue and cause infection (Grimes, 1972).

OTHER CONCOMITANT INJURIES

Diaphragm

Rupture of the diaphragm is uncommon following blunt trauma and seldom accounts for more than two admissions to our unit each year.

Andrus and Morton (1970) reported only 32 cases in 3 different hospitals over approximately 40 years with half of these occurring in the last 10 years.

The common sites for rupture are in the posterior half of the left leaf and in the postero-central portion of the diaphragm. Chest X-ray may be required to demonstrate the hernia. The diagnosis may be delayed as associated injuries often require I.P.P.V., which prevents the abdominal contents from entering the thorax. Only on resumption of spontaneous respiration does the hernia appear. Persistent atelectasis of the left lower lobe should make one suspicious. An E.C.G. may also be helpful as herniation can occur into the pericardial cavity with evidence of pericarditis. The treatment is always surgical repair.

Table 2. Indications for ventilation

1. Abnormal blood gases
2. Paradoxical respiration
3. Tachypnoea
4. Exhaustion
5. Associated head and or abdominal injuries
6. Pre-existing diseases
7. Inability to cough, breathe deeply or co-operate

Oesophagus

Oesophageal injuries are rare following closed chest trauma but can occur following penetrating or perforating injuries. They may be hard to diagnose but the presence of fever, subcutaneous emphysema, mediastinitis and empyema are suggestive. Small tears may close spontaneously with expectant therapy but surgery is usually required. The prognosis is often poor.

Trachea and bronchus

Almost all patients with injury to the tracheo bronchial tree have a fracture involving the first 3 ribs (Paredes, 1975) in association with dyspnoea, haemoptysis, pneumothorax and increasing mediastinal or subcutaneous emphysema. General deterioration of the patient in the presence of a massive air leak with failure of the lung to re-expand despite suction and high concentrations of oxygen should alert one to this possibility. The diagnosis is usually confirmed by bronchoscopy and bronchography but thoracotomy may be required purely on clinical grounds even with a negative endoscopy. Damage may be (1) Complete rupture of the trachea or bronchus with division and separation. (2) Incomplete rupture with partial separation. (3) Complete rupture with communication with the diaphragm. Incomplete rupture can lead to a chronic fibrous stricture with retention of secretions, infection and lung destruction. The diagnosis may initially be missed but suspected if atelectasis occurs months after apparent recovery (Cohn, 1972).

Gun shot wounds
The mortality following bullet injuries to the chest and lungs depends not only on the velocity of the missile but also on the extent of associated injuries. The treatment of low velocity bullet injuries follows conventional lines with the placement of intercostal catheters to drain haemothoraces or pneumothoraces. Supportive therapy includes blood replacement, warm humidified oxygen, antibiotics, analgesia, tracheobronchial suction and chest physiotherapy. Unless there is some preexisting disease or associated injuries involving the head, abdomen or spinal cord, prolonged artificial ventilation is seldom required.

Thoracotomy is indicated if bleeding initially is more than 1500 ml or subsequently becomes greater than 500 ml/h in the presence of a massive air leak, with oesophageal or diaphragmatic injuries, external chest wall damage, metal fragments in the mediastinum, cardiac tamponade or mediastinal shift (Levinsky et al., 1975).

In contrast, direct pulmonary injury from high velocity missiles results in extensive destruction of the lung parenchyma, intra-bronchial bleeding and oedema. There is also a detrimental effect on function in the adjacent, or even the opposite, lung from the site of pulmonary damage due to energy dissipation. If thoracotomy is indicated the main battle for the patient's survival may take place after the operation (Wanebo and van Dyke, 1972). I.P.P.V. and positive end expiratory pressure (P.E.E.P.), in conjunction with steroids and diuretics, are often required to combat the extensive pulmonary oedema. Unfortunately, although the initial prognosis may appear promising, infection and pneumonia often occur and prove resistant to antibiotics.

Damage to heart and great vessels
As pointed out in the Editorial (1975) contusion of the myocardium occurs fairly commonly in blunt injuries to the chest and should be suspected in all crushing injuries, especially with fractures of the sternum. The E.C.G. should be routinely monitored for arrhythmias and changes in T waves and ST segment looked for, indicating myocardial infarction and ischaemia. Survival is extremely rare in the

presence of large wounds of the heart, aorta and pulmonary vessels, as the patient does not live long enough to reach hospital. However, recovery has been described by Goggin *et al.* (1970), in the presence of a slow haemorrhage. The diagnosis is often made by the presence of cardiac tamponade with a raised C.V.P., a low arterial blood pressure, a low pulse pressure and a 'quiet heart' on fluoroscopy. The injection of contrast material into the right atrium may also show a wide shadow between it and the pericardium. Aortic injury usually occurs at two main sites, the aortic root just above the aortic valve and just distal to the left subclavian artery (Love, 1975). Chest X-ray often shows widening of the mediastinal shadow and aortography should be performed.

Injury to the heart and great vessels following gun shot wounds is seldom seen in civilian practice because patients do not survive long enough, despite exceptionally rapid evacuation to hospital. Even in the theatre of war the incidence of survival has not changed much in 25 years being 3.3% in World War II and 2.8% in Vietnam (Gielchinsky and McNamara, 1970).

The diagnosis depends on a high index of suspicion with careful consideration of the trajectory and position of the missile. One must remember however that missiles can ricochet in amazing and un-suspected directions around the chest and abdomen. The patients show signs of cardiac tamponade, haemothorax, dyspnoea and E.C.G. evidence of myocardial injury. Immediate thoracotomy must be undertaken as the pericardium is often filled with large clots which would render pericardiocentesis ineffective. Adequate pericardial drainage, to protect against re-accumulation of blood and permit removal of metallic foreign bodies, is required. Drainage should not be too generous as the heart may herniate out through the pericardium with subsequent strangulation.

BLAST INJURIES OF THE LUNGS

Interest has recently been focused on the effects of bomb explosion on the lungs (McCaughey *et al.*, 1973). Individuals close to the scene of a bomb explosion may be killed immediately or survive only to develop respiratory failure. The majority however escape without any evidence of respiratory insufficiency although the force of the blast can be severe enough to cause loss of limbs.

The clinical effects depend on how high the pressure produced by the explosion rises above atmospheric pressure, on its duration and the

proximity of the patient to the source of detonation. If the pressure rise
slowly to a modest degree there is time for air to flow down through the
trachea and into the alveoli and thus keep pace with the pressure in the
environment. Under these circumstances damage to the lungs rarely
occurs. However, if there is an almost instantaneous rise in environmental pressure of relatively short duration there is no time for an

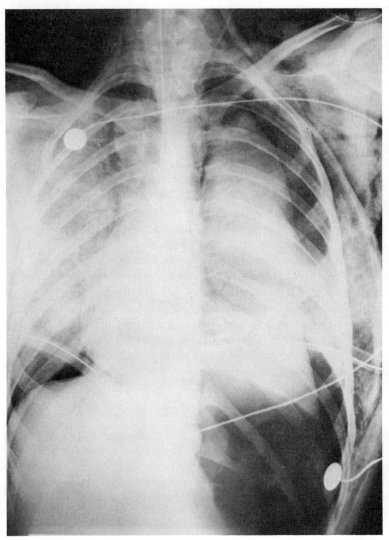

Fig. 1. Bilateral pneumothoraces immediately following bomb explosion.

qualising pressure to be transmitted through the trachea. Under such
ircumstances the direct impact of the blast wave against the body wall
auses severe compression of the chest and abdominal wall. The
liaphragm is thrust upwards and movement of fluid into the thorax
vith rupture of the alveoli and pulmonary vessels occurs with resulting
lveolar rupture, haemorrhage and oedema (White and Richmond,
960). This is referred to as the primary blast effect; lung damage may
lso occur due to missiles energised by blast over-pressure penetrating
he chest wall (secondary effect) and by the individual being thrown
gainst a solid object (tertiary effect).

R espiratory failure may occur immediately following an explosion or

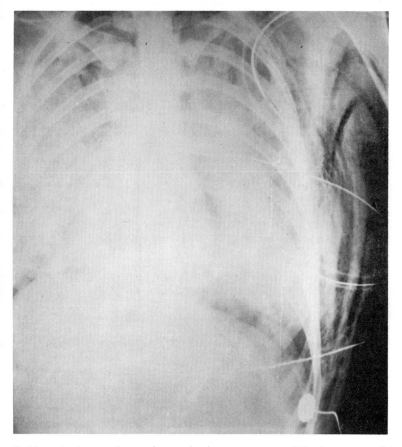

g. 2. Bilateral pulmonary haemorrhage and oedema now apparent following insertion of chest
rains.

be delayed for several days. Patients should be closely observed for 3 to 4 days for signs of respiratory distress. Classically the patient presents with rapid onset of dyspnoea, cyanosis and haemoptysis. Moist sounds may be present in both lung fields but this may not be readily detected i bilateral pneumothoraces are present. Figure 1 shows the chest X-ray o a patient admitted following a bomb explosion. Bilateral pneu mothoraces are present but with the insertion of chest drains and re expansion of the lungs widespread pulmonary haemorrhage and oedema are revealed (Fig. 2).

Treatment of the established condition consists of artificial ventila tion often with oxygen at an F_1O_2 of 1.0, the use of a positive end expiratory pressure (P.E.E.P.), diuretics, albumin and hydrocortisone 500 mg intravenously 4 hourly. The latter often produces dramatic improvement and should be continued for at least two weeks if fata deterioration is to be avoided.

REFERENCES

Andrus, C. H. and Morton, J. H. (1970). Rupture of the diaphragm after blunt trauma Amer. J. Surg. **119**, 686.

Avery, E. E., Morch, E. T. and Benson, D. W. (1956). Critically crushed chests. J Thorac. Surg. **32**, 291.

Ballinger, W. F., Rutherford, R. B., and Zuidema, G. D. (1968). 'The Management o Trauma'. W. B. Saunders.

Bendixen, H. H., Egbert, L. D., Hedley-Whyte, J., Laver, M. B. and Pontoppidan, H (1965). 'Respiratory Care'. C. W. Mosby, St. Louis.

Cohn, R. (1972). Nonpenetrating wounds of the lungs and bronchi. Surg. Clin. N. Amer **52**, 585.

Collie, J. A. and Lloyd, J. W. (1967). Practical points in the treatment of chest injuries Anaesthesiology **22**, 392.

Editorial (1975). Cardiac contusion. Brit. Med. J. **4**, 606.

Franz, J. L., Richardson, J. D., Grover, F. L. and Trinkle, J. K. (1974). Effect o methylprednisolone sodium succinate on experimental pulmonary contusion. J Thorac. Cardiovasc. Surg. **68**, 842.

Gibbons, J., James, O. and Quail, A. (1973a). Management of 130 cases of chest injur with respiratory failure. Brit. J. Anaesth. **45**, 1130.

Gibbons, J., James, O. and Quail, A. (1973b). Relief of pain in chest injury. Brit. J Anaesth. **45**, 1136.

Gielchinsky, I. and McNamara, J. J. (1970). Cardiac wounds at a military evacuatio hospital in Vietnam. J. Thorac. Cardiovasc. Surg. **4**, 603.

Goggin, M. J., Thompson, F. D. and Jackson, J. W. (1970). Deceleration trauma to th heart and great vessels after road traffic accidents. Brit. Med. J. **2**, 767.

Grimes, O. F. (1972). Nonpenetrating injuries to the chest wall and esophagus. Surg Clin. N. Amer. **52**, 597.

James, O., Gibbons, J. and Bissitt, R. (1974). The management of respiratory failur due to combined chest and abdominal injuries. Aust. N.Z. J. Surg. **44**, 277.

Jensen, H. K. (1952). Recovery of pulmonary function after crushing injuries of the chest. *J. Dis. Chest* **22**, 319.

Jones, R. C. (1966). Initial care of the injured patient. *In* 'Care of the Trauma Patient' (Ed. G. T. Shires), p. 187. McGraw-Hill, New York.

Levinsky, L., Vidne, B. Nudelman, I., Salomon, J., Kissin, L. and Levy, M. J. (1975). Thoracic injuries in the Yom Kippur war, experience in a base hospital. *Israel. J. Med. Sci.* **11**, 275.

Lewis, F., Thomas, A. N. and Scholomohm, R. M. (1975). Control of respiratory therapy in flail chest. *Ann. Thorac. Surg.* **20**, 170.

Lloyd, J. W., Smith, A. C. and O'Connor, B. T. (1965). Classification of chest injuries as an aid to treatment. *Brit. Med. J.* **1**, 1518.

Love, J. M. (1975). Chest injuries, *J.A.M.A.* **232**, 385.

McCaughey, W., Coppel, D. L. and Dundee, J. W. (1973). Blast injuries to the lungs. *Anaesthesiology* **28**, 2.

Moore, B. P. (1975). Operative stabilization of nonpenetrating chest injuries. *J. Thorac. Cardiovasc. Surg.* **70**, 619.

Paredes, S. and Hipoma, P. A. (1975). The radiologic evaluation of patients with chest trauma. *Surg. Clin. N. Amer.* **59**, 37.

Powers, J. R. (1975). Management of flail chest. Editorial. *Ann. Thorac. Surg.* **19**, 480.

Roscher, R., Bittner, R. and Stockmann, U. (1974). Pulmonary contusion. *Archs. Surg.* **109**, 508.

Sankaran, S. and Wilson, R. F. (1970). Factors affecting prognosis in patients with flail chest. *J. Thorac. Cardiovasc. Surg.* **60**, 402.

Sykes, M. K., McNichol, M. W. and Campbell, E. J. M. (1969). *In* 'Respiratory Failure' (Ed. M. K. Sykes). Blackwell Scientific Publications, Oxford.

Wanebo, H. and van Dyke, J. (1972). The high velocity pulmonary injury. *J. Thorac. Cardiovasc. Surg.* **64**, 537.

White, C. S. and Richmond, D. R. (1960). Blast biology. *In* 'Clinical Cardiopulmonary Physiology' (Ed. B. L. Gordon). Second Edition. Grune and Stratton, New York.

Section 3: The Management of Head Injuries

D. S. GORDON

INTRODUCTION

In Britain over 100 000 patients are admitted to hospital each year for treatment of head injuries (Lewin, 1967). In some patients a sharp blow causes a depressed fracture of the skull with damage confined to the site of impact. These patients are usually conscious and the only treatment needed is elevation of the depressed fragments. However, a blunt deceleration or acceleration injury is more common in both industrial and road traffic accidents. It causes a closed head injury with diffuse brain damage and the problems of prolonged unconsciousness which often require critical care. In the 1970s a third category of wound has emerged in civilian life – the missile wound of the head; it combines the surgical features of a depressed fracture of the skull with those of widespread brain damage. The compulsory use of crash helmets has decreased the incidence of compound skull fractures, but the expansion of road traffic has led to an increase in closed head injuries, an increase not only in number but in severity. This chapter is concerned with the altered state and the management of the diffusely injured brain.

PATHOLOGY

Primary pathology

The force of a blunt head injury causes momentary deformation of the brain which accounts for the multiple areas of brain damage described by Strich (1961). The radial pressure wave from a bullet traversing the brain creates a transient cavity and causes damage remote from the

398

missile track. Severe and often progressive cerebral oedema character-
ises both types of injury. In addition to the structural damage from
severe brain injury, experimental studies demonstrate an immediate
rise in intracranial pressure, probably the result of vasomotor paralysis
and passive dilatation of cerebral blood vessels.

Secondary pathology

Many patients who survive the impact progressively deteriorate
because of unfavourable conditions in the brain. Tissue acidosis causes
further vasodilatation and cerebral oedema develops. Impaired pulmonary function from bronchial hypersecretion and the aspiration of
blood and gastric contents leads to hypoxia and hypercapnia. Lassen
(1966) suggested that the cerebral vasodilatation caused by hypercapnia encourages shunting of blood from the areas of greatest damage
to relatively intact areas of the brain. This has the twin effect of raising
the intracranial pressure and decreasing perfusion through the damaged tissue. Ischaemia gives rise to further cerebral oedema. Cerebral
blood flow is largely determined by cerebral perfusion pressure
(C.P.P.). C.P.P. is the difference between the mean arterial blood
pressure (M.A.B.P.) and intracranial pressure (I.C.P.), i.e.
M.A.B.P. − I.C.P. = C.P.P. Cerebral blood flow is therefore compromised as I.C.P. rises towards M.A.B.P. (Zwetnow, 1975). Cushing
(1902) described a compensatory rise in blood pressure in response to
rising I.C.P. Unfortunately an abrupt episode of arterial hypertension
can be harmful when there is cerebral vasodilatation; it promotes a
rapid transudation of water and serum protein across the blood-brain
barrier. Shalit and Cotev (1975) believe that this exacerbation of
cerebral oedema actually reduces cerebral blood flow. On the other
hand arterial hypotension, by reducing C.P.P., also reduces cerebral
blood flow. In a patient with cerebral oedema irreparable brain
damage may result. Byrnes et al. (1974) reported that after missile
wounds of the head the prognosis was poor when the systolic blood
pressure was under 90 mm Hg or over 150 mm Hg.

Changes in brain volume brought about by vasodilatation or oedema
can for a time be compensated by reciprocal change in the volume of
intracranial blood vessels and cerebrospinal fluid (Langfitt, 1968).
Unfortunately this compensatory mechanism soon becomes exhausted.
Increasing I.C.P. collapses draining cerebral veins running to the dural
venous sinuses. Back pressure builds up in the capillary bed of the brain.
Under these circumstances cerebral vessels dilate causing further

increase in I.C.P. and the promotion of a vicious circle in which oedema becomes intensified. A sudden rise in central venous pressure can follow minor airway obstruction or even induction of anaesthesia (Tomlinson, 1964). It leads to further increase in I.C.P. and, if cerebral swelling progresses, death occurs from 'coning' at the tentorial opening or at the foramen magnum.

PATIENT MANAGEMENT

The causes of death in head injured patients are:

1. Overwhelming brain damage.
2. Shock, usually from other injuries.
3. Respiratory complications.
4. Progressive brain swelling.

The last three, which contribute to the secondary brain pathology, can be influenced by prompt treatment. The aims of treatment are:

1. To maintain adequate cerebral perfusion by limiting cerebral oedema and maintaining the blood pressure.
2. To improve lung function thus ensuring satisfactory PaO_2 and $PaCO_2$ levels and a normal central venous pressure. According to Wilson (1967) 25% of deaths from head injury result from respiratory obstruction.

Early resuscitation

Hospital critical care, even if it starts within half an hour of injury, may be futile if anoxic brain damage has already taken place. Easton (1968) has shown that general practitioner teams can often institute airway care before the ambulance reaches the scene of the injury. Apart from those areas which operate a flying squad, ambulance treatment is usually limited to the insertion of a pharyngeal airway, placing the patient semiprone and giving oxygen enriched air. Unconscious patients being transported from one hospital to another for critical care should have preliminary tracheal intubation, often supplemented by controlled ventilation under the supervision of an accompanying doctor.

Hospital treatment

The management of severely injured patients is most easily carried out in a central accident unit preferably in a general hospital with thoracic,

orthopaedic, maxillo-facial, plastic and neurological surgical departments. Local circumstances often dictate the details of treatment; a
close grouping of resuscitation room, intensive therapy and neurosurgical units makes for efficient early management. Surgical responsibility should be clearly vested in one surgeon who co-ordinates the
treatment of concomitant injuries and of surgical complications.

Resuscitation procedure

A radio message from the ambulance warns the casualty department to
expect a severe head injury. Often treatment can start within 15 min of
injury (Byrnes *et al.*, 1974). Ideally a very severely injured patient is
received by a team of three doctors: one, usually a surgical registrar or
consultant, to examine, record management and plan surgical treatment; another to start at least two intravenous drips, and the third,
preferably an anaesthetist, takes control of the patient's airway, which
is usually the most urgent measure required.

Clinical examination
In a brief initial examination the extent of the wounds, the level of
consciousness and the adequacy of respiratory function are assessed.
The state of the pupils and any asymmetry of limb function are
recorded. Denny-Brown and Russell (1941) described the paralysis of
pharyngeal and laryngeal muscles which permits inhalation of vomitus
and secretions and blood from the pharynx. The high incidence of early
pulmonary complications accounts for the very unstable neurological
state of many head injured patients, especially those with gunshot
wounds who often vomit.

Transfusion
A low blood pressure is so uncommon in patients with closed head
injuries that it should prompt a search for other injuries. As cerebral
metabolism depends on an adequate C.P.P. and a normal oxygen
carrying capacity of the blood, immediate correction of hypovolaemic
shock is essential. Scalp haemorrhage seldom leads to dangerous blood
loss; but bleeding from the sagittal or transverse sinus can require rapid
transfusion. Arterial blood pressure and central venous pressure
estimations act as a guide to the volume and rapidity of the transfusion.

Airway control
Many patients with only moderate primary brain damage develop
airway obstruction and deteriorate rapidly from the secondary

pathology associated with hypoxia and hypercapnia. Crockard *et al.* (1973) and Byrnes *et al.* (1974) demonstrated in cerebral missile wounds that relief of stertorous breathing and airway obstruction during resuscitation could lead to rapid reduction in intracranial pressure. Most patients who are unconscious should have tracheal intubation (Plewes, 1967). A cuffed endotracheal tube allows tracheal toilet and the administration of humidified oxygen; it almost eliminates the risk of inhalation of gastric contents and pharyngeal blood. When the patient with respiratory difficulty is sufficiently conscious to resent intubation, the anaesthetist may have to use muscle relaxants followed by controlled ventilation. Under such circumstances pancuronium bromide 4 mg is given intravenously and the patient maintained on the ventilator with pancuronium bromide and occasional doses of diazepam 5–10 mg intravenously. The $PaCO_2$ is maintained within the range of 3.3 kPa (25 mm Hg) and 4.0 kPa (30 mm Hg). Levels of $PaCO_2$ less than 2.6 kPa (20 mm Hg) may produce deterioration in cerebral function, most probably secondary to cerebral vasoconstriction. The PaO_2 is initially maintained at around 20 kPa (150 mm Hg) and subsequently reduced to 10.7 kPa (80 mm Hg) to 13.3 kPa (100 mm Hg) after 48 hours artificial ventilation. The early use of controlled ventilation improves alveolar function and corrects hypoxia and hypercapnia. It prevents the sudden and sometimes catastrophic rise in I.C.P. from a bout of coughing. By abolishing abdominal muscle tone it reduces the central venous pressure which in turn reduces I.C.P. Patients with missile wounds benefit from a short period of hyperventilation before operation. Jennett *et al.* (1969) emphasises the importance of avoiding volatile anaesthetic agents which tend to increase I.C.P. through cerebrovasodilation.

Other resuscitation room measures
Rovit and Hagan (1968) found that steroids given to experimental animals before injury seemed to limit the spread of cerebral oedema. In missile wounds steroids given soon after injury probably help reduce intracranial pressure by their action on cell membranes in undamaged brain. Their value in diffuse brain damage is questionable, especially if treatment is delayed. Steroids are generally given for closed head injuries although their value is unproven. An initial dose of dexamethazone (Decadron M.S.D.) 12 mg intravenously is followed by 4 mg 6 hourly by the intramuscular route. A nasogastric tube allows aspiration of gastric contents and the administration of an alkaline solution to reduce the risk of gastric ulceration. If antibiotics are

considered necessary for an open head wound they can be given now along with Tetanus Toxoid. 250 mg ampicillin and 250 mg flucloxacillin (Magnapen) is generally given 6 hourly intramuscularly.

X-rays

The patient should be moved to an X-ray department only when resuscitation is complete. However an early portable X-ray of the chest is a valuable addition to clinical examination in detecting pneumothorax which requires immediate attention. X-rays of the skull are followed by X-rays of the cervical and thoracic spine.

Early prognosis

The decision on further management is made after adequate transfusion and respiratory care (Crockard *et al.*, 1973). If the patient recovers sufficiently to reject his endotracheal tube he can go to the admitting ward or the intensive nursing area of the neurosurgical ward for further observation. Patients with open wounds proceed to the operating theatre. If the neurological signs suggest the presence of an intracranial haematoma it must be sought by burr holes, angiography or computerised tomographic scan (C.T. Scan), depending on the facilities available and the urgency of the case. The C.T. Scan (or E.M.I. scan) provides the most accurate localisation of extradural, subdural or intracerebral haematomata and should be used in all patients suspected to be suffering from an intracranial bleed.

Brown (1971) found that persisting fixed pupils in a patient with decerebrate rigidity carries a hopeless prognosis. Gordon and Crockard (1974) reached the same conclusion in patients with missile injuries.

Critical care in an intensive therapy unit is reserved for a group of patients who are unconscious and require continuous supervision of pulmonary function by anaesthetists. Children and young adults respond best to this system.

Intensive therapy unit

The procedures followed in the intensive therapy unit are a continuation of those started in the resuscitation room – maintenance of lung function and control of cerebral oedema. The most important clinical observations are the level of consciousness, the state of the pupils and the function of the limbs. Most patients admitted for intensive therapy will not be sufficiently conscious to obey commands. However, changes in the level of consciousness can be detected by repeated observations of

Table 1. Chart used by the Institute of Neurological Sciences, Glasgow for sequential observation of the patient with head injury. (Reproduced by kind permission of Teasdale and Galbraith, 1975)

SGH 172

NAME

RECORD No.

		DATE																			
		TIME																				
C	Eyes open	Spontaneously																				
O		To speech																				
M		To pain	Eyes closed by swelling = C																			
		None																				
A	Best verbal response	Orientated																				
S		Confused																				
		Inappropriate Words	Endotracheal tube or tracheostomy = T																			
		Incomprehensible Sounds																				
C		None																				
A	Best motor response	Obey commands																				
L		Localise pain	Usually record the best arm response																			
E		Flexion to pain																				
		Extension to pain																				
		None																				

240
230
220
210
200
190
180
170

40
39
38
37
36 Temperature
35 ° C
34

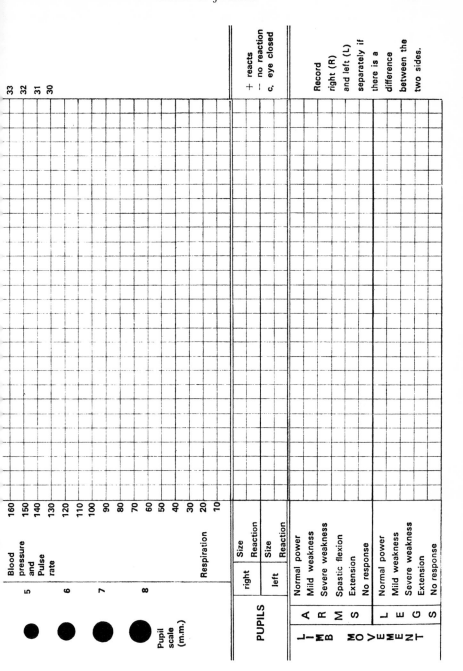

reaction to noise, reaction to visual menace and the patient's response to painful stimuli. On examination of the limbs assessment should be made as to whether there are spontaneous purposeful movements or spontaneous purposeless movements. The reaction to painful stimuli will vary from a purposeful pushing away of the stimulus to a withdrawal from the stimulus or a purposeless generalised extensor reaction. The actual posture of the limbs is a further guide. The limbs may be relaxed or they may be spastic with the arms flexed (decorticate state) or with arms and legs extended (the so called decerebrate state).

The pupils are often small with sluggish reactions. Bilateral changes in pupil size especially in children are not necessarily significant but a record of the pupil size carefully noting asymmetry is important. Increasing size of one pupil may be the earliest indication of an intracranial haematoma.

Increasing blood pressure and decreasing pulse rate are frequently found with intracranial haematomas and are often among the earliest signs to appear.

A chart embracing all these observations, which enables requested observations to be made in an orderly fashion and charted in such a way that is easily seen has been described by Teasdale and Jennett (1974); see Table 1.

In a centre with a neurosurgical department, information on the patient's progress and prognosis can be obtained from intracranial pressure recording (Hulme *et al.*, 1971) and C.S.F. lactate estimations (Crockard *et al.*, 1973). The advantages of intracranial pressure monitoring are:

1. It is a guide to variations in I.C.P. and therefore may provide the earliest evidence of a developing haematoma.
2. It acts as a guide to the effectiveness of therapy, for example a falling pressure with hyperventilation, mannitol or steroids.
3. It provides a guide to prognosis as noted by Troupp (1974).

The disadvantages include a small risk of infection and lack of reliability in any of the present methods. Obstruction of the catheter in the lateral ventricle may give false readings, likewise many of the indwelling transducers are affected by temperature and require frequent calibration.

Intracranial pressure change is detected by a sensor on the dura mater or in the lateral ventricle; a transducer converts the pressure change to an electrical impulse which is converted to a readable output on a chart recorder.

Our preference is for the Richmond screw. This is easily inserted even in a dressing room. It is not suitable for the very thin skull of a small child but it gives satisfactory results in most patients and even if the surrounding tissues become infected, this is not likely to be serious. Cerebral perfusion pressure (M.A.B.P. – I.C.P.) can now be calculated. A perfusion pressure of greater than 30 mm Hg is essential to prevent hypoxia, tissue acidosis and increasing cerebral oedema. Troupp (1974) found that, in the absence of a haematoma, an intracranial pressure greater than 60 mm Hg had a bad prognosis.

Research is at present being undertaken in the assessment of brain compliance by fluid challenge. A small volume, for example 1 ml of saline is injected; usually this will not increase the I.C.P. If, however, I.C.P. is raised a point is reached at which a small injection will give a very striking rise (a state of low compliance). The test is not altogether safe. However, recent experience with injections via a Richmond screw have been encouraging.

Patients with a C.S.F. lactate level greater than 5.5 mmol/l (55 mg/100 ml) on admission all died (Crockard et al., 1973), but those with levels below 2.8 mmol/l (25 mg/100 ml) survived. This information is helpful in determining the benefit to be expected from critical care.

The supportive treatment started on admission may be supplemented by the following.

Hypertonic solutions

Urea has now been supplanted by mannitol. Mannitol, having a greater molecular size, does not so readily penetrate the blood-brain barrier. It has a rapid effect on areas of undamaged brain but probably little or no effect where the blood-brain barrier is impaired (Pappius, 1967). When the intracranial pressure is rising mannitol can be given as a 20% solution, 1.5 gm/kg body weight infused in less than 15 min. Its effect lasts only 3–4 h. As it can lead to marked dehydration, careful control of osmolality is important. The 'rebound' effect seldom occurs with mannitol; it can be prevented by limiting the fluid infusion to about one-third of that lost by diuresis (Shapiro, 1975).

Hypothermia

Rosomoff et al. (1960) found that hypothermia started before experimental head injury, helped to limit brain swelling. Hypothermia now tends to be used simply to combat hyperthermia. Yet a treatment which reduces oxygen requirement may provide some protection for hypoxic brain cells when the adequacy of cerebral perfusion is in doubt.

Intravenous fluids

Hooper (1969) considers that patients with severe head injuries tend to retain water in the first 24 h unless hypertonic solutions are given. A suitable supply for the first day is 1500 ml of 5% glucose. On the second day gastric tube feeding can usually start.

Barbiturates

Smith *et al.* (1974) suggest that barbiturates protect the brain from the effects of hypoxia. Shapiro *et al.* (1974) are investigating the use of barbiturates in conjunction with hypothermia in the management of intracranial hypertension.

Respiratory care

Patients who breathe adequately after resuscitation and maintain normal blood gas tensions are given humidified oxygen-enriched air and have routine tracheal care. Brown (1971) described a state of shallow hyperventilation in which hypocapnia is often accompanied by hypoxia. Hypoxia is aggravated by the oxygen demands of rapid respiration and muscle hypertonus. Hypercapnia accompanies hypoxia when aspirated secretions or vomitus block small air passages in the lung. Cerebral oedema is then intensified. If the PaO_2 remains under 9.3 kPa (70 mm Hg), especially when the intracranial pressure is over 30 mm Hg, controlled ventilation must be considered. Furness (1957) showed that reduction of $PaCO_2$ by hyperventilation reduced the brain volume during neurosurgical operations. Lundberg *et al.* (1959) applied controlled ventilation to the treatment of raised I.C.P. in head injury. Alexander and Lassen (1970) advocated the deliberate reduction of $PaCO_2$ in head injuries, hoping that the resulting vasoconstriction in relatively unaffected areas of the brain would reduce brain volume and I.C.P. with restoration of adequate perfusion in hypoxic areas.

The chief benefits from 'respirator therapy' are:

1. Reduction of oxygen demand and reversal of cerebral metabolic acidosis (Gordon and Rossando, 1968) by preventing stertorous breathing and coughing.
2. Reduction of intracranial pressure by reducing impedance of cerebral venous drainage.
3. Maintenance of high oxygen tension in the blood for the first 48 h.

4. Reduction of cerebral blood volume by hypocapnia. The $PaCO_2$ is maintained between 3.3–4.0 kPa (25–30 mm Hg).

The use of muscle relaxants and sedation in controlled ventilation interferes at times with the assessment of the level of consciousness and limb responses; the state of the pupils and the blood pressure are unaffected. The loss of some neurological signs must be weighed against the advantage of reducing I.C.P. and preventing hypoxia; the conscious level can be assessed at intervals if minimal sedation is used and the relaxant drugs reversed. The diagnosis of traumatic intracranial haematoma in patients undergoing controlled ventilation requires a more liberal use of burr holes, arteriography and the C.T. scan. The E.E.G. is non-specific in acute head injury and the echo-encephalogram is unreliable.

Between 24 and 48 h after admission the patient's condition is reassessed. If there has been a rapid fall in I.C.P., adequate breathing often follows withdrawal of the relaxant drugs and the endotracheal tube can be removed. If improvement is less rapid, ventilation is continued for a few days or, occasionally, in young patients, for over one week. Vapalhati and Troupp (1971) advise against continued mechanical ventilation in patients over 20 years old who have Cheyne-Stokes respiration and decerebrate rigidity. A persistently high intracranial pressure, increasing pulse rate and falling blood pressure are further signs of a poor prognosis. Rossanda et al. (1975) attribute a low incidence of vegetative survival after respirator treatment to the early prevention of hypoxia.

EARLY COMPLICATIONS

Epilepsy. Convulsions usually respond to the intravenous injection of 10 mg diazepam followed, if necessary, by an intravenous infusion of 50 mg diazepam in 500 ml saline. Occasionally one must resort to intravenous thiopentone or even curarisation and controlled ventilation.

Pulmonary oedema. Neurogenic pulmonary oedema, quite distinct from aspiration pneumonitis or fluid overload, was described by Sevitt (1968). Ducker (1968) found that reduction of intracranial pressure decreases the oedema. In such cases mechanical ventilation with a positive end expiratory pressure helps restore oxygenation of the blood.

Meningitis. Occasionally meningitis causes clinical deterioration within 24 h of injury. Meningitis may occur in patients who have neither C.S.F. rhinorrhoea nor a radiologically demonstrable fracture of the base of the skull. It is often signalled by tachycardia, pyrexia, stiff neck and unexplained deterioration of the level of consciousness. Treatment by intravenous chemotherapy must be prompt and vigorous.

It is difficult to define statistically the benefits of treating patients with severe head injuries in intensive therapy units staffed by anaesthetists and physicians with a special interest in critical care. However the importance of prompt reduction of I.C.P. and prevention of hypoxia is self-evident.

REFERENCES

Alexander, S. C. and Lassen, N. A. (1970). Cerebral circulatory response to acute brain disease. *Anesthesiology* **32**, 60.

Brown, A. S. (1971). Intermittent positive pressure ventilation in the management of severe head injuries. *In* 'International Symposium on Head Injuries', p. 266. Churchill Livingstone, London and Edinburgh.

Byrnes, D. P., Crockard, H. A., Gordon, D. S. and Gleadhill, C. A. (1974). Penetrating craniocerebral missile injuries in the civil disturbances in Northern Ireland. *Brit. J. Surg.* **61**, 169.

Crockard, H. A., Coppel, D. L. and Morrow, W. F. K. (1973). Evaluation of hyperventilation in treatment of head injuries. *Brit. Med. J.* **4**, 634.

Cushing, H. (1902). Some experimental and clinical observations concerning states of increased intracranial tension. *Amer. J. Med. Sci.* **124**, 375.

Denny-Brown, D. and Russell, W. R. (1941). Experimental cerebral concussion. *Brain* **64**, 93.

Ducker, T. B. (1968). Increased intracranial pressure and pulmonary oedema. *J. Neurosurg.* **28**, 112.

Easton, K. (1968). Blind oral intubation in the deeply unconscious patient. *Brit. Med. J.* **3**, 252.

Furness, D. N. (1957). Controlled respiration in neurosurgery. *Brit. J. Anaesth.* **29**, 415.

Gordon, D. S. and Crockard, H. A. (1974). Early management of the severe head injury. *Proc. roy. Soc. Med.* **67**, 8.

Gordon, E. and Rossanda, M. (1968). Importance of cerebrospinal fluid acid-base status in the treatment of unconscious patients with brain lesions. *Acta anaesth. scand.* **12**, 51.

Hooper, R. (1969). *In* 'Patterns of Acute Head Injury', p. 76. Edward Arnold, London.

Hulme, A., Chawla, J. C. and Cooper, R. (1971). Continuous monitoring of intracranial pressure in patients with closed head injuries. *In* 'International Symposium on Head Injuries', p. 287. Churchill Livingstone, London and Edinburgh.

Jennett, W. B., Barker, J., Fitch, W. and McDowall, D. G. (1969). Effect of anaesthesia on intracranial pressure in patients with space-occupying lesions. *Lancet* **1**, 61.

Langfitt, T. W. (1968). Increased intracranial pressure. *Clin. Neurosurg.* **16**, 436.

Lassen, N. A. (1966). The luxury-perfusion syndrome and its possible relation to acute metabolic acidosis localized within the brain. *Lancet* **2**, 1113.

Lewin, W. (1967). Severe head injuries. *Proc. roy. Soc. Med.* **60**, 1208.

Lundberg, L., Kjallquist, A. and Bien, C. H. (1959). Reduction of increased intracranial pressure by hyperventilation. *Acta psychiat. neurol. scand.* **34** (Suppl.), 139.

Pappius, H. M. (1967). Biochemical studies on experimental oedema. *In* 'Brain Oedema' (Ed. I. Klatz and F. Seitelberger) p. 445. Springer Verlag, New York.

Plewes, L. W. (1967). Early treatment of multiple injuries. *Proc. roy. Soc. Med.* **60**, 945.

Rosomoff, H. L., Shulman, K., Raynor, R. and Grainger, W. (1960). Experimental brain injury and delayed hypothermia. *Surg. Gynec. Obstet.* **110**, 27.

Rossanda, Marina, Collice, M., Porta, M. and Boselli, L. (1975). Intracranial pressure in head injury. *In* 'Intracranial Pressure II' (Ed. N. Lundberg, U. Ponten and M. Brock) p. 475. Springer Verlag, Berlin, Heidelberg and New York.

Rovit, R. L. and Hagan, R. (1968). Steroids and cerebral oedema: The effect of glucocorticoids on abnormal capillary permeability following cerebral injury in cats. *J. Neuropathol. Exp. Neurol.* **27**, 277.

Sevitt, S. (1968). Fatal road accidents. *Brit. J. Surg.* **55**, 481.

Shalit, M. N. and Cotev, S. (1975). The Cushing response – a compensatory mechanism or a dangerous phenomenon. *In* 'Intracranial pressure II' (Ed. N. Lundberg, U. Ponten and M. Brock) p. 307. Springer Verlag, Berlin, Heidelberg and New York.

Shapiro, H. M., Wyte, S. R. and Loeser, J. (1974). Barbiturate – augmented hypothermia for reduction of persistent intracranial hypertension. *J. Neurosurgery* **40**, 90.

Shapiro, H. M. (1975). Intracranial hypertension. *Anaesthesiology* **43**, 445.

Smith, A. L., Hoff, J. T. and Nielsen, S. (1974). Barbiturate protection in acute focal cerebral ischaemia. *Stroke* **5**, 1.

Strich, S. J. (1961). Shearing of nerve fibres as a cause of brain damage due to head injury. *Lancet* **2**, 443.

Teasdale, G. and Galbraith, S. (1975). Acute impairment of brain function, II. Observation record chart. *Nursing Times* **71**, 972.

Teasdale, G. and Jennett, B. (1974). Assessment of coma and impaired consciousness. *Lancet* **2**, 81.

Tomlinson, B. E. (1964). *In* 'Acute Injuries of the Head'. (Ed. G. F. Rowbotham) p. 116. Churchill Livingstone, Edinburgh.

Troupp, H. (1974). Ventricular fluid pressure recording after severe brain injuries. *Europ. Neurol.* **II**, 227.

Vapalahti, M. and Troupp, H. (1971). Prognosis for patients with severe head injuries. *Brit. Med. J.* **3**, 404.

Wilson, D. (1967). Early treatment of multiple injuries. *Proc. roy. Soc. Med.* **60**, 1946.

Zwetnow, N. N. (1975). Interrelations between I.C.P. and blood circulation within the intracranial space. *In* 'Intracranial Pressure II' (Ed. N. Lundberg, U. Ponten and M. Brock) p. 249. Springer Verlag, Berlin, Heidelberg and New York.

Section 4: The Management of Spinal Injuries

P. G. JOHNSON

INTRODUCTION

The management of spinal injuries demands accurate assessment of both skeletal and neurological damage.

The patient with possible spinal injuries must, from the time of the accident, be moved 'in one piece', to avoid causing or increasing cord damage. When removing the patient from a confined space, the head and trunk must remain in line, the cervical spine being protected by a collar if possible. Once free, traction is applied to the patient's head and legs with the chest and pelvis supported in a straight line. This requires a minimum of three people.

Spine fractures may be stable or unstable. Stability depends on the integrity of the posterior ligament complex, comprising the supraspinous and interspinous ligaments, the ligamentum flavum and the capsules of the facet joints (Holdsworth, 1963). On the stretcher the natural curves of the spine are supported by blankets or pillows. When the site of the fracture is known, padding should maintain slight hyperextension. In cervical spine injuries, small sand bags are placed on either side of the head to prevent rotation.

A spinal injury may be missed in a patient found unconscious with or without evidence of trauma. Such patients must be handled as though the spine were unstable.

Life may be threatened by respiratory or circulatory problems in cervical or high thoracic injuries. At the acute phase of injury – particularly if there has been lung or chest wall trauma, pulmonary aspiration or collapse, artificial ventilation may be required. Intubation in these patients demands skill if further damage to the spinal cord is to be avoided. High spinal cord injuries interrupt the sympathetic outflow, predisposing to orthostatic hypotension and reflex bradycardia. Nasopharyngeal or tracheal stimulation e.g. by suction through an endotracheal or tracheostomy tube may easily precipitate reflex bradycardia and cardiac arrest. These risks are minimised in an adequately ventilated patient but atropinisation may be necessary (Part 2, ch. X, p. 695).

Patients with suspected high spinal injury should be moved in a slight head-down position and their pulse rate carefully recorded.

CERVICAL INJURIES

General comments

The patient with cervical spine injury may also have injured his chest or abdomen and their treatment may be more urgent than that of the spine. Hypotension alone does not necessarily imply hypovolaemia, and when solely related to the cervical cord injury, is associated with a good pulse volume, normal right atrial pressure, and generally a brady-cardia.

Evidence of inadequate ventilation may necessitate urgent intubation and hand ventilation. The pulse rate must be carefully observed during intubation (see above). A planned tracheostomy may be indicated over the subsequent few days due to chest injury, pulmonary collapse, aspiration or infection, or where assisted respiration needs to be continued for a long time. Persistent bradycardia or periods of asystolic arrest related to bronchial or nasopharyngeal suction may necessitate continuous atropinisation (Part 2, ch. X, p. 695).

Lacerations of the face and scalp or an abnormal position of the head, may suggest bony injury. Movements of the neck should be examined only in the conscious patient and performed with caution, stopping immediately if producing pain or paraesthesia.

A complete neurological examination (including the sacral dermatomes) is essential; cord damage governs recovery and changes in the physical signs indicate prognosis (Stauffier, 1975; Hardy and Rossier, 1975). The clinical patterns vary, but two important syndromes are the Acute Anterior Cord Syndrome and the Acute Central Cord Syndrome.

The Acute Anterior Cord Syndrome (Schneider, 1955) results from direct damage to the anterior part of the cervical cord, or its blood supply. There is both upper and lower motor neurone paralysis of the upper limbs and upper motor neurone paralysis of the lower limbs. Pain and temperature sensation are lost on each side, though touch and joint position sensation are preserved in the lower limbs.

The Acute Central Cord Syndrome (Schneider *et al.*, 1954) is caused by haematomyelia and oedema of the central parts of the cord when compressed between a disc anteriorly and the ligamentum posteriorly (Taylor and Blackwood, 1948; Taylor, 1951). There is lower motor neurone paralysis resulting from damage to the anterior horn cells at the site of the injury, and upper motor neurone paralysis below, from involvement of the central fibres of the lateral cortico-spinal tracts at the same level. The sacral fibres being more peripheral are often preserved; hence the importance of examining the sacral dermatomes.

Radiography

High quality radiographs are essential.

1. *Lateral views*

(*a*) In the normal cervical spine only the anterior arch of the atlas projects beyond a line formed by the anterior edges of the vertebral bodies, lines formed by their posterior edges and the bases of the neural spines form a smooth cone (Johnson and Apley, 1976). A haematoma resulting from injury may produce a visible forward displacement of the pharynx or trachea. A displacement of 5 mm or more at the level of the antero-inferior border of the third cervical body suggests cervical spine injury (Weir, 1975).

(*b*) The distance between the odontoid peg and the posterior surface of the anterior arch of the atlas is constant in flexion or extension, and not more than 3 mm in adults or 4.5 mm in children.

(*c*) Displacement forward of one vertebra on another is important, less than half the width of a vertebra suggests unilateral facet dislocation and more, indicates bilateral facet dislocation (Beatson, 1963). Oblique views confirm the side and degree of displacement.

(*d*) The vertebrae must always be counted, because C7 or even C6 may not be visible. Consequently injuries at these levels are often missed. Views of the lower cervical spine may require the shoulder to be depressed by pulling on the arm, a procedure to be performed only by a doctor. Good radiographs, especially in a stout person, are difficult to obtain and the assistance of a radiologist is often essential.

(*e*) To demonstrate dislocation without fracture, flexion and extension films are needed. These are taken under the supervision of a doctor after fracture of the odontoid process has been excluded. The examination must stop should the patient experience symptoms in the arms or legs.

2. *Anteroposterior views*

These may reveal malalignment of the spinous processes, suggesting unifacet dislocation.

An anteroposterior view through the mouth will be needed to demonstrate a fractured odontoid process, though confirmation may require tomography. The same view will reveal displacement of the lateral masses in the bursting type of atlas fracture (Jefferson, 1920).

Individual fractures

Atlas fractures

These are caused by a vertical force, for example a fall onto the head and occur where arches and lateral masses join. Neurological signs may be minimal in patients surviving this injury. The treatment is a collar worn for three months. If there is significant displacement of the lateral masses, suggesting a torn transverse ligament, fusion is indicated (Spence *et al.*, 1970). (Figs 1 and 2.)

Axis fractures

Road traffic accidents and severe falls may result in fracture of the odontoid process, usually through the base (Figs 3–5). Through-the-mouth views and possibly tomograms are needed. Ossification centres of the process should not be confused with fractures (Bhattacharyya, 1970).

Cord damage is often absent or mild in survivors. There may be only

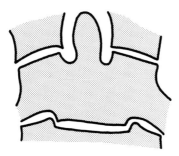

Fig. 1. Normal anteroposterior view of atlas and axis.

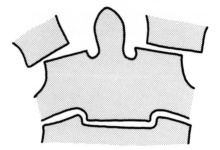

Fig. 2. Displaced lateral masses of atlas.

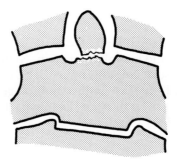

Fig. 3. Fractured odontoid process: antero-posterior view through the mouth of basal fracture.

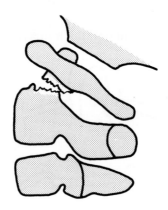

Fig. 4. Fractured odontoid process: lateral view in extension.

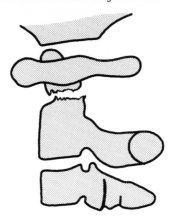

Fig. 5. Fractured odontoid process: lateral view in flexation.

painful limitation of movement and pain over the distribution of the greater occipital nerve.

In treatment accurate reduction is important. Skull traction is generally indicated (Andersen, 1971). The caliper used may be of the Crutchfield, Blackburn or Vinke type. The bed should be one in which the patient can be turned while maintaining traction, for example, a Stryker or Stoke Mandeville bed (Hardy and Elson, 1976). Each day the caliper is checked to see that the locking nuts are secure and the skin in the region of the incisions is inspected and kept clean. Traction is maintained for six weeks followed by an external plaster support for another six weeks.

Union can be expected in ten to twelve weeks (Blockey and Purser, 1956), though the incidence of non-union in some series has been high. This may be related to the level of the fracture (Anderson and D'Alonzo, 1974), to the degree of displacement (Schatzker *et al.*, 1971) or to delay in treatment.

Non-union may lead to instability which is a considerable hazard in an active person and is an indication for posterior fusion, usually between C_1 and C_2. Fusion is also indicated to prevent the onset of late myelopathy, where re-displacement has occurred or in those cases seen late.

Traumatic spondylolisthesis and Hangman's fracture also result from falls or road traffic accidents but these affect the body of the axis. They have similar radiological appearances though their mechanisms differ (Williams, 1975). Hangman's fracture is usually lethal, whereas spondylolisthesis requires only support in a collar, and exhibits few neurological signs. Skull traction should be avoided (Cornish, 1968).

Dislocation without fracture

Posterior dislocation of the axis without fracture has been reported following severe accidents (Haralson and Boyd, 1969; Potzakis *et al.*, 1974; Sassard *et al.*, 1974). These patients had few neurological signs and recovered well, though all required traction and some required fusion.

Anterior wedge fracture

These are rare, stable and lack neurological signs. A collar is worn until symptoms subside.

Burst fractures

These are stable. Though very painful they may have few neurological signs. They require support in a collar until fusion is shown radiologically (Fig. 6).

Severe displacement of the bony fragments may damage the cord, resulting in acute anterior cord syndrome, acute central cord syndrome, or tetraplegia. Such cases require skull traction. Considerable recovery

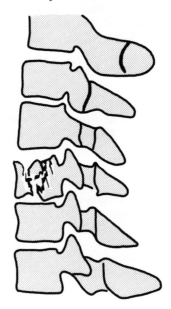

Fig. 6. Burst fracture, C_5.

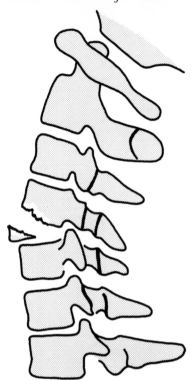

Fig. 7. Hyperextension injury C_4/C_5: avulsion fragment from C_4.

can be anticipated, traction is maintained until callus appears, when support can be continued with a collar.

Hyperextension injuries
Facial trauma and the history may suggest this injury.

The lateral radiographs may appear normal, or a small fragment be avulsed from the lower anterior edge of the vertebra above the level of instability (Fig. 7). Extension films demonstrate the instability. These fractures are, however, stable in the neutral position.

Neurological damage is variable, from transient to permanent paralysis, but generally the prognosis is good.

Support in the neutral position by a collar is needed.

Forward dislocations
Unless the articular facets become locked these injuries are unstable because the posterior ligament complex is disrupted. The lateral

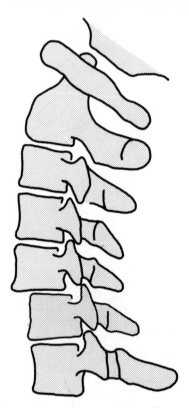

Fig. 8. Forward dislocation: uni-facet dislocation of C_5 on C_6.

radiographs may show whether there is uni- or bilateral dislocation of the posterior articulations (Fig. 8). Oblique views are needed to demonstrate the involved side in unifacet dislocations. The safest method of reduction is skull traction with gradually increasing weights, beginning with 5–10 lb. Check X-rays are taken and if necessary the weights increased by increments of 5 lb, X-rays are repeated 1–2 h after each increment. Usually 10–15 lb affects a reduction but weights up to 35 lb may be necessary. Should this not succeed, traction and manipulation under a general anaesthetic is usually advised (Evans, 1966; Holdsworth, 1970; Burke and Berryman, 1971). Reduction is held by traction for three weeks, when fusion is performed as ruptured ligaments heal poorly.

Tetraplegia may occur though most commonly neurological damage is minimal.

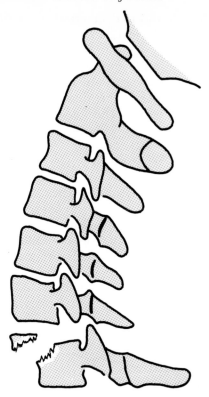

Fig. 9. Fracture-dislocation of C_6/C_7 : avulsion fragment of C_7 ; commonly the facets are fractured also.

Fracture-dislocations

These form the great majority of serious neck injuries, the commonest sites being the C_5/C_6 and C_6/C_7 levels. They have the highest incidence of neurological involvement, including the severest damage. Examination soon after injury and repeated regularly identifies recognised syndromes and changes in signs indicate prognosis.

They are extremely unstable fractures (Fig. 9), caused in the majority of cases by road traffic accidents, falls and sports injuries.

Some surgeons begin treatment by manipulation under general anaesthetic, but a safer method is probably continuous skull traction. This must be done cautiously, under X-ray control, and with due regard to the degree of neurological injury and the build of the patient.

Too great a weight will lead to distraction at the site of injury and a possible increase in neurological damage (Guttman, 1973).

Traction is maintained for four to six weeks. If there is then radiological evidence of satisfactory callus formation, traction can be discontinued and a collar worn until interbody fusion is complete. Should there be little callus at this time fusion is performed as late displacement sometimes occurs (Durbin, 1956).

Cervical injuries in the aged

Damage to the cervical cord can occur in the aged from quite minor injuries. Clinical and radiological evidence of bony and soft tissue injury may be lacking, though the patient has severe pain and obvious neurological signs. The radiograph may demonstrate only degenerative changes, though direct injury to the cord or its blood supply, within the rigid spine has taken place. With vascular injury the changes may be progressive. Protection with a collar and observation of the neurological state is required. Skull traction in a patient with severe degenerative changes is not without hazard.

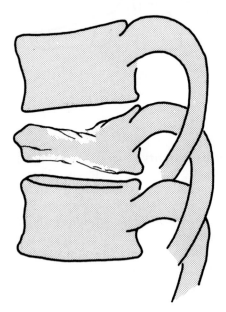

Fig. 10. Thoracic spine: anterior wedge fracture.

THORACIC SPINE INJURIES

From T_1 to T_9 there is great stability and injury is rare.

Anterior wedge fractures
These are stable and are treated symptomatically (Fig. 10). Many occur in vertebrae the site of either osteoporosis or malignant deposits.

Fracture-dislocations
These are caused by severe forces at right angles to the spine. The displacement is irreducible, and treatment consists in managing the paraplegia which invariably results.

THORACO-LUMBAR INJURIES

General comments

These are common and occur at the junction of the rigid thoracic and mobile lumbar spines.

At this level the vertebral canal contains the spinal cord, which ends at the lower border of the first lumbar vertebra, and is surrounded by the obliquely running roots of T_{11}, T_{12} and the lumbar and sacral nerves (Fig. 11). Both cord and roots may be injured. Comparison of the levels of bony injury and neurological lesion distinguishes root from cord damage. This was emphasised by Holdsworth (1963) who stressed the importance of early careful neurological examination, repeated regularly. He maintained that immediate complete paraplegia from cord injury, without any motor or sensory recovery within twenty-four hours is irreparable. Root damage may persist for weeks and still recover. The preservation of voluntary control over the sacral motor segments and sparing of perianal sensation indicates an incomplete lesion and is a good prognostic sign. The greater the extent of motor and sensory sparing below the lesion, and the more rapid its recovery, the better the prognosis (Holdsworth, 1970).

Return of reflex activity, for example, cremasteric, anal or bulbocavernosus reflexes, signify the end of spinal shock. Such changes, unaccompanied by voluntary motor or sensory recovery, are a bad omen indicating isolation of the segments below the lesion.

Palpation of the midline is essential. If the posterior ligament complex has been torn, a gap is felt between two spinous processes. The resistance is less and the finger sinks in. This is a reliable sign of instability.

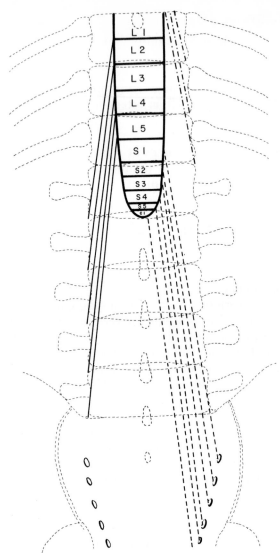

Fig. 11. Lumbar spinal cord: relationship of cord and roots: thoracic roots, —··—··—; lumbar roots, —————————; sacral and coccygeal roots, — — — — — —.

An anteroposterior and two lateral radiographs, one centred over the bodies and one over the spinous processes, are needed. Shift or angulation of the column and changes in shape of the individual

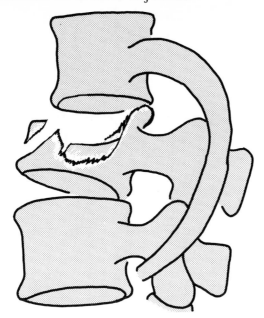

Fig. 12. Fracture-dislocation of T_{12}/L_1: lateral view.

vertebrae, may be seen (Fig. 12). Oblique views are sometimes required.

Individual fractures

Anterior wedge fracture
These result from flexion, are stable and without neurological signs (Fig. 13). Treatment is by analgesics and mobilisation.

Burst fractures
These too are stable, but may be associated with considerable pain. Therefore a plaster jacket for six weeks is wise, followed by a corset for a further six weeks (Fig. 14).

Unstable fractures without paraplegia

Further damage by movement must be prevented. Fixation can be achieved by plates. This method is probably indicated when open reduction is needed because posture and manipulation methods have failed to achieve a reduction. Should the injury be mainly ligamentous,

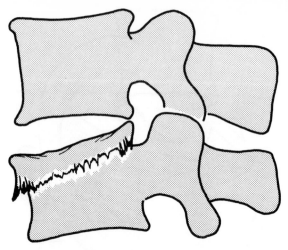

Fig. 13. Lumbar spine: anterior wedge fracture.

bone grafts are added. Such surgery should be performed as soon as the general condition of the patient allows.

Skin sensation is normal, consequently the patient can be safely treated without operation in a plaster bed. Six weeks is usually long enough, after when he can be allowed up wearing a corset until the fracture is stable.

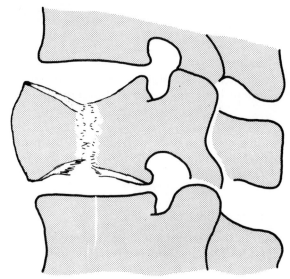

Fig. 14. Lumbar spine: burst fracture.

Unstable fractures with paraplegia

Paraplegia dominates the management and the anaesthetic skin prevents the use of plaster. Such cases are best nursed in spinal centres and should be transferred as soon as their general condition allows, preferably within the first twenty-four hours after injury.

Where the sympathetic outflow has been interrupted and there is evidence of cardiovascular instability, patient transfer should be delayed until stabilisation has occurred. In such cases, and in patients where maintenance of the airway is inadequate, a tracheostomy performed prior to transfer is wise (see also preceding comments, p. 413).

At these centres the damaged spine may be managed conservatively as advocated by Guttman (1973), or more actively by open reduction and plating (Holdsworth and Hardy, 1953; Holdsworth 1970; Lewis and McKibbin, 1974).

Bladder care

From the beginning care should be exercised to avoid over distension and infection.

The eventual type of bladder function depends on the neurological lesion and may take a long time to become fully established. Where the cord lesion occurs above the sacral segments, though voluntary control is lost, the reflex arcs remain and an upper motor neurone, reflex, or automatic bladder results. Where sacral segments or roots are damaged, both voluntary and reflex control ceases and the lower motor neurone, or autonomous bladder results.

Bladder drainage may be intermittent or continuous. The former is used in specialised centres and requires great skill if infection is to be avoided. Normally an indwelling catheter with closed drainage is preferable. Aseptic handling of the catheter is mandatory. It should be changed twice weekly at first, then once a week. Daily oral fluid intake should be 2–3 litres. When being changed weekly the catheter may be left out for a few hours to assess bladder function.

Skin care

Prevention of bed sores demands a high standard of nursing care, with an optimum staff/patient ratio. Day and night the patient must be turned two hourly, and meticulous attention paid to the general hygiene of the skin, the patient's toilet and the condition of the bed linen.

Physiotherapy

The physiotherapist supervises regular breathing and coughing exercises, usually after the two hourly changes of position.

Where patient co-operation allows, self-assisted coughing efforts are
taught. Chest infection calls for added supervision from the physiotherapist, including postural drainage.

Paralysed joints are put through a full range of passive movements
several times each day, to prevent contractures.

Weakened and normal muscles require active graduated exercises to
increase their strength to ensure the greatest independence for the
patient. Where muscle spasms cause discomfort relief may follow
strengthening the antagonistic muscles.

REFERENCES

Anderson, L. D. and D'Alonzo, R. T. (1974). Fractures of the odontoid process of the axis. *J. Bone and Joint Surg.* **56**A, 1663.

Anderson, L. D. (1971). *In* 'Campbells' Operative Orthopaedics' (Ed. A. H. Grenshaw). Fifth Edition, Vol. I, 618. The C. V. Mosley Company, Saint Louis.

Beatson, T. R. (1963). Fractures and dislocations of the cervical spine. *J. Bone and Joint Surg.* **45**B, 21.

Bhattacharyya, S. K. (1974). Fractures and displacement of the odontoid process in a child. *J. Bone and Joint Surg.* **56**A, 1071.

Blockey, N. J. and Purser, D. W. (1956). Fractures of the odontoid process of the axis. *J. Bone and Joint Surg.* **38**B, 794.

Burke, D. C. and Berryman, D. (1971). The place of closed manipulations in the management of flexion-rotation dislocations of the cervical spine. *J. Bone and Joint Surg.* **53**B, 165.

Cornish, B. L. (1968). Traumatic spondylolisthesis of the axis. *J. Bone and Joint Surg.* **50**B, 31.

Durbin, F. C. (1956). Fractions and dislocations of the cervical spine. *J. Bone and Joint Surg.* **38**B, 773.

Evans, D. K. (1966). *In* 'Clinical Surgery. Fractures and Dislocations' (Ed. R. Furlong) p. 15. Butterworths, London.

Guttmann, L. (1973). 'Spinal Cord Injuries: Comprehensive Management and Research.' Blackwell Scientific, Oxford.

Haralson, R. H. III and Boyd, H. B. (1969). Posterior dislocation of the atlas on the axis without fracture. *J. Bone and Joint Surg.* **51**A, 561.

Hardy, A. G. and Elson, R. (1976). 'Practical Management of Spinal Injuries: A Manual for Nurses.' Churchill Livingstone, Edinburgh.

Hardy, A. G. and Rossier, A. B. (1975). 'Spinal Cord Injuries: Orthopaedic and Neurological Aspects'. Goerg Thiemie, Stuttgart. (This book contains an exhaustive review of the literature on spinal cord injuries.)

Holdsworth, F. W. and Hardy, A. G. (1953). Early treatment of paraplegia from fractures of the thoraco-lumbar spine. *J. Bone and Joint Surg.* **35**B, 540.

Holdsworth, F. W. (1963). Fractures, dislocations and fracture-dislocations of the spine. *J. Bone and Joint Surg.* **45**B, 6.

Holdsworth, F. W. (1970). Review article: fractures, dislocations and fracture-dislocations of the spine. *J. Bone and Joint Surg.* **52**A, 1534.

Jefferson, G. (1920). Fracture of the atlas vertebra. Report of four cases and a review of those previously recorded. *Brit. J. Surg.* **1**, 407.

Johnson, P. G. and Apley, A. G. (1976). Fractures of the spine. *Brit. J. Hosp. Med.*, January 1976, 8.

Lewis, J. McKibbin (1974). The treatment of unstable fracture-dislocations of the thoraco-lumbar spine accompanied by paraplegia. *J. Bone and Joint Surg.* **56**B, 603.

Potzakis, M. J., Knop, A., Elfering, M., Hoffer, M. and Harnog, J. P. (1974). Posterior dislocation of the atlas on the axis. *J. Bone and Joint Surg.* **56**A, 1260.

Sassard, W. R., Heinig, C. F. and Pitts, W. R. (1974). Posterior allanto axial dislocation without fracture. *J. Bone and Joint Surg.* **56**A, 625.

Schatzker, J., Rorabeck, C. H. and Waddell, J. R. (1971). Fractures of the dens (odontoid process). *J. Bone and Joint Surg.* **53**B, 392.

Schneider, R. C. (1955). Syndrome of acute anterior spinal cord injury. *J. Neurosurgery* **12**, 95.

Schneider, R. C., Cherry, G. and Pantek, H. (1954). The syndrome of acute central cervical spinal cord injury, with special reference to the mechanisms involved in hyperextension injuries of the cervical spine. *J. Neurosurgery* **11**, 546.

Spence, K. F., Decker, S. and Sell, K. W. (1970). Bursting atlantal fracture associated with rupture of the transverse ligament. *J. Bone and Joint Surg.* **52**A, 543.

Stauffier, E. S. (1975). Diagnosis and Prognosis in Acute Cervical Spinal Cord Injury. *In* 'Symposium Spinal Cord Injuries'. *Clinic Orthopaedics and Related Research* Number 112, 9.

Taylor, A. R. (1951). The mechanism of injury to the spinal cord in the neck without damage to the vertebral column. *J. Bone and Joint Surg.* **33**B, 543.

Taylor, A. R. and Blackwood, W. (1948). Paraplegia in hyperextension cervical injuries with normal radiographic appearances. *J. Bone and Joint Surg.* **30**B, 245.

Weir, Don C. (1975). Rodentgenographic signs of cervical injury. *Clin. Orth. and Rel. Research* **109**, June, p. 9.

Williams, T. G. (1975). Hangman's fracture. *J. Bone and Joint Surg.* **57**B, 82.

Section 5: The Management of Soft Tissue Injuries

G. W. ODLING-SMEE

PATHOPHYSIOLOGY

When an object travelling with a given velocity (V) makes contact with living tissue there is a dynamic transfer of energy from the object to the living tissue, which is in a lower energy state. The wounding capacity of a moving object is directly proportional to its kinetic energy, and this is in turn proportional to its velocity and mass [$KE = \frac{1}{2}MV^2$]. Because kinetic energy increases with the square of velocity, high-velocity objects do substantially greater damage to living tissues than do low velocity missiles. A car travels at 88 ft/s (60 m.p.h), a bullet from a hand gun at 500 ft/s, a high velocity rifle bullet at 2000 ft/s, and fragments from bombs may exceed 8500 ft/s (Fischer *et al*, 1974) (Figs 1a–c). Although variation of the mass of the object causes a much smaller transfer of energy, where the mass is very large as in a motor car, the amount of kinetic energy may approach that in a bullet from a hand gun, but will never reach the kinetic energy of a high velocity rifle bullet. Experimental evidence shows that as a low velocity missile traverses soft tissues it leaves a permanent track. However, a high velocity missile cuts a track, and this is followed by a shock wave, which may damage gas filled viscera. Finally a temporary pulsating cavity is formed (Hopkinson and Watts, 1963), and it is this cavitation which damages most tissues by shearing, stretching and finally rupturing of small blood vessels (Fig. 2). Larger arteries and veins may be pushed aside, and nerves usually suffer axonotmesis. There finally follows a negative pressure phase during which the tissue violently recoils causing more cell disruption and a certain amount of extravasation (Hopkinson and Marshall, 1967). During this phase foreign bodies, clothing and consequently organisms are sucked into the track of the missile and therefore all such injuries are contaminated.

430

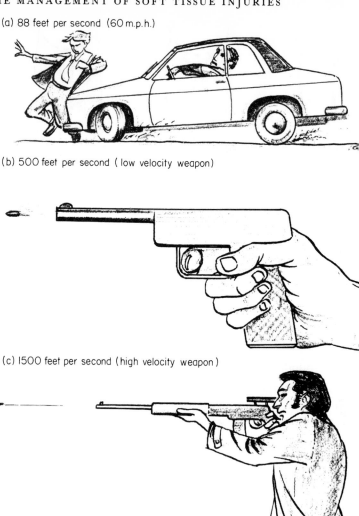

(a) 88 feet per second (60 m.p.h.)

(b) 500 feet per second (low velocity weapon)

(c) 1500 feet per second (high velocity weapon)

Fig. 1. A comparison of the velocity developed by various wounding agents. (a) Road traffic accident. (b) Low velocity weapon. (c) High velocity weapon.

The mechanism described here is that for a high velocity penetrating injury. Clearly the mechanisms of a blunt blow by a large object such as a motor car are similar, but are not completely understood. However, as

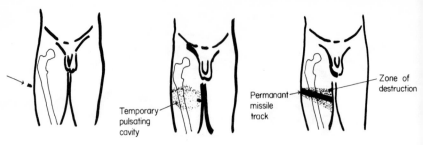

Fig. 2. The formation of a temporary pulsating cavity in a high velocity wound.

the velocity is so small, the amount of tissue destruction is proportionately smaller.

THE TREATMENT OF SOFT TISSUE WOUNDS

Wounds should be divided into two categories: 1. clean, with minimal tissue damage (examples are surgical incisions or wounds caused by glass), and 2. wounds in which there is much tissue destruction and contamination.

1.   Clean wounds

Despite the fact that these wounds may be sutured primarily, great care must be exercised in their treatment to prevent them becoming infected. An adequate anaesthetic must be used, so that the patient feels no pain during manipulation of the wound, and therefore does not inhibit the surgeon. It must be thoroughly cleaned and foreign bodies removed. The sutures should be inserted so that the skin edges are accurately opposed and everted without undue tension.

2.   Traumatised wounds

When much tissue damage has been sustained there is an accumulation of tissue fluid causing profound tissue oedema which may take up to 24 hours to develop to its fullest extent. Inevitably pathogenic organisms will have been carried into the wound (Fig. 3a). Infection will increase the interstitial oedema, and if sutures have been inserted, an increase in intra-wound tension. This may lead to more tissue necrosis, more tissue oedema and a further rise in intra-wound tension (Figs 3b, c). Sutures must, therefore, not be inserted primarily in this type of wound.

(a)

(b)

(c)

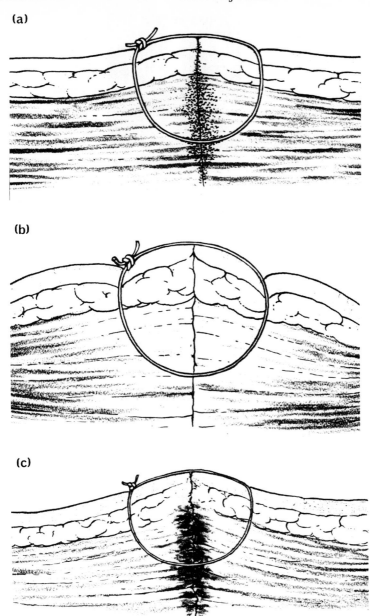

Fig. 3. Pathological factors in contaminated wounds. (a) Wound contaminated with pathogenic organisms. (b) Interstitial oedema causing swelling in the wound. (c) Necrotic muscle causing suppuration in the wound.

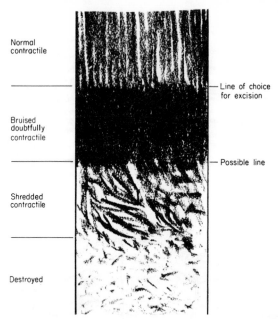

Normal
contractile

———————————— — Line of choice
for excision

Bruised
doubtfully
contractile

———————————— — Possible line

Shredded
contractile

———————————

Destroyed

Fig. 4. The excision of destroyed muscle. It is difficult to recognise dead muscle. Removal of destroyed and shredded muscle will leave a layer of doubtfully contractile muscle. The line of choice for excision is beyond this layer.

Treatment of the traumatised wound should be as follows:

(*a*) *Inspection*. The wound should be carefully inspected under general anaesthesia, and foreign bodies removed. Damage to blood vessels, nerves and bones should be assessed, and the wound laid open so that the interior parts can be examined.

(*b*) *Excision*. Skin is valuable and so only obviously dead skin should be excised. Fat has a poor blood supply, is easily contaminated and so it should be removed freely. Dead muscle must be excised. This is done by excising it until the muscle tissue remaining bleeds freely and contracts when pinched with dissecting forceps (Fig. 4). Deep fascia must be widely incised and left open to allow injured tissue to swell without tension.

(*c*) *Cleaning*. Mechanical cleaning must be thorough. Cetrimide 15% or hexachlorophane 10% aqueous solutions are effective cleaning agents, but mechanical rubbing is more important in loosening dirt than is the agent used. A scrubbing brush is useful in removing embedded grit and other particles.

(d) *Dressing and suture.* The wound is packed with dry gauze and held in place with a pad and crepe bandage. Three to five days later under general anaesthesia, the dressings are removed and the wound inspected. Any necrotic areas that might have been missed should be excised. The skin is then closed, undermining the edges if necessary. It is not necessary to freshen the skin edges, as epithelium is already growing out from them (War Office, 1962). The wound will then heal quickly and the sutures can be removed after seven to ten days.

This process is known as delayed primary suture. It is the treatment of choice for all wounds which are badly traumatised, or where it is certain that much damage has occurred as in high velocity missile injuries.

REFERENCES

Fischer, R. P., Geiger, J. P. and Guernsey, J. M. (1974). Pulmonary resections for severe pulmonary contusions secondary to high velocity wounding. *Injury* **14**, 293–302.

Hopkinson, D. A. W. and Marshall, J. C. (1967). Firearm Injuries. *Brit. J. Surg.* **54**, 344.

Hopkinson, D. A. W. and Watts, J. C. (1963). Studies in experimental missile injuries of skeletal muscle. *Proc. Roy. Soc. Med.* **56**, 461.

War Office (1962). 'A Field Surgery Pocket Book', p. vii. H.M.S.O.

Section 6: The Management of Abdominal and Visceral Injuries

G. W. ODLING-SMEE

ABDOMINAL INJURIES: DIAGNOSIS AND MANAGEMENT

Abdominal injuries may be penetrating or non-penetrating. Penetrating injuries present very little difficulty in diagnosis, but blunt injuries are a greater problem, because of the difficulty of deciding when to open the abdomen.

Blunt injuries

Petty (1973) believes that damage to abdominal organs is manifest at differing times, and he describes a time scale (Fig. 1). There are three

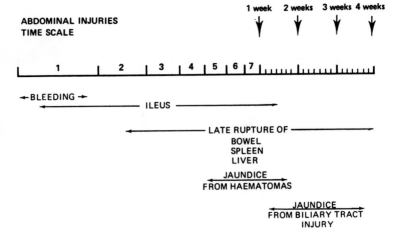

Fig. 1. Time scale in abdominal injuries.

436

phases following blunt injury: the first lasts some hours and is dominated by the problems of bleeding and its control: the second phase lasts some days, and may extend to several weeks, and is dominated by the problems of ileus, late bleeding and delayed rupture of the spleen and other organs: the third phase lasts months and is mostly concerned with rehabilitation.

Diagnosis of a damaged viscus requires care. It is important to realise that injuries can overlap both structure and function in such a way as to distort and disguise the separate clinical signs (London, 1964), and those elicited may, in themselves, be misleading (Proctor, 1967; London, 1969; Shepherd, 1971; Gissane, 1962). Marks of clothing and bruising on the skin of the abdominal wall may suggest underlying visceral damage (Proctor, 1967), and movements of the abdominal wall may be helpful if there is no evidence of chest injury. Abdominal tenderness and muscle guarding are probably the most reliable physical signs (Cooke and Southwood, 1964; Lewis, 1961). Perhaps the most important clinical finding is that of deterioration, and repeated examination is mandatory where there remains a doubt (Petty, 1973).

Investigations may contribute something to diagnosis. An abdominal X-ray in the erect position showing gas under the diaphragm will suggest a ruptured hollow viscus, and fractured ribs may point to a lacerated kidney or spleen. Obliteration of the psoas shadow suggests a retroperitoneal collection of fluid and may be due to a ruptured kidney or duodenum. If the patient's condition permits, barium studies of the gastro-intestinal tract, and angiography of the coeliac, superior and inferior mesenteric vessels may be of use. An intravenous pyelogram is essential if there is a likelihood that the kidneys have been injured. These investigations however take time and are best reserved for the case in which there is doubt. Some surgeons have made use of diagnostic peritoneal lavage, and claim that it makes diagnosis much more accurate (Root et al., 1965; Engrav et al., 1975). This may be associated with enzyme analysis of the lavage fluid for anatomical accuracy (Delany et al., 1976).

The most difficult decision in blunt injuries is whether and when to operate. Shock, the presence of free gas on X-ray, gradual increasing abdominal distension and increasing abdominal pain, tenderness and rigidity, indicate that the abdomen should be explored. The decision is difficult if the signs are equivocal and delay is seldom advantageous. Rutherford Morison is said to have told his students, 'It is better to look and see than to wait and see'. This is still true today.

Perforating injuries

These are easy to recognise, and no great skill is required in making a diagnosis. As a general rule, all perforating injuries should be explored, and a laparotomy performed to ascertain if any viscus has been damaged. Wounds in the upper thighs, buttocks and back, may well be associated with a visceral injury, and if there is doubt exploration should be undertaken. Tangential wounds and laceration of the anterior abdominal wall can also be confusing. Increasing shock, tenderness at a site other than the wound, and guarding spreading over the abdomen, are signs of visceral damage. An X-ray is necessary to see if the missile is still in the abdominal cavity and if there is any of the signs referred to above.

VISCERAL INJURIES: DIAGNOSIS AND MANAGEMENT

Before starting to explore, it is important to make sure that the patient is adequately resuscitated, or if this is impossible due to intra-abdominal bleeding, to make sure that adequate intravenous cannulae are in position, and that plenty of cross-matched blood is to hand.

Vertical incisions are better than transverse ones, for they may be extended up and down and into the chest if necessary. It is important not to miss any damage in the initial exploration, and so the contents should be inspected methodically, and every part of them visualised as far as is possible.

Solid organs

Spleen
Ruptured spleens tend to bleed profusely and immediately on rupture, but the delayed rupture caused by a sub-capsular haematoma must be remembered although it is a rare occurrence (Benjamin *et al.*, 1976).

Liver
The liver is often wounded in penetrating injuries. The injuries may vary from a small furrow to the shattering of the whole liver. In the Belfast series, liver injury has been the second commonest cause of death, and where patients have died it has usually been caused by a torn hepatic vein. These are very difficult to expose and ligature, especially as the bleeding is profuse. Suturing of deep lacerations may control bleeding, but packing with gauze is not advised (Ward-McQuaid, 1969). When major lacerations have separated large portions of the

liver from the porta hepatis, partial or complete lobectomy is necessary and has been used successfully in Belfast. High velocity wounds may disrupt large areas of liver and require resection.

Pancreas

Pancreatic injury is rare; most cases are caused by penetrating wounds rather than by blunt trauma (Heyse-Moore, 1976). It is easy to overlook damage to the pancreas, and it is often very difficult to detect severance of the duct. In most cases, if it is suspected, simple drainage only should be employed, but if the divided duct can be seen, an attempt to repair it may be made. If there is severe damage to the body or the tail, a formal distal pancreatectomy is the treatment of choice (Back and Frey, 1971; Weitzman and Rothschild, 1968).

Kidney

Kidney damage is best handled conservatively. Excretion urography may be useful in making a diagnosis. The only indication for immediate nephrectomy is continued bleeding (Petty, 1973), but a functioning kidney with extravasation of urine may need repair. If when exploring a retroperitoneal haematoma a ruptured kidney is discovered, a repair may be attempted, or a polar nephrectomy performed. If only one kidney is present a repair may be attempted earlier than if two are present. It is possible that the pressure from a retroperitoneal haematoma may cause oliguria, but it is not possible to be sure whether the extrinsic pressure, or the low renal perfusion pressure that usually accompanies it, contributes more to the low urine output (Hanson, 1976).

Hollow organs

Tears of the stomach are not common in non-penetrating injuries but may occur when blunt trauma follows a heavy meal (Yajko *et al.*, 1975; Vassey *et al.*, 1975; Asch *et al.*, 1975; Bussey *et al.*, 1975). Duodenal trauma has an evil reputation whether it occurs in penetrating or blunt injuries. If the rupture is retroperitoneal it is easily overlooked (Cohn *et al.*, 1952). If the damage is overlooked or an early laparotomy is not performed the mortality is very high, and should delay have occurred it is safer to oversew the tear and to fashion a gastrojejunostomy (Lucas *et al.*, 1975). Reinforcing patches do not improve the result (McInnis *et al.*, 1975).

Injuries to the biliary system are rare. There have been a few reports of avulsed gall bladders (Ali, 1975; Brown, 1932; Halker, 1963) and injuries of the common duct are even rarer (Maier *et al.*, 1968). They are best treated by a by-pass using a loop of jejunum. Occasionally this injury is not suspected in blunt trauma, and jaundice will appear on the seventh to fourteenth day (Fielding and Strachan, 1975). These cases have been reported when the patient is drunk, and it has been pointed out by Pirola and Davis (1968) that alcohol causes a rise in pressure in the biliary system.

Injury to the small bowel is usually obvious at operation, and is common in blunt trauma. Aristotle knew that 'the intestine of a deer can easily rupture without injury to the skin'. It commonly occurs at the junction of fixed and mobile parts (the duodeno-jejunal flexure and the ileocaecal region), but may occur from compression against the spine of where there is pathological fixation, such as an adhesion (Razali and Thomas, 1975). It may also occur from a bursting injury (Williams and Sargent, 1963). These injuries may need resection if a length has been badly torn, but otherwise heal very well with simple closure.

The colon is commonly injured and is the commonest viscus injured by penetrating missiles in Belfast. In colonic wounds the classical teaching has always been '. . . one must never omit to establish a colostomy' (War Office, 1962). Several authors have suggested that with modern antibiotics and good surgical technique it might be possible to avoid this (Odling-Smee, 1970; Lo Cicero *et al.*, 1975), but there have been several other reports to suggest that either exteriorisation or defunctioning must be performed (Mulherin *et al.*, 1975). Experience in Belfast suggests that although there is no change in mortality between the two groups, the morbidity caused by infection is much greater when this is not done (Table 1). When the right side of the

Table 1. The results of a survey of infection in gun-shot wounds of the colon in Belfast treated by different methods

	% with resection or defunctioning	% without resection or defunctioning	Total
Wound infection	41.2	42.0	42.0
Chest infection	23.5	20.3	21.0
Urinary infection	17.6	2.8	9.0
Intraperitoneal infection	17.6	29.7	27.1
Total infection rate	20.98	79.01	100.0

colon is damaged a hemicolectomy is a good alternative to repair as exteriorisation is difficult and defunctioning hardly possible. Damaged colon should therefore either be resected or repaired and defunctioned or exteriorised.

REFERENCES

Ali, M. (1975). Avulsion of the gall bladder in blunt abdominal trauma. *Injury* **6**, 334.

Asch, M. J., Coran, A. G. and Johnston, P. W. (1975). Gastric perforation secondary to blunt trauma in children. *J. Trauma*, **15**, 187–189.

Back, R. D. and Frey, C. F. (1971). Diagnosis and treatment of pancreatic trauma. *Amer. J. Surg.* **121**, 20–29.

Benjamin, C. I., Engrav, L. H. and Perry, J. F. Jr. (1976). Delayed rupture or delayed diagnosis of rupture of the spleen. *Surg. Gynaec. Obstet.* **142**, 171–172.

Brown, H. P. (1932). Traumatic cholecystectomy. *Ann. Surg.* **92**, 952.

Bussey, H. J., McGehee, R. N. and Tyson, K. R. T. (1975). Isolated gastric rupture due to blunt trauma. *J. Trauma*, **15**, 190–191.

Cohn, I. Jr., Hawthorne, H. R. and Frobese, A. S. (1952). Retroperitoneal rupture of the duodenum in non-penetrating abdominal trauma. *Amer. J. Surg.* **84**, 293–301.

Cooke, R. V., and Southwood, W. F. W. (1964). Closed abdominal injuries. *Brit. J. Surg.* **51**, 767–769.

Delany, H. M., Moss, C. M. and Carnevale, N. (1976). The use of enzyme analysis of peritoneal blood in the clinical assessment of abdominal organ injury. *Surg. Gynaec. Obstet.* **142**, 161–167.

Engrav, L. H., Benjamin, C. I., Strate, R. G. and Perry, J. F. (1975). Diagnostic peritoneal lavage in blunt abdominal trauma. *J. Trauma*, **15**, 854–859.

Fielding, J. W. L. and Strachan, C. J. L. (1975). Jaundice as a sign of delayed gall-bladder perforation following blunt abdominal trauma. *Injury* **7**, 66–67.

Gissane, W. (1962). The basic surgery of major road injuries. *Ann. roy. Coll. Surg. Eng.* **30**, 281–298.

Halker, E. (1963). Avulsion of the gall bladder. *Dan. Med. Bull.* **10**, 8, 262.

Hanson, G. C. (1976). Personal communication.

Heyse-Moore, G. H. (1976). Blunt pancreatic and pancreaticoduodenal trauma. *Brit. J. Surg.* **63**, 226–228.

Lewis, I. (1961). Non-penetrating injuries of the abdomen. *Proc. roy. Soc. Med.* **54**, 562–563.

Lo Cicero, J., Tajima, T. and Drapanas, T. (1975). A half-century of experience in the management of colon injuries. *J. Trauma* **15**, 575–579.

London, P. S. (1964). Clinical Surgery *In* 'Accident Surgery' (Ed. Rob and Smith) Vol. 3, p. 95. Butterworths, London.

London, P. S. (1969). The management of serious injuries of the trunk. *Proc. roy. Soc. Med.* **62**, 248–250.

Lucas, C. E. and Ledgerwood, A. M. (1975). Factors influencing outcome after blunt duodenal injury. *J. Trauma* **15**, 839–846.

McInnis, W. D., Aust, J. B., Cruz, A. B. and Root, H. D. (1975). Traumatic injuries of the duodenum: a comparison of primary closure and the jejunal patch. *J. Trauma* **15**, 847–851.

Maier, W. R., Lightfoot, W. P. and Rosemond, W. P. (1968). Extrahepatic biliary ductal injury in closed trauma. *Amer. J. Surg.* **116**, 103–108.

Mulherin, J. L., Sawyers, J. L. (1975). Evaluation of three methods for managing penetrating colon injuries. *J. Trauma* **15**, 580–587.

Narasimhan, M. J. and Day, S. B. (1975). Biological perspectives of some trauma injuries. *In* 'Trauma' (Ed. S. B. Day). Plenum, London and New York.

Newton, E., McMullen, J. H., Butler, E. G. *et al.* (1962). 'Mechanisms of Wounding'. (Ed. J. B. Coates). Wound Ballistics, Medical Department, U.S. Army, U.S. Govt. Printing Office.

Odling-Smee, G. W. (1970). Ibo civilian casualties in the Nigerian civil war. *Brit. Med. J.* **2**, 592–596.

Petty, A. H. (1973). Abdominal injuries. *Ann. roy. Coll. Surg. Eng.* **53**, 167–177.

Pirola, R. C. and Davis, A. E. (1968). Effects of ethyl alcohol on sphincteric resistance at the choledochoduodenal junction in man. *Gut* **9**, 557–60.

Proctor, H. (1967). Abdominal injuries. *Proc. roy. Soc. Med.* **60**, 950–951.

Razali, H. and Thomas, W. M. C. (1975). Isolated jejunal injuries arising from blunt abdominal trauma. *Injury* **6**, 33–35.

Root, H. D., Hauser, C. W., McKinley, C. R., LaFave, J. W. and Mendiola, R. P. (1965). Diagnostic peritoneal lavage. *Surgery* **57**, 633–37.

Shepherd, J. A. (1971). Trauma to the abdomen: diagnosis. *Ann. roy. Coll. Surg. Eng.* **48**, 11.

Vassey, L. E., Kledier, R. L., Koch, E. and Morse, T. S. (1975). Traumatic gastric perforation in children from blunt trauma. *J. Trauma* **15**, 184–186.

War Office (1962). 'A Field Surgery Pocket Book', p. vii. H.M.S.O.

Ward-McQuaid, J. N. (1969). Massive trunk injuries. *Proc. roy. Soc. Med.* **62**, 250–253.

Weitzman, J. J. and Rothschild, P. D. (1968). Surgical management of traumatic rupture of the pancreas due to blunt trauma. *Surg. Clin. N. Amer.* **48**, 1347–1353.

Williams and Sargent (1963). Mechanism of intestinal injury in trauma. *J. Trauma* **3**, 288–294.

Yajko, R. D., Seydel, F. and Trimble, C. (1975). Rupture of the stomach from blunt abdominal trauma. *J. Trauma* **15**, 177–183.

Section 7: The Management of the Critically Ill Patient with Extensive Burns

J. W. L. DAVIES

INTRODUCTION

The amount of heat absorbed by tissues from very hot water, steam or burning materials is frequently sufficient to cause full thickness skin loss destruction. When this injury is extensive (i.e. covering more than one third of the body surface) it initiates a sequence of potentially lethal changes involving not only the loss of body fluids and ions but also the ingress of pathogenic micro-organisms. Unlike most other forms of injury extensive burns may remain unhealed for many weeks and thus require intensive care for a long period.

The degree of hazard to life is dependent upon both the severity of the burn and the age of the patient. This hazard was high prior to 1940, it remained relatively constant at a lower level during the following 25 years and has since decreased again. A recent survey (Bull, 1971) of mortality probability in 1922 patients using probit analysis has shown the estimates contained in Fig. 1. While it should be appreciated that the values in the figure are averages and an individual patient may have a prognosis which is better or worse than the average, the table gives a guide to which patients may show the best response to intensive care and those in which it is unlikely to do more than prolong life by a few hours or days.

443

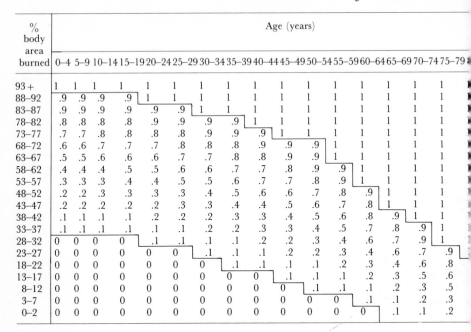

Fig. 1. Mortality probability chart (1965–1970) relating area of body surface burned and age of the patient. Taken with permission from Bull (1971).

THE EXTENT OF INJURY

The severity of a burn is dependent upon both the depth and the extent of the injury, this latter being usually expressed as a percentage of the total body surface area. The precise estimates of the area of various parts of the body described by Lund and Browder (1944) (Table 1) are usually modified into the easily remembered 'rule of nines' (Wallace, 1951). The area of the palmar surface of the patient's outstretched hand and fingers is approximately 1% of the body surface. In patients with very extensive burns it is easier to assess the area of unburned skin and subtract from 100% to give the area of the burn. Babies and young children have lower limbs which are proportionately smaller and heads which are proportionately larger in surface area than those of adults (Table 1).

The depth of burning is normally divided into three categories (Fig. 2):

1. Erythema is redness of the skin without blistering which spon-

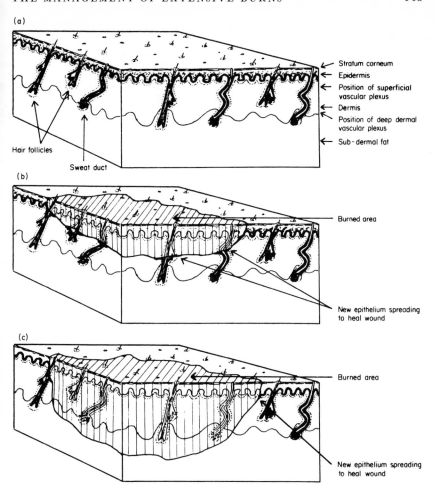

(a)

Stratum corneum
Epidermis
Position of superficial vascular plexus
Dermis
Position of deep dermal vascular plexus
Sub-dermal fat

Hair follicles
Sweat duct

(b)

Burned area

New epithelium spreading to heal wound

(c)

Burned area

New epithelium spreading to heal wound

Fig. 2. Diagrams illustrating the structure of normal skin (a) (the position of the vascular system is indicated), partial thickness skin loss burn (b) (healing can occur from below the burn as well as the wound edge), and full thickness skin loss burn (c) (healing can only occur from the edge of the wound). Taken with permission from Lawrence and Bull (1976).

taneously disappears within 1–2 days. It is usual not to include erythema burning in the assessment of total area burned.
2. Partial thickness skin loss implies that some of the deep epithelial elements of the skin are viable, and a new epithelium will form from the hair follicles and sweat ducts beneath the eschar of dead dermis in 1–4 weeks.

Table 1. Contribution of various body areas to total body surface at different ages (as %). (Adapted from Lund and Browder, 1944)

Area	Years				
	0–1	1–4	5–9	10–16	Adult
Head and neck	21	19	15	13	9
Trunk	32	32	32	32	32
Upper limbs	19	19	19	19	19
Lower limbs	28	30	34	36	40

3. Full thickness skin loss implies that virtually all hair follicles and sweat glands have been destroyed. Healing of such a burned area can only occur by slow epithelial ingrowth from the edges of the burn and by wound contraction. The destruction of nerve endings in deep dermal and full thickness burns renders them analgesic, a factor which is used to determine the depth of burning at the time of the primary assessment on admission to hospital (Bull and Lennard-Jones, 1949). In a co-operative patient, pricking of the burned area with a sterile hypodermic needle differentiates those areas which are pain sensitive and partial thickness skin loss from the analgesic areas which are deep partial or full thickness skin loss. If the location and extent of these areas are drawn on a pictorial chart, a comparison can be made subsequently between the analgesic areas and those which granulate and need skin grafting.

TYPES OF INJURY

Burns may be caused by contact with any solid, liquid or gas which has a temperature greater than about 50°C. The duration of contact is also an important determinant of the depth of burning (Fig. 3). From this figure it may be seen that a one second exposure to a conducting metal surface at temperatures between 70°C and 100°C will cause a partial thickness skin burn while higher temperatures will cause full thickness skin burns. A one minute exposure will cause partial thickness burns when the temperature is between 55°C and 65°C, at all higher temperatures the burn will be full thickness skin loss. Temperatures of less than −1°C can also cause skin damage through freezing of the tissues (Ward, 1974), again the severity of the 'frostbite' increases with the duration of exposure.

Hot liquids or gases containing a variety of chemical agents such as

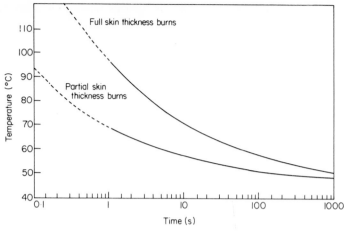

Fig. 3. The relationship between temperature and duration of contact causing partial or full thickness skin loss burns. Taken with permission from Lawrence and Bull (1976).

acids, alkalis, oxidising agents and most heavy metal salts may cause more severe burns than expected from the temperature or the duration of exposure. When there may be absorption of toxic chemicals irrigation with specific antidotes as well as water is required to minimise the severity of injury. The problems associated with the treatment of extensive industrial chemical burns have been described by Cason (1959), and those associated with the inhalation of hot gases sometimes containing toxic chemical compounds are discussed by Mellins and Park (1975). Burns may also be caused by electrical contact, electric flash, arcing or a combination of current and heat as when a child puts a hand on the bar of an electric fire. There is further discussion of electrical injuries in Part 2, ch. III, p. 467 of this book.

FLUID RESUSCITATION

Types of fluid used

An important effect of heat is to destroy the keratin layer in the skin which makes normal skin virtually impermeable to water. The damage also increases the capillary permeability which allows loss of plasma into the extravascular space with the formation of oedema and the appearance of exudate on the burned surface. The quantity of exudate is variable – a partial skin thickness scald may produce many litres of exudate per day whereas a deep flame burn with charring of the skin may appear almost dry.

The loss of fluid from the circulation by this leakage is more rapid than the venous and lymphatic return of extracellular fluid and causes a rapid fall in plasma volume. As erythrocytes do not normally pass into the extravascular fluid the haematocrit and the viscosity of the blood in the vascular system will rise. A fall in plasma volume occurs in all burned patients but only becomes sufficiently severe to require active treatment in children with burns covering more than 10%, and in adults with burns covering more than 15% of the body surface. The most suitable fluid to replace the plasma loss is the subject of some debate.

According to some workers patients with burns covering up to 30% of the body surface may be adequately treated with an oral input of water containing a mixture of approximately equal parts of sodium chloride and sodium bicarbonate at an isotonic concentration (Markley et al., 1956, 1959). Some patients however required an intravenous infusion since the oral input became less than adequate due to vomiting. The constituents of intravenous forms of therapy vary widely between units treating burned patients. Some use isotonic balanced electrolyte solutions such as Ringer's lactate (Baxter, 1974) while others use a hypertonic lactate solution with a sodium concentration around 225 mmol/l (Monafo, 1970; Monafo et al., 1973). However, as plasma-like fluid is lost from the circulation, plasma is considered to be the most suitable replacement solution in many burn units (Artz, 1971; Birke and Liljedahl, 1968; Burke and Constable, 1965; Davies, 1975a; Reiss et al., 1953). In the absence of fresh, frozen or reconstituted freeze-dried plasma an albumin solution may be used. In the United Kingdom at present, human plasma protein fraction (P.P.F.) is being substituted for freeze-dried plasma. It is a solution containing 95% albumin and is free from the hepatitis virus. In centres where protein colloid is unavailable, too costly or considered undesirable the carbohydrate dextran in saline may be used as an alternative. Some units use dextran 70, others use dextran 110 with a larger average molecular weight and therefore greater persistence in the plasma. The undoubted effectiveness of plasma volume restoration and maintenance by dextran is offset by its relative *in vivo* chemical stability. Its removal from the plasma to the reticulo endothelial system and subsequent slow renal excretion with little metabolic breakdown does not provide the body with either energy or amino acids – as follows from the catabolism of albumin. The albumin solution is however about 20 times more expensive than dextran.

When the main aim of treatment is to restore and maintain the plasma volume at levels which are as near normal as possible (or at above normal levels when red cell destruction is marked) the intravenous infusion of colloidal solutions is undoubtedly more effective than the oral or intravenous administration of isotonic crystalloid solutions (Davies, 1968). With the colloidal solutions the relatively large molecular weight molecules persist in the plasma for longer periods than the ions contained in the crystalloid solutions, which are quickly distributed throughout the extracellular fluid volume. Therapy with crystalloid solutions therefore only increases the plasma volume in proportion to a rise in the extracellular fluid volume. The undesirable effects of a greatly enlarged extracellular fluid volume, presenting as oedema, prompted the use of hypertonic crystalloid solutions by Monafo *et al.* (1973). A recent detailed comparative review of the most commonly used forms of therapy (Davies, 1975a, b) indicates that all forms of therapy result in approximately similar inputs of the sodium ion per kilogram body weight per 1% burn. The total volumes of fluid given are variable but result in most patients receiving therapy which is slightly less than isotonic with respect to the sodium ion. Exceptions are the patients receiving only hypertonic balanced lactate saline solutions. When colloid is considered essential some units treating burned patients give large volumes during the first 24 hours after burning and smaller volumes later (Davies, 1975a) while others give large volumes of crystalloid therapy during the first day and colloid in volumes up to 2 litres during the second 24 h after burning (Baxter, 1974). As it has been shown that most forms of therapy are almost equally effective when controlled by skilled hands there has been a welcome trend in units treating burned patients to select what they consider to be the best form of treatment and then to stick to its use.

Principles of treatment

The following method using a mixture of colloid and crystalloid solutions has been adopted by the Burns Unit of Birmingham Accident Hospital. Patients with burns covering over 10% (children) or 15% (adults) of the body surface receive oral therapy consisting of isotonic bicarbonate saline solution, chilled or with added fruit juice or flavouring to make it more palatable, at hourly intervals in volumes which are about three-quarters of the water input consumed in normal health (Aberdeen, 1961). In addition to this oral input the patients receive intravenously a mixture of equal volumes of electrolyte solution (usually Plasmalyte 148) and colloid. Recently this colloid input has changed from reconstituted freeze dried plasma to H.P.P.F. alone and then (for economic reasons) to alternate bottles of H.P.P.F. and dextran 110. The rate of infusion of the combined colloid plus electrolyte solution is guided by the venous haematocrit for the first 12–16 h and by the rate of urine production subsequently. When vomiting prevents an adequate oral input of salt and water the intravenous component of the crystalloid solution is increased appropriately. The haematocrit of venous or capillary blood is measured as soon as possible after admission to hospital using a high speed centrifuge (10 000 r.p.m. for 5 min).

From values of body height and weight measured on admission to hospital, the expected normal haematocrit, red cell, plasma and blood volume are noted from either a table of normal values (Topley and Jackson, 1957) or calculated from equations described by Nadler *et al.* (1962). The initial plasma volume deficit is calculated from the value of the initial measured haematocrit and the expected normal value for the plasma volume using the following equation:

$$PV \text{ loss} = PV_1 - \frac{PV_1 \times 100 - H_1}{100 - H_N}$$

where H_1 = measured haematocrit value, H_N = expected normal haematocrit value, PV_1 = expected normal plasma volume.

While the infusion of a volume of plasma equal to the calculated plasma volume deficit should increase the plasma volume and thus reduce the haematocrit to the expected normal value, the blood volume will only be restored to its normal value if the red cell volume has remained unchanged. This will not be true if the patient was anaemic prior to burning or shows haemoglobinaemia indicating red cell destruction arising from the direct effect of heat. The continuing loss of plasma may be corrected by the continuous infusion of colloid at rates which may be altered following hourly measurements of the venous haematocrit. The aim of the colloid infusion is to keep the plasma volume normal, and this will be done when the haematocrit is returned to normal in burns covering up to about one third of the body surface. In patients with more extensive burns it should be assumed that some red cell destruction has occurred, the rate of colloid infusion is then adjusted to keep the haematocrit about 10% below the expected normal value. If haemoglobinaemia and haemoglobinuria are present to a significant extent the colloid infusion is adjusted to keep the venous haematocrit about 20% below normal until the transfusion of whole blood or packed red cells returns the subnormal red cell volume to near the expected normal value. The duration of the diminishing rate of plasma and crystalloid infusion may be only 24 hours in patients with burns covering up to one quarter of the body surface, more than 48 hours may be required for burns exceeding two thirds of the body surface.

Volumes of resuscitation fluid when colloid is included

Experience with the above formula to calculate the initial fluid administration and with other criteria to indicate the subsequent fluid requirements suggests the following guide lines:

1. During the first hour after admission to hospital adults receive 60–90 ml colloid per 10% of burn, the lower values are more applicable to patients of lower body weight and the higher values for patients with body weights of over 70 kg. These values are derived from the observed requirements which lie between 1 and 1.5 litres of colloid per 10% of burn in 24 hours, or half these volumes in the first 8 hours after burning. Children receive 0.06 times their normal plasma volume of colloid per 15% of burn derived from the observed requirements expressed as one plasma volume of colloid per 15% of burn in 24 hours, or half this volume during the first 8 h after burning. If the time between burning and admission to hospital is delayed by 2 or 3 hours these inputs may need to be doubled or tripled.

2. During the subsequent few hours the rates of administration of colloid are continued as given initially until the venous haematocrit is returned to normal, or subnormal values if red cell loss is suspected. The rate of colloid administration is then adjusted to keep the venous haematocrit at near constant values until diuresis commences. This is often around the 16th hour in patients with burns of less than 50%, it may be delayed to around the 30th hour with very extensive burns. The urine volume during this period of stabilisation will often lie around 0.5 ml per hour per kg body weight.

3. After the onset of diuresis the rate of administration of colloid and crystalloid is regulated to maintain the rate of urine flow at between 0.5 and 1.0 ml per hour per kg body weight; other physical signs and symptoms and the level of the venous haematocrit are then of less importance.

4. During the second day after burning in patients with burns covering less than 50% of the body surface, or during the third day in the more extensively burned patients the intravenous fluid input can usually be decreased to zero. Concomitantly the oral fluid input is

increased to compensate for the fluid losses in urine, exudate and by evaporation from the burned tissues. It is normally possible to include milk and other nutritious foods in the oral input by the end of the second day.

In circumstances where no protein containing colloid solution is available dextran 110 (or 70) can be used in the same way as just described for plasma. Past experience suggests that smaller volumes of dextran than plasma may be required to satisfy the various clinical criteria described above because of the greater water binding capacity of the dextran.

Volumes of resuscitation fluids when only crystalloid solutions are used

Body weight is the main criterion used in most burn units to control the volumes of crystalloid solutions given. The level of the venous haematocrit is almost always ignored and only a few units make an allowance for the severity of the burn. The method of resuscitation described by Moyer *et al.* (1944 and 1965) recommends the administration of electrolyte solutions by mouth and if necessary also intravenously at a steady rate in volumes which are double those of the patients' water input in normal health (which is weight dependent) and irrespective of the severity of the burn. Most burned patients would then receive between 75 and 150 ml/h. An allowance is made for severity of burning by Baxter (1974) who gives isotonic Ringer's lactate solution intravenously at a steady rate during the first 24 h after burning in volumes which are close to 4 ml per kg body weight per one per cent burn. Only abnormal urine volumes or abnormal clinical signs and symptoms are followed by an appropriate change in the rate of input of the crystalloid solution.

Measurements of central venous pressure made during the period of intensive fluid therapy have been shown to be an unsatisfactory guide to the quantities of fluid given or the rate at which it should be given (Rubin and Bongiovi, 1970).

Aids to the interpretation of the effectiveness of resuscitation

In the Birmingham Burns Unit records of the volumes and nature of the fluids infused, the urine volumes and changes in the venous haematocrit are considered essential for the treatment of patients with extensive burns. These records, kept hour by hour until the end of the phase of intensive care, are plotted on 'shock charts' using different colours to denote different fluids. Patient examples of two such charts are illustrated in Figs 4 and 5. All inputs and outputs are summated at 8 h, 24 h and 48 h after burning. Records should also be kept by the nursing staff of hour by hour assessments of the patient's condition, details of administered drugs and the standard clinical measurements of body temperature, pulse rate, respiration rate and blood pressure. All these records allow an assessment of the progress of resuscitation to be made at any time. During the weeks after burning until the burned area is healed precise records of nutrition, body weight and modes of therapy should also be kept.

Depending upon the facilities and personnel available the following additional measurements aid the treatment of selected patients, particularly those with the most extensive burns.

Urine osmolality

This should be measured on each hourly urine sample if the volume is unexpectedly small or intensely stained with haemoglobin or otherwise appears to have a low solute content. If the osmolality of one or more samples is unexpectedly high tests should be made for carbohydrate. Osmolality measurements are of little use if either dextran or mannitol has been infused since both may be excreted in large amounts in urine. If renal function appears to be adequate by 24 h after burning the urine passed during the second and subsequent days can be pooled into 12 or 24 h samples prior to the measurement of osmolality and the concentrations of urea, sodium, potassium, chloride and creatinine.

Detailed studies by Eklund *et al.* (1970), Eklund (1970a, b) and Settle (1974) have shown that burned patients often show short periods of impaired renal function with urine volumes which may be either high, normal or low and with a solute content which may be normal or low. The combination of low volume and low osmolality is particularly ominous. While short episodes of renal impairment usually resolve spontaneously anuria associated with more severe renal failure has a grave prognosis, in spite of active peritoneal or haemodialysis. Part 1, ch. IV discusses the management of renal failure in more detail.

Red cell volume

Estimates using the radioactive chromate method (Davies, 1960) allow accurate (within ±5%) replacement of those red cells absent from the circulation because of pre-existing anaemia or post-burn losses due to the early direct effect of heat or subsequent red cell destruction. During the first two days after burning the timing and magnitude of these losses

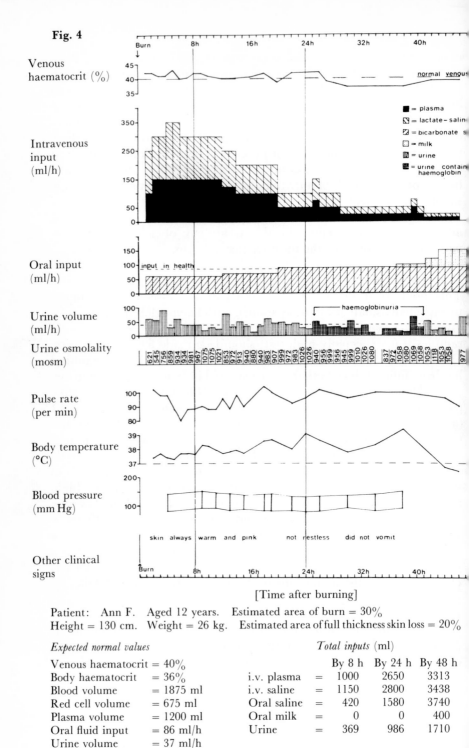

Fig. 4

[Time after burning]

Patient: Ann F. Aged 12 years. Estimated area of burn = 30%
Height = 130 cm. Weight = 26 kg. Estimated area of full thickness skin loss = 20%

Expected normal values

Venous haematocrit = 40%
Body haematocrit = 36%
Blood volume = 1875 ml
Red cell volume = 675 ml
Plasma volume = 1200 ml
Oral fluid input = 86 ml/h
Urine volume = 37 ml/h

Total inputs (ml)

	By 8 h	By 24 h	By 48 h
i.v. plasma =	1000	2650	3313
i.v. saline =	1150	2800	3438
Oral saline =	420	1580	3740
Oral milk =	0	0	400
Urine =	369	986	1710

Fig. 5

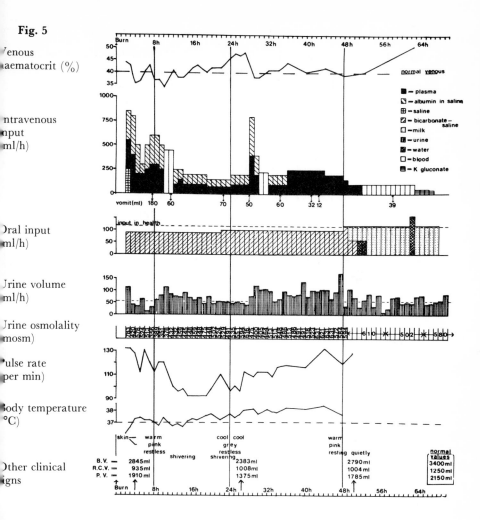

[Time after burning]

Patient: Pat B. Aged 15 years. Estimated area of burn = 55%
Height = 155 cm. Weight = 47 kg. Estimated area of full thickness skin loss = 47%

Expected normal values   *Total inputs* (ml)

			By 8 h	By 24 h	By 48 h
Venous haematocrit	= 40%				
Body haematocrit	= 36%	i.v. plasma =	1650	3325	7525
Blood volume	= 3400 ml	i.v. albumin =	1550	3300	4700
Red cell volume	= 1250 ml	i.v. saline =	250	250	250
Plasma volume	= 2150 ml	Blood =	0	900	1350
Oral input	= 117 ml/h	Oral saline =	540	2000	4400
Urine volume	= 54 ml/h	Oral milk =	0	0	0
		Oral water =	0	0	0
		Urine =	292	1386	3466

of red cells have been described in detail by Topley *et al.* (1962). In occasional patients there is an acute episode of gross red cell destruction causing marked haemoglobinaemia and haemoglobinuria with a marked deterioration in the patients clinical condition, a prompt blood transfusion of adequate volume is then essential. During the subsequent weeks, or months in patients with the most extensive burns the red cell volume steadily falls, the treatment of which may require red cell transfusions at the rate of a litre of blood a week.

Blood acid base balance and oxygen content
These measurements are often of great importance in the treatment of patients who sustained their injury in a confined space. These patients may have inhaled steam or smoke containing a variety of noxious compounds derived from the combustion of material such as furnishing plastics. Patients with burns of the face sometimes develop respiratory obstruction due to laryngeal oedema. The management of patients who require artificially assisted respiration is dealt with in more detail in Part 1, ch. II, and Part 2, ch. V, p. 539.

The transient metabolic acidosis observed in some patients can readily be treated by the administration of sodium bicarbonate solutions.

MEDICAL ASPECTS OF BURN SURGERY

Soon after admission to hospital the patient should be seen by the surgical team who will be responsible for the repair of areas of full thickness skin loss. This repair by excision of the eschar and skin-grafting (usually with autograft but in very extensive burns it may be part autograft and part homograft or heterograft) can take place at any time after burning depending on the extent and depth of the burn and the condition of the patient.

Within a few hours of burning

Surgical repair of the wound at this time is usually confined to the treatment of well defined areas of full thickness and deep partial skin loss which are relatively small in area (a few per cent of the body surface) such as those caused by splashes of molten metal. Medical care of these patients is routine, involving a thorough history and examination, and tests for haemoglobin level and sickle-cell trait in appropriate patients to rule out pre-existing anaemia. Large excisions are usually delayed until after the period of intensive fluid therapy.

Some patients with circumferential burns of the trunk experience difficulty with respiration, or have impaired blood flow in limbs when the coagulated skin contracts and the tissues beneath become oedematous. The relief of shallow respiration or impaired circulation may require decompression incisions through the skin and sometimes the deep fascia. These incisions will be through analgesic tissue in patients with full thickness skin loss burns. Urgent action may also be required in those patients sustaining deep facial burns since oedema may cause marked interference with respiration. An endotracheal tube will ensure an adequate airway for several days, but a tracheotomy may then be needed in spite of the infection hazards involved if the overlying skin is burned. The neck wound will require extraordinary care if infection with *Pseudomonas aeruginosa* is to be avoided.

On the third or fourth day after burning

That is after the period of intensive fluid therapy, extensive excisions and grafting may be carried out involving as much as 20–30% of the body surface. Like the smaller burns these excisions may be down to deep fascia or superficial tangential excisions as described by Janžekovič (1970) and Jackson and Stone (1972). Medical care prior to these operative procedures consists of ensuring that the patients' red cell and plasma volumes are at normal levels and that ample compatible blood is available to cover the anticipated blood loss arising from the excision of the burned and autograft skin. Medical contraindications to surgical procedures at this time after burning include cardiac insufficiency, blood or tissue hypoxia arising from burns affecting any part of the respiratory tract, impaired renal function or grossly infected burned areas. The presence of Group A streptococci is a contraindication to skin grafting and *P. aeruginosa* is a contraindication to both tangential excision and skin grafting.

By the third or fourth day after burning the patient may be at the peak of the hypercatabolic phase which follows all forms of injury and thus in need of adequate (i.e. supranormal) inputs of energy and amino acid nitrogen. These can and should be given intravenously during the period of pre- and postoperative oral starvation using commercially available parenteral nutrient solutions (see Part 1, ch. IX).

By the fourth week after burning

The partial thickness skin loss burns will have healed leaving well defined areas of full thickness skin loss. In patients with very extensive burns the healed partial thickness skin loss burn provides additional autograft donor area. The medical care of the patient during this period is vitally important since not only will metabolic activity be high requiring intensive nutrition, but also the burned area may well become infected with pathogenic microorganisms. Strict barrier nursing, monitoring of the organisms on the burn and appropriate antibiotic therapy are needed to minimise the risk of a fatal septicaemia.

METABOLIC CHANGES OCCURRING DURING THE PROLONGED PHASE OF INTENSIVE CARE

All patients with burns covering more than a few per cent of the body surface show metabolic rates which rise to supranormal levels during the first few days after burning. The observed rates appear to be directly related to the severity of the burn with almost twice normal resting metabolic rates in patients with very extensive burns. This increased metabolic activity will require an increased input of energy-rich materials, if the energy needs are not to be derived from the body stores causing a loss of body weight. The inputs of energy rich materials shown in Table 2 allow for body size and severity of burning and appear to be adequate for patients treated in burn units with environmental temperatures around 22°C. The inputs can be reduced by 25% if the environmental temperature surrounding the patient is maintained above 30°C. While some units prefer (or have to give) the energy inputs shown in Table 2 based entirely on carbohydrate, it is generally considered better treatment if half the energy input is derived from fat and half from carbohydrate.

Unfortunately during this period between burning and operation most patients suffer some degree of anorexia so that their dietary intake may be less than their normal requirements in health (of between 6 and 7 MJ (1450 kcal and 1650 kcal) per day for an adult) and nowhere near

Table 2. Minimal desirable energy inputs per day. (Data taken from Davies and Liljedahl, 1971)

Adults
0.08 MJ (20 kcal) per kg body weight plus 0.30 MJ
(70 kcal) per 1% burn

Children*
0.25 MJ (60 kcal) per kg body weight plus 0.15 MJ
(35 kcal) per 1% burn

---

* Patients up to 25 kg in body weight

their actual requirements which may exceed 10 MJ (2400 kcal) per day in patients with burns covering about one-third of the body surface or 15 MJ (3600 kcal) per day in patients with burns covering over 75% of the body surface. Marked losses of body weight can then only be limited by alternative modes of nutrition.

A high protein, high energy diet given as a steady slow infusion down a fine bore nasogastric tube is often effective and will ensure in most patients that their net input is near to that considered desirable. Allison and Woolfson (1976) have found the high protein high energy solution given in Table 3 a useful oral supplement.

The limit to the usefulness of a high protein high energy oral input may be offset by nausea, vomiting or diarrhoea, all of which can significantly reduce the net input. If these conditions persist or are associated with an intermittent ileus, adequate nutrition may then only be possible using the intravenous route. Intravenous nutrition using a peripheral vein can provide 0.84 MJ (200 kcal) per litre of fluid administered using 5% glucose solution and 8.4 MJ (2000 kcal) per litre using the fat emulsion Intralipid – 20%. Markedly hypertonic

Table 3. General purpose tube feed based on a glucose polymer (Caloreen[R]) and milk protein (Complan[R]) as described by Allison and Woolfson (1976)

Nutrient	Weight	Non-protein energy	Protein	Nitrogen	Sodium	Potassium
Caloreen	250 g	4.2 MJ (1000 kcal)	—	—	—	—
Complan	300 g	4.5 MJ (1070 kcal)	60 g	9.6 g	46 mmol	53 mmol
Totals	550 g	8.7 MJ (2070 kcal)	60 g	9.6 g	46 mmol	53 mmol

The Caloreen/Complan mixture is normally made up to 3 litres with water, but only two litres may be used if large water inputs are contraindicated. More sodium or potassium may be added as clinically indicated. Patients with extensive burns require high energy and nitrogen intakes as shown in Tables 2 and 4. Provided the same proportions of energy to g nitrogen are observed the amounts of Caloreen and Complan may be increased to the limit of tolerance of the patient. There is sufficient fat in Complan to prevent fatty acid deficiency. The vitamin, mineral and trace element content are probably sufficient for most patients.

The feed is given down a fine bore Ryles tube (8 or 10 FG, unless the 550 g of feed are diluted in only 2 litres of water when a larger bore tube may be required to ensure an adequate flow of the higher viscosity fluid) by continuous drip at half strength during the first 24 h and thereafter at full strength. Diarrhoea may be induced by a too rapid rate of infusion. It may also be induced by the use of broad spectrum antibiotics. The symptom can be controlled by codeine phosphate syrup 60–120 mg daily. The occasional symptom of nausea in the early stages can be controlled by Maxolon.

Caloreen[R] – Milner Scientific and Medical Research Co., Liverpool, U.K. Complan[R] – Glaxo-Farley Food, Plymouth, Devon, U.K.

solutions of glucose (25 or 50%) can provide a greater carbohydrate energy input in a smaller administered fluid volume but their administration requires the use of a central venous catheter and may require the simultaneous infusion of substantial quantities of insulin (Allison *et al.*, 1968), (see Part 1, ch. IX, p. 263).

In most burned patients however the role of intravenous nutrition is that of a supplementary input. While its use may sometimes be lifesaving particularly in patients with the most extensive burns, the maintenance of a patient intravenous line for many weeks requires intensive care of a very high quality. This is particularly true if the site of entry of the cannula is through burned tissue which may become infected. The risk of cannula blockage is not small when the fluids passing through it are as diverse as fat emulsions, solutions of carbohydrates, amino acids, electrolytes and blood.

Two methods may be used to assess whether a patient is receiving adequate nutrition. The simpler method depends on frequent measurements of body weight. With adequate nutrition weight losses of less than 5% of that on admission to hospital should be attainable in patients with burns covering up to 50% of the body surface. Weight losses of up to 10% may sometimes be inevitable in very extensively burned patients during periods of bacteraemia or septicaemia. The main limitation to the use of body weight measurements is uncertainty concerning the contribution made by accumulations of fluid. Certainly during the first week after burning oedema is prevalent in most patients since much of the fluid given during the first 48 h after burning remains in tissues. Due to this, body weights are often 20% above normal by 48 h after burning and only return to normal some 7–10 days later. A more precise method of controlling nutritional needs comes from measurements of resting metabolic rate using standard spirometric methods to determine oxygen consumption. The energy production implied by the observed value of the resting metabolic rate can be calculated from the patient's age, body height and body weight (to give body surface area). An adequate energy input can then be assured if the measured energy production in a 24 hour period is followed by an input of energy-rich materials during the next 24 hours in amounts which would in theory at least offset the energy produced during the previous day.

The optimal input of amino acid nitrogen cannot be determined by reference to the urinary nitrogen excretion because of recycling within the body. Apparently adequate nitrogen inputs allowing for body size and severity of burning are shown in Table 4. Whatever input of amino

Table 4. Daily desirable inputs of protein (or as nitrogen). (Data taken from Davies and Liljedahl, 1971)

Adults

1 g protein per kg body weight plus 3–4 g protein per 1% burn

Children*

3 g protein per kg body weight plus 1 g protein per 1% burn

As nitrogen

Adults 0.06 g per kg body weight plus 0.20–0.25 g per 1% burn
Children* 0.20 g per kg body weight plus 0.06 g per 1% burn

---

* Patients up to 25 kg body weight

acid nitrogen is attained it is essential that sufficient energy-rich materials are provided to give optimal utilisation of the administered amino acid nitrogen. The energy to nitrogen ratio should be at least 0.84 MJ (200 kcal) per g of nitrogen.

Normal body heat production is balanced by heat loss by radiation, convection and conduction. In hot environments these routes of heat loss may be insufficient to prevent a rise in body temperature and thus the onset of sweating. In contrast in cold environments body heat loss by these routes may be excessive which is corrected by shivering thermogenesis. The conversion of skin to a freely water permeable state by heat ensures that a burned patient is in a state of 'uncontrolled sweating'. The appearance of exudate on the skin surface is followed by evaporation of water unless the environmental humidity is saturated with water. As the latent heat of evaporation of water is approximately 2.42 MJ (580 kcal) per litre the drain on a patient's rate of heat production, if he provides all the energy, will be at this rate for every litre of water lost by evaporation. Studies in a series of patients treated by the exposure method have shown that the evaporative water loss is approximately 0.30 ml/cm^2 (or 3 litres/m^2) of burned area per day (Davies *et al.*, 1974). The actual area of the burn can be calculated from its percentage area multiplied by the actual body surface area (m^2) derived from body height and weight and standard tables (e.g. DuBois and DuBois, 1916), see also Part 1, ch. VII, p. 169, Table 11.

The increased heat requirements associated with this evaporative water loss may initiate persistent shivering unless the patient is kept very warm. Measurements made in burn units where the temperature of the patient's room can be controlled by the patient indicates that extensively burned patients treated exposed are only comfortable at environmental temperatures above 30°C. At these high room temperatures the ambient relative humidity should be maintained below 25% to ensure that the patient's burned areas remain dry enough to limit the growth of bacterial contaminants, and to provide acceptable working conditions for nursing and medical staff.

Many studies have demonstrated the beneficial effects of treating burned patients in warmer environmental conditions (Barr *et al.*, 1968, 1969; Wilmore *et al.*, 1975). The patients show metabolic rates, rates of body protein catabolism and dietary energy inputs which are reduced nearly to normal values. They show significantly smaller losses of body weight and their general clinical condition appears much improved over that observed in patients treated in a cooler (22°C) environment (Davies *et al.*, 1969). More recent studies suggest that treating patients beneath infrared heaters, the heat output from which can be controlled by the patients, makes it possible to eliminate the hypermetabolism which is seen in burned patients treated by all other methods (Danielsson *et al.*, 1976; Liljedahl, 1976). This method of directing the heat energy onto the patient saves the expense of heating the whole room and ensures that the medical and nursing staff have more comfortable environmental conditions.

The large evaporative water losses shown by extensively burned patients requires treatment with large daily inputs of water. An approximate guide to these requirements can be calculated from the equations given above (of 3 litres per m² of burned area per day) plus 1.5–2.0 litres per day for urine production in adults or 1 litre in children. Many patients will therefore require water inputs of at least 5 litres per day to prevent dehydration. The daily urine volume will be a reasonable guide to the adequacy of the water input except in patients with impaired renal function.

The control of the patient's electrolyte balance may be difficult. The very large amounts of sodium given in the first 48 hours after burning, often amounting to a 50% increase in body content acts as a reservoir for the losses of this ion in exudate and urine. The daily exudate losses appear to be fairly constant until full thickness burns are grafted, or show a steady decline as partial thickness burns heal. In contrast the daily urine losses of sodium are variable. Over the first two to three weeks after burning the cumulative losses of sodium in urine and exudate may exceed 150 mmol per day when the burned area covers about one third of the body surface and may exceed 250 mmol per day in patients with very extensive burns. Such losses will initially come from the raised body content but must later be replaced by a similar daily input if hyponatraemia is to be avoided. A substantial daily input of potassium (at least 100 mmol per day for an adult, and less in proportion to body weight in children) is required during the weeks following burning to offset the early (and continuing) losses by leakage from heat damaged cells.

OTHER ASPECTS OF THE INTENSIVE CARE OF PATIENTS WITH EXTENSIVE BURNS

Infection

It is standard practice in many burn units to give protection against tetanus by a 'booster' injection of toxoid if the patient is already actively immunised. Non-immunised patients should have Human Antitetanus Globulin (A.T.G.) or protection by systemic antibiotics (Erythromycin or Cloxacillin).

There is some divergence of opinion concerning the need for topical antibacterial agents applied to the burned surface. In small burn units where patients can be nursed in single bedded rooms with sufficient nursing personnel to ensure that cross-infection can be controlled, even patients with burns covering over 80% of the body surface have been nursed to recovery without the application of any topical antibacterial agents to the burned surface (Davies et al., 1977). In the larger burn units it is more difficult to control cross infection mainly because of a lower nursing staff to patient ratio. As a single infected patient can be a reservoir from which other extensively burned patients may acquire a potentially lethal infection, barrier nursing and topical antibacterial agents are required if episodes of septicaemia are to be minimised. Many antibacterial agents have been applied to burned tissue with varying degrees of effectiveness. The most recent effective agents are Sulfamylon (mafenide) (Moncrief et al., 1966; Lowbury and Jackson, 1970), 0.5% silver nitrate (Moyer et al., 1965; Cason et al., 1966; Lowbury and Jackson, 1968), silver sulfadiazine (Stanford et al., 1969; Lowbury et al., 1971a, b) and cerium nitrate (Monafo et al., 1977). These agents are more effective for prophylaxis than therapy so invasive infections should be treated with systemic antibiotics appropriate to the sensitivity of the organisms.

CONCLUSIONS

The duration of intensive care required by a patient with burns depends on the severity of the burn.

(a) Burns covering up to 10% (children) or 15% (adults) of the body surface will usually only require intensive care if the burns are complicated by damage to the eyes, hands, kidneys or the respiratory tract.

(*b*) All patients with burns of greater severity will require intensive care for at least 24 h and for at least 48 h if the burn covers more than one third of the body surface. The intensive care of these patients during this time will be mainly concerned with the control of fluid resuscitation.

(*c*) Patients with burns covering over 50% of the body surface and some of lesser area may continue to require intensive care for weeks, and those with burns covering more than 70% of the body surface for months if they are to survive their injury.

During these weeks and months of intensive care it will be necessary to keep a very close watch on metabolism and nutrition, fluid and electrolyte balances including the requirements for blood, and the harmful effects of pathogenic organisms contaminating the burn wound both before and after the application of autograft skin.

ACKNOWLEDGEMENTS

The clinical management of patients with burns described in this chapter is that of the Birmingham Burns Unit under the direction of the surgeon in charge Mr D. M. Jackson. The author acknowledges with gratitude the helpful comments, assistance and advice given by both Mr Jackson and Dr J. P. Bull, director of the M.R.C. Industrial Injuries and Burns Unit.

REFERENCES

Aberdeen, E. (1961). Average fluid values and electrolyte needs: an introduction to a 'guessing chart'. *Lancet* **1**, 1024.

Allison, S. P., Hinton, P. and Chamberlain, M. J. (1968). Intravenous glucose tolerance, insulin and free-fatty-acid levels in burned patients. *Lancet* **2**, 1113.

Allison, S. P. and Woolfson, A. M. J. (1976). Personal communication.

Artz, C. P. (1971). The Brooke formula. *In* 'Contemporary Burn Management' (Ed. H. C. Polk and H. H. Stone) pp. 43–52. Little, Brown & Co., Boston.

Barr, P.-O., Birke, G., Liljedahl, S.-O. and Plantin, L.-O. (1968). Oxygen consumption and water loss during treatment of burns with warm dry air. *Lancet* **1**, 164.

Barr, P.-O., Birke, G., Liljedahl, S.-O. and Plantin, L.-O. (1969). Studies on Burns. X. Changes in B.M.R. and evaporative water loss in the treatment of severe burns with warm dry air. *Scand. J. Plast. Reconstr. Surg.* **3**, 30.

Baxter, C. R. (1974). Fluid volume and electrolyte changes of the early postburn period. *Clinics in Plast. Surg.* **1**, 693.

Birke, G. and Liljedahl, S.-O. (1968). The influence of different types of early treatment on the prognosis of severe burns. *Ann. N.Y. Acad. Sci.* **150**, 711.

Bull, J. P. and Lennard-Jones, J. E. (1949). The impairment of sensation in burns and its clinical application as a test of the depth of skin loss. *Clin. Sci.* **8**, 155.

Bull, J. P. (1971). Revised analysis of mortality due to burns. *Lancet* **2**, 1133.

Burke, J. F. and Constable, J. D. (1965). Systemic changes and replacement therapy in burns. *J. Trauma* **5**, 242.

Cason, J. S. (1959). Report on three extensive industrial chemical burns. *Brit. Med. J.* **1**, 827.

Cason, J. S., Jackson, D. M., Lowbury, E. J. L. and Ricketts, C. R. (1966). Antiseptic and aseptic prophylaxis for burns: Use of silver nitrate and of isolators. *Brit. Med. J.* **2**, 1288.

Danielsson, U., Arturson, G. and Wennberg, L. (1976). The elimination of hypermetabolism in burned patients: a method suitable for clinical use. *Burns* **2**, 110.

Davies, J. W. L. (1960). A critical evaluation of red cell and plasma volume techniques in patients with burns. *J. clin. Path.* **13**, 105.

Davies, J. W. L. (1968). Blood volume changes and sodium distribution in patients with burns. *Ann. N.Y. Acad. Sci.* **150**, 659.

Davies, J. W. L. (1975a). The fluid therapy given to 1027 patients during the first 48 hours after burning. I. Total fluid and colloid output. *Burns* **1**, 319.

Davies, J. W. L. (1975b). The fluid therapy given to 1027 patients during the first 48 hours after burning. II. The inputs of sodium and water and the tonicity of therapy. *Burns* **1**, 331.

Davies, J. W. L., Liljedahl, S.-O. and Birke, G. (1969). Protein metabolism in burned patients treated in a warm (32°C) or cool (22°C) environment. *Injury* **1**, 43.

Davies, J. W. L. and Liljedahl, S.-O. (1971). 'Contemporary Burn Management' (Ed. H. C. Polk and H. H. Stone) pp. 151–169. Little, Brown & Co., Boston.

Davies, J. W. L., Lamke, L.-O. and Liljedahl, S.-O. (1974). A guide to the rate of non-renal water loss from patients with burns. *Brit. J. Plastic Surg.* **27**, 325.

Davies, J. W. L., Lamke, L.-O. and Liljedahl, S.-O. (1977). Metabolic studies during the successful treatment of three adult patients with burns covering 80–85% of the body surface. *Acta chir. scand. Suppl.* *468*, 25–60.

DuBois, D. and DuBois, E. F. (1916). Clinical calorimetry: a formula to estimate the approximate surface area if height and weight is known. *Arch. intern. Med.* **17**, 863.

Eklund, J., Granberg, P.-O. and Liljedahl, S.-O. (1970). Studies on renal function in burns. I. Renal osmolal regulation, glomerular filtration rate and plasma solute composition related to age, burned surface area and mortality probability. *Acta chir. scand.* **136**, 627.

Eklund, J. (1970a). Studies on renal function in burns. II. Early signs of impaired renal function in lethal burns. *Acta chir. scand.* **136**, 735.

Eklund, J. (1970b). Studies on renal function in burns. III. Hyperosmolal states in burned patients related to renal osmolal regulation. *Acta chir scand.* **136**, 741.

Jackson, D. M. and Stone, P. A. (1972). Tangential excision and grafting of burns. *Brit. J. Plastic Surg.* **25**, 416.

Janžekovič, Z. (1970). A new concept in the early excision and immediate grafting of burns. *J. Trauma* **10**, 1103.

Lawrence, J. C. and Bull, J. P. (1976) Thermal conditions which cause skin burns. *Eng. Med.* **5**, 61.

Liljedahl, S.-O. (1976). Personal communication.

Lowbury, E. J. L. and Jackson, D. M. (1970). Further trials of chemoprophylaxis for burns. *Injury* **1**, 204.

Lowbury, E. J. L. and Jackson, D. M. (1968). Local chemotherapy for burns with gentamicin and other agents. *Lancet* **1**, 654.

Lowbury, E. J. L., Jackson, D. M., Ricketts, C. R. and Davis, B. (1971a). Topical chemoprophylaxis for burns: Trials of creams containing silver sulphadiazine and trimethoprim. *Injury* **3**, 18.

Lowbury, E. J. L., Jackson, D. M., Lilly, H. A., Bull, J. P., Cason, J. S., Davies, J. W. L. and Ford, P. M. (1971b). Alternative forms of local treatment for burns. *Lancet* **2**, 1105.

Lund, C. C. and Browder, N. C. (1944). The estimation of areas of burns. *Surg. Gynec. Obstet.* **79**, 352.

Markley, K., Bocanegra, M., Bazan, A., Temple, R., Chiappori, M., Morales, G. and Carrion, A. (1956). Clinical evaluation of saline solution therapy in burn shock. *J. Amer. Med. Ass.* **161**, 1465.

Markley, K., Bocanegra, M., Bazan, A., Temple, R., Chiappori, M., Morales, G. and Carrion, A. (1959). Clinical evaluation of saline solution therapy in burn shock. II. Comparison of plasma therapy with saline. *J. Amer. Med. Ass.* **170**, 1633.

Mellins, R. B. and Park, S. (1975). Respiratory complications of smoke inhalation in victims of fires. *J. Pediat.* **87**, 1.

Monafo, W. W. (1970). The treatment of burn shock by the intravenous and oral administration of hypertonic lactated saline solutions. *J. Trauma* **10**, 575.

Monafo, W. W., Chuntrasakul, C. and Ayvazian, V. H. (1973). Hypertonic sodium solutions in the treatment of burn shock. *Amer. J. Surg.* **126**, 778.

Monafo, W. W., Tandon, S. N., Ayvazian, V. H., Tuchschmidt, J., Skinner, A. M. and Deitz, F. (1976). Cerium nitrate—new topical antiseptic for extensive burns. *Surgery* **80**, 465.

Monafo, W. W., Ayvazian, V. H. and Skinner, A. M. (1977). Control of infection in major burn wounds by cerium nitrate/silver sulphadiazine. *Burns* **3**, 104.

Moncrief, J. A., Lindberg, R. B., Switzer, W. E. and Pruitt, B. A. (1966). Use of topical antibacterial therapy in the treatment of the burn wound. *Archs. Surg.* **92**, 558.

Moyer, C. A., Brentano, L., Gravens, D. L., Margraf, H. W. and Monafo, W. W. (1965). Treatment of large human burns with 0.5% silver nitrate solution. *Archs. Surg.* **90**, 812.

Moyer, C. A., Coller, F. A., Iob, V., Vaughan, H. H. and Marty, D. (1944). A study of the interrelationship of salt solutions, serum and defibrinated blood in the treatment of severely scalded anaesthetized dogs. *Ann. Surg.* **120**, 367.

Nadler, S. B., Hidalgo, J. U. and Bloch, T. (1962). Prediction of blood volume in normal human adults. *Surgery* **51**, 224.

Reiss, E., Stirman, J. A., Artz, C. P., Davis, J. H. and Amspacher, W. H. (1953). Fluid and electrolyte balance in burns. *J. Amer. Med. Ass.* **152**, 1309.

Rubin, L. R. and Bongiovi, J. (1970). Central venous pressure – an unreliable guide to fluid therapy in burns. *Archs. Surg.* **100**, 269.

Settle, J. A. D. (1974). Urine output following severe burns. *Burns* **1**, 23.

Stanford, W., Rappole, B. W. and Fox, C. L. (1969). Clinical experience with silver sulfadiazine. A new topical agent for control of pseudomonas infection in burns. *J. Trauma* **9**, 377.

Topley, E. and Jackson, D. M. (1957). The clinical control of red cell loss in burns. *J. clin. Path.* **10**, 1.

Topley, E., Jackson, D. M., Cason, J. S. and Davies, J. W. L. (1962). Assessment of red cell loss in the first two days after severe burns. *Ann. Surg.* **155**, 581.

Wallace, A. B. (1951). The exposure treatment of burns. *Lancet* **1**, 501.

Ward, M. (1974). Frostbite. *Brit. Med. J.* **1**, 67.

Wilmore, D. W., Mason, A. D., Johnson, D. W. and Pruitt, B. A. (1975). Effect of ambient temperature on heat production and heat loss in burn patients. *J. Appl. Physiol.* **38**, 593.

Section 8: The Management of Electrical and Lightning Injuries

GILLIAN C. HANSON

INTRODUCTION

Approximately 1000 people die yearly in the United States from electrical current excluding lightning and more than 100 people are killed and 300 people injured by lightning. About 12 people a year are struck by lightning in Britain.

Electric current of 1000 volts or less is considered low tension current and above 1000 volts, high tension current. High tension wires usually carry alternating current of high voltage and amperage. Alternating current is more dangerous than direct current of similar intensity. As the number of cycles is increased in an alternating current, the danger decreases, since muscle and nerves are less sensitive to high frequencies. Domestic 50 H (G.B.) and 60 H (U.S.A.) alternating current is likely to affect the respiratory centre and heart. The degree of tissue damage in an electric injury is proportional to the intensity of the current which passes through the body.

$$\text{Amps (intensity)} = \frac{\text{Volts}}{\text{Resistance}} \quad \text{(tension or potential difference)}$$

The lightning strike is a complex strike with different constituent parts. The leader forms a path from cloud to earth, followed by the main return stroke discharging along the same path in the opposite direction. There may be as many as 40 successive current peaks of 10 000–200 000 amps occurring within a fraction of a second, with a potential difference of up to 20 million volts.

467

The resistance of body tissues to the flow of a current is variable and in order of decreasing magnitude is: bone, fat, tendon, skin, muscle, blood and nerve.

The tissue damage produced in an electric or lightning injury may be the result of any one, or a combination of three mechanisms – (1) electrical heating producing a thermal burn, (2) electric current passing through the body, leaving entrance and exit areas of coagulative necrosis, and (3) the effects of an electric arc when high voltage sparks bridge the gap between the conductor and the body.

PATHOPHYSIOLOGY

In low tension injuries the victim often becomes locked to the contact. Low tension burns are generally of the contact type and rarely is there damage to the brain, heart or other viscera. The only low tension burn which may create urgent complications is that involving the mouth and face.

In high tension accidents, locking to the contact is uncommon and the patient may be thrown away from the contact developing serious injuries. In this group systemic complications are common (Table 1) and most of the patients are rendered unconscious. The most severe local lesions which have a higher incidence of complications are found in the pathway of greatest resistance, i.e. from hand to hand, or from hand to foot, while current flow through the lowest resistance pathway (in and out of the same extremity) causes less serious damage. Detection of the inflow and outflow sites in a patient admitted with electrical or lightning injury is important, since knowledge of the current pathway will enable one to suspect areas which may be damaged.

In accidents where the current passes through the head, injury is generally confined to the scalp and skull. These patients may however sustain severe brain damage requiring artificial ventilation and may die several days later secondary to coagulative necrosis or cerebral vessel thrombosis (Skoog, 1970).

EMERGENCY TREATMENT

Advice on management will be confined to the immediate care and no attempt will be made to discuss the treatment of long-term complications.

If a group of people are struck by lightning, some may be stunned but continue spontaneous ventilation and a few may fall unconscious, become pulseless and stop breathing. Generally the apnoea and cardiac

Table 1. Urgent complications which may arise following an electrical or lightning injury

Cardiac	Ventricular fibrillation
	Cardiac dysrhythmias including bradyarrhythmias
Respiratory	Respiratory arrest
	Oral and nasal burns producing oedema and airway obstruction
	Pulmonary aspiration
	Pulmonary contusion
Central	Loss of consciousness – respiratory arrest
nervous	Convulsions
system	Cerebral oedema
	Subarachnoid or intracerebral haemorrhage
Bone	Fractures
	Dislocation of joints
	Lesions of the cervical spine producing quadraplegia
Bowel	Gastrointestinal dilatation – vomiting and fluid loss
	Gastric haemorrhage
Deep tissues	Muscle necrosis and soft tissue oedema – producing loss of intra-vascular volume.
Skin	Second and third degree burns with fluid loss
Blood vessels	Vessel occlusion with subsequent tissue and muscle necrosis
Kidneys	Tubular necrosis
Metabolic	Metabolic acidosis
	Depletion of intravascular volume
	Exposure hypothermia

arrest is temporary. Persons who are apnoeic should not be taken as dead but mouth to mouth resuscitation and external cardiac massage should be instituted immediately. Patients who have sustained severe lightning injury appear to withstand prolonged periods of apnoea (Ravitch *et al.*, 1961; Nesmith, 1971). Taussig (1968) postulated that after lightning strike, the cessation of metabolism in all cells is so instantaneous that the onset of degenerative processes is delayed.

Cardiac resuscitation

On arrival at hospital, full resuscitation should be instituted (refer to Part 2, ch. I). The patient should be intubated and hand ventilated and the cardiac activity assessed. Ventricular fibrillation should be cardioverted with d.c. shock. Cardiac asystole is relatively common and is regarded by some workers as a sequel of severe irritation of the vagus nerve (Lynch and Shorthouse, 1949). Intracardiac adrenaline may stimulate pulsation or precipitate ventricular fibrillation which can be

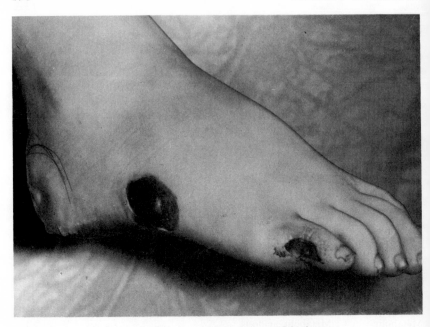

Fig. 1. Current exit sites on the little toe and lateral aspect of the foot.

treated by d.c. shock. A severe bradyarrhythmia should be treated with intravenous isoprenaline. After initial cardiac resuscitation – assessment of the site of current inflow and outflow (Fig. 1) and the area of the body affected by flashburns (Fig. 2), will give some indication of the organs and tissues that are likely to have been damaged (Fig. 3). The myocardium may be affected by lightning or electrical injury leading to either contusion or muscle fibre necrosis. The myocardial damage which generally shows an infarct pattern on the E.C.G. (Fig. 4) may be associated with cardiac dysrhythmias and these should be appropriately treated. Hanson and McIlwraith (1973) reported a high level of catecholamines in a child suffering from lightning injury. A persistent tachycardia may therefore justify the use of a β-adrenergic blocking agent.

Respiratory resuscitation

Cardiac arrest may be complicated by pulmonary aspiration. Gastric dilatation and ileus has been noted in patients with lightning injury;

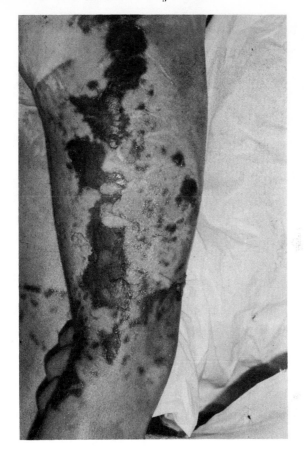

Fig. 2 Lightning injury, flash burns over the right flank.

this predisposes the patient to aspiration (Hanson and McIlwraith, 1973). Maintenance of the airway is therefore vital in the unconscious patient; the stomach should be drained and 15 ml of 0.3 molar sodium citrate put down the tube after aspirating to dryness. Evidence of lung contusion, pulmonary aspiration or cerebral oedema secondary to hypoxia, is an indication for intubation and ventilation. Cerebral oedema is an indication for hyperventilation; a pulmonary end expiratory pressure should be used if there is evidence of aspiration (see Part 2, ch. V, p. 568). Extensive burns to the mouth and lips may necessitate a tracheostomy.

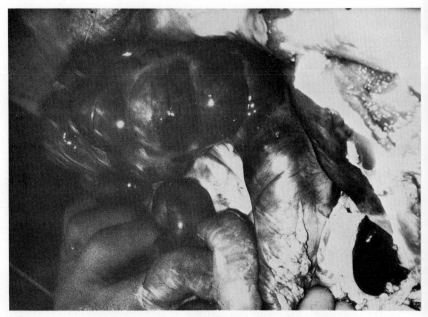

Fig. 3. Post mortem appearances of the ascending colon following lightning shock. Severe bruising presumably due to blast injury.

Metabolic and fluid control

The unpredictable damage to muscle, bone, tendons, subcutaneous fat and other deep tissues, makes clinical estimation of fluid volume loss impossible. It has been recommended in electrical injuries that the volume of fluid required is estimated by multiplying the extent of the surface injury by three if under 20% and by two or less as the extent of the surface injury increases (Baxter, 1970).

Volume requirements can be more accurately gauged by monitoring the central venous pressure. The fluid used should preferably contain protein, such as purified protein fraction or dried plasma, or blood in the case of blood loss. Because of damage to vessels and the danger of arterial thrombosis, the haematocrit should be maintained around 30%. Skin and core temperature should be taken early. Exposure hypothermia is common and may be one of the factors producing a refractory cardiac dysrhythmia or persistent metabolic acidosis. A severe metabolic acidosis is common – probably due to acid washout from the devascularised tissue, however the decrease in pH

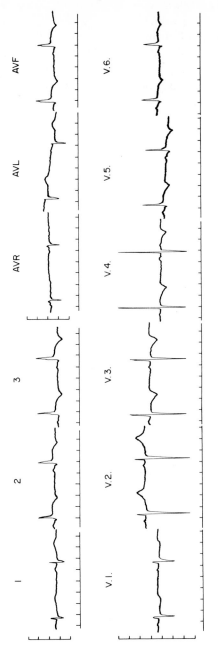

Fig. 4. Electrocardiographic changes in a child 12 years, four days following a lightning injury.

does not necessarily correlate with the extent of injury. Astrup analyses should be performed 2–4 hourly after a severe lightning or electrical injury since a pH which is at first normal may fall several hours later. Sodium bicarbonate should be given according to the Astrup analysis, correcting to a base deficit of 8.

Acute renal failure may be a complication and is commonly associated with myoglobinuria (Yost and Holmes, 1974). Mannitol (0.2 g/kg B.W. infused over 2–3 min) should be infused routinely once the central venous pressure is normal; should myoglobinuria be detected, more aggressive mannitol therapy is indicated. Kay and Boswick (1973) recommend 5–10 g of mannitol infused hourly over several days – given in conjunction with careful electrolyte and fluid volume control.

Nervous system management

The significance of cerebral oedema after electro-trauma has been emphasised by Jellinek (1928); his findings suggest that it can develop rapidly. Cerebral oedema should be managed along the usual lines (see p. 407), intubation and ventilation is indicated if there is respiratory

Table 2. Summary of urgent management of a patient suffering from electrical or lightning injuries

System involved	Treatment
Cardiac	
Cardiac arrest	Treatment of cardiac arrest
Supraventricular tachycardia	Consider β-blockade if persistent
Respiratory	
Respiratory arrest	Ventilation
Lung contusion	If severe for artificial ventilation
Aspiration	Artificial ventilation with P.E.E.P.
Metabolic and fluid volume	
Metabolic acidosis	Sodium bicarbonate
Fluid volume depletion	P.P.F. or plasma, or blood
	Maintain Hct at 30%
Hypothermia	Slowly rewarm
Gastrointestinal	
Stomach	Aspirate – put down 15 ml 0.3 molar sodium citrate
Gastric haemorrhage	? Surgery

depression secondary to the use of drugs for control of convulsions. Electro-trauma may be complicated by cerebral or subarachnoid haemorrhage – sequestial neurological examinations are therefore important. Respiratory depression may be secondary to injury of the cervical spine.

Gastrointestinal

'Electro-ileus' and bowel contusion is well documented. Intestinal ulceration and bleeding may necessitate emergency surgery. Should surgery be necessary there is apparently a high incidence of complications which may gravely affect the ultimate prognosis (Kay and Boswick, 1973).

Soft tissue and muscle injury

Vascular occlusion secondary to oedema in an extremity affected by an electrical injury, is fairly common. If an escharotomy does not restore the distal circulation, then a fasciotomy is indicated. Burn injuries to the mouth may require urgent surgery in order to stop bleeding from the labial artery.

Sepsis

Prophylactic antibiotics are not indicated. Deep necrotic areas should be debrided early to prevent the onset of anaerobic sepsis.

ELECTRICAL OR LIGHTNING INJURY IN THE PREGNANT MOTHER

Foetal maceration and death has been reported (Rees, 1965). Electrical or lightning injuries in the pregnant mother may be complicated by 'premature' onset of labour (Chan and Sivasamboo, 1972), or even rupture of the uterus (Samsoenario, 1959).

SUMMARY

The immediate management of a patient suffering from severe lightning or electrical injuries has been described, this is summarised in Table 2. Subsequent management has been discussed in considerable detail by Kay and Boswick (1973), Skoog (1970) and Sturim (1971).

REFERENCES

Baxter, C. R. (1970). Management of major electrical injury. *Surg. Clin. N. Amer.* **50**, 1401.

Chan, Y. W. and Sivasamboo (1972). Lightning accidents in pregnancy. *J. Obstet and Gynec.* **79**, 761.

Hanson, G. C. and McIlwraith, G. (1973). Lightning injury: two case histories and a review of management. *Brit. Med. J.* **4**, 271.

Jellinek, S. (1928). Über die Heilwirkung der Lumbalpunktion bei schweren elektrischen Unfällen. *Wein, klin. Wschr.* **41**, 622.

Kay, N. R. M. and Boswick, J. A., Jr. (1973). The management of electrical injuries of the extremities. *Surg. Clin. N. Amer.* **53**, 1459.

Lynch, M. J. G. and Shorthouse, P. H. (1949). Injuries and death from lightning. *Lancet* **I**, 473.

Nesmith, M. A. (1971). A case of lightning stroke. *J. Florida Med. Assoc.* **58**, 36.

Ravitch, M. M., Lane, R., Satar, P., Steichen, F. M. and Knowles, P. (1961). Lightning stroke. Report of a case with recovery after cardiac massage and artificial respiration. *New Engl. J. Med.* **264**, 36.

Rees, W. D. (1965). Pregnant woman struck by lightning. *Brit. Med. J.* **I**, 103.

Samsoenario (1959). Rupture of a pregnant uterus by a lightning strike. *Madj. Kedokt. Indonesia* **9**, 420.

Skoog, T. (1970). Electrical Injuries. *J. Trauma* **10**, 816.

Sturim, H. S. (1970). The treatment of electrical injuries. *J. Trauma* **11**, 959.

Taussig, H. B. (1968). 'Death' from lightning – and the possibility of living again. *Ann. Int. Med.* **68**, 1345.

Yost, J. W. and Holmes, F. F. (1974). Myoglobinuria following lightning stroke. *JAMA* **228**, 1147.

IV

The Management of Infection

Section 1: Infection and the I.T.U.

J. C. STODDART

INTRODUCTION

In a short chapter it is impossible to do more than summarise an extensive subject, but the most important points will be emphasised. Every patient who is admitted to an intensive therapy unit is at risk both from his underlying disease and because of the methods of treatment employed. It has been recognised for many years that infection with gram negative organisms is a particular problem for such patients. There are several reasons for this. In the first place, it is believed that major physical trauma interferes with the normal immune response to infection (Alexander, 1968; Miller *et al.*, 1973). Secondly, manipulations which destroy the continuity of mucous membranes and muco-cutaneous junctions such as catheterisation, intubation, tracheostomy and many surgical manoeuvres increase the likelihood of local infection (Lowbury *et al.*, 1970; Gaya, 1976).

Probably more important than either of these is the well recognised fact that hospitalisation causes the bacterial population of the patient's gastrointestinal tract to change (Gaya, 1976). The bacteria listed in Table 1 are those which are most frequently incriminated in intensive therapy unit infection and sepsis, with Pseudomonas and Klebsiella being the most important.

477

Table 1. Organisms responsible for
gram negative infections

E. coli	Proteus
Pseudomonas	Enterobacter
Klebsiella	Bacteroides

These organisms, which are normally found in the human gastrointestinal tract are usually of low virulence. It is essential to realise that the
identification of one or more of them from secretions is not automatically an indication for the use of antibiotics, for in many cases they are
commensals (Price and Sleigh, 1970; Burns, 1973). Finally, the
widespread use of broad spectrum antibiotics, which are more effective
against gram positive organisms, and the use of other antibiotics in
inadequate dosage, increases the likelihood that an antibiotic-resistant
gram negative bacterial flora will emerge. This last point will be
mentioned again later.

CROSS-INFECTION

The concentration of critically ill, dependent patients in a confined
space can obviously lead to disastrous cross-infection and every
intensive therapy unit must have a policy aimed at its prevention. In the
first instance this means there must be enough well trained nurses so that
they do not have to move between patients without time for handwashing and if necessary, garment changing (Kominos et al., 1972).

Casual visitors to the unit must be discouraged, and all visitors made
to wear clean gowns and shoe covers. Patients who present a risk to
others, such as those with infected burns, discharging fistulae etc., or
who are at risk themselves because of depression of their immune
response due to disease or drugs (corticosteroids, azothioprine etc.)
should be nursed in isolation. Equipment which has been used and
which could become infected must be cleaned and sterilised before
being re-used. Ventilators, humidifiers and suction units are particularly likely to become contaminated (Phillips and Spencer, 1965;
Cartwright and Hargreave, 1970). They should be bacteriologically
checked at short intervals while in use and sterilised after use.

These and other inanimate sources of infection are listed in Table 2.

The sterilisation of ventilators may be a difficult problem since many
have very complex valve systems and devious gas pathways. The more

Table 2. Sources of infection

Taps, sinks, overflows
Ventilators, humidifiers, nebulisers
Suction apparatus
Air conditioning units
Tubes of lubricating jelly
Food stuffs, food mixers, water jugs
Local anaesthetic solutions, stock bottles
Detergent and antiseptic solutions
Intravenous solutions and intravenous catheters

complex gas driven devices such as the Bird and the Bennett are probably best sterilised with ethylene oxide gas. The more simple machines such as Cape and the Engstrom can be readily sterilised either with ethylene oxide, formaldehyde or hydrogen peroxide vapour. The Radcliffe and similar machines are usually sterilised by the use of liquid antiseptics such as glutaraldehyde. The subject has been reviewed recently (Lumley, 1976). Although it is difficult to substantiate cross-infection or auto-reinfection from ventilators and humidifiers the risk is such that these machines should be monitored bacteriologically at least twice each week while in use and replaced by sterile machines as often as possible during long-term ventilation. Lumley and her co-workers (Holdcroft et al., 1973; Lumley et al., 1976) make out a very good case for the routine use of heated bacterial filters on both the inspiratory and expiratory gas pathways. Although most of these filters are very efficient it is important to recognise that failure can occur and the use of such filters does not relieve the medical attendant of the responsibility of bacteriological monitoring.

Wash-hand basins may be particularly difficult to clean and sterilise and in particular the overflow and wastepipes may be persistently colonised. It is possible to heat the outflow and U-bend from wash-hand basins (Econa Products Limited, Solihull, Warwickshire) so that pathogenic organisms do not grow. Unfortunately such waste traps tend to emit an unpleasant smell. It is not certain that such sites are an important source of infection but a wash-hand basin has been incriminated in at least one outbreak (Teres et al., 1973). The faucet may also become infected and it should be monitored regularly and heated to red heat with a plumber's blow torch if contamination is identified.

Intravenous infusion fluids and intravenous catheters have also been found to give rise to serious systemic infections, both bacterial and fungal (Freeman and King, 1972; Goldman *et al.*, 1973; Editorial, 1974). This can only be minimised if all such equipment is inserted with an aseptic technique and thereafter handled with great care (see p. 256). When intravenous cathers are removed it is usual for the tip or the entire catheter to be sent for bacteriological examination. Frequently fibrin is noted to be adherent to the tip of the catheter. In many such cases bacteria are isolated. It is difficult to evaluate the significance of this finding (Freeman and King, 1975). If the patient has systemic sepsis the responsible organism will almost invariably be found in the catheter tip. This does not mean that the catheter was the originator of the infection. However, if the systemic infection is caused by a common skin commensal such as *Staphylococcus aureus* or *S. albus* or if no other source for the infection can be found the catheter must bear the blame. In most intensive therapy units, if a patient develops pyrexia while an indwelling venous catheter is in place and no other source can be incriminated it is usual to remove the catheter (see also p. 257).

Drugs should not be added to intravenous infusion bottles nor injected into intravenous lines unless absolutely essential, and then only with the appropriate precautions. Drip sets must be changed every 24 h and because the infusion fluid may become contaminated, any which remains after 8 h should be discarded.

AUTOGENOUS INFECTION

It was stated earlier that the natural habitat of the organisms involved was the human gastrointestinal tract, and it is now widely believed that auto-infection plays an important role in the very sick patient (Stoddart, 1974; Gaya, 1976). Access from the gastrointestinal tract to other sites is gained via soiled linen, skin transfer, vomitus and other secretions.

The prevention of this route of infection is very difficult. It is impossible to sterilise the gut, even if sufficient time is available, although encouraging results have been reported (Goldring *et al.*, 1975). The nursing staff must be taught how to minimise the risk by keeping the patient and his bedding clean at all times, changing dressings when indicated, discouraging the patient from touching himself and always washing their hands thoroughly after performing wound or rectal toilet. It is probable that the use of rectal thermometers increases the risk of gram negative infections particularly if the unit is busy and the nursing staff rushed. This practice should therefore be abandoned in favour of other systems (Part 2, ch. II, p. 312).

THE ANTIBIOTIC PROBLEM

Gram negative infection is a major problem because of the relative effectiveness of antibiotics against gram positive organisms. However, there are good grounds for believing that a contributory cause of gram negative sepsis is the use of broad spectrum antibiotics either prophylactically or for the treatment of bacteriologically unidentified fevers. A further cause is the use of the correct antibiotic in inadequate dosage. Such therapy causes the resident bacterial flora to change and allows resistant strains to emerge (Editorial, 1970; Lowbury *et al.*, 1970; Price and Sleigh, 1970; Bryant *et al.*, 1972; Garrod, 1972; Stoddart, 1974; Darrell and Uttley, 1976; Gaya, 1976). Price and Sleigh abolished a persistent Klebsiella infection from a neurosurgical unit by stopping all prophylactic antibiotics. In another survey (Editorial, 1970) 64% of 76 patients who developed Pseudomonas infections had been receiving broad spectrum antibiotics.

The isolation of an organism from the body does not necessarily mean that significant sepsis is present. As the result of a survey of patients in a chest unit, Burns (1973) established that Pseudomonas was acting as an acute pathogen in only 5 out of 63 patients with positive cultures.

One of the most difficult tasks in medicine today is to decide if a patient has a significant bacterial infection and to identify its cause. Tests such as the limulus plasma assay (Levin *et al.*, 1970) and the nitroblue tetrazolium test (Park *et al.*, 1968; Freeman and King, 1972) are neither widely available nor generally acceptable and the institution of antibiotic therapy has to be determined by the clinician's overall assessment of the situation. Obviously if a patient has a positive blood culture and is acutely ill, there is no difficulty, but when a patient has a lingering pyrexia and is potentially at risk it is tempting to give an antibiotic without awaiting bacterial confirmation.

Many intensive therapy units have an antibiotic policy which is based upon experience of the type of infection patients bring into the unit and its site of origin. This should be reviewed from time to time and in any case antibiotic treatment should be changed as soon as the offending organism is identified.

There are few real indications for the use of prophylactic antibiotics. Vascular surgery on the lower limbs carries a hazard of clostridial infection and penicillin may be given prophylactically for 48 h. Other indications are debatable and in no case should a broad spectrum antibiotic be given prophylactically.

If a patient develops the clinical signs of gram negative septicaemia

then a pre-selected regime of treatment may be embarked upon
provided that blood and secretions are taken for culture before its
commencement. If antibiotics have been given before the appearance of
these signs the chances of obtaining bacteriological identification are
negligible.

REFERENCES

Alexander, J. W. (1968). Neutrophil function in selected surgical disorders. *Ann. Surg.*
   168, 447.
Bryant, L. R., Trinkle, J. K. and Mobin-Uddin, K. (1972). Bacterial colonization
   profile with tracheal intubation and mechanical ventilation. *Arch. Surg.* **104**, 647.
Burns, M. W. (1973). Significance of pseudomonas in sputum. *Brit. Med. J.* **2**, 382.
Cartwright, R. Y. and Hargreave, P. R. (1970). Pseudomonas in ventilators. *Lancet* **1**,
   40.
Darrell, J. H. and Uttley, A. H. C. (1976). Antibiotics in the perioperative period. *Brit.
   J. Anaesth.* **48**, 13.
Editorial (1970). Prophylactic antibiotics. *Lancet* **2**, 1231.
Editorial (1974). Microbiological hazards of intravenous infusion. *Lancet* **1**, 543.
Freeman, R. and King, B. (1972). Infective complications of intravenous catheters and
   the monitoring of infections by the nitroblue tetrazolium test. *Lancet* **1**, 992.
Freeman, R. and King, B. (1975). Isolations of aerobic spore bearing bacilli from the
   tips of indwelling intravascular catheters. *J. Clin. Path.* **2**, 28, 146.
Garrod, L. P. (1972). Causes of failure of antibiotic therapy. *Brit. Med. J.* **2**, 473.
Gaya, H. (1976). Infection control in intensive care. *Brit. J. Anaesth.* **48**, 9.
Goldman, D. A., Martin, W. T. and Workington, J. W. (1973). Growth of bacteria and
   fungi in total parenteral nutritional solutions. *Am. J. Surg.* **129**, 314.
Goldring, J., Scott, A., McNaught, W. and Gillespie, G. (1975). Prophylactic oral
   antimicrobial agents in elective colonic surgery. *Lancet* **2**, 997.
Holdcroft, A., Lumley, J. and Gaya, H. (1973). Why disinfect ventilators? *Lancet* **1**, 240.
Kominos, D. S., Copeland, C. E. and Grosiak, B. (1972). Mode of transmission of
   Pseudomonas aeruginosa in a burns unit and an intensive care unit in a general
   hospital. *Appl. Microbiol.* **23**, 309.
Levin, J., Poore, T. E., Zanbert, N. B. and Oser (1970). Detection of endotoxin in
   human blood. *New Eng. J. Med.* **283**, 1313.
Lowbury, E. J. L., Thorn, B. T., Lilly, H. A., Babb, J. R. and Whitall, K. (1970).
   Sources of infection with Pseudomonas aeruginosa in patients with tracheostomy.
   J. Med. Microbiol. **3**, 39.
Lumley, J. (1976). Decontamination of anaesthetic equipment and ventilators. *Brit. J.
   Anaesth.* **48**, 3.
Lumley, J., Holdcroft, A., Gaya, H., Darlow, H. M. and Adams, D. J. (1976).
   Expiratory bacterial filters. *Lancet* **2**, 22.
Miller, R. W., Polakavetz, S. U., Horrick, R. B. and Cowley, R. A. (1973). Analysis of
   infections acquired by the severely injured patient. *Surg. Gynec. Obstet.* **137**, 1, 7.
Park, B. N., Fikrig, S. M. and Smith, E. M. (1968). Infection and nitroblue tetrazolium
   reduction by neutrophils. *Lancet* **2**, 532.

Phillips, I. and Spencer, G. (1965). Pseudomonas aeruginosa cross infection due to contaminated respiratory apparatus. *Lancet* **2**, 1325.

Price, D. J. E. and Sleigh, J. D. (1970). Control of infection due to Klebsiella aerogenes in a neurosurgical department by withdrawal of all antibiotics. *Lancet* **2**, 1213.

Stoddart, J. C. (1974). Gram negative infection in the I.C.U. *Critical Care Medicine* **2**, 1, 17.

Teres, D., Schweers, P., Bushnell, L. S., Hedley-Whyte, J. and Feingold, D. S. (1973). Sources of Pseudomona aeruginosa infection in a respiratory/surgical intensive therapy unit. *Lancet* **1**, 415.

Section 2: The Management of Infections of the Nervous System

J. M. OXBURY

The infections of the central nervous system can be subdivided into meningitis, abscess and encephalomyelitis. Many cases require specialist neurological or neurosurgical care, though treatment may be initiated outside specialist units.

MENINGITIS

The commonest bacterial causes of meningitis in the United Kingdom are *Neisseria meningitidis*, *Streptococcus pneumoniae* and *Haemophilus influenzae*. They are responsible for the large majority of adult and childhood cases. Pneumococcal meningitis predominates amongst the elderly in the United Kingdom, but not necessarily elsewhere. Haemophilus predominates amongst children. The organisms commonly responsible for neonatal meningitis are *E. coli*, Proteus, Pseudomonas, Streptococci and Staphylococci. The other common cause of meningitis is virus infection particularly due to mumps and enteroviruses. Less common causes of meningitis include: Mycobacterium tuberculosis; Streptococci (other than Pneumococcus) and Staphylococci, especially following head injury, or in association with sinusitis and ear infections, or secondary to ruptured intracerebral abscess; Listeria monocytogenes; *Cryptococcus neoformans*; syphilis.

Meningitis typically presents as an acute febrile illness with severe headache, vomiting, photophobia and neck stiffness. The progress can be very rapid, especially with meningococcal and pneumococcal meningitis, producing death within hours. Examination usually reveals neck stiffness and a positive Kernig's sign, but the latter may be absent as, indeed, may the former, particularly in neonates and the elderly.

484

The patient may be delirious, drowsy or comatose. Cranial nerve palsies may occur but signs of focal cerebral hemisphere involvement are unusual and, if present, suggest the possibility of cerebral abscess or focal encephalitis. These various features apply to all forms of acute meningitis. Occasionally the clinical presentation may give some indication of the aetiology. A petechial or purpuric rash suggests the possibility of meningococcal meningitis, but similar rashes sometimes occur in viral meningitis. Choroidal tubercles indicate a tuberculous origin.

Cerebrospinal fluid examination

Lumbar puncture at a very early stage is mandatory. The number and type of cells should be determined, the protein and glucose content should be estimated and the latter should be compared with that of a blood specimen obtained at the same time as the lumbar puncture, a gram-stained film should be examined by an experienced bacteriologist, a Ziehl–Neelson preparation should be similarly examined if there is any possibility of tuberculosis, and appropriate cultures should be set up. The C.S.F. contents vary according to the aetiology of the meningitis (see Table 1). Typically the pyogenic meningitides (most commonly meningococcal, pneumococcal and *Haemophilus influenzae*) produce a purulent C.S.F. which is turbid and contains thousands of white cells, predominantly polymorphs. Meningococci and pneumococci are usually visible on the gram-stained preparation and the C.S.F. glucose is usually absent or markedly reduced compared to the blood level. However, the picture may be confused if the patient has been partially treated with antibiotics before being admitted to hospital; then the cell count may be lower, there may be a greater proportion of lymphocytes, and organisms may not be detected on microscopic examination. When the cells are predominantly lymphocytes, particularly in a patient who has not received antibiotics, the main differential diagnosis is between viral meningo-encephalitis, cerebral abscess and tuberculous meningitis. Examination of Ziehl-Neelson preparations may detect the presence of acid-fast bacilli, and establish the diagnosis of tuberculous meningitis, but several examinations may be required before they are found. This should be confirmed (but only after several weeks) by the results of culture. If the clinical picture and the C.S.F. suggest tuberculous meningitis but acid-fast bacilli are not detected, it is wise to administer anti-tuberculous chemotherapy at least initially. When the patient has focal cerebral signs or epileptic seizures

Table 1. Cerebrospinal fluid in C.N.S. infections

Condition	Cells (per mm³)	Protein (mg/100 ml)	Sugar	Microscopy
Meningococcal meningitis	$2-10 \times 10^3 +$ 95% polys.	200 – 400 +	Usually ↓ or absent	Intra- and extracellular gram negative diplococci
Pneumococcal meningitis	$2-10 \times 10^3 +$ 95% polys.	200 – 400 +	Usually ↓ or absent	Gram positive diplococci
H. influenzae meningitis	$2-10 \times 10^3 +$ 95% polys.	200 – 400 +	Usually ↓ or absent	May appear 'sterile'
Tuberculous meningitis	Up to 400 mostly lymphos.	Up to 400 +	Usually ↓	Acid-fast bacilli on Ziehl-Neelson
Cerebral abscess	Up to 200 mostly lymphos.	Usually <200	Normal	'Sterile'
Viral meningitis (e.g. mumps)	Up to 1000 mostly lymphos.	Normal or slightly ↑	May be ↓	'Sterile'
Herpes simplex encephalitis	Up to 1000 mostly lymphos. but also polys.	Up to 500	Normal	'Sterile'

with a predominantly lymphocytic pleocytosis in the C.S.F., the possibility of cerebral abscess and herpes simplex virus encephalitis must be considered and a specialist neurological opinion should be obtained with a view to neuroradiological investigation.

If the diagnosis remains in doubt, other possibilities should be considered including: infection outside but in proximity to the meninges (e.g. paravertebral abscess, epidural abscess), brucellosis, leptospirosis, cryptococcus, Behcets, sarcoid, etc.

Treatment

The planning of an effective antibiotic regime depends upon rapid and accurate bacteriological diagnosis. In what follows the doses recommended are (unless otherwise stated) for adults and they must be modified for children. Severely ill patients from whom turbid C.S.F. is obtained should be given intrathecal crystalline penicillin 10 000–20 000 units at the initial lumbar puncture without awaiting bacterial diagnosis. The dose of intrathecal penicillin should never exceed 20 000 units because there is a considerable risk of dangerous side effects.

Meningococcal meningitis
The treatment should commence with benzyl-penicillin 2–4 mega units 4-hourly administered by intravenous bolus injection. The total daily dose should not exceed 24 mega units and particular care should be taken in patients with renal failure because of the danger of a penicillin-induced encephalopathy. (Intravenous cephaloridine 1 g 6 hourly should be given to patients allergic to penicillin; renal function must be carefully monitored especially in patients in whom it is already impaired.) The treatment may be changed to sulphonamides (sulphadiazine 1–2 g 6 hourly) if the organism is shown to be sensitive. Patients with meningococcal meningitis may suffer severe pain in the head and neck and they may be extremely agitated. It is important that they be heavily sedated and given adequate analgesia with chlorpromazine, sodium amytal and codeine phosphate as necessary. Vital functions must be monitored closely and care taken to maintain the airway.

Meningococcal septicaemia may produce severe shock (Waterhouse–Friderichsen syndrome) with profound hypotension, tachycardia, a petechial rash and thrombocytopoenia, all at a stage before meningeal signs become apparent. The administration of intravenous hydrocortisone 500 mg stat. followed by 500–1000 mg 4 hourly may be life saving. The value of heparin in combating the consumption coagulopathy is less certain.

Pneumococcal meningitis
Benzyl-penicillin 2–4 mega units should be given every 2–4 h by intravenous bolus injection as with meningococcal meningitis, and patients who are allergic to penicillin should be given cephaloridine 1 g intravenously every 6 h. Intrathecal penicillin (pure crystalline) 10 000–20 000 units may be given at the initial lumbar puncture if the C.S.F. is turbid. The dangers in the use of cephaloridine and intrathecal penicillin have been mentioned previously (p. 487).

Haemophilus influenzae *meningitis*
The treatment of choice lies between intravenous ampicillin 150–400 mg/kg body weight/24 h in 6 divided doses, and chloramphenicol given to children in doses of 100 mg/kg body weight/24 h in 4 divided doses. The disadvantages of ampicillin is that some strains of *Haemophilus influenzae* are insensitive and these are becoming more common. The disadvantage of chloramphenicol is the occasional complication of agranulocytosis.

Pyogenic meningitis of undetermined aetiology
In thirty per cent of cases of acute pyogenic meningitis the responsible organism cannot be established on the initial gram stain. Opinions differ as to the most satisfactory initial antibiotic regime for such patients. In children there is a considerable chance that *Haemophilus influenzae* is responsible so it is reasonable to use chloramphenicol (100 mg/kg body weight/24 h in 4 divided doses) together with benzyl-penicillin (6–12 mega units per day in divided doses) even though this has the theoretical disadvantage of combining a bacteriostatic and a bactericidal agent. Alternatively, ampicillin (loading dose of 50 mg/kg body weight followed by 150 mg/kg body weight/24 h intravenously in 6 divided doses), possibly combined with cloxacillin (1 g 6 hourly by intravenous injection) may be used.

Tuberculous meningitis
Treatment should be started with three antituberculous drugs combined (streptomycin 0.5–1.0 g/day intramuscularly, isoniazid 100 mg 8 hourly with pyridoxine 10 mg and rifampicin 450–600 mg is a satisfactory regime). Isoniazid 50 mg and streptomycin 50 mg may be

administered intrathecally. The patient should be transferred to a unit specialised in the management of tuberculous meningitis.

Viral meningitis
No specific chemotherapy is available for viral meningitis and treatment is simply supportive. Sedation with chlorpromazine and amytal may be necessary and headache may need treatment with codeine phosphate. The prognosis is usually good. It is worth checking that the patient has been immunised against poliomyelitis.

CEREBRAL ABSCESS

Abscesses may be situated either within the substance of the brain, subdurally over the brain, or epidurally in relation to the brain or the spinal cord. Such abscesses require specialist neurological or neuro-surgical care and their management will not be discussed in detail.

The possibility of an intracerebral abscess should be considered if the symptoms of meningitis (headache, vomiting, impaired consciousness and delirium) are accompanied by epilepsy, evidence of focal cerebral damage (e.g. hemiparesis, hemisensory impairment, hemianopia, aphasia or papilloedema), or if there is a predisposing cause for cerebral abscess such as local infection (middle ear, mastoid, nasal sinus), septicaemia particularly secondary to intrathoracic infection, or a history of skull fracture. When intracerebral abscess is suspected, lumbar puncture should be delayed until an urgent specialist neurological or neurosurgical opinion has been obtained. Of the more readily available investigations an isotope brain scan is as good as any for detecting a cerebral abscess although no doubt this will be replaced by computerised axial tomography.

VIRAL ENCEPHALOMYELITIS

The viral encephalomyelitides can be broadly divided into 2 groups. In one the virus invades and multiplies in the central nervous system, e.g. Herpes simplex, poliomyelitis, rabies, coxsackie A and B, and echo viruses.

In the other form encephalitis appears to arise from an immune response without direct invasion of nerve tissue by the virus, e.g. mumps, acute measles encephalitis, chicken pox, influenza.

In general, encephalitis produces manifestations of diffuse brain disease arising acutely or subacutely. There is drowiness and mental confusion, often progressing to coma. Epileptic seizures are common and the cerebrospinal fluid usually shows a pleocytosis especially with lymphocytes.

Herpes simplex virus encephalitis requires special mention as it is the most commonly recognised cause of sporadic encephalitis in the United Kingdom. It is an acute focal necrotising encephalitis with a very poor prognosis. During the prodromal phase of the illness, lasting a few days, there is headache, fever, general malaise and vomiting. This is followed by the neurological phase characterised by epileptic seizures, mental confusion, impaired consciousness and signs of focal cerebral hemisphere dysfunction particularly aphasia and mild hemiparesis. There is usually a C.S.F. pleocytosis involving lymphocytes more than polymorphs but the C.S.F. can be normal even in fulminating cases. The presence of pathology in one or both temporal lobes may be revealed by carotid angiography, computerised axial tomography or less reliably by isotope brain scans.

Although specific chemotherapy has been attempted with both idoxuridine and cytosine arabinoside there is little to indicate that either is effective. The epilepsy should be controlled with adequate doses of anticonvulsants. Approximately 50% of patients die within one month of the onset and autopsy reveals severe cerebral oedema.

Raised intracranial pressure

Cerebral oedema should be treated with intravenous infusions of mannitol 20% solutions, 400 ml administered in 2 h once every 24 h and followed by frusemide 40–80 mg i.v. 4 h later and 12 h later. A careful watch must be kept on electrolytes but the blood urea may be allowed to rise to 20–30 mmol/l as the patient becomes dehydrated. Dexamethasone, so valuable in the control of cerebral oedema caused by tumours, seems ineffective in the treatment of focal encephalitis.

Section 3: The Management of Established Tetanus

J. H. KERR

INTRODUCTION

Widespread immunisation is making tetanus an increasingly rare disease, but the management of a severe case still represents an enormous therapeutic challenge. When a patient first presents with tetanus, it is not possible to predict with any certainty the ultimate severity of the attack, although, in general terms, the more rapid the appearance and progression of the symptoms, the more widespread, severe and prolonged are they likely to be. An interval of less than two days between the appearance of the first symptom and that of the first generalised spasm augers badly, although a considerably longer onset period is no guarantee that severe symptoms may not follow. Patients can be categorised as mild, moderate or severe (Table 1) only when the disease is fully developed and hence it is prudent to treat all patients as potentially severe cases.

Consideration should be given to the possible transfer of the tetanus patient to a regional centre in which a continuing experience of the disease has been maintained. Patients may be moved with least risk soon after diagnosis but must be accompanied by a physician skilled and equipped to deal with generalised or laryngeal spasms. If there appears to be a chance that these symptoms may be provoked during transfer, the patient should be intubated before departure and sedated, paralysed and artificially ventilated during the journey.

DIAGNOSIS AND GENERAL THERAPEUTIC MEASURES

Tetanus should be suspected in any patient who presents with trismus and local or generalised muscle stiffness, especially if symptoms appear

Table 1. Symptoms, treatment and classification of tetanus

Symptoms	Specific treatment	Retrospective classification of severity

Trismus
Increased muscle
  tone
	Diazepam
	  (Chlorpromazine)
		Mild

Dysphagia Laryngeal spasms	Tracheostomy	Moderate

Severe generalised
  muscle spasms
	Therapeutic
	  paralysis and
	  I.P.P.V.
		Severe

Autonomic
  disturbances
	Anti-adrenergic
	  therapy	

within a few weeks of injury. The symptoms of phenothiazine sensitivity may present a similar picture although they respond rapidly to an injection of an anti-Parkinsonian drug such as benztropine (1–2 mg).

Treatment in tetanus is essentially symptomatic but all patients with the disease should receive antibiotics, active and passive immunisation and undergo wound excision. In order to detect the appearance of severe muscular or laryngeal spasms, they should be nursed in a well-lighted intensive therapy unit rather than placed in a darkened side-room. Treatment with penicillin (1 mega unit 6 hourly i.m.) or tetracycline (100 mg 6 hourly i.m.) should be commenced as early as possible to ensure that all Clostridia are killed. Human antitetanus immunoglobulin (e.g. Wellcome Humotet 3000–10 000 units i.m.) should be administered since it avoids the anaphylactic side effects that often followed the horse antisera and because it remains active in the circulation for much longer. If a focus of infection is found, surgical debridement should be carried out shortly after administration of the antitoxin so that any toxin released into the circulation at surgery is neutralised. An attack of tetanus does not confer immunity so that active immunisation with a full course of absorbed toxoid injections should be given during the recovery period.

SYMPTOMATIC MEASURES

Muscular hypertonicity

The trismus and increased muscle tone of the mild case of tetanus can usually be controlled adequately with diazepam (10 mg 3–4 hourly orally or parenterally), but the dose and frequency of administration may have to be increased if spasms appear. Chlorpromazine has also been widely and effectively employed against these symptoms.

Dysphagia and airway management

Trismus is a common early symptom in tetanus and is frequently accompanied by inco-ordination of the swallowing and laryngeal protective reflexes. Correct management of the airway is of crucial importance because lethal laryngeal spasm may occur spontaneously or be induced by attempts to swallow saliva or to pass a naso-gastric tube. In addition, inhalation of infected material from the mouth will produce atelectasis and pneumonia; the latter remains a common cause of death in tetanus.

To minimise pulmonary complications, protection of the airway by intubation with a cuffed tube is advocated as soon as dysphagia is suspected. The symptom may be demonstrated as a tendency to cough and clear the throat after swallowing a mouthful of water, and, in more advanced form, as an inability to swallow saliva so that the patient drools or spits it out. Oro-tracheal intubation should be performed after induction of general anaesthesia with thiopentone (250–400 mg i.v.) and after muscle relaxation with suxamethonium (75–100 mg i.v.), which acts normally even in the presence of severe trismus. Tracheostomy with a cuffed tube should be carried out electively with full sterile precautions and meticulous pulmonary care instituted and maintained until normal pharyngo-laryngeal function returns.

Muscle spasms

Muscle spasms in tetanus can be either localised or generalised and of varying severity. Sustained contraction of the muscles is exhausting, painful and, if the respiratory muscles become involved, dangerous. When large doses of diazepam or Chlorpromazine are employed in attempts to control severe spasms, over-sedation produces hypoventilation between spasms. In this situation, and when muscle spasms themselves interfere with ventilation, therapeutic paralysis with curare (15–30 mg i.m. or i.v.) and I.P.P.V. is indicated. Curare is given sufficiently frequently to allow ventilation to proceed freely and to keep the patient comfortable. The results of this treatment have improved prognosis when used early in the disease rather than after prolonged attempts to manage the patient with sedative agents. Smythe *et al.*

(1974) have reported remarkable success in neonates with similar techniques.

Once curarisation and I.P.P.V. have commenced, anxiety in the conscious but paretic patient should be minimised by frequent reassurance from the nursing staff and by mild hypnosis from diazepam (10 mg 4–6 hourly i.m. or down the naso-gastric tube) or pentobarbitone (100 mg 6–8 hourly down the naso-gastric tube). Some of the most severe cases, however, become unresponsive and appear comatose for periods of 1–3 weeks during the critical phase of their illness. They recover consciousness during the recovery phase and appear normal apart from amnesia. In these patients sedative agents and muscle relaxants should be kept to a minimum (Kerr et al., 1974). During recovery, curare requirements decrease and treatment with diazepam may be re-instituted to reduce muscle stiffness during weaning from I.P.P.V.

Over the few days after the withdrawal of curare, patients should be encouraged to resume spontaneous ventilation for gradually increasing periods of time. These should be limited to 10–15 min initially to avoid exhaustion and a full night's sleep on the ventilator should be allowed until weaning is complete. The ventilator may safely be dispensed with once the patient can achieve a vital capacity of 1.5–2 litres and he can sleep comfortably without artificial ventilation. If available, a ventilator which permits intermittent mandatory ventilation (I.M.V.) may be employed to ease the transition between controlled and spontaneous ventilation, although few problems are normally encountered with this group of patients.

Nutrition

Patients with mild tetanus may be fed orally but once dysphagia develops a naso-gastric tube should be inserted while the patient is anaesthetised for tracheostomy. The considerable caloric (approximately 2500 cal/day) and fluid requirements of the tetanus patient can be satisfied effectively over the 2–4 week period of dysphagia by naso-gastric feeding and, since tube feeds normally contain milk, the chance of gastro-intestinal bleeding is reduced. Paralytic ileus occurs fairly frequently in severe tetanus but it usually responds to intermittent gastric drainage followed by the instillation of antacids and gut stimulants (e.g. metoclopramide).

Fluid balance

Fluid balance must be carefully maintained since overhydration will increase the likelihood of pneumonia, while underhydration may lead to deep venous thrombosis and subsequently to pulmonary embolism, another common cause of death in tetanus. Complete fluid balance studies, which include daily weighing of the patient, indicate that insensible fluid losses, especially from sweating and loss of saliva, may total several litres each day. Tetanus patients sweat most profusely during the second and third weeks of the disease and particularly at night, when several changes of bedding may be required. Enough i.v. or naso-gastric fluid should be given to produce a daily urine output of at least 1.5–2 litres and to maintain the urine specific gravity at or below 1.015. Daily weighing is desirable although some loss of weight is to be expected because of tissue catabolism especially in curarised patients.

Although anticoagulation with warfarin has been carried out in some tetanus units without serious complications (Kerr *et al.*, 1968), avoidance of dehydration is an equally valuable prophylactic measure against pulmonary embolism.

Cardiovascular complications

Autonomic disturbances occur frequently in severely affected tetanus patients and may be fatal. Younger patients often develop a fluctuating hypertension and increasing tachycardia after a few days of treatment. Exaggerated responses to tracheal suction, high cardiac outputs with reduced oxygen extraction, high metabolic rates in paralysed patients and raised serum and urine catecholamine levels suggest that the sympathetic nervous system is overactive and have been followed by cardiac dysrhythmias, peripheral vasoconstriction and unresponsive hypotension (Keilty *et al.*, 1968; Kerr *et al.*, 1968; Corbett *et al.*, 1969). The addition of adrenergic blocking agents to conventional treatment has been advocated (Prys-Roberts *et al.*, 1969) and promising results reported after its use from several centres (e.g. Lazar, 1970; Kanarek *et al.*, 1973).

In the presence of an unexplained and persistent tachycardia, propranolol (5–20 mg 4–8 hourly) should be given down the naso-gastric tube and, if hypertension persists, bethanidine (5–20 mg 6–8 hourly) should be added. For the emergency treatment of cardiac dysrhythmias, practolol (1–5 mg i.v.) is recommended rather than intravenous propranolol.

Elderly patients, however, may have a transient hypertensive phase lasting 1–4 days before the appearance of episodes of profound hypotension, which may be rapidly fatal if coronary perfusion proves inadequate. These episodes differ from classical shock in that the blood pressure, pulse rate and central venous pressure fall rapidly together, the patient remains warm and well perfused and urine flow continues. They usually occur in association with coma and become less common when consciousness is regained. The cardiovascular status can be improved temporarily but repeatedly if endogenous catecholamine release is induced by stimuli such as vigorous passive movements of the limbs, aspirating secretions from the trachea, and increasing the arterial carbon dioxide level. In these circumstances, sedative agents, analgesics and muscle relaxants raise the threshold level of stimulation required to produce an increase in blood pressure and should therefore be administered only if clearly indicated (Corbett *et al.*, 1973; Kerr *et al.*, 1974).

Continuous direct monitoring of cardiovascular variables is recommended to allow rational therapy for the different autonomic complications which may occur. Long acting sedative or antiadrenergic agents should be avoided in elderly patients to permit the radical change of treatment which becomes necessary if hypotension develops.

REFERENCES

Corbett, J. L., Kerr, J. H., Prys-Roberts, C., Crampton Smith, A. and Spalding, J. M. K. (1969). Cardiovascular disturbances in severe tetanus due to overactivity of the sympathetic nervous system. *Anaesthesia* **24**, 198.

Corbett, J. L., Spalding, J. M. K. and Harris, P. J. (1973). Hypotension in tetanus. *Brit. Med. J.* **3**, 423.

Kanarek, D. J., Kaufman, B. and Zwi, S. (1973). Severe sympathetic hyperactivity associated with tetanus. *Arch. Int. Med.* **132**, 602.

Keilty, S. R., Gray, R. C., Dundee, J. W. and McCullough, H. (1968). Catecholamine levels in severe tetanus. *Lancet* **2**, 195.

Kerr, J. H., Corbett, J. L., Prys-Roberts, C., Crampton Smith, A. and Spalding, J. M. K. (1968). Involvement of the sympathetic nervous system in tetanus. *Lancet* **2**, 236.

Kerr, J. H., Travis, K. W., O'Rourke, R. A., Sims, J. K. and Uhl, R. R. (1974). Autonomic complications in a case of severe tetanus. *Amer. J. Med.* **57**, 303.

Lazar, M. (1970). Zur pathogenese and therapie des tetanus. *Schweiz. Med. Wschr.* **100**, 1486.

Prys-Roberts, C., Corbett, J. L., Kerr, J. H., Crampton Smith, A. and Spalding, J. M. K. (1969). Treatment of sympathetic overactivity in tetanus. *Lancet* **1**, 542.

Smythe, P. M., Bowie, M. D. and Voss, T. J. V. (1974). Treatment of tetanus neonatorum with muscle relaxants and intermittent positive pressure ventilation. *Brit. Med. J.* **1**, 223.

Section 4: The Management of Gas Forming and Anaerobic Infections and Dermal Gangrene

GILLIAN C. HANSON

INTRODUCTION

Gas forming infections may be produced by strict anaerobes or facultative anaerobes. Anaerobes are organisms using bound oxygen or organic compounds as final hydrogen acceptors, the hydrogen ion being donated by a substrate with its transfer resulting in energy production (Van Beek *et al.*, 1974). Facultative anaerobes are capable of using an anaerobic pathway if the metabolic conditions in the tissue are appropriate.

Gases of varying solubility are produced (carbon dioxide and hydrogen sulphide which are soluble, and nitrogen and hydrogen which are relatively insoluble) through denitrification, fermentation and deamination.

The presence of gas should alert the clinician to the presence of tissue hypoxia extensive enough to support anaerobic bacterial growth. Such a situation implies extensive tissue damage and a form of infection which not recognised early, or appropriately treated, is associated with a high mortality.

Anaerobic sepsis is not always associated with gas production.

Acute dermal gangrene is a curious and frequently lethal condition which should be considered as a separate entity. The condition can be divided into two types, necrotising fasciitis and progressive bacterial gangrene.

GAS FORMING AND ANAEROBIC INFECTIONS

The non-clostridial gas forming infections have been classified by Van Beek and co-workers (1974). Gas forming infections can be reasonably

497

classified as follows:

1. Caused by facultative anaerobes:
   Coliforms
   Other gram negative rods – e.g. Serratia
   Streptococci
   Staphylococci
   Others – Klebsiella, Pseudomonas.
2. Caused by strict anaerobes:
   Clostridia
   Streptococci
   Bacteroides.

Anaerobic surgical sepsis, a review of the organisms involved and the bacteriological methods for diagnosis have been reviewed by Nichols and Smith (1975). Endogenous anaerobes are located in the oral cavity, colon and vagina, Actinomyces and *Bacteroides oralis* being present only in the mouth where the *B. fragilis* and Clostridium are absent. Most of the other endogenous anaerobes including the various other species of Bacteroides, Clostridium, Fusobacteria, Lactobacillus and Streptococci are found in all three sites.

Presentation

The important indication of possible anaerobic sepsis is the history that the infection follows surgery of the oral cavity, the vagina or the colon, or a deep-seated wound has become contaminated with soil or faeculent material, or a relatively ischaemic area (e.g. an amputation stump) has become similarly contaminated. Other vulnerable sites of infection where surgery has not been involved include anal fissures, sinuses, torn haemorrhoids, tooth root infections and intra-uterine death.

Many of the conditions present with abscess formation, the pus being putrid or foul smelling. Pus production is often extensive and when involving the abdominal wall (generally following bowel surgery) there may be multiple loculated subcutaneous abscesses. Crepitus is frequently absent when localised abscess formation is present, the patient may be toxic but frequently after surgical drainage rapidly recovers. Such patients may recover with adequate surgical drainage and no antibiotics. Shock is rare. In the more serious anaerobic infections there is no true pus formation, spread is rapid and the mortality high.

The organisms most frequently involved are the Clostridia, Pseudomonas, Coliforms, Klebsiella, anaerobic Streptococcus and

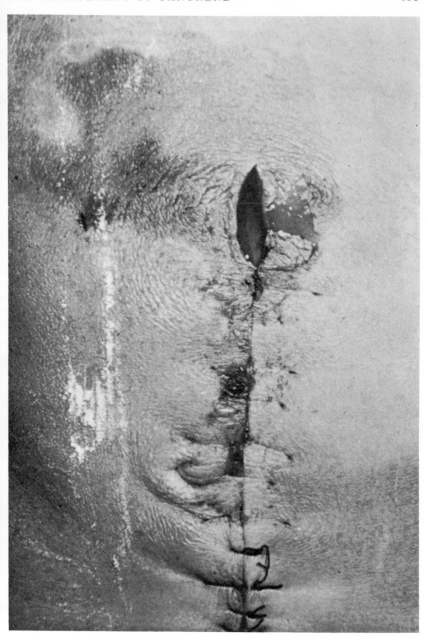

Fig. 1. Clostridial cellulitis involving the laparotomy site for bowel perforation.

occasionally the Bacteroides species. The severity of the infection and hence the treatment largely depends upon a clinical classification.

Wound contamination and dominant anaerobic wound infection

Anaerobes may be found as incidental contaminants of healthy looking superficial wounds: this need not cause alarm. However, if heavily infected the wound may have a foul smell, show greenish black sloughs in the deeper parts and have a brownish seropurulent discharge. There may be fever and toxaemia but provided treatment is rapid the patient does not become shocked. Treatment consists of irrigation of the wound with hydrogen peroxide, wound debridement if sloughs are present and hyperbaric oxygen if the dominant organism is clostridial (see p. 504). Antibiotics are rarely required provided local treatment is thorough. The wound should be looked at carefully daily in order to exclude the onset of anaerobic cellulitus.

Anaerobic cellulitus

In this condition the anaerobes multiply in the depths of the wound and spread along fascial planes: the muscles are not involved. Gas escapes into the tissue spaces opening them up and further aiding the diffusion of organisms. The onset is more gradual (3–4 days) than in gas gangrene and there may be little systemic disturbance until the cellulitus is extensive or is complicated by muscle involvement (Fig. 1). The organism involved is generally clostridial but occasionally (in our experience) an anaerobic Streptococcus. The condition must be distinguished from necrotising fasciitis, where gas formation is absent, toxaemia severe, a dominant organism rarely isolated and where the process may develop some distance from the initial surgical incision.

Cellulitis should be treated similarly to anaerobic myonecrosis.

Anaerobic myonecrosis

This is essentially an infection of living muscle and one or more of the toxigenic clostridia is generally involved. Clostridial gas gangrene usually presents as a sudden acute infection with a short incubation period. Symptoms may develop within a few hours or days of wound contamination, and the earliest symptom is nearly always pain or a sense of heaviness in the affected part. The pain becomes intense and is associated with progressive swelling, oedema, and local tenderness. There may be a thin watery discharge and a peculiar sweetish smell is

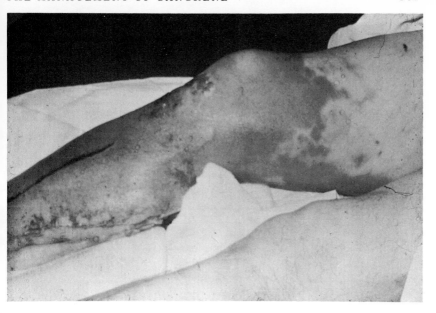

Fig. 2. Clostridial myonecrosis involving the lower limb following compound traumatic fracture of the tibia.

often noted. Later, with increasing swelling and tension, the skin becomes brawny or white and marbled. In very severe infections massive discoloration with formation of blebs and bullae occurs (Fig. 2). The temperature is seldom high. The patient is often pale and sweaty; a flushed appearance is rare.

Jaundice may be present and is either related to intravascular haemolysis, portal thrombophlebitis or hepatocellular failure. Disorientation, hallucinations and even mania may be evident. Renal failure is common. The mortality is high, and death may occur within 24 h of the initial diagnosis, hiccoughing and vomiting being frequent terminal events. Anaerobic myonecrosis due to non-clostridial organisms is most commonly related to the Streptococcus (Fig. 3), Coliform and Klebsiella. Gas production is rarely pronounced, the muscle usually more haemorrhagic and not characterised by the mousy smell of clostridial myonecrosis. The temperature is often high and in our experience the mortality as high as that due to clostridial infection. Toxaemia (unlike that due to Clostridia) is not relieved with hyperbaric oxygen.

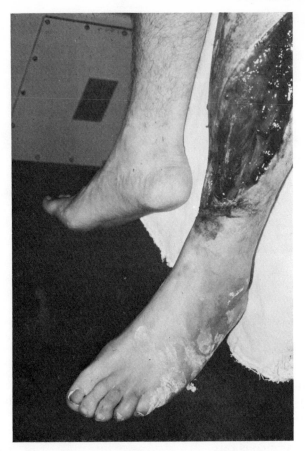

Fig. 3. Myonecrosis secondary to an anaerobic streptococcal infection.

Anaerobic uterine infection

This condition is distinguished from myonecrosis in that (*a*) if the clostridium is involved the organisms may be isolated from the blood stream, (*b*) the blood stream may be infected with anaerobic and aerobic organisms, and (*c*) these patients have a greater tendency to develop coagulation abnormalities and renal failure. The management of uterine infections is discussed in Part 2, ch. XI, p. 735.

Diagnosis and treatment of anaerobic cellulitus and myonecrosis

Material from the source of infection should be taken either directly or by needle aspiration and examined (see Table 1). By this means the

Table 1. Diagnosis of infection

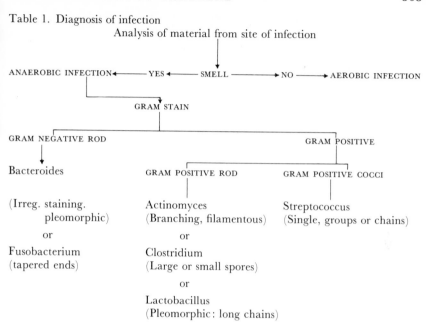

main infecting organism can generally be identified and appropriate antibiotic therapy instituted prior to surgery. The Bacteroides species should be treated with intravenous clindamycin and intravenous metronidazole, the Clostridia with benzyl penicillin G and the Streptococcus with a cephalosporin. On the bacteriological plate the streptococcus may be sensitive to ampicillin but the response clinically appears less effective than with a cephalosporin. A dominant facultative anaerobe occasionally is the cause and under such circumstances either a cephalosporin may be used or where a resistant organism is suspected, gentamicin. This should always be combined with clindamycin until a Bacteroides infection has been excluded. Combined anaerobic and aerobic infections will require antibiotic combinations according to the gram stain and bacterial predominance, the combination may have to be changed once bacterial sensitivities are available.

The treatment of shock and toxaemia is described in Part 2, ch. II, p. 355. There are certain aspects of management which play an important role in the treatment of the patient suffering from anaerobic sepsis.

1. The diabetic, whether diagnosed or unknown, has an increased susceptibility to anaerobic infections. A deep-seated infection may

develop following trauma in a patient with diabetic peripheral neuropathy, the initial trauma passing unnoticed until overt gangrene has developed. There is an increased incidence of anaerobic sepsis in diabetic patients with peripheral vascular disease. Treatment of diabetic ketoacidosis may therefore form part of patient management and may also be a factor in timing the optimum period for surgery. Surgery should not be contemplated until the base deficit is 8 or less and the pH 7.3 or more.

2. Intravascular haemolysis is common in particular with clostridial and streptococcal infections. Blood transfusion in clostridial infections should be delayed if possible until after treatment with hyperbaric oxygen (H.B.O.): H.B.O. seems to arrest the haemolysis. In other infections where H.B.O. is not indicated, care has to be taken not to overload the patient during transfusion, and exchange transfusion may be indicated – particularly in patients with renal failure.

3. Hyperbaric oxygen is indicated in all patients suffering from clostridial cellulitus, clostridial myonecrosis or clostridial uterine infection. Patients suffering from a suspected clostridial infection should be transferred as early as possible to an H.B.O. unit. The onset of shock and toxaemia is rapid and time should not be wasted in confirming the diagnosis by culture.

Patients may be treated in a compressed air chamber while breathing oxygen from a close-fitting face-mask or be treated in a single person transparent hyperbaric oxygen chamber. The patient alone is enclosed within the chamber which is filled and ventilated with 100% oxygen at raised ambient pressure. This system has the advantage that the patient does not have to wear a face mask and rapid decompression is possible because nitrogen bubbling is eliminated. The physiological basis of hyperbaric oxygen therapy is described elsewhere (Lamphier et al., 1966).

Hyperbaric oxygen and antibiotics are essentially complementary in treatment (Slack et al., 1969). Gas gangrene antiserum is probably more dangerous than helpful and its use is contraindicated.

Patients with clostridial myonecrosis are generally extremely toxic and this, plus a metabolic acidosis, may predispose these patients to convulsions whilst receiving H.B.O. treatment. Prior to H.B.O. therapy, metabolic and volume imbalance should be corrected. It is rare for patients with clostridial toxaemia to have PaO_2 values sufficiently low to warrant artificial ventilation. Under such rare circumstances, H.B.O. may have to be foregone and as high a PaO_2 as possible achieved with 100% F_IO_2 for 30 minutes preoperatively. A chest X-ray must always be performed before H.B.O.; a pneumothorax is an absolute indication for continuous drainage before and during H.B.O. Patients with severe chronic airways disease must be compressed with care since the irritant effect of oxygen and the increased gas density may induce bronchospasm and respiratory distress.

4. Radical surgery with postoperative capillary oozing is common. It is therefore important to adhere to the rules for massive haemorrhage (p. 335) and to prepare the patient preoperatively as mentioned on p. 377.

5. Acute dilatation of the stomach and toxic ileus with extensive haemorrhage is common. Pulmonary aspiration is a complication. Stomach bleeding may be successfully arrested with cimetidine, given either orally or intravenously. Surgery is rarely required, haemorrhage resolving once toxaemia is eliminated.

6. Surgery forms an essential part of management, and should ideally be performed after a session of H.B.O. therapy in patients with suspected or proven clostridial sepsis. H.B.O. is particularly indicated preoperatively in patients who are severely toxic, appearing to reduce temporarily the severity of toxaemia and shock. On rare occasions surgery may have to be performed in a patient with a systolic pressure of less than 100 mm Hg, surgical removal of the gangrenous area generally producing dramatic clinical improvement. This in particular applies to patients suffering from non-clostridial myonecrosis. Surgery must be radical and frequently requires more extensive tissue excision or amputation than originally contemplated. It must be realised that H.B.O. in clostridial infection cannot save dead tissue and that radical surgery is generally lifesaving in patients with anaerobic gangrene. Massive blood transfusion is often required.

7. A high percentage of patients develop renal failure requiring dialysis.

8. A high percentage of these patients following surgery require intensive therapy for many days. Oozing from the areas of debridement is common and potent analgesia is generally required for wound dressings. Extensive areas of debridement should be taken down daily to twice daily, cleaned with hydrogen peroxide and then exposed to hyperbaric oxygen. The areas should then be packed with eusol.

9. Once the areas are clean, plastic surgery is commonly required, in particular when the anterior abdominal wall, chest or thigh has been involved.

10. Patients suffering from clostridial infection complicating trauma may develop further complications, such as the fat embolism syndrome,

or may require treatment of vascular injuries or fractures. Differentiation of a disordered mental state subsequent to anaerobic toxaemia from a delayed traumatic intracerebral bleed may on occasions be difficult.

Our experience has been that non-clostridial myonecrosis is associated with a higher mortality than clostridial myonecrosis, provided diagnosis and treatment of the latter is made early. Early diagnosis and appropriate management of clostridial infections is rarely complicated by prolonged pulmonary failure.

ACUTE DERMAL GANGRENE

Acute dermal gangrene is a relatively rare condition which has been given a variety of names by various authors, thus confusing terminology (Fournier, 1883; Meleney, 1933 and Crosthwait, 1964). Ledingham and Tehrani (1975) classified the condition into two categories – necrotising fasciitis (Wilson, 1952) and progressive bacterial gangrene.

Necrotising fasciitis

Necrotising fasciitis is a rapidly progressive necrotising process which affects the subcutaneous fat, superficial fascia and upper surface of the deep fascia. The condition most commonly follows abdominal surgery, but may also follow drainage of a perineal infection, and rarely involves the extremities. There may be some delay between the initial surgical procedure and onset of skin involvement, averaging in one series 11 days (range 6–31 days) (Ledingham and Tehrani, 1975). The patient is often toxic and febrile before there is evidence of skin involvement. The skin initially shows redness, swelling and oedema, the subcutaneous tissues feel indurated on palpation and the area of induration is palpable beyond the area of erythema. If the skin is left, blister formation occurs and subsequently gangrene with sloughing of the skin. After skin-sloughing, fascial necrosis can be seen undermining apparently normal skin (Fig. 4).

The organisms involved are generally mixed and rarely is the clostridial organism solely responsible. In the past, the streptococcus was most commonly implicated but now a colifirm is commonly isolated in varying combination with Streptococci, Pseudomonas, Proteus, Staphylococci and/or Bacteroides species.

A high temperature accompanied by a tachycardia, delerium and drowiness occurs rapidly if the condition is not recognised. Fluid and

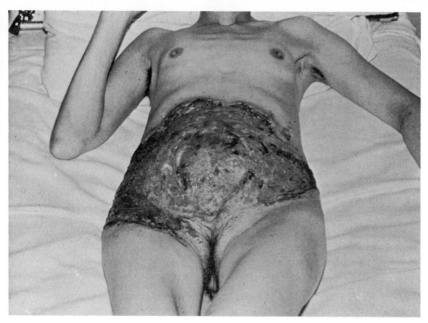

Fig. 4. Necrotising fasciitis involving the anterior abdominal wall. The skin has partially sloughed, the rest removed by surgery. The condition developed following hysterectomy for fibroids; there was no intra-abdominal sepsis.

electrolyte loss may be considerable, and is largely due to a commonly associated ileus and lack of gastrointestinal absorption, and fluid loss into the affected area.

Early surgical debridement is essential and should be performed preferably before the onset of toxaemia. Extensive areas of necrosed fascia has to be excised and healthy looking tissue approximately three centimetres outside the affected area should be removed. Considerable areas of skin may be healthy and can be undercut or excised and used for subsequent skin grafting. During the surgical procedure drainage sites should be looked at carefully to exclude any subcutaneous tracking of fluid from the peritoneal cavity. Should there be faecal contamination of the affected area, a proximal colostomy or ileostomy should be performed, the outlet being positioned through healthy tissue.

Extensive blood and serum loss may occur postoperatively and should be adequately replaced. The operation should be covered with antibiotics, but provided all necrotic areas have been excised, are rarely indicated postoperatively. H.B.O. postoperatively is valuable in preventing superinfection with Pseudomonas, Proteus, or Clostridial organisms and appears to accelerate granulation of the affected area. The affected area should be irrigated with hydrogen peroxide and following H.B.O. therapy covered with packs soaked in eusol. Pigskin grafts can often be placed on the area within 48 hours and skin grafting started within 7 days following operation. Healing and recovery is generally rapid.

The condition may develop in patients predisposed to sepsis, e.g. the diabetic, the patient with leucopenia, hypoalbuminaemia or on steroids. These conditions should be appropriately treated. An adequate supply of calories is mandatory and may necessitate parenteral feeding. In spite of the frequency of hypoalbuminaemia and hypergammaglobulinaemia, immunological studies in three patients demonstrated no abnormality. Provided the condition is diagnosed early and radical surgery instituted prior to the onset of toxaemia, the mortality is low, except in the elderly, or the patient with underlying disease such as leukaemia or carcinoma.

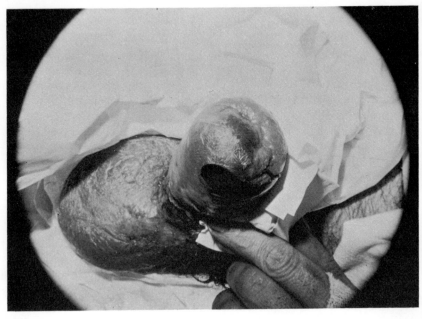

Fig. 5: Progressive bacterial gangrene involving the penis perineum and posterior surface of the scrotum.

Progressive bacterial gangrene

This condition most commonly involves the perineum but on rare occasions may develop in other areas, in particular the lower limbs in association with peripheral vascular disease. The whole skin thickness is primarily involved and there is little involvement of the subcutaneous tissues. The type involving the male genitalia appears to fit the description by Fournier in 1883.

The disease starts as an area of erythema, rapidly changing to purplish gangrene. Spread is rapid and within 5 days (in the perineal form) involves the scrotum and occasionally the penis (Fig. 5). Spread onto the anterior abdominal wall is rare. Toxaemia occurs early, is rarely as severe as a necrotising fasciitis and the aetiology (because of the site of involvement) may not be noticed for several days unless the condition is suspected. In a high percentage of patients, no portal of entry can be demonstrated, but minimal trauma and poor hygienic conditions are common in the elderly. In the remainder, blunt trauma, or a perineal abscess may be the initiating factor. Multiple organisms may be involved, including the Proteus, Pseudomonas, *E. Coli*, Staphylococcus, Clostridia, anaerobic Streptococci and Bacteroides species.

Treatment includes replenishment of blood volume, appropriate treatment of electrolyte and acid base imbalance, antibiotics, surgery and H.B.O. A broad spectrum antibiotic should be used, including clindamycin (until a bacteroides infection has been excluded) but is probably of minor importance in contrast to the surgical management. Surgical debridement consists of removal of the gangrenous skin and excision of healthy skin to about 3 cm beyond the affected area. Castration is rarely indicated. Postoperative management should be similar to that of necrotising fasciitis. Epithelisation is extremely rapid and skin grafting rarely required.

REFERENCES

Crosthwait, R. W., Jnr., Crosthwait, R. W. and Jordan, G. L., Jnr. (1964). Necrotising fasciitis. *J. Trauma* **4**, 148.

Fournier, J. A. (1883). Gangrene foudroyante de la verge. *Sem. Med.* (Paris) **3**, 345.

Lamphier, E. H. and Brown, I. W., Jnr. (1966). Fundamentals of Hyperbaric Medicine. Publ. No. 1298, Washington D.C. Nat. Acad. Sci. Nat. Res. Council.

Ledingham, I. McA. and Tehrani, M. A. (1975). Diagnosis, clinical course and treatment of acute dermal gangrene. *Brit. J. Surg.* **62**, 364.

Meleney, F. L. (1933). A differential diagnosis between certain types of infectious gangrene of the skin. *Surg. Gynec. Obstet.* **56**, 847.

Nichols, R. L. and Smith, J. W. (1975). Modern approach to the diagnosis of anaerobic surgical sepsis. *Surg. Clin. N. Amer.* **55**, 21.

Slack, W. K., Hanson, G. C. and Chew, H. E. R. (1969). Hyperbaric oxygen in the treatment of gas gangrene and clostridial infection. *Brit. J. Surg.* **56**, 505.

Van Beek, A., Zook, E., Yaw, P., Gardner, R., Smith, R. and Glover, J. L. (1974). Nonclostridial gas-forming infections. *Archs. Surg.* **108**, 552.

Wilson, B. (1952). Necrotising fasciitis. *Am. Surg.* **18**, 416.

Section 5: The Management of Severe Chronic Intra-abdominal Sepsis

GILLIAN C. HANSON

INTRODUCTION

Patients initially admitted to the intensive therapy unit with intra-abdominal sepsis associated with shock, malnutrition, or severe electrolyte imbalance, may be initially resuscitated and then proceed to a prolonged toxic illness punctuated by various crises generally related to intra-abdominal infection, electrolyte imbalance, or organ failure (Fig. 1).

These patients offer a tremendous challenge to the intensive 'therapist' and it is only by careful attention to details in treatment, constant assessment with periodic changes in management, that some of these patients survive.

MANAGEMENT

Their management can be summarised under the following headings: Metabolic and fluid control, Nutrition, Maintenance and support of vital organ function, Control of infection, Surgery.

Metabolic and fluid control

Patients with intra-abdominal sepsis readily become fluid depleted, either secondary to ileus and large volumes of gastric aspirate being inadequately replaced with intravenous fluid, or subsequent to chronic loss from diarrhoea or fistula sites.

Fluid volume control is therefore one of the most important aspects of management and has been discussed in Part 1, ch. VI, p. 158. It must be

511

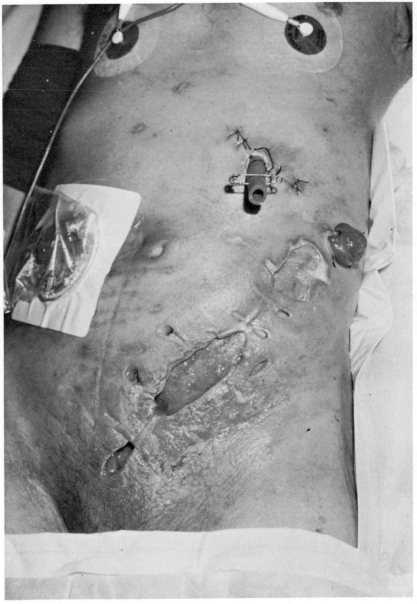

Fig. 1. Chronic intra-abdominal sepsis. Patient with multiple fistula sites opening onto the anterior abdominal wall. Treatment included management of 3 episodes of septic shock, laparotomy on two occasions for drainage of loculated pus, intravenous fluid, metabolic and nutritional control for 6 weeks and ventilation for 4 weeks.

recalled that differentiation of sodium from predominant water depletion by assessment of skin turgor is impossible in wasted patients, since loss of subcutaneous fat may be mistaken for a decrease in interstitial fluid. Careful fluid balance recordings, daily weighing and right atrial pressure monitoring is therefore essential.

In the absence of careful fluid balance control, such patients may become sufficiently fluid depleted to present with shock. Once these patients become shocked, large volumes of appropriate fluid may be required to restore blood volume; severe volume depletion if unde-tected may be complicated by acute renal failure – especially in the elderly. During rapid volume replacement, potassium monitoring and adequate potassium replacement is essential. Central venous pressure monitoring is particularly important in the elderly who tend to develop pulmonary oedema subsequent to sodium overload. E.C.G. monitoring is also important during rapid volume replacement, since cardiac dysrhythmias are common and T-wave changes may signify alterations in the intracellular/extracellular potassium ratio.

Volume replacement in a patient who has been in negative nitrogen balance for a week or more should include albumin containing solutions such as blood, plasma, purified protein fraction, or salt-free albumin. The serum albumin level in such patients is generally less than 25 g/l and it is known that the interstitial space accumulates large quantities of oedema fluid when the plasma albumin falls below 25 g/l (Cervera and Moss, 1974).

Electrolyte imbalance is common, its correction is described in Part 1, ch. VI. Fluid and metabolic abnormalities should be corrected over the first 2–3 days following admission, intravenous feeding being left until all abnormalities have been corrected. Maintenance of electrolyte balance during intravenous feeding is described on p. 250.

Nutrition

The techniques used for intravenous nutrition and the solutions to be used are described in Part 1, ch. IX.

Intravenous feeding may be required for up to 3 months – the use of intravenous sites has therefore to be carefully considered at the onset. These patients are particularly predisposed to catheter sepsis, generally being hypoalbuminaemic and malnourished at the onset of treatment. Nutrition solutions can generally be infused through the side arm of a three-way tap the main line being used for right atrial pressure monitoring. Right atrial pressure monitoring is essential during ventilation, when fluid balance control is difficult, whilst the patient remains toxic and pre- and postoperatively. Catheters should be changed once every 10 days and whenever there is evidence of catheter sepsis.

Patients with chronic fistula losses or diarrhoea rapidly become calcium and magnesium depleted. Phosphate depletion is also common. Replacement and maintenance is described on p. 252.

The requirements for trace metals in long term nutrition in adults is uncertain. It is probable that trace metal supply is of particular importance during the intravenous feeding of infants and young children and when intravenous feeding is continued for more than two weeks in adults. Wretlind (1972) used the 'Addam Electrolyte Solution' to replace trace metals* but other workers (Wilmore and Dudrick, 1968; Lee, 1974) have successfully used plasma for this purpose. Plasma or fresh blood (500 ml) infused weekly should supply an adequate quantity of trace metals in adults on intravenous nutrition. Aminosol 10% also contains trace metals and should therefore be used in preference to pure crystalline L-amino-acids for long term nutrition in adults, unless its use is contra-indicated.

Vitamins and haematinics to be given during intravenous feeding are shown in Table 5, p. 254. Folic acid, vitamin B_{12} and iron should be started after one week of parenteral nutrition, and folic acid should be started immediately in patients on dialysis, patients receiving products containing trimethoprim and in patients receiving ethanol as a calorific source (Wardrop et al., 1975).

During intravenous feeding and/or oral feeding via the Ryles tube, magnesium trisilicate mixture should be put down the Ryles tube 4 hourly. This technique seems, in our hands, to eliminate the complication of acute gastrointestinal bleeding.

Ileus in patients with chronic intra-abdominal sepsis may continue for many weeks, changing from an intravenous feeding regime to oral feeding, therefore, has to be done gradually. These patients rapidly become nitrogen depleted and it must be ensured that adequate daily protein and calories are given during the transition phase. Ileus may be intermittent and the clinical course may be punctuated by a series of laparotomies – during this period a return to intravenous feeding is essential.

Maintenance and support of vital organ function

Pulmonary insufficiency has been recognised for many years as a serious

* Now available as Addamel solution (KabiVitrum Ltd).

complication arising in patients with extensive nonthoracic sepsis – its management is discussed in greater detail in Part 2, p. 552.

At the height of intra-abdominal sepsis these patients generally require artificial ventilation and since the course is frequently protracted, should be tracheostomised if respiratory assistance is required for more than one week.

Pulmonary shunting, miliary atelectasis and particularly basal atelectasis, is characteristic. A deterioration in pulmonary function may be related to intra-abdominal abscess formation, an intestinal crisis (e.g. perforation), or secondary pulmonary infection. Pulmonary function does not subside until the intra-abdominal sepsis is under control and ventilation often has to be continued for many weeks in order to maintain an adequate PaO_2. P.E.E.P. should be applied routinely (because of the high incidence of atelectasis) and except in patients with severe pulmonary failure, can be maintained at 2–4 cm H_2O. The PaO_2 should be maintained at 10.7–13.3 kPa (80–100 mm Hg) and the F_IO_2 50% or less. It is essential to examine the chest daily, pneumothorax, pulmonary collapse and secondary infection must be detected early and treated appropriately.

The timing for patient weaning is important and should not be contemplated if further surgery is likely over the next few days. Laparotomy or operation may lead to a further period of deterioration in pulmonary function and artificial ventilation should be continued for at least two days postoperatively. Patients should be weaned off slowly once the PaO_2 is 9.3 kPa (70 mm Hg) or above on an F_IO_2 of 35% or less on 2 cm P.E.E.P., and be allowed to breathe spontaneously against an expiratory resistance of 2 cm H_2O. Weaning in these patients may take a week to two weeks and should not be rushed.

Patients with severe sepsis characteristically have a high cardiac output in association with a low pulmonary vascular resistance (Clowes et al., 1974). It is unusual for septic patients to be able to maintain this high output throughout their illness and one of the many factors producing clinical deterioration is the onset of right heart or biventricular failure. It is probable that a high pulmonary vascular resistance is one of the major factors causing right heart failure in sepsis (Clowes et al., 1975). Pulmonary shunting can be reduced by improving cardiac output and therefore where there is a high alveolar-arterial oxygen difference, digitalis should be considered. Glucose potassium and insulin may not only provide calories but may also improve cardiac output (McNamara et al., 1970).

2,3-Diphosphoglycerate deficiency leads to a compensatory increase in cardiac output – this may precipitate cardiac failure when the cardiac output is already high secondary to sepsis. Sepsis itself has no effect on oxygen dissociation but decreased levels of 2,3-D.P.G. may be found in hypophosphataemia and transfusion of old blood (Clowes *et al.*, 1974). It is essential in these patients to optimise the oxyhaemo-globin dissociation curve by maintaining a normal red cell 2,3-D.P.G. A normal serum phosphate should therefore be ensured.

A sustained tachycardia of 100–120/min is common and the incidence of dysrhythmias high; it may be related to digoxin toxicity (precipitated by renal failure or hypokalaemia), potassium imbalance, a metabolic acidosis, hypoxia, ventricular failure, hypovolaemia or severe sepsis related to intraperitoneal accumulation of pus. A supraventricular tachycardia of over 140/min in the absence of any correctable factor may be halted by the use of verapamil hydrochloride or a partial β-blocker such as oxyprenalol. Total β-blockade is dangerous in these patients since it may be complicated by a prolonged period of bradycardia or asystole. Ventricular extrasystoles are best treated with intravenous lignocaine and a ventricular tachycardia is most rapidly and effectively treated with d.c. cardioversion.

Patients with chronic intra-abdominal sepsis frequently have a diminished creatinine clearance, which is further diminished during periods of severe stress. Renal function should be observed carefully and factors such as hypovolaemia, cardiac failure, potassium imbalance, hyperosmolality or hypoxia, likely to precipitate deterioration should be avoided. Repeated operative procedures are likely to produce deterioration in the creatinine clearance postoperatively, volume control pre- and postoperatively is therefore essential. Mannitol should be used routinely postoperatively once fluid volume deficits have been corrected.

Monitoring antibiotic levels when using a potentially nephrotoxic antibiotic is essential. Diuretic therapy during the use of a nephrotoxic antibiotic may precipitate renal failure.

Control of infection

It is essential, before using antibiotics, to take swabs for culture from the relevant sites and to take blood cultures routinely. Antibiotics should be used for short periods only and have no part to play in the management of intra-abdominal abscess formation which requires good surgical drainage.

Peritoneal dialysis is valuable in the immediate postoperative management of extensive nonlocalised peritonitis and this is combined with instillation of 200 ml 2% noxythiolin solution twice daily for the first three days after operation. The noxythiolin should be left in the peritoneal cavity for one hour before draining out (Pickard, 1972). Extensive skin sloughing over fistula sites requires frequent changes of dressings which may be associated with extreme distress to the patient, pain may be relieved by the inhalation of Entonox (50% oxygen with nitrous oxide) for 5 min prior to, and during the dressing procedure. Irrigation of the fistula site with hydrogen peroxide followed by Milton (sodium hypochlorite 0.5%) packs where application of a colostomy or ileostomy bag has not been possible, has been found to give maximum success. Hyperbaric oxygen in conjunction with plastic surgery may be valuable in increasing the percentage take of a skin graft or accelerate skin healing once the fistula has been closed. Hyperbaric oxygen at $2\frac{1}{2}$ atmospheres absolute is indicated (in conjunction with surgical excision) where fistula sites have been complicated by *Clostridium welchii* infection of the anterior abdominal wall.

Antibiotics should always be used where there has been a positive blood culture – should be given in high doses either intravenously or intramuscularly, and should be stopped once two sets of blood cultures on consecutive days have been negative. Gentamicin should be used as the last resort, should always be combined with carbenicillin (to cover the Streptococcus and prevent the emergence of resistant strains of *Pseudomonas pyocyaneus*) and the dose should be regulated according to peak and trough blood levels. Where bacterial resistance to gentamicin is possible tobramycin should be substituted. A positive blood culture for the Bacteroides species may take several days and when septicaemia is suspected, the initial antibiotic therapy should always include intravenous clindamycin. A low grade pyrexia 39°C or less with a pulse of 100–110/min is common and does not necessarily require antibiotic therapy.

Surgery

Patients with intra-abdominal sepsis must be frequently assessed for any evidence of clinical deterioration. Sepsis may have spread from the original site, or the preceding surgical procedure may have contributed to dissemination of infection and abscess formation. Occult collections of intraperitoneal pus are often the major factor precipitating multiple organ failure and death. When treating the chronically septic patient it is therefore imperative to maintain an aggressive surgical attitude, frequent consultations being made between the surgeon in charge of the case and the I.T.U. medical team. Drainage of pus and even on occasions more dramatic surgery (e.g. bowel resection) may be life-saving, and a desperately ill patient is not a contraindication for surgery if the procedure itself may save the patient.

A fluctuating pyrexia and leucocytosis may not be present in patients on steroids, in the elderly or malnourished patient. Pleuritic pain may suggest subdiaphragmatic irritation, mucous diarrhoea may be consistent with a pelvic collection of pus.

Seriously ill patients when operated upon for generalised peritonitis, may continue postoperatively with generalised peritonitis for several weeks, loculation ultimately occurring between loops of bowel.

Indications for laparotomy are multiple and include: pyrexia, in particular fluctuating, associated with a persistent tachycardia and jaundice. Clinical evidence of pus collection, a palpable mass in the abdomen or on pelvic examination, or evidence of fluid loculation by X-ray, ultrasound or radio-isotope scan.

On occasions the indication for laparotomy may be less obvious and be related to a persistent ileus, and/or clinical deterioration of the patient with evidence of increasing pulmonary and renal failure. A fluctuating pyrexia with repeatedly positive blood cultures which recur after an adequate course of antibiotics, indicates loculation of pus. A period of septic shock may necessitate an emergency laparotomy when an acute intra-abdominal crisis is suspected, e.g. perforation, or rupture of an abscess producing generalised peritonitis.

Persistent fistula discharge, in particular when on X-ray the fistula is close to the surface, or where toxaemia is thought to be related to intraperitoneal leakage of fistula fluid, may on occasions justify a laparotomy.

In chronic intra-abdominal sepsis, leakage from an anastomis performed several weeks previously may occur suddenly and produce acute toxaemia and shock. This is clearly an indication for laparotomy; a peritoneal tap under such circumstances may not be diagnostic.

On occasions, chronic sepsis may be complicated by bowel infarction, producing a rise in pulse rate and increasing toxaemia. Should this condition be suspected, laparotomy and appropriate surgery may be life-saving.

CONCLUSION

Management of the patient with chronic intra-abdominal sepsis is based upon metabolic, nutritional, and fluid control, and maintenance of vital organ function.

Antibiotic therapy should be limited to short periods of appropriate therapy. The patient should be constantly assessed for any evidence of deterioration which would warrant an exploratory laparotomy.

REFERENCES

Cervera, A. L. and Moss, G. (1974). Crystalloid distribution following haemorrhage and haemodilution. *J. Trauma* **6** (14), 506.

Clowes, G. H. A. Jr., O'Donnell, T. F. Jr., Ryan, N. T. and Blackburn, G. L. (1974). Energy metabolism in sepsis. Treatment based on different patterns in shock and high output. *Ann. Surg.* **175**, 684.

Clowes, G. H. A. Jr., Hirsch, M. F. E., Williams, L., Kwasnik, E., O'Donnell, T. F., Cuevas, P., Saini, V. K., Moradi, I., Farizan, M., Saravis, C., Stone, M. and Kuffler, J. (1975). Septic lung and shock lung in Man. *Ann. Surg.* **5**, 681.

Lee, A. (1974). Intravenous nutrition. *Brit. J. Hosp. Med.* **11**, 719.

McNamara, J. G., King, J. A. C. and Drucker, W. R. (1970). Effect of hypertonic glucose on haemorrhagic shock in rabbits. *Ann. Thorac. Surg.* **9**, 116.

Pickard, R. G. (1972). Treatment of peritonitis with pre and postoperative irrigation of the peritoneal cavity with Noxythiolin solution. *Brit. J. Surg.* **59**, 642.

Wardrop, C. A. J., Heatley, R. V., Hughes, L. E. and Tennant, B. (1975). Acute folate deficiency in surgical patients on amino-acid/ethanol intravenous nutrition. *Lancet* **2**, 640.

Wilmore, D. W. and Dudrick, S. J. (1968). Growth and development of an infant receiving all nutrients exclusively by vein. *J.A.M.A.* **203**, 140.

Wretlind, A. (1972). Complete intravenous nutrition. *Nutr. Metab.* **14** (Suppl. 1) 57.

V

The Management of Specific Forms of Respiratory Failure

Section 1: Respiratory Failure in Chronic and Acute Chest Disease

M. W. McNicol

RESPIRATORY FAILURE IN CHRONIC CHEST DISEASE

Introduction

The overall prognosis of patients with severe chronic chest disease has probably improved in recent years, and they tend to present at a later stage with more advanced disease (Howard, 1974). The reasons for this change are not clear, but it may account for the fact that there has, with few exceptions (O'Donohue *et al.*, 1970), been little improvement in survival rates for patients in acute episodes of respiratory failure even in increasingly well equipped and sophisticated respiratory intensive care units (Martin and Marshall, 1973; Petty *et al.*, 1975; Burk and George, 1973; Asmundsson and Kilburn, 1974; Sluiter *et al.*, 1972). Older patients with more advanced diseases are not easy to treat, despite the ready availability of techniques such as mechanical ventilation. It is not clear exactly which factor determines prognosis – age, severity of chronic chest disease, or intercurrent disease – but in the older patient many of these may exert an unfavourable influence.

521

Management of infection, fluid retention and airway obstruction

Infection

There has been no significant development in antibiotic therapy. Infection should be assumed to be due to *H. influenza* or *Strep. pneumonia* unless there is good reason to believe another pathogen may be present. One of the following antibiotics should be given: ampicillin 500 mg six hourly, cotrimoxazole tabs, 2 twice daily, tetracycline 250 mg six hourly, cephalexin 500 mg six hourly, or benzyl penicillin 1 mega unit intramuscularly six hourly with streptomycin 1 g intramuscularly daily.

Antibiotic treatment should not be delayed for the results of sputum culture. Specimens should be sent if there is any uncertainty about the possible organism or if there is any delay in response.

It is generally agreed that the effective treatment of infection requires good clearance of secretions from the respiratory tract; vigorous and frequent coughing should be encouraged with this in mind. The physiotherapist often offers considerable help with this. There is no evidence that the more advanced forms of physiotherapy have any significant benefit (American Review Respiratory Disease, 1974).

Fluid retention

The importance of fluid retention remains uncertain (Editorial, 1975) but where there is oedema, diuretics should be given (e.g. Frusemide 40 mg daily). Over-vigorous diuretic therapy should be avoided, as not only may the patient be somewhat resistant to diuretics but electrolyte problems, particularly potassium depletion, may be produced and massive diuresis may cause reduction in cardiac output.

Bronchodilator therapy

Though the airway obstruction in these patients is largely irreversible there is a small reversible component and bronchodilators should be used (see p. 529).

All patients should receive this initial therapy. In those who are acutely ill or who fail to respond promptly, further treatment should be considered.

Oxygen therapy

These patients tolerate arterial hypoxaemia relatively well and are at considerable risk from carbon dioxide narcosis after oxygen therapy. Careful control of inspired oxygen concentration is essential. Oxygen should be used on specific medical prescription only. There is unfortunately considerable uncertainty about the precise indications for the use of oxygen. In acute respiratory failure and chronic chest disease the patient's major adaptive mechanism is probably a change in distribution of blood flow which can maintain oxygen supply to vital tissues in the face of severe arterial hypoxaemia (Flenley, 1975). Change in the dissociation curve of haemoglobin is probably of little importance (Flenley et al., 1975). There is no single good index of dangerous hypoxia and if any single measurement is to be made mixed venous oxygen is probably the best available indicator (Mithoefer et al., 1974), but is considered imperfect by some workers (Lee and Wright, 1972) and a routine use of mixed venous oxygen saturation measurement which requires pulmonary artery catheterisation is probably not justified.

A decision on whether oxygen therapy is required depends on an assessment of the available oxygen, the product of the arterial oxygen content and cardiac output. In these patients cardiac output is usually normal and arterial oxygen content can be either measured or derived from arterial oxygen tension. Few measurements have been made of oxygen consumption but those which are available do not suggest that it is markedly elevated (normally less than 300 ml/min).

When arterial oxygen saturation falls below 70% corresponding to an arterial PO_2 of 4.7 kPa (35 mm Hg), available oxygen has fallen to 700 ml/min and the patient is on the steep part of the dissociation curve where a slight further fall in PO_2 would produce a significant reduction in oxygen content. He is clearly at risk from inadequate oxygen supply and supplementary oxygen should be given. If the PO_2 is above 4.7 kPa (35 mm Hg) oxygen therapy is not essential but may be helpful in the relief of symptoms such as dyspnoea and can be given on that basis if its hazards are borne in mind.

Prediction of response to oxygen therapy remains imprecise. Patients with the lowest pre-treatment PaO_2 usually show the poorest response (Lopez-Majanio et al., 1973) although others have suggested that the mechanisms determining pre-treatment PaO_2 are different from those determining response to oxygen therapy (King et al., 1973). Although the problem of underventilation following oxygen therapy has been recognised for many years, its mechanism is still uncertain. It is increasingly recognised that not only is there central respiratory depression from loss of hypoxic drive, but also, as has been demonstrated on theoretical grounds (West, 1971) and has been shown in other conditions (Sykes and Finlay, 1971), there is significant increase in dead space ventilation as a result of change in ventilation–perfusion relationships. It is a generally reasonable assumption that the patient with the highest pre-treatment $PaCO_2$ and the lowest pre-treatment PaO_2 are most at risk, being most likely to have a rise in $PaCO_2$ and most vulnerable to its effects. The more vigorously oxygen therapy is pursued the greater the risk of carbon dioxide narcosis and therefore the greater the possibility of the need for mechanical ventilation. Thus 2 of the 7 patients studied by Warrell *et al.* (1970) who received meticulous oxygen therapy required mechanical ventilation, a higher proportion than might have been expected from the information available about their pre-treatment condition. In the less fit elderly patients this raises acutely the need to plan the total pattern of management and to exercise great care in the giving of oxygen. A suggested scheme for oxygen therapy and the monitoring of response to it is shown in Table 1.

The initial concentration of oxygen therapy should be 24% and a mask which delivers this concentration at a high flow rate should be used. If the rise in arterial oxygen following 24% oxygen therapy is inadequate 28% should be employed. It should virtually never be necessary to use 32% and this should only be used with great caution. Oxygen must be given continuously for at least the first 24 h and should normally be continued until such time as there has been an unequivocal response with fall in $PaCO_2$ and rise in PaO_2. Thereafter the concentration can be reduced and treatment with oxygen discontinued

Table 1. Summary of the management of a patient with chronic chest disease

All patients	Dangerously hypoxaemic (PaO_2) < 4.7 kPa (35 mm Hg) or not improving	
Infection Antibiotics Drain sputum Bronchodilators Diuretics if oedematous	Additional oxygen 24% Monitor 1 h, 24 h or clinical deterioration ? Adequate PaO_2 achieved ⟶ ? Excessive rise of $PaCO_2$ PaO_2 inadequate 28% oxygen PaO_2 rise excessive	CO_2 narcosis Fit + acute illness Facilities to ventilate available → Mechanical ventilation Less fit Facilities poor No good acute cause → Doxapram

relatively rapidly. With concentrations up to 32% there is no risk of oxygen toxicity, higher concentrations should not normally be employed in these patients through a mask. Occasionally a ventilated patient receives an inspiratory oxygen percentage above 50. This should be avoided because of the hazard of oxygen toxicity. The precise importance of oxygen toxicity is as yet uncertain (Editorial, 1970; Clark, 1974) but the risk is such that it is prudent to avoid the use of higher concentrations. With effective mechanical ventilation, adequate clearance of secretions, and the use of positive end expiratory pressure, it should virtually never be necessary to employ a higher concentration to obtain an arterial PO_2 of above 8.0 kPA (60 mm Hg) which is a reasonable level.

There is good evidence that oxygen therapy is beneficial. Mixed venous oxygen rises significantly although to a considerably lesser extent than arterial oxygen (Flenley et al., 1973) indicating improved tissue oxygen delivery.

Long-term oxygen therapy

It is clearly established that in patients with pulmonary hypertension secondary to chronic chest disease, oxygen therapy for more than 15 h/day will lower the pulmonary artery pressure (Stark et al., 1972), and there is some evidence that this treatment may produce clinical benefit (Stewart et al., 1975; Anderson et al., 1973; Stark et al., 1973; Block et al., 1974). Carbon dioxide retention appears to be largely a problem of the acute illness (Brundin, 1974), and there have been no real problems with long-term oxygen therapy. Treatment is complex and expensive, and methods such as the use of the oxygen concentrator are being explored (Stark et al., 1973). No adequate information on controlled assessment is yet available, but preliminary results are encouraging, apparently particularly in reducing numbers of hospital admissions.

Respiratory stimulants

The role of respiratory stimulants remains uncertain. If an effective stimulant were available it could antagonise central respiratory depression following loss of hypoxic drive. It would of course have no effect on under-ventilation due to an increase in dead space ventilation. There is not as yet any really effective respiratory stimulant. The majority of the drugs are analeptics and produce arousal and stimulation of a variety of other centres in the central nervous system. There are variable and usually not striking effects on respiration. Of the drugs available, Doxapram is probably the most effective and least toxic. It is generally effective (Moser *et al.*, 1973; Riordan *et al.*, 1975) and has been shown to be effective in salvage therapy of patients underventilating acutely on oxygen therapy (Riordan *et al.*, 1973).

Respiratory stimulants should be used in patients who develop actual or potential carbon dioxide narcosis following oxygen therapy ($PaCO_2$ greater than 10.7 kPa (80 mm Hg) when mechanical ventilation is thought to be contraindicated. Following Doxapram infusion significant improvement in clinical condition and arterial blood gases with rise in PaO_2 and some fall in $PaCO_2$ should be apparent within an hour. Treatment may be continued for up to 3 to 4 days. Infusion can be given in rates of up to 3 mg/min; higher doses are liable to be associated with increase in side effects and the additional response obtained probably does not routinely justify the use of a dose greater than 2 mg/min.

Widely differing views on respiratory stimulants are still held and are well set out in two articles in *Chest* (Woolf, 1970; Bickerman and Chusid, 1970).

Mechanical ventilation
This is a more complex form of therapy which should be used on specific indication of an acute, potentially reversible episode in a patient with a worthwhile prognosis who has failed to respond to other forms of therapy, or in the salvage of a patient with respiratory failure whose management has been complicated by therapeutic mishap, such as the administration of opiates on a misdiagnosis of left ventricular failure. A decision on whether the patient should be ventilated or not ought to be made early in treatment, preferably at the start of treatment and subsequent management planned in the light of that, in particular the energy with which oxygen therapy is pursued. It is bad practice to have to assess the patient's suitability for mechanical ventilation when there is an urgent need to carry this out. The decision will in general depend on the fitness of the patient before hospital admission and acuteness of the precipitating factor of the episode of respiratory failure.

There are no major advances in techniques. Several reports suggest that positive end expiratory pressure may be beneficial (Barat and Asuero, 1975; Suter *et al.*, 1975). High levels of P.E.E.P. must not be used because of the increased risk of pneumothorax. P.E.E.P. up to 15 cm of water is relatively safe and pneumothorax only an occasional complication. In the early stages ventilation rarely presents any problems, but the difficulties are in weaning the patient off the ventilator. These problems will be greatest when patient selection is poor. Many patients can be managed with endotracheal intubation alone but a proportion still require tracheostomy. This will almost always be necessary in patients who have difficulty in weaning from the ventilator. The more severe the preceding chronic chest disease, the longer will the period of ventilation have to be and the greater the difficulty in weaning (Jessen et al., 1967). There are now a few reports on the physiological changes following the cessation of mechanical ventilation (Gilbert et al., 1974; Feeley and Hedley Whyte, 1975) but as yet there are no clearly established criteria for attempting weaning, and the indications must be largely clinical. These are mainly control of infection with reduction in volume and purulence of secretions and clearing of abnormalities on chest X-ray, and improvement in the underlying function as assessed by fall in the ventilator pressure required and rise in PaO_2. It is not normally difficult to assess patient's response by close observation at times when ventilation has to be discontinued such as for endotracheal tube suction. This is often poorly tolerated initially but as the underlying condition improves, this becomes much better tolerated and the patient will show readiness to come off the ventilator by making satisfactory spontaneous respiratory efforts during this time and by showing considerable improvement in cough.

There are no dangers in mechanical ventilation specific to respiratory failure in patients with chest disease other than the problems of infection and functional capability of the lungs.

Other forms of therapy

Patients in respiratory failure from chronic chest disease are often middle aged or elderly and not particularly fit, especially in those whose function is poor and where there may be problems in weaning from the ventilator, vigorous attention to other medical illnesses is essential. Cardiac failure normally responds to diuretics and improvement in oxygenation and airway function. Digoxin is of no specific benefit but may be useful for supraventricular tachycardias which not uncommonly complicate respiratory failure. If these do not respond to digoxin and require treatment, cardioversion should be used. Beta-blockers are contraindicated. Many of these patients are polycythemic but in the acute stages venesection is probably contraindicated. There is a tendency for the polycythemia to improve rapidly with the resolution of the acute episode. Venesection should only be used if it persists after recovery. In the acute phases significant venesection is liable to lower cardiac output and contribute to the problems of tissue oxygenation.

RESPIRATORY FAILURE IN ACUTE CHEST DISEASE
Asthma

There has been an increasing recognition of the relatively slow evolution of the majority of severe attacks of asthma and therefore of the importance of early recognition by both patient and physician of the need for intensification of treatment (Sherwood Jones, 1971). Measures such as direct access for patients to a specialised unit have been described (Crompton and Grant, 1975) and appear to offer some benefit. The risks of the period of major reduction in steroid dose or steroid withdrawal are increasingly emphasised (Fraser *et al.*, 1971). A recent analysis of deaths from asthma (McDonald *et al.*, 1976) however notes that a proportion of the deaths remain sudden and unpredictable and that part of the mortality still appears unavoidable. A survey of hospital deaths (Cochrane and Clark, 1975) suggests that many were avoidable and that objective assessment was inadequate.

The physiological abnormalities have been reviewed by Rees *et al.* (1968); Meisner and Jones (1968) and Rebuck and Read (1971). The basic problem is a marked though potentially reversible increase in expiratory air flow resistance. This leads to over-inflation of the lung with increases in lung volume and, as it is patchy in its distribution, it causes severe ventilation-blood flow disturbance in the lung. This in turn leads to hypoxemia. Respiratory efforts are usually forceful and in the early and moderately severe stages of the attack of asthma over-ventilation is a normal response with fall in $PaCO_2$; in the later stages of the severe attack the $PaCO_2$ may rise. In contrast in the patient with respiratory failure from chronic chest disease the cardiac output is often low, largely as a result of reduced venous return from increased intrathoracic pressure and the intense respiratory effort, with perhaps some complicating loss in circulating volume from the dehydration. Anxiety is a common feature and sympathetic over-activity with tachycardia and in the early stages hypertension is not uncommon.

Management of acute bronchial asthma

The acute attack responds normally within 24 hours but once the patient is in status asthmaticus response may take as long as 2 to 3 days. Treatment is essentially with bronchodilators and cortico-steroids to reverse the airway obstruction, supportive therapy includes oxygen and

Table 2. Summary of the management of a patient with bronchial asthma

All patients	No response	
Bronchodilators 　Aminophylline 500 mg i.v. 　　6 hourly 　Inhaled salbutamol 4 hourly Corticosteroids Antibiotics if infected Oxygen if hypoxic 　$PaO_2 < 8.0$ kPa (60 mm Hg) Fluid replacement if inadequate 　circulating volume Bicarbonate if acidotic (pH <7.2)	$PaCO_2 \uparrow$ Exhaustion Clinical Increasing tachycardia 　　　　+ Falling B.P. Persistent low PaO_2 Persistent low or falling P.E.F. (Peak Expiratory Airflow)	Intubate and Ventilate

correction of electrolyte and fluid balance. Should respiration fail, mechanical ventilation has to be employed. A table summarising management of bronchial asthma is shown in Table 2.

Bronchodilators
It was thought in the early 1960s that isoprenaline might have been responsible for the increase in mortality in asthma which then occurred. This increase has since disappeared (Inman and Adelstein, 1969). The general consensus of opinion now appears to be that the problems were related to more inadequate and inappropriate therapy rather than bronchodilators. Furthermore newer β_2-specific adrenergic agonists, rimiterol, salbutamol and terbutaline (Kingsley and Volans, 1973; Marlin and Turner, 1975; May *et al.*, 1975; Spiro *et al.*, 1975) have now largely replaced isoprenaline. They are as potent as isoprenaline for bronchodilatation but have a much weaker action on the cardiovascular system, which when given by inhalation is clinically insignificant. They differ in duration of action, rimiterol having the shortest, terbutaline the longest. There is now good evidence of their value by inhalation but their role in intravenous use is uncertain. A single controlled comparison with intravenous aminophylline and salbutamol showed a marginal but significant fall in pulse rate with aminophylline and no change in salbutamol. Side effects with salbutamol however were fewer (Williams *et al.*, 1975).

There is some evidence that the mode of action of the adrenergic agonists is different from that of aminophylline. The effect of the two drugs is at least additive and there may be some potentiation. The optimum regime for bronchodilatation in the severe asthmatic would appear to be a combination of intravenous aminophylline by a slow infusion (500 mg six hourly) and an aerosol of either rimiterol, salbutamol or terbutaline. There appears to be no good ground for choice between these and this must remain essentially a matter for individual preference. Inhalation can be given intermittently four to six hourly. There is a dearth of reports to confirm the supposed greater efficacy of I.P.P.B. as a means of administering bronchodilator aerosols and any efficient aerosol generator appears to be effective (Gold, 1975; Webber *et al.*, 1974; Shenfield *et al.*, 1974). It is possible that I.P.P.B. may be harmful (Karetzky, 1975; Gold, 1975).

Both intravenous aminophylline and inhaled bronchodilator should be used with greater caution in the presence of severe tachycardia (pulse rate above 140 beats/min). This is not an absolute contraindication but is a clear indication for reduction in dose, careful observation of response and titration of dose accordingly. At one time it was thought that adrenergic drugs might aggravate arterial hypoxemia and this may be clinically significant. Evidence for this is not strong; and the tendency to produce this effect is much less marked with the specific β_2-agonists and the presence of arterial hypoxemia need not be taken as a contraindication to bronchodilator therapy.

Cortico-steroids

While it is generally agreed that steroid dose in status asthmaticus should be high, there is no agreement on what constitutes a high dose (Editorial, 1975a). There is no evidence of abnormal steroid handling or responsiveness in severe asthma (Cayton and Howard, 1973). Asthmatics in status, not previously treated with steroids, have been shown to respond as rapidly to tetracosactrin as to hydrocortisone (Collins *et al.*, 1975). In the dose used plasma cortisol levels did not exceed 100 µg/ml and these levels can be achieved with smaller doses of hydrocortisone than had previously been thought necessary. The same study suggests that continuous infusion may be more effective than intermittent doses; the authors recommend a dose of hydrocortisone 3 mg/kg/6 hourly. There is still not a great deal of information about the time course of response to steroid therapy. Such information as is available suggests that it is relatively slow. In chronic asthma Ellul-Micallef *et al.* (1974) found improvement at 5 hours after oral prednisolone and Ellul-Micallef and Fenech (1975a, b) subsequently reported a more rapid response to intravenous prednisolone, but

Collins *et al.* (1975) found no real change for 6 hours and relatively small improvement at 24 h in acute asthma.

Other supportive therapy

Oxygen should be given in an attempt to relieve arterial hypoxaemia. This is frequently relatively resistant to treatment and higher concentrations have to be employed; it is probably not worthwhile starting below 28% and concentrations of up to 50% may be necessary to achieve arterial oxygen saturation over 80% which is desirable. Underventilation is not normally a problem but may occur and arterial $PaCO_2$ should be monitored closely during the first two hours after the start of oxygen therapy, particularly when higher concentrations are being used. In patients who have been severely breathless for some time dehydration and loss of circulating volume is not uncommon and this should be corrected by intravenous infusion. Acidosis is not infrequently present and it has been suggested that this impairs the response to bronchodilators. There is some evidence that correction of acidosis by sodium bicarbonate may improve the response (Mithoeffer *et al.*, 1968). Antibiotics should be given only on specific indication of infection which is uncommon in status asthmaticus. Prophylactic antibiotic therapy combined with high dose steroid therapy runs a major risk of secondary infection.

Sedation of a patient in status asthmaticus is absolutely contra-indicated unless a decision has been made to undertake mechanical ventilation and the equipment for doing so is at hand and fully ready. Rapid depression of respiration frequently follows sedation with carbon dioxide narcosis and severe, not infrequently fatal, hypoxaemia.

All patients with a severe attack of asthma should be treated initially in an intensive therapy unit; if this is not available, close observation is essential until there is unequivocal evidence of improvement. Deterioration can be very rapid. Regular observations of pulse rate, blood pressure and urine output are essential. Some assessment of expiratory airflow obstruction such as peak expiratory flow must be made 4–6 hourly and arterial blood gas analysis must be freely available and readily used to assess progress and response to therapy. If the pulse rate exceeds 120/min, cardiac monitoring is required and full resuscitation facilities should be available.

Mechanical ventilation

Although the emphasis of treatment is increasingly on avoidance of mechanical ventilation by earlier and more energetic conservative treatment, it remains the final form of salvage therapy. Widely varying results are reported indicating widely differing criteria for selection. The optimum timing of intervention remains unclear, and mechanical ventilation of the severe asthmatic remains a difficult and hazardous undertaking. Not only may it be difficult to ventilate the patient adequately in the face of his very severe airway obstruction but these hypoxic patients with low cardiac output (Knowles and Clark, 1973; Straub et al., 1969) often compensate poorly for the cardiovascular stress at the initiation of ventilation, when synchronisation is poor and high ventilatory pressures are required. Severe falls in blood pressure and consequent tissue hypoxia can be readily precipitated.

The indications for ventilation are: exhaustion, progressive rise in $PaCO_2$ and failure of response to therapy in the severely ill patient. There is no good index of exhaustion other than clinical judgement, except perhaps a rising pulse rate in the absence of other cause. The exhausted patient may very quickly abandon the effort of breathing and is at risk of rapid deterioration with an anoxic cardiac arrest. Mechanical ventilation should always be started before this stage is reached. In the small number of patients who underventilate on oxygen mechanical ventilation should always be considered when the $PaCO_2$ exceeds 8.0 kPa (60 mm Hg) and must be undertaken if the $PaCO_2$ exceeds 10.7 kPa (80 mm Hg). A decision to ventilate for failure to respond to conventional therapy is a particularly difficult one. A patient in status asthmaticus may take as long as three days to recover although some demonstrable effect from cortico-steroids and bronchodilators is normally seen within 24 hours. If despite maximal therapy the patient's condition assessed clinically seems to be unchanged, if there is no significant reduction in tachycardia, no major improvement in simple indices of expiratory air flow, e.g. peak flow rate and no significant improvement in arterial blood gas pressures, ventilation should always be considered. A decision to undertake it in those circumstances should be made jointly by an experienced physician and anaesthetist.

When it has been decided to undertake mechanical ventilation, treatment should normally be instituted without further delay. The patient should be oxygenated effectively as possible. Endotracheal intubation should be carried out by a skilled operator with the minimum of delay using muscle relaxants and mild sedation. The heavier the sedation the greater the risk of a cardiovascular problem. Relaxants should be continued to suppress as much as possible the patient's voluntary respiratory efforts which frequently add to the difficulty of establishing satisfactory ventilation. The respirator setting chosen should use a relatively low inspiratory flow rate and high inspiratory pressure should be available (not less than 80 cm water). An intravenous line should always be available so that additional fluids or drugs can be administered as required through it. Synchronisation with the ventilator must always be achieved and continuing sedation and the use of muscle relaxants may be necessary. Triggering of the ventilator or any respiratory effort by the patient is contraindicated since it increases oxygen consumption, and impairs the efficacy of ventilation. When ventilation is established other therapy should be continued. The period on the respirator required is not normally longer than three to four days. Once improvement starts it is usually rapid. Inspiratory pressures fall, arterial blood gases improve and there is usually little difficulty in weaning from the respirator.

Bronchial lavage
There is a lack of further information on the place, if any, of bronchial lavage (Ambiavagar and Sherwood Jones, 1967). This technique assists in the removal of mucus plugs but it is unsafe except in skilled and experienced hands and can only be carried out when a patient is well established on a ventilator and adequately oxygenated. An injection of even warm buffered saline down the endotracheal tube disturbs the pattern of respiration and often precipitates respiratory effort and may aggravate broncho-constriction so that hypoxemia is increased. Unless the operator is very competent and is able to ventilate effectively and manage this situation, the hazards outweigh the benefit. The technique is not suitable for general use.

RESPIRATORY FAILURE IN PNEUMONIA

Respiratory failure may complicate any severe pneumonia from the fulminating influenzal pneumonia in the healthy young adult to the widespread patchy basal pneumonia in the elderly post-operative patient. The specific problems are usually related to a difficulty in secretion management, to hypoxemia from ventilation, blood flow abnormality and to general toxemia. These patients are often febrile, acutely ill and have an increased metabolic rate and oxygen requirement. If effective cough is lost, secretions cannot be adequately cleared. If there is severe hypoxemia not responsive to oxygen therapy, mechanical ventilation should always be considered and should normally be employed. The specific features of the pneumonic illness may complicate management, particularly if mechanical ventilation is to be used in pneumonia where breakdown is a prominent feature, e.g. staphlococcal pneumonia. There is then a considerably increased risk of pneumothorax, pneumomediastium, etc. which require particular care. For the treatment of infection the co-operation of the micro-biologist is essential. If there is no information on the infecting organism, examination of a gram stain smear of the sputum is frequently helpful but effective antibiotic therapy normally requires frequent sputum culture and regular consultation with the microbiologist about the sensitivity of the infecting organism.

EXTRA-CORPOREAL OXYGENATION IN RESPIRATORY FAILURE

There are now several reports of the use of membrane oxygenators in respiratory failure (Hill *et al.*, 1972; Bartlett *et al.*, 1974; Heiden *et al.*, 1975; Kolobow *et al.*, 1975; Cooper *et al.*, 1976; Newball *et al.*, 1975). These have been mainly in fulminating acute conditions, which are potentially largely reversible and early results are disappointing. Although it is likely that this technique will be restricted to specialised centres, it may well represent a significant advance in the management of the acute episode (see Part 4, ch. IV, p. 965).

REFERENCES

Ambiavagar, M. and Sherwood Jones, E. (1967). Resuscitation of the moribund asthmatic. *Anaesthesia* **22**, 375.

Anderson, P. B., Cayton, R. M., Holt, P. J. and Howard, P. (1973). Long term oxygen therapy in cor pulmonale. *Quart. J. Med. New Series* **42**, 563.

Asmundsson, T. and Kilburn, K. (1974). Survival after acute respiratory failure. *Annals Int. Med.* **80**, 54.

American Review of Respiratory Diseases (1974). **110**, Part 2. Proceedings of the Conference on the Scientific Basis of Respiratory Therapy. Petty, T. L. Physical therapy. p. 129. Jones, N. C. Physical therapy – present state of the art. p. 132. Mellins, R. B. Pulmonary physiotherapy in the paediatric age group, p. 137. Bryan, A. C. Comments. p. 143. Grimby, G. Aspects of lung expansion in relation to pulmonary physiotherapy. p. 145; Respiratory muscle fixation in patients with chronic obstructive pulmonary disease. p. 145. Sharp, J. T. Resp. muscle fixation in patients with chronic obstructive pulmonary disease; its relationship to disability and to respiratory therapy. p. 154.

Barat, G. and Asuero, M. S. (1975). Positive end-expiratory pressure. *Anaesthesia* **30**, 183.

Bartlett, R. H., Gazzaniga, A. B., Fong, S. W. and Burns, N. E. (1974). Prolonged extracorporeal cardiopulmonary support in man. *J. Thoracic and Cardiovascular Surgery* **68**, 918.

Bickerman, H. A. and Chusid, E. L. (1970). The case against the use of respiratory stimulants. *Chest* **58**, 53.

Block, A. J., Castle, R. J. and Keitt, A. S. (1974). Chronic oxygen therapy. *Chest* **65**, 279.

Brundin, A. (1974). Arterial blood gases in respiratory insufficiency in the clinically stable state and during acute exacerbations of respiratory failure. *Scand. J. Resp. Dis.* **55**, 181.

Burk, R. H. and George, R. B. (1973). Acute respiratory failure in chronic obstructive pulmonary disease. *Arch. Int. Med.* **132**, 865.

Cayton, R. M. and Howard, P. (1973). Plasma cortisol and the use of hydrocortisone in the treatment of status asthmaticus. *Thorax* **28**, 567.

Clark, J. M. (1974). The toxicity of oxygen. *Amer. Rev. Resp. Dis.* **110**, 40.

Cochrane, G. M. and Clark, T. J. H. (1975). A survey of asthma mortality in patients between ages 35 and 64 in the Greater London hospitals in 1971. *Thorax* **30**, 300.

Collins, J. V., Clark, T. J. H., Brown, D. and Townsend, J. (1975). The use of corticosteroids in the treatment of acute asthma. *Quart. J. Med.* **174**, 259.

Cooper, J. D., Duffin, J., Glynn, M. F. X., Nelems, J. M., Teasdale, S. and Scott, A. A. (1976). Combination of membrane oxygenator support and pulmonary lavage for acute respiratory failure. *J. of Thoracic and Cardiovascular Surgery* **71**, 304.

Crompton, G. K. and Grant, I. W. B. (1975). Edinburgh emergency asthma admission service. *Brit. Med. J.* **4**, 680.

Gold, M. I. (1975). The present status of I.P.P.B. therapy. *Chest* **67**, 469.

Editorial (1970). Lung damage by oxygen. *Lancet* **2**, 1292.

Editorial (1975a). Corticosteroids in acute severe asthma. *Lancet* **2**, 166.

Editorial (1975b). Oedema in cor pulmonale. *Lancet* **2**, 1289.

Ellul-Micallef, R., Borthwick, R. C. and McHardy, G. J. R. (1974). The time course of response to prednisilone in chronic bronchial asthma. *Clin. Science and Mol. Med.* **47**, 105.

Ellul-Micallef, R. and Fenech, F. F. (1975a). Intravenous prednisilone in chronic bronchial asthma. *Thorax* **30**, 312.

Ellul-Micallef, R. and Fenech, F. F. (1975b). Effect of intravenous prednisilone in asthmatics with diminished adrenergic responsiveness. *Lancet* **2**, 1269.

Feeley, T. W. and Hedley Whyte, J. (1975). Weaning from controlled ventilation and supplementary oxygen. *New Eng. J. Med.* **292**, 903.

Flenley, D. C. (1975). 'Oxygen Measurements in Biology and Medicine'. (Ed. J. P. Payne and D. W. Hill) p. 181. Butterworths, London.

Flenley, D. C., Fairweather, L. J., Cooke, N. J. and Kirby, B. J. (1975). Changes in haemoglobin binding curve and oxygen transport in chronic hypoxic lung disease. *Brit. Med. J.* **1**, 602.

Flenley, D. C., Miller, H. C., King, A. J., Kirby, B. J. and Muir, A. L. (1973). Oxygen transport in acute pulmonary oedema and in acute exacerbations of chronic bronchitis. *Brit. Med. J.* **1**, 78.

Fraser, P. M., Speizer, F. E., Waters, S. D. M., Doll, R. and Mann, N. M. (1971). The circumstances preceding death from asthma in young people in 1968–1969. *Brit. J. Dis. Chest* **65**, 71.

Gilbert, R., Auehemloss, J. H., Peppi, D. and Ashutosis, K. (1974). The first few hours of a respirator. *Chest* **65**, 152.

Gold, M. I. (1975). The present status of I.P.P.B. therapy. *Chest* **67**, 469.

Harris, L. (1975). Comparison of cardiorespiratory effects of rimiterol and terbutaline aerosols. *Bull. de Physiopathologie Respiratoire* **11**, 801.

Heiden, D., Mielke, C. H., Rodvien, R. and Hill, J. D. (1975). Platelet hemostasis and thromboembolism during treatment of acute respiratory insufficiency with extracorporeal membrane oxygenation. *J. Thoracic and Cardiovascular Surgery* **70**, 644.

Hill, J. D., Fallat, R. J., Eberhart, R. C., Osborn, J. J. and Gerbode, F. (1972). Acute respiratory insufficiency. *J. Thoracic and Cardiovascular Surgery* **64**, 551.

Howard, P. (1974). Changing face of chronic bronchitis with airways obstruction. *Brit. Med. J.* **2**, 89.

Inman, W. H. W. and Adelstein, A. M. (1969). Rise and fall of asthma mortality in England and Wales in relation to use of pressurised aerosols. *Lancet* **2**, 279.

Jessen, O., Kristensen, H. S. and Rasmussen, K. (1967). Tracheostomy and artificial ventilation in chronic lung disease. *Lancet* **2**, 9.

Karetzky, M. S. (1975). Asthma mortality associated with pneumothorax and intermittent positive pressure breathing. *Lancet* **1**, 828.

King, T. K. C., Ali, N. and Briscoe, W. A. (1973). Treatment of hypoxia with 24 per cent oxygen. *Amer. Rev. Resp. Dis.* **108**, 19.

Kingsley, P. J. and Volans, G. N. (1973). A comparison of the $\beta 1$ and $\beta 2$ effects of subcutaneous isoprenaline, salbutamol and terbutaline in adult man. *Eur. J. Clin. Pharmac.* **7**, 263.

Knowles, G. K. and Clark, T. J. H. (1973). Pulsus paradoxus as a valuable sign indicating severity of asthma. *Lancet* **2**, 1356.

Kolobow, T., Stool, E. W., Sacks, K. L. and Vurek, G. G. (1975). Acute respiratory failure. *J. Thoracic and Cardiovascular Surgery* **69**, 947.

Lee, J. and Wright, F. (1972). Central venous oxygen saturation in shock. *Anaesthesiology* **36**, 472.

Lopez-Majano, V. and Dutton, R. E. (1973). Regulation of respiration during oxygen breathing in chronic obstructive lung disease. *Amer. Rev. Resp. Dis.* **108**, 232.

Marlin, G. E. and Turner, P. (1975). Comparison of the $\beta 2$-adrenoceptor selectivity of rimiterol, salbutamol and isoprenaline by the intravenous route in man. *Brit. J. Clin. Pharmac.* **2**, 41.

Martin, L. V. H. and Marshall, R. L. (1973). Survival of chronic bronchitics after intermittent positive pressure ventilation. *Anaesthesia* **28**, 10.

May, C. S., Paterson, J. W., Spiro, S. G. and Johnson, A. J. (1975). Intravenous infusion of salbutamol in the treatment of asthma. *Brit. J. Clin. Pharmac.* **2**, 503.

McDonald, J. B., Seaton, A. and Williams, D. A. (1976). Asthma deaths in Cardiff 1963–1974: 90 deaths outside hospital. *Brit. Med. J.* **1**, 1493.

Meisner, P. and Hugh-Jones, P. (1968). Pulmonary function in bronchial asthma. *Brit. Med. J.* **1**, 470.

Mithoefer, J. C., Holford, F. D. and Keighley, J. F. (1974). The effect of oxygen administration on mixed venous oxygenation in chronic obstructive pulmonary disease. *Chest* **66**, 122.

Moser, K. M., Luchsinger, P. C., Adamson, J. S., McMahon, S. M., Schluiter, D. P., Sfivack, M. and Weg, J. C. (1973). Respiratory stimulation with intravenous doxapram in respiratory failure: a double-blind cooperative study. *New Engl. J. Med.* **288**, 427.

Newball, H. H., Stool, E. W. and Kolobow, T. (1975). Follow up respiratory function of a patient treated with a membrane lung. *Amer. Rev. Resp. Dis.* **112**, 725.

O'Donohue, W. J., Baker, J. P., Bell, G. M., Muren, O. and Patterson, J. L. (1970). The management of acute respiratory failure in a respiratory intensive care unit. *Chest* **58**, 603.

Petty, T. L., Lakshminarayan, S., Sahn, S. A. and Zwillich, C. W. (1975). Intensive respiratory care unit. *JAMA* **233**, 34.

Rebuck, A. S. and Read, J. (1971). Assessment and management of severe asthma. *Amer. J. Med.* **51**, 788.

Rees, H. A., Millar, J. S. and Donald, K. W. (1968). A study of the clinical course and arterial blood gas tensions of patients in status asthmaticus. *Quart. J. Med. New Series* **37**, 541.

Riordan, J. F., Sillett, R. W. and McNicol, M. W. (1974). Response to a respiratory stimulant (doxapram) in severe respiratory failure. *Brit. J. Dis. Chest* **68**, 39.

Riordan, J. F., Sillett, R. W. and McNicol, M. W. (1975). A controlled trial of doxapram in acute respiratory failure. *Brit. J. Dis. Chest* **69**, 57.

Shenfield, G. M., Evans, M. E. and Paterson, J. W. (1974). The effect of different nebulizers with and without intermittent positive pressure breathing on the absorption and metabolism of salbutamol. *Brit. J. Clin. Pharmac.* **1**, 295.

Sherwood Jones, E. (1971). Intensive therapy of asthma. *Proc. roy. Soc. Med.* **64**, 1151.

Sluiter, H. J., Blokzijl, E. J., van Dijl, W., van Haeringen, J. R., Hilvering, C. and Steenhuis, E. J. (1972). Conservative and respirator treatment of acute respiratory insufficiency in patients with chronic obstructive lung disease. *Amer. Rev. Resp. Dis.* **105**, 932.

Spiro, S. G., Johnson, A. J., May, C. S. and Paterson, J. W. (1975). Effect of intravenous injection of salbutamol in asthma. *Brit. J. Clin. Pharmac.* **2**, 495.

Stark, R. D. and Bishop, J. M. (1973). New method for oxygen therapy in the home using an oxygen concentrator. *Brit. Med. J.* **2**, 105.

Stark, R. D., Finnegan, P. and Bishop, J. M. (1972). Daily requirement of oxygen to reverse pulmonary hypertension in patients with chronic bronchitis. *Brit. Med. J.* **3**, 724.

Stark, R. D., Finnegan, P. and Bishop, J. M. (1973). Long term domiciliary oxygen in chronic bronchitis with pulmonary hypertension. *Brit. Med. J.* **3**, 467.

Stewart, B. N., Hood, I. C. and Block, A. J. (1975). Long term results of continuous oxygen therapy at sea level. *Chest* **68**, 486.

Straub, P. W., Buhlmann, A. A. and Rossier, P. H. (1969). Hypovolaemia in status asthmaticus. *Lancet* **2**, 923.

Suter, P. M., Fairley, B. and Isenberg, M. D. (1975). Optimum end-expiratory airway pressure in patients with acute pulmonary failure. *New Engl. J. Med.* **292**, 284.

Sykes, M. K. and Finlay, W. E. I. (1971). Dead space during anaesthesia. *Anaesthesia* **26**, 22.

Wang, P. and Clausen, T. (1976). Treatment of attacks in hyperkalaemic familial periodic paralysis by inhalation of salbutamol. *Lancet* **1**, 221.

Warrell, D. A., Edwards, R. H. T., Godfrey, S. and Jones, N. L. (1970). The effect of controlled oxygen therapy on arterial blood gases in acute respiratory failure. *Brit. Med. J.* **2**, 452.

Webber, B. A., Shenfield, G. M. and Paterson, J. W. (1974). A comparison of three different techniques for giving nebulized albuterol to asthmatic patients. *Amer. Rev. Resp. Dis.* **109**, 293.

West, J. B. (1971). Causes of carbon-dioxide retention in lung disease. *New Engl. J. Med.* **284**, 1232.

Williams, S. J., Parrish, R. W. and Seaton, A. (1975). Comparison of intravenous aminophylline and salbutamol in severe asthma. *Brit. Med. J.* **4**, 685.

Woolf, C. R. (1970). The use of 'respiratory stimulant' drugs. *Chest* **58**, 49.

Section 2: Pulmonary Failure following Sepsis and Trauma

GILLIAN C. HANSON

INTRODUCTION

Post-traumatic respiratory distress syndrome became well recognised during the management of combat casualties in the Vietnam war (Proctor et al., 1970; Bredenberg, 1974). Since then an enormous volume of literature has appeared regarding its pathogenesis and management (Barnes and Merendino, 1972; Blaisdell and Schlobohm, 1973). Ashbaugh in a series of articles (Ashbaugh et al., 1967; Ashbaugh and Petty, 1972) described the respiratory distress syndrome and emphasised that 19 of his series of 31 patients who died of the lesion had pulmonary sepsis. Eiseman (1975) showed in his paper that the immediate post-injury period if treated vigorously is generally no longer fatal but that instead, respiratory distress syndrome of late onset associated with generalised or pulmonary sepsis was the life-threatening lesion. They concluded that respiratory insufficiency still existed following injury but that careful attention to fluid therapy, diuretics and adequate mechanical ventilation now prevented early death. They noted that the late onset of respiratory distress syndrome was frequently characterised by the lack of serious ventilatory problems immediately post-injury and common to them was sepsis, which could have been primary or a complication to other pulmonary problems. Fulton and Jones (1974) reviewed the admissions to their hospital for trauma and found that pulmonary insufficiency developed in only 7% of their patients with hypovolaemic shock; on the other hand sepsis was present in 91% of those who had pulmonary failure requiring respiratory support and of all patients who became septic, 42% had serious respiratory problems. Clowes *et al.* (1975) compared data on haemodynamic and respiratory function from patients after experiencing severe haemorrhagic shock with the data from patients who suffered fulminating non-thoracic sepsis. The mild respiratory dysfunction induced by severe haemorrhagic shock and massive blood transfusion contrasted markedly with the severe prolonged pulmonary insufficiency which accompanied extensive sepsis. Their findings supported the views of the preceding authors, that sepsis was of major importance in the induction of the so called 'shock lung'.

It would appear that regardless of the nature of the insult, the lung has essentially the same response, namely the formation of septal oedema. Drinker (1945), Clowes (1974) and Blaisdell *et al.* (1970) have reviewed the sequence of events. Characteristically, the post-shock lesion consists of septal oedema, vascular congestion with trapped platelet emboli and some alveolar collapse. The Stage I lesion of sepsis in addition to oedema and congestion, is characterised by leucocytic infiltration and more diffuse collapse (focal atelectasis). Clinically the Stage 1 lesion is manifested by hypoxia and shunting and the lungs on

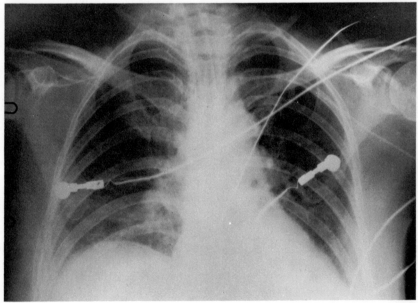

Fig. 1. Pulmonary failure following sepsis. Stage I. Patient with intraperitoneal sepsis. Ground glass appearance on X-ray.

X-ray are clear or have a slight ground glass appearance (Fig. 1). Considerable lung oedema may be present before there are X-ray changes (Vito *et al.*, 1974). Should the condition not be appropriately treated, the lesion may progress to Stage II bronchopneumonia with polymorphonuclear leucocytes in the alveoli and septa accompanied by areas of consolidation giving a mottled appearance on X-ray (Fig. 2). Clowes *et al.* (1975) noted that only the secondarily infected post-shock traumatised patients developed severe hypoxia and shunting, whereas the extent of shunting in the septic patients was significantly greater even if the lesions remained in Stage I. The duration of shunting was prolonged in the septic patients and rarely subsided until the septic focus was eliminated. Pulmonary compliance was decreased to a greater extent in pulmonary failure associated with sepsis suggesting a greater degree of alveolar collapse and oedema in Stage I than experienced in the patients developing pulmonary failure following trauma. Cardiac function also differed in the two groups. Cardiac function was found to be excellent in the majority of post-shock traumatised patients, being high initially and subsiding to normal by the fourth day. Only 20 of the 38 septic patients however, successfully

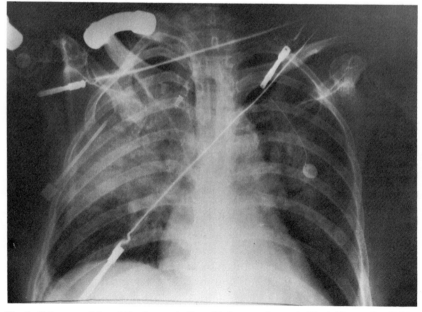

Fig. 2. Pulmonary failure following sepsis. Stage II. Same patient as in Fig. 1. X-ray taken 9 days later showing extensive lung infiltration.

maintained a high cardiac output throughout their illness in response to a characteristically low peripheral vascular resistance (Shoemaker *et al.*, 1973). Clowes *et al.* (1975) found that those patients who failed to maintain a high cardiac output were those who showed the greatest degree of shunting and loss of compliance. Shunt appears to decrease once cardiac output improves. It was also noted that a raised pulmonary vascular resistance was characteristic of pulmonary failure secondary to sepsis and that there was a significantly greater gradient from mean P-A pressure to left atrial pressure in the septic than in the post-traumatic shock patients (Clowes *et al.*, 1975).

Thus shunting, compliance and pulmonary vascular resistance all seem greater and last longer in the septic patient than in the patient who has sustained haemorrhagic shock followed by massive blood replacement. With improved techniques in respiratory care – death is unlikely to occur immediately in pulmonary failure following non-thoracic trauma, but may develop later if complicated by thoracic or non-thoracic sepsis.

FACTORS WHICH MAY CONTRIBUTE TO PULMONARY FAILURE FOLLOWING TRAUMA AND ACCENTUATE PULMONARY FAILURE ASSOCIATED WITH SEPSIS

The causes of progressive pulmonary insufficiency in surgical patients was discussed by Collins (1969) and many other authors have discussed the aetiological factors in relation to various clinical situations, e.g. Connell *et al.* (1975) and Brown *et al.* (1974) in haemorrhagic and traumatic shock, Clowes *et al.* (1975) in relation to generalised sepsis and Robb *et al.* (1972) in endotoxic shock.

The aetiological factors precipitating or producing further deterioration in pulmonary failure are numerous.

Fluid overload

Fluid overload can generally be prevented during rapid volume replacement by central venous pressure monitoring, careful observation of urine output and avoidance of excessive sodium administration. The catabolic response to stress is sodium retention, and excessive quantities of sodium containing solutions should be avoided during resuscitation. The dose of bicarbonate ions initially administered to a patient with a metabolic acidosis should be 50 mmol – bearing in mind that during volume replacement peripheral and renal perfusion should improve and adequate ventilation will correct hypercarbia and/or hypoxia. Subsequent doses should be given according to the Astrup analysis (see p. 203). It must be remembered that steroids, in particular when used in massive dosage as for shock associated with sepsis, produce sodium retention.

The fluid to be used for volume replacement is important (see p. 341). It is known that the interstitial space rapidly accumulates fluid once the serum albumin falls below 25 g/l and the major fear is that this decrease in serum albumin may lead to pulmonary oedema (Cervera and Moss, 1974). It is therefore important in patients who develop severe to profound haemorrhagic shock or in patients who become hypovolaemic and are already hypoalbuminaemic that volume should be replaced with blood (when the haematocrit is less then 30%) or a protein containing solution such as plasma protein fraction or salt-free albumin. Even the albumin molecule may not be large enough to prevent pulmonary oedema in the face of increased alveolar capillary permeability. Perhaps the use of high molecular weight dextrans should be considered for plasma expansion in patients who already have, or are particularly predisposed to this condition.

The use of non-filtered blood

Reul *et al.* (1973) showed that post-traumatic pulmonary insufficiency had been radically reduced by finescreen filtration (Ultipor, Pall, Fenwal). Fibrin platelet and leucocyte aggregates, denatured protein fat and cellular stroma accumulate in stored blood (Swank, 1970; McNamara *et al.*, 1971 and 1972). Cullen and Ferrara (1974) recommended that finescreen filtration should be employed when transfusion of more than two units of blood is anticipated. When platelets are required, fresh blood should be used without filtration, methods of blood component therapy such as packed cells with cell washing also eliminate the problem of particulate matter infusion (Reul *et al.*, 1974).

For further details on blood filtration see Part 4, ch. III, p. 948.

Metabolic factors

Sodium overload has already been mentioned – the onset of the hypernatraemic hyperosmolar syndrome may lead to expansion of the intravascular space (especially when renal tubular function is impaired) and left ventricular failure may be complicated by the onset of a pulmonary diffusion defect secondary to interstitial and interalveolar oedema.

Brown and co-workers (1974) noted that an increase in pulmonary vascular resistance was one of the earliest dynamic responses to injury and that the magnitude of the increase appeared to be related to the severity of the injury. Kim and Shoemaker (1972) noted that the pulmonary vascular resistance increase in the early stages of shock was pH dependent and that approximately two-thirds of the resistance could be abolished by maintaining venous pH in the normal or slightly alkalotic range during the hypotensive period. Brown and co-workers (1974) from their study concluded that the interaction of pH, pulmonary vascular resistance and the volume of blood supplying the pulmonary circulation, was of major significance in the development of pulmonary shunting.

Potassium deficiency is relatively common following haemorrhagic shock or during volume replacement with potassium free solutions – this may lead to a decrease in myocardial contractility and a tendency towards cardiac dysrhythmias. Clowes and co-workers (1975) found that patients with severe non-pulmonary sepsis who failed to maintain a high cardiac output exhibited the greatest degree of pulmonary shunting and loss of compliance.

Hyponatraemia secondary to inappropriate release of antidiuretic hormone has been well documented following brain trauma, especially in association with subdural haematomata (Fichman and Bethune, 1968; Maroon and Campbell, 1970). These patients have an increased tendency to pulmonary oedema. Moss and co-workers (1972) postulated that the entire pathophysiological sequence of the 'shock lung syndrome' could be explained by autonomically mediated pulmonary venospasm initiated by hypovolaemic hypoxia during the period of shock.

Organ failure

The onset of organ failure may precipitate pulmonary oedema – monitoring of renal, hepatic, and cardiac function is therefore essential in the critically ill post-traumatic or septic patient. Renal failure may be complicated by fluid overload and hepatic failure by hypoalbuminaemia and a predisposition to sepsis. The onset of left ventricular failure may be missed if monitoring is confined to pulmonary artery and/or right atrial pressure. Civetta and Gabel (1975) stressed that the onset of pulmonary oedema is an indication for careful monitoring in critically ill patients. Pulmonary artery wedge pressure monitoring was essential in order to correct the erroneous though seemingly well founded suspected diagnosis of left ventricular failure in their patients. Clowes *et al.* (1975) found that circulatory insufficiency was one of the major causes for pulmonary shunting in severe sepsis and postulated that the two principal causes were fluid translocation and hypovolaemia. Nevertheless, the elderly patient under stress is predisposed to left ventricular failure and appropriate antifailure therapy rapidly reverses the pulmonary diffusion defect.

Shock

Connell and co-workers (1975) showed experimentally that hypotension and hypovolaemia are attended by aggregation of platelets and leucocytes which microembolise to the microcirculation and cause destruction of the vascular endothelium and other structures of the lungs. The production of hypovolaemia insufficient to cause hypotension was also shown to cause identical lesions. It was further observed that the re-infusion of the withdrawn blood without filtration increased the severity of the pulmonary lesions. Pulmonary failure following trauma in humans is generally preceded by a period of hypotension treated with blood transfusion; in pulmonary failure following sepsis however the syndrome may develop in patients who have never been hypotensive, or become hypotensive after the syndrome has developed (McLean *et al.*, 1968; Rosoff *et al.*, 1967). The unexpected appearances of pulmonary insufficiency after resuscitation from haemorrhagic shock is often a sign of the development of major sepsis (Clowes *et al.*, 1975; Civetta and Gabel, 1975; Wilson *et al.*, 1969). The term shock lung for this syndrome is therefore inappropriate, and should preferably be replaced by pulmonary failure secondary to sepsis, or very occasionally to pulmonary failure secondary to extensive non-thoracic trauma.

Problems relating to the lungs

Any pulmonary factor which occurs in the presence of pulmonary failure is likely to perpetuate the condition. Intermittent positive pressure ventilation under high airways pressure may be complicated by acute pneumothorax or pneumomediastinum, the likelihood is increased when a positive end expiratory pressure of 10 cm of water or more is applied (Powers *et al.*, 1972). The application of a high positive end expiratory pressure (generally greater than 10 cm of water) in the presence of cardiac instability may decrease cardiac output thereby reducing pulmonary perfusion and accentuating the hypoxia (Lenfant and Howell, 1960). Careful monitoring prior to and after the introduction of P.E.E.P. is therefore important (see p. 327).

Lung collapse may complicate artificial ventilation especially when there are large quantities of pulmonary aspirate, such collapse may be difficult to re-expand and may be complicated by sepsis. Pulmonary sepsis may complicate artificial ventilation and may be the factor precipitating pulmonary failure following trauma. Experimentally it has been found both in post-shock states and in sepsis that synthesis and secretion of surfactant (principally L-dipalmitoyl phosphatidyl choline) is reduced (Clowes, 1974). Surfactant action is further impaired by the presence in the alveoli of protein which inhibits the surface activity of the phospholipids. These effects promote alveolar collapse, and the loss of the bacteriostatic activity of surfactant may contribute to the advent of bronchopneumonia (Clowes et al., 1975). The experimental and clinical evidence for circulating agents producing pneumonitis in non-thoracic sepsis has been reviewed by Clowes (1974) and include endotoxin, fibrinopeptides secondary to disseminated intravascular coagulation (D.I.C.), kinins, serotonin, prostoglandins and ATP-ase released from platelets, and vasoactive peptides released from lysis of protein from damaged tissues. It would appear that septic patients have one or more agents circulating which are capable of inducing pulmonary oedema and a rise in pulmonary vascular resistance. Their presence seems to precede the development of A-V shunting, oedema and reduced compliance (Clowes et al., 1975). Hypoxia may produce central nervous depression, loss of the cough reflex, and pulmonary aspiration, thereby accentuating the already existing pulmonary shunt. Oxygen produces toxic effects on the lung by reducing the synthesis of lecithin and the total amount of pulmonary surface lipids (Norman et al., 1971). Damage to the alveolar lining by exposure to an inspiratory oxygen percentage of greater than 60% for short periods or possibly greater than 50% for longer periods, may kill the patient through oxygen toxicity alone. It is only by careful attention to the percentage of oxygen inspired in pulmonary failure that this can be eliminated as the ultimate factor producing death from hypoxia.

Pulmonary aspiration

This is a known hazard in the management of the critically ill and may be an important factor contributing towards pulmonary failure in states where the cough reflex is impaired. It is a particular hazard in patients suffering from multiple trauma and may complicate intubation for pulmonary failure or induction of anaesthesia (for further details see p. 563).

Generalised infection

Circulating agents which may precipitate pneumonitis in patients suffering from generalised sepsis have been referred to above. Neely and co-workers (1971) have shown that the mortality rate associated with septic shock varied widely with the source of infection, intraperitoneal sepsis being the most lethal. Patients with intraperitoneal sepsis are particularly susceptible to pulmonary failure and this is frequently the major factor precipitating death – the patient dying terminally of right ventricular failure secondary to an increasing pulmonary vascular resistance, biventricular failure, or increasing hypoxia frequently associated with bronchopneumonia. It is probable that microthrombosis in the pulmonary microcirculation may be an important aetiological factor in pulmonary failure associated with generalised sepsis. Milligan and co-workers (1974) noted a marked reduction in platelet count with associated coagulation deficiencies consistent with disseminated intravascular coagulation in nineteen patients with septic shock. The observation that the platelet count fell prior to the full development of the pulmonary disturbance was in favour of a causal relationship. On the other hand, Robb and co-workers (1972) showed that showers of microemboli could be demonstrated by cinematography to lodge in the portal and pulmonary microcirculation during an early and terminal phase of experimentally produced endotoxin shock. The platelet count fell when the platelets becamse sequestered from the circulation as pulmonary microemboli. They suggested that muscle tissue was the greatest potential source of emboli.

Miscellaneous factors

Generalised anaesthesia is followed by hypoxaemia lasting several days in the majority of patients. Laver and Bendixen (1966) consider this is related to military atelectasis. The degree of hypoxia produced is rarely serious unless superimposed upon hypoxia due to various factors, in particular generalised sepsis or thoracic trauma.

Operation

Significant deleterious changes in respiratory mechanics may follow laparotomy or thoracotomy (Eisman and Ashbaugh, 1968; Okinaka, 1967). These changes may precipitate pulmonary failure in a patient who has preceding interstitial pulmonary oedema.

Embolism

Thromboembolism and microthrombosis. The familiar form of thrombo-embolism certainly may occur in supine patients with inadequate hydration and slow peripheral blood flow. Eeles and Sevitt (1967) have found pulmonary macro- and microthrombi to be common in injured and burned patients.

Disseminated intravascular coagulation commonly occurs in clinical shock states – the question is how much it contributes to the deterioration in pulmonary function. Microembolism may be an important contributory factor in the development of pulmonary failure following endotoxin shock (Robb *et al.*, 1972).

Fat embolism. The analysis of pulmonary morphological findings in patients who die from septic and traumatic-haemorrhagic shock show similar changes, namely microthrombi, and interstitial and peri-vascular oedema. Fat globuli appear on microscopic examination in 55% of patients following trauma and in only 8% of patients with septic shock (Zimmermann *et al.*, 1972). Fat embolism therefore appears to play an important role in the development of pulmonary failure following trauma. It has been stated that 0.8–6% of patients with severe traumatic injuries will develop the fat embolism syndrome (Wilson and Salisbury, 1944; Newman, 1948).

THE FAT EMBOLISM SYNDROME

Definition

Gurd and Wilson (1974) have drawn attention to the difficulty in distinguishing between the existence of embolic fat in the lungs of patients who have suffered trauma, and the true syndrome in which a chemical interstitial pneumonitis is a prominent feature associated with a series of characteristic symptoms and signs. The pulmonary disorder is characterised by hypoxia.

Pathophysiology

Since the role which fat plays in this condition is uncertain, it is wise to term the condition the fat embolism syndrome as opposed to pulmonary fat embolism.

Peltier (1956) suggested that neutral triglycerides embolising to the lungs were converted there to unsaturated fatty acids by the action of lipase. Unsaturated fatty acids are known to be irritant and result in congestion, oedema and intra-alveolar haemorrhage. This theory is supported experimentally in that intravenous injection of unsaturated fatty acids produces a similar syndrome whereas neutral fat does not (Benatar *et al.*, 1972). It is probable that intravascular aggregation of red cells and fat embolism both play an important role in the production of the syndrome. Intravascular coagulation is thought to be initiated by thromboplastin released from the fat, and the presence or absence of fibrin is dependent on the fibrinolytic response to clotting (Saldeen, 1970).

Clinical features of the fat embolism syndrome

The syndrome generally develops following fracture of the long bones or pelvis but may follow cracking injuries or minimal fractures such as that of the calcaneum or patella. In all cases there is a latent period between injury and onset of symptoms, the average time being forty-six hours (Gurd and Wilson, 1974). In patients who have sustained a long bone fracture, symptoms may develop during or following surgical manipulation of the fracture site.

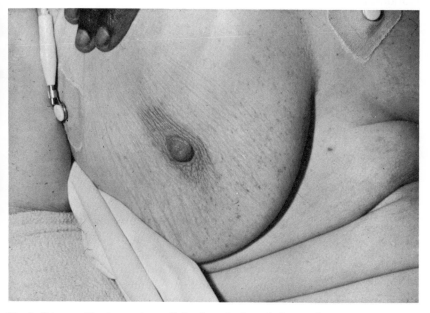

Fig. 3. Skin petechiae in a patient suffering from the fat embolism syndrome.

Respiratory involvement manifested by dyspnoea and tachypnoea is the commonest initial manifestation. Cyanosis is often absent even when arterial hypoxia is marked. The patient may present with a pyrexia or cerebral signs such as confusion, lack of co-operation, restlessness, memory deterioration or drowsiness, the tachypnoea being missed. The petechial rash (see Fig. 3) is found in approximately 50% of patients and may be found on the chest anterior axillary fold and the root of the neck; retinal exudates and haemorrhages may be seen and occasionally fat droplets in the retinal vessels. Mild jaundice may be noted and some degree of renal failure is common.

Investigations

The haemoglobin level frequently falls by 50% and thrombocytopenia is common and may be present in the absence of any deficiency in coagulation. Disseminated intravascular coagulation occasionally complicates the fat embolism syndrome. Gurd (1970a) described a diagnostic procedure for fat embolism. After filtration of the serum through a microfilter, he found greater differences between serum and filtrate in trauma cases and in patients with clinical signs of fat embolism. According to Gurd's description it should be possible to stain the retained fat globules on the filter paper, their size being greater than 8 microns. Nolte and co-workers (1974) found that the technique was difficult to standardise and concluded that the method was not diagnostic and in cases of clear cut fat embolism syndrome could even be misleading.

Prys-Roberts (1974) described in detail the respiratory changes associated with the fat embolism syndrome. When emboli of fat or any other material enter the pulmonary circulation and occlude the flow of blood to discrete or diffuse groups of alveoli whose ventilation is maintained, then these areas behave functionally as increased alveolar dead space (Bruecke et al., 1971) and have a ventilation perfusion ratio ($\dot{V}_{A/Q}$) approaching zero. Hyperventilation is common in the early stages of the syndrome and is increased above that required to compensate for the increased dead space; low arterial $PaCO_2$ levels therefore tend to detract from the true defect in gas exchange.

Following the initial phase the alveolar dead space tends to return to normal and there develops a period of interstitial pneumonitis. The ventilation of the areas of lung involved becomes reduced although blood flow continues, thereby producing hypoxia during air breathing and a markedly increased alveolar-arterial oxygen difference. Patients

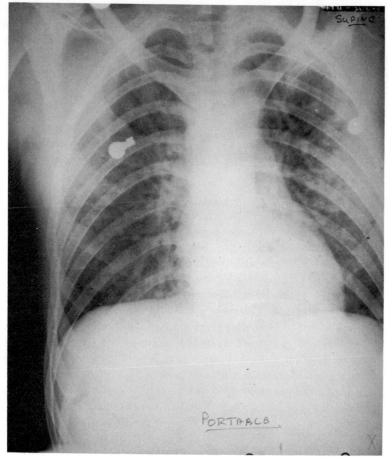

Fig. 4. Classical chest X-ray appearances in a patient suffering from the fat embolism syndrome.

at this stage, especially when ventilated, are markedly predisposed to pulmonary infection.

The chest X-ray is characteristic at the phase of interstitial pneumonitis (Fig. 4) showing a snowstorm appearance; there may be auscultatory signs of pulmonary oedema.

Fat embolism in sickle cell disease

Fat embolism is a known complication of marrow infarction in patients with sickle cell disease and should be considered in sickle cell crisis when there is deterioration in respiratory function, a fall in PaO_2, and normoblastaemia associated with thrombocytopenia in the blood (Hutchinson *et al.*, 1973). Evidence of disseminated intravascular coagulation should be looked for. It is essential in such patients to start heparin early and ensure a PaO_2 of 12–13.3 kPa (90–100 mm/Hg) with restoration of haemoglobin to a level which maintains the haematocrit around 30%.

DIAGNOSIS AND TREATMENT OF PULMONARY FAILURE SECONDARY TO SEPSIS AND TRAUMA (other than the fat embolism syndrome)

The diagnosis of pulmonary failure has already been discussed – the condition is characterised by a recent traumatic incident generally associated with haemorrhagic hypotension and treated with massive transfusion of non-filtered old blood, or a patient suffering from extensive sepsis. Hyperventilation is characteristic in the patient who is sufficiently fit to compensate for the increasing hypoxia. The alveolar-arterial oxygen gradient is high and is commonly associated with a rising airways pressure. The right atrial and pulmonary artery pressure is commonly high but the pulmonary capillary wedge pressure (P.C.W.P.) is generally normal until terminally, when left ventricular failure may develop. P.C.W.P. may not, however, reflect left ventricular function when the intrathoracic pressure is high. The chest X-ray in Stage I generally is clear or shows a slight ground glass appearance (Fig. 1) but in Stage II the chest X-ray shows extensive mottling due to pulmonary sepsis (Fig. 2). Chest aspirate at this stage is commonly purulent.

The various factors which may contribute towards deterioration in pulmonary failure has been stressed. It is important, once the condition has been diagnosed, to attempt to prevent any of these factors occurring and to recognise and treat them appropriately should they arise.

Early diagnosis of pulmonary failure following trauma or sepsis is essential in order to prevent the effect of factors which may produce further deterioration. The object of management is a series of sequential steps designed to increase and maintain the functional residual capacity. The patient's arterial oxygen tension should be observed whilst breathing spontaneously on air and the indication for artificial ventilation may be an increasing respiratory rate in a patient whose PaO_2 is slowly falling, or a patient whose PaO_2 on 35% oxygen via a face mask is 9.3 kPa (70 mm/Hg) or less. It is essential not to assume that the mask used will deliver the oxygen percentage stated by the manufacturers. The inspiratory oxygen percentage should be checked inside the mask with an oxygen analyser. It is unlikely that an inspiratory oxygen percentage above 35% will be achieved with a nonocclusive mask in a hyperventilating patient. Benatar and co-workers (1973) made use of iso-shunt lines for control of oxygen therapy. This facilitates rapid determination of the optimal inspired oxygen for patients hypoxaemic due to venous admixture and limited the number of blood gas analyses required for patient management. J. H. Kerr (1975 and personal communication) is at present investigating the effect of different inspired oxygen concentrations (performed in quick succession) on the shunt values (Fig. 5). In the majority of patients the shunt value increased as the F_IO_2 was increased (hyperoxic shunt) but in the patients with severe lung damage the shunt value decreased as the F_IO_2

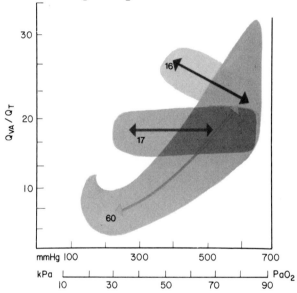

Fig. 5. I.P.P.V. with N_2/O_2 mixtures: 93 sets of observations on 44 patients. Patterns of response of oxygenating efficiency (expressed as % venous admixture – Q_{VA}/Q_T) with changing alveolar tensions (PaO_2) during I.P.P.V. in 44 patients. Each set of observations includes two or more estimations of oxygenating efficiency made after short exposures to different inspired oxygen concentrations while ventilation remained unchanged.

On the majority of occasions (60/93), venous admixture increased as PaO_2 increased (hyperoxic shunt). Where lung damage was most severe and efficiency most impaired, venous admixture decreased as inspired oxygen was increased while during recovery the response to oxygen altered in that venous admixture initially remained unchanged (iso-shunt pattern) and eventually the hyperoxic shunt pattern reappeared. (Reproduced by kind permission of J. H. Kerr, Nuffield Department of Anaesthetics, Oxford.)

increased. As the patient's lung condition improved, the shunt pattern changed from the latter to an iso-shunt pattern and finally to a hyperoxic pattern. It is suggested that this change may indicate steady improvement in pulmonary failure and may therefore be a guide to assessing the optimum time for patient weaning.

The alveolar arterial-oxygen difference may be calculated. Woo and Hedley-Whyte (1973) recommend that the calculation be made after the patient has breathed 100% oxygen for 5 min; the alveolar oxygen tension then equals the barometric pressure minus 6.3 kPa (47 mm Hg) (water vapour pressure at 37°C). A normal alveolar-arterial oxygen gradient with a person breathing 100% oxygen is 4–9.3 kPa (30–70 mm Hg). When the alveolar arterial oxygen gradient is greater than 46.7 kPa (350 mm Hg) breathing 100% oxygen, controlled ventilation is required and the dosage of oxygen should be redetermined after another set of blood gas measurements. The scheme for oxygen therapy based on alveolar arterial oxygen gradients (measured on 100% oxygen) recommended by Woo and Hedley-Whyte is shown in Table 1. The degree of pulmonary shunting – as previously described – may be affected by exposure of the lungs to different oxygen percentages and it is therefore preferable to calculate the $A\text{-}aDO_2$ gradient on the

Table 1. Scheme for oxygen therapy based on alveolar arterial oxygen gradients (measured on 100% oxygen). (Reproduced with kind permission from Woo and Hedley-White, 1973.)

Alveolar arterial oxygen gradient on 100% oxygen kPa (mm Hg)	Suggested method of treatment	Suggested fraction of inspired oxygen for therapy
4–9.3 (30–70)	None	0.21 (room air)
9.3–16 (70–120)	None	0.21 (room air)
16–33.3 (120–250)	Face-mask or cannula	0.35
33.6–46.7 (250–350)	Face-mask	0.4
46.7–60 (350–450)	I.P.P.V	0.5
60–73.3 (450–550)	I.P.P.V.	0.6
73.3–86.7 (550–650)	C.P.P.V.	0.6 (titrate P.E.E.P. up to 17 cm H_2O)

inspiratory oxygen percentage the patient is receiving. Subsequent to these recommendations, Goldfarb and co-workers (1975) have modi-fied the alveolar-arterial gradient by dividing the PaO_2 in mm Hg and producing a respiratory index (R.I.). They found that any patient who had an R.I. as high as 2 required intubation and patients with an R.I. of over 7 rarely survived. The equation suggested to them by Siegel and Farrell (1973) was the following:

$$\frac{[(P_B - P_{H_2O}T)F_IO_2 - PaCO_2] - PaO_2}{PaO_2} = \frac{P(\text{A-a}DO_2)}{PaO_2}$$

Where P_B = barometric pressure in mm Hg, $P_{H_2O}T$ = alveolar water vapour pressure at the patient's temperature (T) (approximately 47 mm Hg), $PaCO_2$ = arterial partial pressure of carbon dioxide assumed to be equal to the alveolar partial pressure of the carbon dioxide $(PaCO_2)$ in mm Hg, F_IO_2 = fractional concentration of oxygen in inspired gas, PaO_2 = arterial partial pressure of oxygen in mm Hg.

The respiratory index has been found to be an excellent method of tracking progress in the patient suffering from pulmonary failure subsequent to sepsis or trauma.

On rare occasions it is possible to raise the PaO_2 in a patient where assisted ventilation is considered necessary with the introduction of an end expiratory resistance, allowing the patient to breathe spon-taneously. Walling and Savage (1974) have found this system valuable in a small series of patients – it must be stressed, however, that the patient may become exhausted and that oxygen used up during the process of breathing is prevented by C.P.P.V. (artificial ventilation with an end expiratory pressure).

The use of I.P.P.V. with a volume-cycled ventilator is often sufficient to produce an increase in oxygen tension to 10.7–13.3 kPa (80–100 mm Hg) with the use of an inspiratory oxygen percentage of 40 or less. The $PaCO_2$ should be kept at or slightly below normal. Should the PaO_2 not rise above 9.3 kPa (70 mm Hg) on the above measures, a pulmonary end expiratory pressure should be applied.

The monitoring systems recommended before and following the introduction of P.E.E.P. are summarised in Part 2, ch. II, p. 327.

P.E.E.P. is of value in reduction of alveolar collapse and restoration of a normal ventilation perfusion ratio (Clowes et al., 1975). Dangers exist in its use and Clowes and co-workers advise (1975) that P.E.E.P. of 15 cm or more should not be employed unless pulmonary haemo-dynamics and cardiac output can be monitored.

It must be stressed that P.E.E.P. must be employed with extreme caution in a patient who is known to suffer from chronic respiratory failure. A patient with a low functional residual capacity with a consequent potential for recruitment of collapsed alveoli may benefit, but a patient whose alveoli are near maximum expansion may be harmed. It has been suggested by Suter *et al.* (1975) that failure to discriminate between these modalities may be the reason for inconsistent results being obtained in the therapeutic use of P.E.E.P. (King *et al.*, 1973).

Ventilation should be continued until a PaO_2 of 10 kPa (75 mm Hg) or more can be maintained on an inspiratory oxygen percentage of 35% and P.E.E.P. of 2.5 cm H_2O. Weaning should be gradual and should be commenced by allowing the patient to breathe against an end expiratory resistance in conjunction with I.M.V.

There are many other factors that are vitally important during the period of ventilation. Suction of the bronchial tree should be performed by a strictly aseptic technique, sputum for anaerobic and aerobic cultures should be sent 3 times weekly and antibiotics should not be used for the pulmonary condition unless there is evidence of sepsis. Patients on broad spectrum antibiotics for disseminated infection are markedly predisposed to secondary lung infection from anaerobes (such as Bacteroides) *Pseudomonas pyocyaneus*, Proteus, Klebsiella, or fungal species.

Patients who require ventilation for intra-abdominal sepsis frequently require it for over one week. We have found a nasal endotracheal tube under such circumstances unsatisfactory and find a tracheostomy easier to maintain, easier for bronchial toilet and easier for patient weaning.

Many other factors contribute to the maintenance of pulmonary function – maintenance of an adequate right ventricular cardiac output being of particular importance. Inotropic agents, or glucose potassium and insulin may on occasions be required in pulmonary failure following extensive sepsis (Clowes *et al.*, 1974). Other important factors include adequate protein nutrition for antibacterial defence and surfactant synthesis (Alexander, 1972) and maintenance of normal metabolic balance.

Heparin has been suggested for the treatment of disseminated intravascular coagulation secondary to sepsis (Corrigan *et al.*, 1968). It is unlikely however that heparin will ameliorate the lung condition which is generally well established before the haematological abnormalities become sufficiently severe to warrant its use.

Pre-medication of experimental cats and dogs with methylprednisolone sodium succinate has been reported to be beneficial in preventing some of the deleterious lung effects of haemorrhagic shock (Wilson, 1972). At the present time there appears to be little justification for their use in patients with post-traumatic pulmonary failure and should only be used for patients with extensive sepsis where shock treated by the usual measures fails to resolve (see Part 2, ch. II, p. 367).

THE TREATMENT OF PULMONARY FAILURE SECONDARY TO THE FAT EMBOLISM SYNDROME

The diagnosis of the fat embolism syndrome has been described on p. 549. The management of the hypoxia is similar to that described for pulmonary failure following trauma (where there is no evidence of the fat embolism syndrome) but there are certain aspects of drug management which should be considered.

The affected part should be immobilised and further surgery should be delayed until pulmonary function has improved to the extent that the patient is able to breathe spontaneously. Occasionally the fracture cannot be adequately immobilised and there is evidence after 4 days' ventilation of deterioration in pulmonary function, this may be associated with increased patchiness on the chest X-ray. Under such circumstances if secondary pulmonary infection is unlikely, immobilisation of the fracture by pinning may have to be considered, keeping in mind that there may be further deterioration in pulmonary function at the time or within four days of the operation. Various drugs have been considered in the treatment of the fat embolism syndrome. *Intravenous alcohol* has been advocated to decrease the action of serum lipase on the assumption that lipolysis of the neutral fat emboli is harmful (Adler *et al.*, 1961). Its use is not universally accepted as large doses are required and clinical results unimpressive (Benatar *et al.*, 1972). *Dextran 40*—The efficacy of low molecular weight dextran in the treatment of fat embolism has been suggested in a case report by Bergentz (1961) and by Denman and co-workers (1964). Subsequent reports however have not mentioned its use in treatment (Dines *et al.*, 1972; Gurd and Wilson, 1974), or have advised against it because extravasation into already oedematous lung parenchyma might further enhance the retention of fluid in lung tissue (Scott, 1973). *Heparin* has been recommended by many authors largely because it may inhibit the platelet-fibrinogen consumption process, and has been shown by Adler and co-workers (1961) to activate lipase and expedite the fat clearing process. Scott

(1973) has suggested, however, that this agent may be disadvantageous in elevating free fatty acid levels and may encourage spontaneous bleeding from unrecognised sites of trauma. Heparin rarely has to be used for disseminated intravascular coagulation alone, and should be used with caution and under thrombin control in patients with chest trauma because of the danger of an intrathoracic bleed. It is advisable not to use it for the first 48 h after an operation and it should be avoided in hypertensive patients. Heparin should be considered in patients likely to be ventilated for more than 5 days (because of the danger of pulmonary embolism) and in patients where the syndrome is severe and requires 50% or more inspiratory oxygen to maintain an adequate PaO_2. It should be titrated intravenously by continuous infusion and rigidly controlled by maintaining the thrombin time at two to three times normal.

Zimmermann and co-workers (1972) in controlled trials with protase inhibition in patients with the shock lung syndrome and the fat embolism syndrome, found a reduced mortality when Trasylol was used in conjunction with heparin. Gurd (1970b) also found a reduction in mortality from 27% in 33 patients receiving supportive therapy alone to 5.4% in 37 patients receiving Trasylol in addition to supportive therapy.

In view of these findings, it is wise to add Trasylol to the heparin therapy should the PaO_2 (in the absence of P.E.E.P.) not be maintained at an adequate level on an inspiratory oxygen percentage of 60. It should be used without heparin where its use is contraindicated.

Steroids have been advocated for the treatment of the fat embolism syndrome (Fischer et al., 1971; Dines et al., 1972) but to date the results have not been wholly convincing and their use if prolonged may predispose the patient to infection. Perhaps it would be reasonable to use one dose (30 mg methylprednisolone hemisuccinate per kg body weight as an intravenous stat dose) should pulmonary function continue to deteriorate after the use of appropriate ventilation, metabolic and fluid volume control, and heparin and/or Trasylol. The use of steroids under such circumstances will be extremely rare since the majority of patients treated with more conventional treatment will survive provided secondary pulmonary infection does not arise.

Antibiotics. Patients with the fat embolism syndrome who require ventilation are markedly predisposed to infection. Prophylactic anti-biotics should not be used but should be prescribed if a dominant organism is isolated from the sputum with additional evidence of infection – purulent sputum – deterioration in the chest X-ray. Pyrexia and tachycardia in the presence of the fat embolism syndrome is not a reliable indicator of sepsis unless the temperature remains high after 4 days from the onset of the clinical symptoms and signs.

Calcium. Volz (1966) suggested that hypocalcaemia can be severe enough to result in tetany – serum calcium levels should be carefully observed but rarely fall to dangerously low levels.

Platelets. Platelets frequently fall to levels around 100 000 mm³ – a haemorrhagic diathesis due to thrombocytopenia in association with the fat embolism syndrome has not been personally encountered.

REFERENCES

Adler, F., Lai, S. P. and Peltier, L. (1961). Fat embolism. Prophylactic treatment with lipase inhibitors. *Surg. Forum* **12**, 453.

Alexander, J. W. (1972). Host defense mechanisms against infection. *Surg. Clin. N. Amer.* **52**, 1367.

Ashbaugh, D. G., Bigelow, D. W., Petty, T. L. and Levine, B. E. (1967). Acute respiratory distress in adults. *Lancet* **1**, 319.

Ashbaugh, D. G. and Petty, T. L. (1972). Sepsis complicating the acute respiratory distress syndrome. *Surg. Gyn. Obstet.* **135**, 865.

Barnes, R. W. and Merendino, C. A. (1972). Post traumatic pulmonary insufficiency syndrome. *Surg. Clin. N. Am.* **52**, 625.

Benatar, S. R., Ferguson, A. D. and Goldschmidt, R. B. (1972). Fat embolism – some clinical observations and a review of controversial aspects. *Quart. J. Med. New Series* **41**, 85.

Benatar, S. R., Hewlett, A. M. and Nunn, J. F. (1973). The use of iso-shunt lines for control of oxygen therapy. *Brit. J. Anaesth.* **45**, 711.

Bergentz, S. E. (1961). Studies on the genesis of post traumatic fat embolism. *Acta Chir. Scand.* **282** (Suppl.), 1.

Blaisdell, F. W. and Schlobohm, R. M. (1973). The respiratory distress syndrome. A review. *Surgery* **74**, 251.

Blaisdell, F. W., Lion, R. C. and Stallone, R. J. (1970). The mechanisms of pulmonary damage following traumatic shock. *Surg. Gynec. Obstet.* **130**, 15.

Bredenberg, C. E. (1974). Acute respiratory distress. *Surg. Clin N. Amer.* **54**, 5.

Brown, R. S., Kim, S. E. and Shoemaker, W. C. (1974). Haemodynamic mechanisms in the development of pulmonary venous admixture (shunting). *J. Surg. Res.* **17**, 192.

Bruecke, P., Burke, J. F., Lam, K., Shannon, D. C. and Kazemi, H. (1971). The pathophysiology of pulmonary fat embolism. *J. Thorac. and Cardiovasc. Surg.* **61**, 949.

Cervera, A. L. and Moss, G. (1974). Crystalloid distribution following haemorrhage and haemodilution. *J. Trauma* **14**, 506.

Civetta, J. M. and Gabel, J. C. (1975). 'Pseudocardiogenic' pulmonary oedema. *J. Trauma* **15**, 143.

Clowes, G. H. A. Jr. (1974). Pulmonary abnormalities in sepsis. *Surg. Clin. N. Amer.* **54**, 5.

Clowes, G. H. A. Jr., O'Donnell, T. F. Jr., Ryan, N. T. and Blackburn, G. L. (1974). Energy metabolism in sepsis treatment based on different patterns in shock and high output states. *Ann. Surg.* **179**, 684.

Clowes, G. H. A. Jr., Hirsch, M. F. E., Williams, L., Kurasnik, E., O'Donnell, T. F., Cuevas, P., Saini, V. K., Moradi, I., Farizen, M., Saravis, C., Stone, M. and Kuffler, J. (1975). Septic lung and shock lung in Man. *Ann. Surg.* **181**, 681.

Collins, J. C. (1969). The causes of progressive pulmonary insufficiency in surgical patients. *J. Surg. Res.* **9**(12), 685.

Connell, R. S., Swank, R. L. and Webb, M. C. (1975). The development of pulmonary ultrastructural lesions during haemorrhagic shock. *J. Trauma* **15**, 116.

Corrigan, J. J. Jr., Ray, W. L. and May, N. (1968). Changes in the blood coagulation system associated with septicaemia. *New Engl. J. Med.* **279**, 851.

Cullen, D. J. and Ferrara, L. (1974). Comparative evaluation of blood filters: a study in vitro. *Anaesthesiology* **41**, 568.

Denman, E. E., Cairns, C. S. and Holmes, C. M. (1964). Case of severe fat embolism. Treated by intermittent positive-pressure respiration. *Brit. Med. J.* **2**, 101.

Dines, D. E., Linscheid, R. L., Didier, E. P. (1972). Fat embolism syndrome. *Mayo Clin. Proc.* **47**, 237.

Drinker, C. L. (1945). 'Pulmonary Edema and Inflammation.' Harvard University Press, Cambridge.

Eeles, G. H. and Sevitt, S. (1967). Microthrombosis in injured and burned patients. *J. Pathol. Bacteriol.* **93**, 275.

Eisman, B. and Ashbaugh, D. C. (1968). Pulmonary effects of nonthoracic trauma. *J. Trauma* **8**, 623.

Eiseman, L. W. B. (1975). The changing pattern of post-traumatic respiratory distress syndrome. *Ann. Surg.* **5**, 693.

Fichman, M. B. and Bethune, J. E. (1968). The role of adrenocorticoids in the inappropriate antidiuretic hormone syndrome. *Ann. Intern. Med.* **68**, 806.

Fischer, J. E., Turner, R. H., Herndon, J. H. and Riseborough, E. J. (1971). Massive steroid therapy in severe fat embolism. *Surg. Gynec. and Obstet.* **132**, 667.

Fulton, R. L. and Jones, C. E. (1974). 'The Etiology of Post-Traumatic Pulmonary Insufficiency in Man.' Presented to Amer. Coll. of Surgeons.

Goldfarb, M. A., Churej, T. F., McAsian, T. C., Sacco, W. J., Weinstein, M. A. and Cowley, R. A. (1975). Tracking respiratory therapy in the trauma patient. *Amer. J. Surg.* **129**, 255.

Gurd, A. R. (1970a). Fat embolism: an aid to diagnosis. *J. Bone and Joint Surg.* **52B**, 732.

Gurd, A. R. (1970b). The treatment of fat embolism. Preliminary communication symposium. Melbourne, Sydney.

Gurd, A. R. and Wilson, R. I. (1974). The fat embolism syndrome. *J. Bone and Joint Surg.* **56B**, 408.

Hutchinson, R. M., Merrick, M. V. and White, J. M. (1973). Fat embolism in sickle cell disease. *J. Clin. Path.* **26**, 620.

Kerr, J. H. (1975). Oxygen transfer during I.P.P.V. in Man. *Brit. J. Anaesth.* **47**, 695.

Kim, S. I. and Shoemaker, W. C. (1972). The role of acidosis in the development of increased pulmonary vascular resistance and shock lung in experimental haemorrhagic shock. *Surgery* **73**, 723.

King, E. G., Jones, R. L. and Patakas, D. A. (1973). Evaluation of positive end-expiratory pressure therapy in the adult respiratory distress syndrome. *Can. Anaesth. Soc. J.* **20**, 546.

Laver, M. B. and Bendixen, E. H. (1966). Atelectasis in the surgical patient: recent conceptual advances. *Progr. Surg.* **5**, 1.

Lenfant, C. and Howell, B. J. (1960). Cardiovascular adjustments in dogs during continuous positive pressure breathing. *J. Appl. Physiol.* **15**, 425.

McLean, A. P. H., Duff, J. H. and MacLean, L. D. (1968). Lung lesions associated with septic shock. *J. Trauma* **8**, 891.

McNamara, J. J., Boatright, D., Burran, E. L., Molot, M. D., Summers, E. and Stremple, J. F. (1971). Changes in some physical properties of stored blood. *Ann. Surg.* **174**, 58.

McNamara, J. J., Burran, E. L., Larson, E., Omiya, G., Suchiro, G. and Yamase, H. (1972). Effect of debris in stored blood on pulmonary microvasculature. *Ann. Thorac. Surg.* **14**, 133.

Maroon, J. C., Campbell, R. C. (1970). Subdural haematoma. *Arch. Neurol.* **22**, 235.

Milligan, G. F., MacDonald, J. A. E., Mellon, A. and Ledingham, I. McA. (1974). Pulmonary and haematologic disturbances during septic shock. *Surg. Gynec. and Obstet.* **138**, 43.

Moss, G., Staunton, C. and Stein, A. A. (1972). Cerebral aetiology of the 'shock lung syndrome'. *J. Trauma* **12**, 885.

Neely, W. A., Berry, D. W., Rushton, F. W. and Hardy, J. D. (1971). Septic shock: clinical physiological and pathological survey of 244 patients. *Ann. Surg.* **173**, 657.

Newman, P. H. (1948). The clinical diagnosis of fat embolism. *J. Bone and Joint Surg.* **30B**, 290.

Nolte, W. J., Olafsson, T., Scherslen, T. and Lewis, D. H. (1974). Evaluation of the Gurd test for fat embolism. *J. Bone and Joint Surg.* **56B**, 417.

Norman, J. N., MacIntyre, J., Ross, R. R. and Smith, G. (1971). Etiological studies of pulmonary oxygen poisoning. *Am. J. Physiol.* **220**, 492.

Okinaka, A. J. (1967). The pattern of breathing after operation. *Surg. Gynec. Obstet.* **125**, 785.

Peltier, L. F. (1956). Fat embolism III. The toxic properties of neutral fat and free fatty acids. *Surgery* **40**, 665.

Powers, S. R. Jr., Burdge, R., Leather, R., Monaco, V., Newell, J., Sardar, S. and Smith, E. S. (1972). Studies of pulmonary insufficiency in nonthoracic trauma. *J. Trauma* **12**, 1.

Proctor, H. J., Ballantine, T. V. N. and Broussard, N. D. (1970). Analysis of pulmonary function following non-thoracic trauma with recommendation for therapy. *Ann. Surg.* **172**, 2.

Prys-Roberts, C. (1973). Respiratory problems of the seriously injured patient. *Injury* **5**, 67.

Prys-Roberts, C. Editorial (1974). Fat embolism and post-traumatic hypoxaemia. *J. Bone and Joint Surg.* **56B**, 405.

Reul, G. J., Greenberg, S. D., LeFrak, E. A., McCollum, W. B., Beall, A. C. Jr. and Jordan, J. L. Jr. (1973). Prevention of post traumatic pulmonary insufficiency. *Archs. Surg.* **106**, 386.

Reul, G. J., Beall, A. C. and Greenberg, S. D. (1974). Protection of the pulmonary microvasculature by fine screen blood filtration. *Chest* **66**, 4.

Robb, H. J., Margulis, R. R. and Jabs, L. M. (1972). Role of pulmonary microembolism in the haemodynamics of endotoxin shock. *Surg. Gynae. and Obstet.* **135**, 777.

Rosolf, L., Weil, M., Bradley, E. C. and Berne, C. J. (1967). Haemodynamic and metabolic changes associated with bacterial peritonitis. *Am. J. Surg.* **114**, 180.

Saldeen, T. (1970). The importance of intravascular coagulation and infiltration of the fibrinolytic system in experimental fat embolism. *J. Trauma* **10**, 287.

Scott, A. A. (1973). Fat embolism: a rational approach to treatment. *Canad. Med. Assoc. J.* **109**, 867.

Shoemaker, W. C., Montgomery, E. S., Kaplan, E. and Elwyn, D. H. (1973). Physiologic patterns in surviving and non-surviving shock patients. *Archs. Surg.* **106**, 630.

Siegal, J. H. and Farrell, E. J. (1973). A computer simulation model to study the clinical observability of ventilation and perfusion abnormalities in human shock states. *Surgery* **73**, 898.

Suter, P. M., Fairley, H. B. and Inenberg, M. D. (1975). Optimum end-expiratory airway pressure in patients with acute pulmonary failure. *New Engl. J. Med.* **292**, 284.

Swank, R. L. (1970). Alteration of blood on storage: Measurement of adhesiveness of 'aging' platelets and leucocytes and their removal by filtration. *New Engl. J. Med.* **265**, 728.

Vito, L., Dennis, R. C., Weisel, R. D. and Hechtman, H. B. (1974). Sepsis presenting as acute respiratory insufficiency. *Surg. Gynec. Obstet.* **138**, 896.

Volz, R. G. (1966). Current concepts of fat embolism. *Rocky Mountain Med. J.* **63**, 39.

Walling, P. T. and Savage, T. M. (1974). Preliminary experience with a circuit to increase the airways pressure in adults breathing spontaneously. *Brit. J. Anaesth.* **46**, 379.

Wilson, R. F., Kafi, A., Asuncion, Z. and Walt, A. J. (1969). Clinical respiratory failure after shock or trauma. *Archs. Surg.* **98**, 539.

Wilson, J. W. (1972). Treatment or prevention of pulmonary cellular damage with pharmacologic dose of corticosteroid. *Surg. Gynec. Obstet.* **134**, 675.

Wilson, J. V. and Salisbury, C. V. (1944). Fat embolism in war surgery. *Brit. J. Surg.* **31**, 384.

Woo, S. W. and Professor Hedley-Whyte, J. (1973). Oxygen therapy. *Brit. J. Hosp. Med.* **9**, 487.

Zimmermann, W. E., Vogel, W., Mittermayer, C. H., Walker, F., Kuner, E., Shäfer, H., Birzle, H., Netenjacob, J. and Hirschauer, M. Gas Exchange and Metabolic Disorders in Traumatic-Haemorrhagic and Septic Shock and their treatment. Paper read at a Symposium on Shock. Buenos Aires, S. America. October 1972, p. 141.

Section 3: The Pulmonary Aspiration Syndrome

GILLIAN C. HANSON

INTRODUCTION

Pulmonary aspiration is well recognised as a cause of pulmonary disease and in many clinical settings is probably the most common cause of pulmonary pathology. The clinical situations following aspiration were reported by Cameron and Zuidema (1972). They commented that aspiration may be occult and difficult to diagnose. In liquid aspiration the severity of the pulmonary lesion appears to be closely related to the pH of the gastric contents. It would appear that a pH below 3 should be regarded as the critical level below which aspiration symptoms become severe (Crawford, 1970). Taylor (1975) however presented a case report of severe pulmonary aspiration in a patient whose gastric contents had a pH of 3.5. Morbidity and mortality depend on the volume, nature and acidity and the distribution of the aspirated material. Aspiration of solid material may cause immediate asphyxia and death, smaller particles may cause collapse of a lung or a segment of lung, whereas aspiration of acidic fluid may lead to a subacute-inflammatory reaction in the lungs known as Mendelson's syndrome (Mendelson, 1945).

The mortality from liquid aspiration of acidic fluid remains high. Cameron and Zuidema (1972) reported that 62% of patients died from aspiration, the mortality being 40% if only one lobe was involved and more than 90% if more than one lobe was involved. These results were similar to those of Arms et al. (1974), who in a series of 88 patients reported a mortality of 63%. The mortality from obstetric aspiration is

563

probably high because of the frequency with which a large surface area of lung is involved.

PREVENTION

Because of the high mortality, prevention is of the greatest importance and has been discussed in detail by McCormick (1975).

Appreciation of the risk

All patients who have impaired airway control are at risk – the patient nursed in the intensive therapy unit is therefore particularly vulnerable. Patients particularly at risk in this setting include the tracheostomised patient, the critically ill patient with ileus, the patient about to be intubated, the critically ill patient receiving intragastric feeds via a Ryles tube, the patient being resuscitated and the semiconscious or unconscious patient.

Elective intubation

Elective intubation should be preceded by a period of starvation.

Posture

Any patient with an impaired cough reflex should be nursed head down in the lateral position and suction should be readily available. Transport of critically ill patients is particularly hazardous – the patients should be accompanied by a skilled anaesthetist with equipment and drugs available for emergency intubation and hand ventilation. A powerful sucker and a source of oxygen at adequate pressure to ensure a flow of 14 litres per minute is also essential.

Nasogastric intubation

The stomach and oesophagus should be emptied before emergency intubation by nasogastric aspiration through a Ryles tube (10–12 English gauge: 18–21 French gauge). The stomach should be aspirated to dryness (aided by turning the patient on the left side) and 15 ml of 0.3 molar sodium citrate put down the tube (Lahiri *et al.*, 1973). A single dose of magnesium trisilicate mixture is known not to be sufficient to raise a preceding gastric pH of less than 3 to above this level (Lahiri *et al.*, 1973). Intubation should be performed in the supine position with an experienced assistant and facilities available for emergency suction.

There have been many controversies about the ideal position for intubation in the critically ill patient. McCormick (1967) considered that the supine position in conjunction with other preventive measures is to be preferred and is less likely to cause delay and difficulty in securing the airway. It must be remembered that it is unlikely the stomach has been emptied totally and that retention of the tube in the stomach renders the cardia incompetent. Induction of vomiting with ipecacuanha emetic B.P.C. or the intravenous injection of apormorphine is contraindicated in the critically ill patient. The risk of omission of a nasogastric tube has to be balanced against the skill of the anaesthetist and the urgency of the situation.

DIAGNOSIS

Pulmonary aspiration should be suspected in any semiconscious patient who vomits and such patients should be appropriately investigated. Severe liquid aspiration may cause immediate collapse, dyspnoea, cyanosis and generalised bronchospasm but symptoms of moderate liquid aspiration may only become manifest 6–8 h after the incident. The prognosis for the latter may be serious unless diagnosed and appropriately treated. The condition should be suspected during anaesthesia, if the patient develops bronchospasm for no apparent reason and maintenance of a good colour becomes difficult. Endotracheal suction is often diagnostic – bile stained fluid may be aspirated from the airway or in severe cases profuse sero-sanguineous froth. Chest X-ray (Figs 1a and 1b) will show mottling of the area of lung involved which is usually more marked 24 hours later. Hypoxia is invariable and the $PaCO_2$ is low unless there was preceding respiratory depression. In severe cases the situation is complicated by the onset of hypovolaemia and a metabolic acidosis.

Aspiration of solid contents is generally more dramatic, the patient developing laryngeal obstruction or suddenly becoming breathless and cyanosed after vomiting. Clinical and X-ray findings will confirm an area of lung collapse.

TREATMENT

Aspiration of solids

Where solid or semi-solid gastric contents have been aspirated, urgent bronchoscopy is generally indicated. Preoxygenation is essential and oxygen should be administered during the procedure.

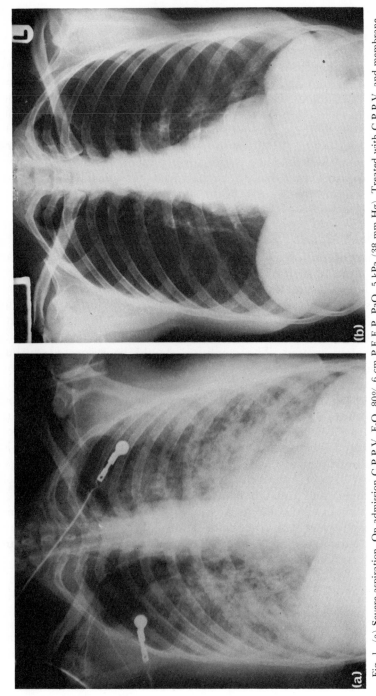

Fig. 1. (a) Severe aspiration. On admission C.P.P.V. F_{IO_2} 80% 6 cm P.E.E.P. PaO_2 5 kPa (38 mm Hg). Treated with C.P.P.V. and membrane oxygenator. (b) Same patient. Resolution after 18 days' treatment. Pulmonary function tests including diffusing capacity (D.L.C.O.) within normal limits 4 weeks after the incident.

Aspiration of liquids

The immediate management of pulmonary aspiration has been summarised by McCormick (1975). The management of severe pulmonary aspiration involves clearance of the airway, the possible use of bronchial lavage, artificial ventilation and the correction of blood volume and acid base balance. Steroids and antibiotics are generally used; various other drugs have been recommended by different authors. Supplemental oxygenation using a membrane oxygenator may have to be considered in patients with severe hypoxia refractory to the usual treatment.

Clearance of the airway

Prompt removal of aspirated material from the bronchial tree is imperative. The pH should be obtained from the pharyngeal or tracheal secretion at the time of aspiration. This should be carried out before the onset of pulmonary oedema which has been known to neutralise the acid within 10 min. If the measurement has not been made at once, the pH of the gastric contents (provided no antacid has been added subsequent to the aspiration) taken within 4 h of the aspiration has been shown to correlate well with mortality (Lewis et al., 1971).

Aspiration should be continued until the airways are clear – over-vigorous suction may lead to bronchial mucosal trauma, subsequent bleeding and a predisposition to infection. In severe pulmonary aspiration, suction may increase the degree of hypoxia – and therefore has to be performed efficiently and for short periods only. The patient should be hand ventilated on oxygen in between periods of suction.

Bronchial lavage

Lavage has been recommended by various authors (Simenstad et al., 1962; Baggish and Hooper, 1974) but it has been found to be of no benefit experimentally and such treatment may lead to additional areas of involvement (Bannister et al., 1961). Pulmonary surfactant is known to play an important role in preventing alveolar collapse and maintaining a near-zero surface tension at the air interface, thereby preventing intra-alveolar oedema (Scarpelli, 1971). Surfactant may be dispersed into the alveoli during bronchial lavage, and may be lifted off its normal position over the epithelial cells during the formation of massive pulmonary oedema (Scarpelli, 1971).

Bronchial lavage is therefore contraindicated in the management of these patients and may indeed be dangerous when used in patients who are already hypoxic. Bronchoscopy is not indicated in the management of a patient with aspiration of liquid gastric contents.

Artificial ventilation

The value of mechanical ventilation in the treatment of the aspiration syndrome has been reported by numerous investigators, both experimentally and clinically (Hamelberg and Bosonworth, 1964; Cameron *et al.*, 1968; Booth *et al.*, 1972). Cameron and his associates (1968) used an aspirate with pH 1 and changed a universally fatal model to one with 100% survival after 6 h intermittent positive pressure ventilation. As a result of their experimental studies they suggested that a clinical trial is warranted in the use of routine positive pressure ventilation after aspiration. They felt that some patients might be placed on a ventilator unnecessarily but this would be justifiable if other patients were salvaged by this procedure.

The use of a positive end expiratory pressure (P.E.E.P.) in order to raise the arterial oxygen tension of severely hypoxic patients on artificial ventilation has now been well accepted. It has been shown to be of value in treating patients with alveolar instability and closure but to be of little use when hypoxaemia is caused by obstructed airways or pneumonitis (McMahon *et al.*, 1973). P.E.E.P. in experimentally induced pulmonary oedema does not facilitate mobilisation of interstitial fluid nor improve lung mechanics, but produces an improvement in gas exchange through inflation of previously collapsed areas (Brown, P. P. *et al.*, 1974).

Chapman *et al.* (1974) ventilated dogs with continuous positive pressure ventilation immediately after aspiration of 2 ml/kg body weight of hydrochloric acid and showed that the lung appearance was normal except for small haemorrhages at the posterior bases, in contrast to those that breathed spontaneously where the lungs were haemorrhagic and congested. Experimental evidence is sufficiently convincing to justify the use of C.P.P.V. in all patients requiring ventilation for the aspiration syndrome. P.E.E.P. may have an adverse haemodynamic effect and therefore the pressure used should be, if at all possible, 10 cm H_2O or less. Experimentally, cardiac output starts to fall at an end expiratory pressure of 10 cm H_2O or more – this is probably the effect of increased intrathoracic pressure impeding venous return (Leonard, 1974).

Quist and co-workers (1975) have shown experimentally that the addition of P.E.E.P. of 12 cm H_2O to normovolaemic dogs during mechanical ventilation produces an acute decrease in cardiac filling pressure – this was associated with a marked increase in right atrial and pulmonary capillary wedge pressure, but calculated transmural pressures shared a decrease. Sustained application of P.E.E.P. did not lead to any circulatory adaptation, but transfusion improved cardiac output. They found that oedema developed after abrupt withdrawal. If these findings can be related to the situation in humans volume replacement may be necessary during the institution of P.E.E.P. and rapid withdrawal may be complicated by pulmonary oedema.

I.M.V. with a low level of P.E.E.P. should be used therefore during weaning since it appears to minimise the increase in intrapulmonary right to left shunt which normally occurs during weaning from controlled ventilation (Feeley et al., 1975), and may prevent reactive pulmonary oedema.

Patients with the aspiration syndrome are frequently hypovolaemic – attention should be paid to the restoration of a normal circulating blood volume since P.E.E.P. will only accentuate the decrease in cardiac output, increase the intrapulmonic shunt and contribute to hypoxaemia. The incidence of pneumothorax is increased when using P.E.E.P., but it appears to be a late rather than an early complication when pressures of 10 cm H_2O or less are used and is generally associated with pulmonary sepsis (Van Haeringen et al., 1974, and also in the discussion following the paper).

Oxygen has to be used during artificial ventilation in order to maintain adequate tissue oxygenation. The amount of oxygen available to the cell is the product of cardiac output and arterial oxygen content (Nunn and Freeman, 1964). The arterial oxygen pressure and hence oxygen saturation is invariably reduced in pulmonary aspiration. Kontos et al. (1967) have demonstrated in man that arterial hypoxia results in a compensatory increase in cardiac output, this compensation may be compromised if the dynamic blood volume is low. Maintenance of cardiac output by appropriate blood volume replacement therefore plays an important role in attaining adequate tissue oxygenation in the aspiration syndrome. Since there are so many variable factors associated with the aspiration syndrome, it is probably wise to maintain a PaO_2 on continuous positive pressure ventilation of 8–13.3 kPa (60–100 mm Hg.). The inspiratory oxygen percentage should be kept if at all possible to 60% or less during the first 24 h of continuous positive pressure ventilation, although there is experimental evidence to suggest that the traumatised lung if exposed to high oxygen percentages within 24 h of trauma has some protective mechanism against oxygen toxicity (Winter *et al.*, 1974). After 24 h the inspiratory oxygen percentage should be lowered to 40–50 when long term therapy is anticipated (Saltzman and Fridovich, 1973; Sevitt, 1974). Guidelines for management of the critically ill patient on mechanical ventilation with P.E.E.P. are summarised in Part 2, ch. II, p. 329, Table 5.

Correction of blood volume and acid base imbalance

It is well recognised both experimentally (Chapman *et al.*, 1974) and clinically (Moseley and Doty, 1970) that severe pulmonary aspiration is associated with a fall in cardiac output. This probably reflects a hypovolaemic state secondary to pulmonary oedema (Awe *et al.*, 1966). In spite of a low dynamic blood volume, the central venous pressure may be raised, thereby giving the impression of normovolaemia; this is probably related to pulmonary venospasm (Booth *et al.*, 1972) and not to bronchospasm (which may be absent) as suggested by Moseley and Doty (1970). A low cardiac output may increase the already existing intrapulmonic shunt, and therefore when this is suspected in the presence of a raised central venous pressure (i.e. greater than 10 cm H_2O at the midaxillary level measured in the horizontal plane) a fluid challenge of 200 ml of an appropriate volume expander should be given (Sykes, 1973). The pulmonary capillary wedge pressure if correctly placed generally accurately reflects left atrial pressure but as the positive and expiratory pressure is increased, may be totally misleading (see Part 2, ch. II, p. 319).

The fluid used for volume replacement should be carefully considered. Although no documented evidence could be found, protein loss into the alveoli will inevitably lead to a fall in serum proteins and a decrease in plasma osmotic pressure. This, in conjunction with destruction of lung surfactant will increase the tendency towards pulmonary oedema. Replacement with crystalloids with resultant haemodilation may increase the tendency towards the 'wet lung syndrome' (Cervera and Moss, 1974) thereby producing further deterioration in a patient who has aspirated. Volume replacement should therefore preferably be with plasma protein fraction, dried plasma, or salt-free albumin. The haematocrit should be maintained at 28–30%. Whole blood should be given if the haematocrit is below this level.

A metabolic acidosis is frequently present in massive pulmonary aspiration and is probably related to poor peripheral perfusion secondary to hypovolaemia; the arterial oxygen level has little effect on the serum lactate until it has reached 4.1 kPa (36 mm Hg) or less (Carey *et al.*, 1971). Brown, R. S. and co-workers (1974) showed that the onset of increase in pulmonary vascular resistance in hypovolaemic shock was pH dependent and that two-thirds of the rise could be abolished by maintaining venous pH in the normal or slightly alkalotic range during the hypotensive period. Timely and appropriate dosage of intravenous sodium bicarbonate is therefore important in the management of the aspiration syndrome (see Part I, ch. VII, p. 203).

Steroids

Parenteral steroids have been recommended as anti-inflammatory agents since 1955 (Dougharty and Schneebeli, 1955) and have consequently been universally used in the management of patients with pulmonary aspiration. All case reports lack a control. The series of 40 patients with recognised aspiration of liquid gastric contents reported by Mendelson (1946) did not receive steroids and all survived. Downs *et al.* (1974) and Chapman *et al.* (1974) have made an excellent evaluation of steroid therapy in experimental aspiration pneumonitis. It appears that once a maximal tissue response has occurred, steroid therapy is not beneficial. Downs *et al.* (1974) found that if steroids play a beneficial role in treatment, it seems to be limited to animals that aspirate material in the narrow pH range of 1.5–2.1. Cameron and co-workers (1973) treated 47 patients suffering from aspiration pneumonia with steroids, there was no apparent effect on the overall mortality. The dosage and type of corticosteroid to be used appears equally controversial, it is probably wise to use a steroid with minimal salt-retaining properties such as methyl prednisolone sodium succinate and to use large doses (30 mg/kg body weight intravenously 8-hourly) for a limited period of 48–72 h. Large doses of prednisolone may lead to an increase in urine output and hypokalaemia; care must be taken to maintain an adequate circulating blood volume – potassium supplements are invariably required.

Antibiotics

Bacterial infection appears to have little part to play in the initial illness (Bannister and Sattilaro, 1961) and it is probably wise to withhold antibiotics until anaerobic and aerobic cultures of the tracheal aspirate are available. Bartlett *et al.* (1974) performed a prospective study on 54 cases of pulmonary infection following aspiration. Specimens were either transtracheal aspirates, empyema fluid or blood. Anaerobic bacteria were recovered in 93% of patients and were the only pathogens in 42%, the predominant species being Bacteroides – indicating that anaerobes play a key role in most cases of infection following aspiration.

Other drugs

Digoxin should be used if there is evidence of cardiac failure and should be particularly considered in patients known to have preceding myocardial damage. Bronchospasm may be a prominent initial feature of pulmonary aspiration and antispasmodics have been widely recommended in treatment (McCormick, 1967); their use, however, has to be carefully considered in relation to their pharmacological activity. Most bronchodilators increase minute volume and alveolar ventilation, but hypoxaemia may become worse as a result of an increase in cardiac output, resultant increase in pulmonary blood flow and an intensification of the ventilation perfusion deficit (Palmer, 1971). This situation has been reported following aminophylline (Rees *et al.*, 1967a), adrenaline (Rees *et al.*, 1967b) and isoprenaline (Knudson and Constantine, 1967). Bronchodilators may also produce an increase in heart rate or cardiac dysrhythmia and therefore are dangerous when used in an hypoxic patient. Salbutamol, however, has been found to increase the F.E.V. to a greater degree than isoprenaline with little increase in heart rate (Paterson, 1971) and an insignificant increase in oxygen uptake in doses up to 1 μg/kg B.W. infused over 5 min (Gibson and Cottart, 1971). Cardiac output has been shown to increase with salbutamol and is probably related to an increase in blood flow through the peripheral circulation (Gibson and Cottart, 1971). Salbutamol, therefore, when carefully titrated intravenously may be of value in the management of bronchospasm in the aspiration syndrome but should only be used once the dynamic blood volume has been restored. Because of its action on the peripheral vasculature, a further 'top-up' of blood volume may be required during its use.

The membrane oxygenator

Should the above treatment fail to produce clinical and biochemical improvement, extracorporeal oxygenation should be considered. Criteria (which may be too rigid and erring on the side of conservatism) have been stated in the Editorial in 'Anaesthesia and Intensive Care' (1974) and also in Part 4, ch. IV, p. 966.

From personal experience (Browne *et al.*, 1977), membrane oxygenation may be life saving in severe pulmonary aspiration and should not be left too late. Evidence of right heart failure, a fall in cardiac output due to diminution of venous return secondary to P.E.E.P., the onset of oliguria (in the presence of an adequate circulating blood volume), or C.P.P.V. complicated by a pneumothorax or secondary pulmonary infection, may also be factors which should be taken into account when considering membrane oxygenation in a young healthy patient with previously normal lungs. Details in the technique and use of the membrane oxygenator are presented on p. 965.

SUMMARY OF MANAGEMENT

In the light of the preceding discussion, the following conclusions can be made.

1. Early diagnosis and appropriate management is essential in order to decrease the mortality from pulmonary aspiration.

2. The ultimate degree of pulmonary destruction cannot be gauged at the time of aspiration and the prognosis does not necessarily correlate (experimentally) with blood gas changes taken during the first 6 hours following aspiration (Cameron et al., 1968).

3. Continuous positive pressure ventilation appears to be one factor that radically alters the prognosis, and experimental data is sufficiently convincing to justify its use in all patients who have aspirated. The inspiratory oxygen percentage should be maximally 60% for the first 24 h and then reduced to 50% or less. The level of P.E.E.P. used should be as low as possible in order to achieve a PaO_2 between 8–13.3 kPa (60–100 mm Hg). When weaning the patient off P.E.E.P., the level should be reduced slowly and the patient should be allowed to breathe spontaneously once the blood gases are 9.3 kPa (70 mm) or more on an inspiratory oxygen percentage of 35% and P.E.E.P. of 2 cm or less. The patient should be allowed to breathe spontaneously initially against an end expiratory pressure of 2–5 cm H_2O which is tailed off over the subsequent 2–5 days. Abrupt stoppage may lead to a recrudescence of pulmonary oedema (Van Haeringen et al., in Discussion, 1974).

4. Hypovolaemia is a well recognised feature of pulmonary aspiration – central venous pressure (C.V.P.) and pulmonary artery wedge pressure (P.C.W.P.) monitoring may not be reliable indications of dynamic blood volume. In the presence of raised C.V.P. – volume replacement can be achieved by a fluid challenge. P.C.W.P. appears to correlate fairly closely with left atrial pressure until P.E.E.P. reaches a level of 10 cm H_2O or above. Correct placement may be difficult – and

an incorrectly placed catheter in the pulmonary artery will reflect pulmonary vascular resistance and not left atrial pressure. Crystalloid solutions should not be used for volume replacement. A metabolic acidosis should be corrected with intravenous sodium bicarbonate – overcorrection is easy and therefore it is wise not to use sodium bicarbonate unless the base deficit is 8 or more.

5. Steroids are not of proven value in the aspiration syndrome, but until there is further evidence should be used in large doses (prednisolone sodium succinate 30 mg/kg B.W. intravenously 8 hourly) for a period of 24 h.

6. Antibiotics should not be used until anaerobic and aerobic cultures of the tracheal aspirate are available. Intravenous clindamycin metronidazole or septrin may have to be used either alone or in combination with another appropriate antibiotic in order to cover the anaerobic organism which may be present. The antibiotic course should be limited to 5 days.

7. Antispasmodics should not be used unless there is overt broncho-spasm at the time of aspiration. Salbutamol titrated intravenously in an adult dosage of 1–5 µg/min so that the pulse rate does not rise above 10/min above the basal value, may be considered. It should be used with caution in patients with pulse rates greater than 130/min and should not be used until hypovolaemia has been corrected.

8. Membrane oxygenator. Membrane oxygenation is indicated if in spite of the above measures the PaO_2 fails to rise or continues to fall below 6.1 kPa (50 mm Hg). It may also be indicated in patients where (because of P.E.E.P. and high ventilatory airway pressures) the PaO_2 cannot be maintained above 6.1 kPa (50 mm Hg) without a fall in cardiac output and resultant inadequate tissue perfusion. The membrane oxygenator in these circumstances allows the lungs to be ventilated at a lower tidal volume and lower level of P.E.E.P. while still maintaining an adequate PaO_2.

REFERENCES

Arms, R. A., Dines, D. E. and Tinstman, T. C. (1974). Aspiration pneumonia. *Chest* **65**, 136.

Awe, W. C., Fletcher, W. S. and Jacob, S. W. (1966). The pathophysiology of aspiration pneumonitis. *Surgery* **60**, 232.

Baggish, M. S. and Hooper, S. (1974). Aspiration as a cause of maternal death. *Obstet. Gynae.* **43**, 327.

Bannister, W. K., Sattilaro, A. J. and Otis, R. D. (1961). Therapeutic aspects of aspiration pneumonitis in experimental aspiration. *Anaesthesiology* **22**, 440–443.

Bartlett, J. G., Gorbach, S. L. and Finegold, S. M. (1974). The bacteriology of aspiration pneumonia. *Amer. J. Med.* **56**, 202.

Booth, D. J., Zuidema, G. D. and Cameron, J. L. (1972). Aspiration pneumonia: pulmonary arteriography after experimental aspiration. *J. Surg. Res.* **12**, 48.

Brown, P. P., Elkins, R. C. and Greenfield, L. J. (1974). Treatment of the isolated oedematous canine lung with graded P.E.E.P. *Chest* **2** (Suppl. Part 2) 24S.

Brown, R. S., Kim, S. I. and Shoemaker, W. C. (1974). Haemodynamic mechanisms in the development of pulmonary venous admixture (shunting). *J. Surg. Res.* **17**, 192.

Browne, C. H., Chew, H. E. R., Clark, E., Edwards, J. M., Hanson, G. C. and Roberts, K. D. (1977). The management of the pulmonary aspiration syndrome. *Intens. Care Med.* **3**, 257.

Cameron, J. L., Sebr, J., Anderson, R. P. and Zuidema, G. D. (1968). Aspiration pneumonia: results of treatment by positive pressure ventilation in dogs. *J. Surg. Res.* **8**, 447–457.

Cameron, J. L. and Zuidema, G. D. (1972). Aspiration pneumonia. Magnitude and frequency of the problem. *J.A.M.A.* **219**, 1194.

Cameron, J. L., Mitchell, W. H. and Zuidema, G. D. (1973). Aspiration pneumonia. Clinical outcome following documented aspiration. *Archs. Surg.* **106**, 49.

Carey, L. C., Lowery, B. D. and Cloutier, C. T. (1971). Current problems in surgery (ed. Ravitch, M. M.) p. 16. Year Book Medical Publishers Inc., Chicago.

Cervera, A. L. and Moss, G. (1974). Crystalloid distribution following haemorrhage and haemodilution. *J. Trauma* **14**, 506.

Chapman, R. L., Modell, J. H., Ruiz, B. C., Calderwood, H. W., Hood, C. I. and Graves, S. A. (1974). Effect of continuous positive-pressure ventilation and steroids on aspiration of hydrochloric acid (pH 1.8) in dogs. *Anesth. Analg.* **53**, 556–562.

Crawford, J. S. (1970). The anaesthetist's contribution to maternal mortality. *Brit. J. Anaesth.* **42**, 70.

Dougharty, T. F. and Schneebeli, G. L. (1955). Use of steroids as anti-inflammatory agents. *Ann. N.Y. Acad. Sci.* **61**, 328.

Downs, J. B., Chapman, R. L., Modell, J. H. and Hood, C. I. (1974). An evaluation of steroid therapy in aspiration pneumonitis. *Anaesthesiology* **40**, 129.

Editorial (1974). II. Extracorporeal oxygenation of the blood in acute respiratory failure. *J. Anaesthesia and Intensive Care* **2**, 106.

Feeley, T. W., Saumarez, R., Klick, J. M., McNabb, T. G. and Skillman, J. J. (1975). Positive end-expiratory pressures in weaning patients from controlled ventilation. *Lancet* **2**, 725–728.

Gibson, D. G. and Cottart, D. J. (1971). Haemodynamic effects of intravenous salbutamol in patients with mitral valve disease: comparison with isoprenaline atropine. *Post. Grad. Med. J.* **47** (Suppl.) 40.

Hamelberg, W. and Bosonworth, P. P. (1964). Aspiration pneumonitis: experimental studies and clinical observations. *Anaesth. and Analg.* **43**, 669.

Kontos, H. A., Levasseur, J. E., Richardson, D. W., Page Mauck, H. Jr., Patterson, J. L. Jr. (1967). Comparative circulatory responses to systemic hypoxia in man and in anaesthetised dog. *J. Appl. Physiol.* **23**, 381–386.

Knudson, R. J. and Constantine, H. P. (1967). An effect of isoproterenol on ventilation-perfusion in asthmatic versus normal subjects. *J. Appl. Physiol.* **22**, 402–406.

Lahiri, S. K., Thomas, T. A. and Hodgson, R. M. H. (1973). Single-dose antacid therapy for the prevention of Mendelson's syndrome. *Brit. J. Anaesth.* **45**, 1143.

Leonard, A. S. (1974). Discussion: correlation of pulmonary wedge and left atrial pressure. *Archs. Surg.* **109**, 276.

Lewis, R. T., Burgess, J. H. and Hampson, L. G. (1971). Cardiorespiratory studies in critical illness. Changes in aspiration pneumonitis. *Archs. Surg.* **103**, 335.

McCormick, P. W. (1967). Pulmonary aspiration in obstetrics. *Hosp. Med.* **2**, 163.

McCormick, P. W. (1975). Thoughts on immediate care. Immediate care after aspiration of vomit. *Anaesthesia* **30**, 658.

McMahon, S. M., Halprin, G. M. and Sieker, H. O. (1973). Positive end-expiratory airway pressure in severe arterial hypoxaemia. *Amer. Rev. Resp. Dis.* **108**, 526.

Mendelson, C. L. (1945). The aspiration of stomach contents into the lungs during obstetric anaesthesia. *Am. J. Obstet. Gynec.* **11**, 191.

Mendelson, C. L. (1946). The aspiration of stomach contents into the lungs during obstetric anaesthesia. *Am. J. Obstet. Gynec.* **52**, 191.

Moseley, R. V. and Doty, D. B. (1970). Physiologic changes due to aspiration pneumonitis. *Ann. Surg.* **171**, 73.

Nunn, J. F. and Freeman, J. (1964). Problems of oxygenation and oxygen transport during haemorrhage. *Anaesthesia* **19**, 206.

Palmer, K. N. U. (1971). Effect of bronchodilator drugs on arterial blood gas tensions in bronchial asthma. *Post. Grad. Med. J.* **47** (Suppl.) 75.

Paterson, J. W. (1971). Human pharmacology: comparison of intravenous isoprenaline and salbutamol in asthmatic patients. *Post. Grad. Med. J.* **47** (Suppl.) 38.

Quist, J., Potoppidan, H., Wilson, R. S., Lowenstein, E. and Laver, M. B. (1975). Haemodynamic responses to mechanical ventilation with P.E.E.P. *Anaesthesiology* **42**, 45.

Rees, H. A., Borthwick, R. C., Millar, J. S. and Donald, K. W. (1967a). Aminophylline in bronchial asthma. *Lancet* **2**, 1167.

Rees, H. A., Millar, J. S. and Donald, K. W. (1967b). Adrenaline in bronchial asthma. *Lancet* **2**, 1164.

Saltzman, H. A. and Fridovich, I. (1973). Editorial. Oxygen toxicity. *Circulation* **48**, 921.

Scarpelli, E. M. (1971). Physiology and pathology of pulmonary surfactants. *Triangle* **10**, 47.

Sevitt, S. (1974). Diffuse and focal oxygen pneumonitis. *J. Clin. Path.* **27**, 21.

Simenstad, J. O., Galway, C. F. and Maclean, L. D. (1962). Tracheo-bronchial lavage for treatment of aspiration and atelectasis. *Surg. Forum.* **13**, 155.

Sykes, M. K. (1963). Venous pressure as a clinical indication of adequacy of transfusion. *Ann. R. Coll. Surg.* **33**, 185.

Taylor, G. (1975). Acid pulmonary aspiration syndrome after antacids. *Brit. J. Anaesth.* **47**, 615.

Van Haeringen, J. R., Blokzijl, E. J., Van Dyl, W., Kleine, J. W., Peset, R. and Sluiter, H. J. (1974). Treatment of the respiratory distress syndrome following nondirect pulmonary trauma with positive end-expiratory pressure with special emphasis on near-drowning. *Chest* **66** (Suppl. part 2) 30 S.

Winter, P. M., Smith, G. and Wheelis, R. F. (1974). The effect of prior pulmonary injury on the rate of development of fatal oxygen toxicity. *Chest* **66** (Suppl. part 2) 1 S.

Section 4: Near-Drowning

GILLIAN C. HANSON

INTRODUCTION

Between 1000 and 1500 people die of accidental drowning each year in Great Britain (Editorial, 1972). Blood alcohol levels are commonly high in patients who have drowned accidentally and may be an important contributory factor (Pleuckhahn, 1972).

Ritchie (1972) defines drowning as a situation where a person has died of asphyxiation by submersion in a liquid medium, whether or not the medium has entered the lungs. The term near-drowning has been applied by Modell (1971) to those who survive submersion. A third category includes the subject who survives near-drowning to die some hours or days later. Survival has been reported after total submersion for 22 min (Kvittingen and Naes, 1963).

PATHOPHYSIOLOGY

Drowning may occur without aspiration in approximately 20% of victims – it is probable that severe glottic spasm leads to asphyxia (Gooden, 1972). This is most likely to arise in patients submersed in irritant liquids – which includes sea-water containing sand and shells and chlorinated fresh water.

Near-drowning may also occur in the good swimmer attempting underwater endurance tests. The subject hyperventilates before diving, thereby reducing the $PaCO_2$ to around 2.7 kPa (20 mm Hg). The $PaCO_2$ may only rise to the normal alveolar level of 5.3–5.9 kPa (40–44 mm Hg) while the PaO_2 has fallen to dangerously low levels leading to loss of consciousness secondary to hypoxia.

577

Water in the alveoli produces a ventilation – perfusion imbalance, and the presence of foreign bodies may produce obstruction of other larger airways. The lung compliance decreases which increases the work of breathing and may produce reflex hyperventilation. The ultrastructural changes produced by saline and fresh water instillation have been well documented (Alexander, 1968). The vascular endothelium is stripped from the alveolar basement membrane, together with oedema of the alveolar cells. Giammona and Modell (1967) showed in experimental total immersion in dogs that distilled water altered the surface tension measurements of lung extracts. Surfactant was washed out of the lungs with isotonic saline and sea water aspiration but normal surface activity remained. Experimental work in animals suggests that the biochemical and respiratory effects from salt water drowning are different from fresh water drowning. The difference, however, in near-drowned humans appears to be minimal. Hypoxia is generally severe and may be associated with mild elevations in carbon dioxide tension.

Electrolyte changes are rarely dramatic in human near-drowning victims. High sodium levels are rarely found in victims drowned in salt water and sodium, chloride and potassium levels are generally within the normal range in fresh water near-drowning (Modell, 1971). Serum magnesium has been noted to rise in sea water drowning (Swann and Spafford, 1951) and potassium may rise in drowning from fresh water due to haemolysis of red cells. Approximately 85% of humans who die of drowning and presumably most of those who survive, aspirate less than 22 ml/kg B.W. of water (Ritchie, 1972). This is the most probable explanation for the minimal electrolyte changes seen in human near-drowning victims.

Cardiovascular function is usually normal except in patients who become hyperkalaemic or hypothermic. A body temperature of 30°C or less is likely to be complicated by ventricular fibrillation. Individuals can generally survive a water temperature of 25°C, but once the temperature drops below 20°C ventricular fibrillation may develop, especially if the subject indulges in heavy exercise. The more obese the subject, the longer the survival period. At temperatures around 0°C the subject may develop cold hyperaemia when it is probable that vascular smooth muscle relaxes and heat loss is facilitated. Death may occur quite suddenly on exposure to cold water (5°C or less) and is probably related to reflex hyperventilation secondary to contact of the chest wall with the water (Keatinge et al., 1969). After prolonged asphyxia, cerebral damage may develop secondary to the period of hypoxia.

Renal failure is also a complication which may arise secondary to a number of factors, namely hypoxia, metabolic acidosis, hypothermia and haemolysis.

TREATMENT

The treatment of near-drowning is summarised in Table 1.

Table 1. Summary of treatment of severe near-drowning

Initial management. Care at the site of accident (see p. 580).

Management on admission to hospital
  I. *Respiratory*
Clinical evidence of cyanosis and/or pulmonary oedema – intubate – aspirate secretions, hand ventilate on 100% oxygen. Take chest X-ray.
  Astrup analysis
  Hb., B.U., electrolytes, B.G.
Chest X-ray – evidence of pulmonary oedema and/or PaO_2–9.3 kPa (70 mm) or less on 35% oxygen or more – ventilate with appropriate oxygen percentage and P.E.E.P. of 2–5 cm H_2O. If patient able to breathe spontaneously without distress, consider allowing the patient to breathe without mechanical assistance using a constant positive airways pressure. Serial blood gases.
  Steroids. Methylprednisolone hemisuccinate 5 mg/kg B.W./24 h give intravenously 4 hourly, continue for 72 h.
  Antibiotics. Culture sputum anaerobically and aerobically.
Salt water drowning – cloxacillin and ampicillin
Fresh water drowning – cephalosporin
Alter according to sputum sensitivities.
  Bronchodilators. Consider if has severe bronchospasm with high airway pressure.
Use i.v. salbutamol (see Part 2, ch. V, p. 574).
Observe for – pneumothorax or pneumomediastinum, pulmonary infection.

  II. *Restoration of cardiac function*
Check core temperature, if <30°C and in V.F. unlikely to cardiovert, commence external cardiac massage. Rewarm rapidly (see p. 136) until temperature 30°C or above, correct acid-base imbalance and cardiovert. Asystole-intracardiac adrenaline and i.v. 10 ml 10% calcium chloride (see Part 2, ch. I).
  Fluid and Metabolic Control
Evidence of cardiac dysrhythmia, hypothermia or respiratory distress, give 50 mmol of sodium bicarbonate i.v.
  Check pH B.D. 30 minutes later, if pH 7.2 or less or B.D. >12, repeat sodium bicarbonate 50 mmol.
Insert C.V.P. catheter – restore C.V.P. to normal with P.P.F.
If B.P. still low and C.V.P. high normal – titrate volume replacement solution by 'fluid challenge'.
C.V.P. high (>15 cm H_2O) B.P. low, consider monitoring P.C.W.P. for assessment of fluid balance and L.V. status.

Table 1. Summary of treatment of severe near-drowning—*continued*

Observe Se K and Hb.
Evidence of haemolysis, give fresh blood.
Evidence of renal failure – estimate time for renal dialysis.

III. *Hypothermia*
Core temperature 32°C or less – *warm actively*. (See Part 1, ch. VI, p. 135.)
Heat humidified gases to 40°C at the mouth.
Warm i.v. fluids to 37°C.
In severe hypothermia with V.F. consider peritoneal dialysis with dialysate warmed to 37°C.
Do not surface rewarm.
Core temperature > 32°C – *warm passively*.
Observe for *secondary drowning* in patients who have apparently recovered.
Treat I and II as above.
Observe core temperature, may have to be cooled.

Initial management

The major aims at the rescue site is provision of adequate ventilation, circulatory assistance and the prevention of any further heat loss from the body.

Many authorities advise that no manoeuvres should be made to drain the lungs of fluid but Modell *et al.* (1974) advise that this should be attempted in near-drowning from sea-water.

Mouth-to-mouth resuscitation in a patient failing to breath adequately spontaneously will often bring back satisfactory cardiac rhythm (Redding *et al.*, 1960). Should the pulse fail to return after mouth-to-mouth ventilation has been established for approximately 30 s, then external cardiac massage should be started. External cardiac massage and mouth-to-mouth resuscitation should be continued until a femoral pulse of good volume is palpable and the patient is breathing spontaneously. Oxygen can be administered via an Ambu bag or rebreathing bag (see ch. I), or the exhaled air of the resuscitator can be reinforced by intraining oxygen via a catheter into the resuscitator's own mouth during inspiration. The victim's body should be covered as far as is possible with clothing in order to prevent further heat loss. On arrival at hospital treatment will depend upon the condition of the patient. All patients who have survived submersion should be admitted to hospital for observation, since their recovery may be complicated by the development of secondary drowning. This may develop in as little as five minutes, or as long as five days, after recovery from initial near-drowning. It is wise therefore to admit apparently well patients to the intensive therapy unit for observation for 24–48 h.

Subsequent management

In the severely ill near-drowned victim, treatment can be categorised into ventilatory management, restoration of cardiac function, fluid and metabolic control, and the treatment of hypothermia.

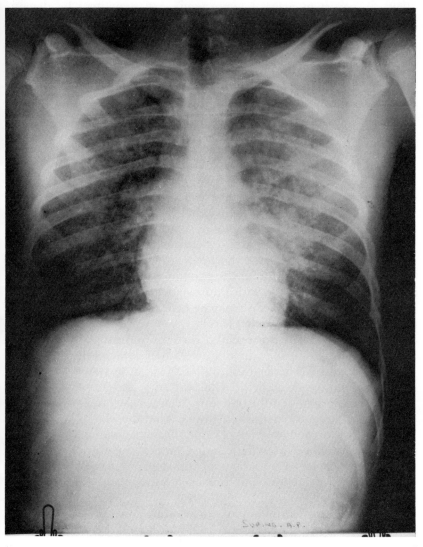

Fig. 1. Boy, 14 years old, admitted 1 h after immersion incident. Chest X-ray at the time of admission.

Ventilatory management

Severely ill patients generally have a high alveolar-arterial oxygen gradient when breathing 100% oxygen consistent with perfusion of nonventilated alveoli and this may persist for 24–48 h (Modell *et al.*, 1968). A persistent arterial hypoxaemia can sometimes be demonstrated for days after the immersion episode in patients breathing room air and may be due to hypoventilation of alveoli (Modell *et al.*, 1968) or to alteration of the normal characteristics of the alveoli and alveolar-capillary interface with production of diffusion problems. It therefore seems reasonable to have a fairly radical approach to the management of near-drowning victims. Patients with evidence of pulmonary oedema on the chest X-ray (see Fig. 1) and/or a PaO_2 of 9.3 kPa (70 mm) or less, where the PaO_2 prior to the incident was assumed to be normal, should be intubated, the secretions aspirated, and the patient ventilated with a P.E.E.P. of 2–5 cm H_2O (Rutledge and Flor, 1972). Should these principles not be applied, the patient's condition may seriously deteriorate as a result of increasing pulmonary oedema (Fig. 2). During this period maintenance of an adequate circulating blood volume, cardiac output and urine output by appropriate adjustment of the ventilatory indices is essential. On occasions, a slightly raised $PaCO_2$ may have to be tolerated for a short period in order to ensure adequate cardiac output (Fig. 3). A diuresis is common over the subsequent 48 h and frequently correlates with improvement in the blood gases and pulse volume. A decrease in pulmonary oedema may lag behind clinical and biochemical improvement.

Glasser *et al.* (1975) successfully treated a patient with salt water near-drowning with introduction of a constant positive airways pressure without mechanical ventilation. This latter system appears to be only applicable where the vital capacity and inspiratory force remain near normal and the only impairment is arterial oxygenation.

The use of steroids remains controversial but the work of Sladen and Zauder (1971) suggests that it is of value. They suggest that the action of steroids is to reduce the inflammatory process thereby resolving the pulmonary oedema. The dosage recommended is 5 mg/kg B.W. per 24 h of methyl prednisolone intravenously given 4 hourly and continued for 72 h. Such a high dosage may be complicated by hypokalaemia and sodium ion retention – central venous pressure monitoring is therefore essential.

Antibiotics are generally advocated. Anaerobic and aerobic culture of the bronchial secretions are essential since the organism isolated may

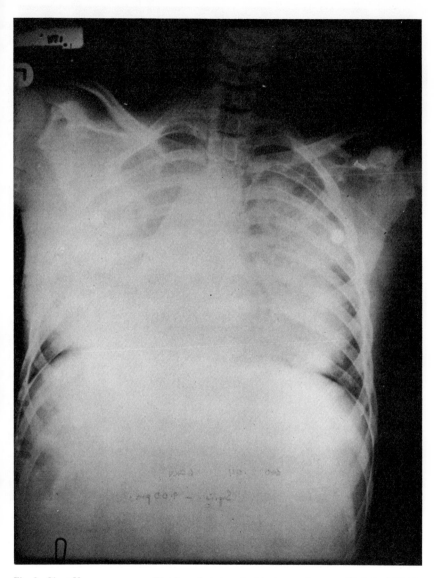

Fig. 2. Chest X-ray appearance 2 h after admission. At this time patient very ill. Pulse 140/min, B.P. 100/60. Resp. rate 50/min. Astrup analysis: pH 7.35, PaO_2 4.6 kPa (34.5 mm), $PaCO_2$ 4.7 kPa (35.3 mm), B.D. 5. Electrolytes: normal.

Patient intubated, ventilated on P.E.E.P. 4 cm H_2O F_IO_2 0.5. Tidal volume had to be kept low over the subsequent 3 h in order to maintain an adequate pulse volume and urine output.

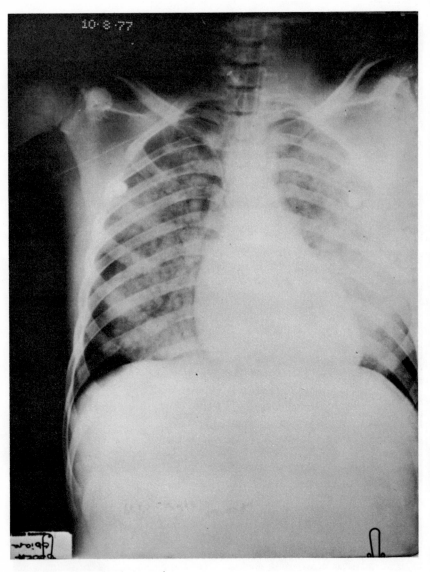

Fig. 3. Chest X-ray showing some improvement.

The clinical condition had improved and it was possible to increase the tidal volume and P.E.E.P. to 6 cm H_2O. Astrup analysis prior to alteration of ventilatory indices: pH 7.24, PaO_2 7.2 kPa (54.0 mm), $PaCO_2$ 5.3 kPa (39.8 mm), B.D. 9.6.

After introduction of P.E.E.P. 6 cm H_2O – Astrup analysis: pH 7.33, $PaCO_2$ 5.3 kPa (39.8 mm), PaO_2 8.6 kPa (64.5 mm), B.D. 4.6.

be unusual. *Pseudomonas putrifaciens* appears to be common in ocean water and a case has been reported of secondary chest infection with this organism following near-drowning in sea water (Rosenthal *et al.*, 1975). The organism is generally resistant to cephalosporins but sensitive to ampicillin, carbenicillin and gentamicin.

It would therefore be reasonable to start a course of ampicillin and cloxacillin in a patient with salt water near-drowning and cephalosporins in fresh water near-drowning. The treatment should be altered according to the bacterial sensitivities: clindamycin or metronidazole should be used for the bacteroides species.

Inhaled liquid may cause irritative bronchospasm. Should a broncho-dilator be indicated, the type used should be carefully selected (see p. 572).

Because of the reduced compliance and high airways pressure – the phase of acute pulmonary oedema may be complicated by a pneumothorax or pneumomediastinum. A sudden rise in airways pressure without evidence of airway obstruction whilst the patient is on C.P.P.V., may be the first sign of pneumothorax. Diagnosis and early drainage is imperative, since a tension pneumothorax may develop extremely rapidly in a patient on a volume cycled ventilator.

Pulmonary function generally improves rapidly with appropriate treatment. Glauser and Smith (1975) reported a case of near-drowning in fresh water which necessitated ventilatory support with P.E.E.P. and high oxygen concentrations. Hypoxia persisted and open lung biopsy on the 26th hospital day showed interstitial fibrosis. Over the ensuing two months pulmonary function returned to normal. The pulmonary fibrosis was attributed to incomplete resolution of the alveolar interstitial pathology, secondary to the near-drowning and exposure to high oxygen mixtures.

Restoration of cardiac function

Adequate oxygenation generally restores cardiac rhythm. Should asystole be present after intubation and hand ventilation, ventricular fibrillation may be precipitated with intracardiac adrenaline and 10 ml of 10% calcium chloride (see p. 283). Ventricular fibrillation is likely to be resistant to d.c. cardioversion if the core temperature is 28°C or less – under such circumstances the patient should be rewarmed rapidly (see Part 1, ch. VI, p. 135).

The victim is likely to be hypothermic if he is wearing a life jacket – since it is impossible for an unsupported immersed subject to achieve a low core temperature (28°C or less) without drowning (Golden and Rivers, 1975). A prolonged period of resuscitation at the site of the accident is also likely to predispose the victim to hypothermia.

Fluid and metabolic control

On arrival at hospital it is reasonable to give the patient with any cardiac dysrhythmia or respiratory embarrassment, 50 mmol sodium bicarbonate intravenously. Further doses of sodium bicarbonate would depend upon the acid base status but should rarely exceed a total of 150 mmol. In patients with a severe near-drowning incident – hypotension and tachycardia may develop secondary to loss of protein-rich exudate into the alveoli. The correct volume replacement solution under such circumstances is plasma protein fraction or dried plasma. The volume should be titrated intravenously according to the central venous pressure, pulse rate and blood pressure. Should the central venous pressure be high and the blood pressure remain low, volume replacement should be gauged by fluid challenge (see Part 2, ch. II, p. 308). On rare occasions accurate volume replacement may necessitate monitoring of the pulmonary capillary wedge pressure (see p. 319).

Diuretics have been suggested (Miles, 1968) but these can only accentuate the depletion in intravascular volume (Editorial, 1972).

There are rarely changes in serum sodium or chloride levels in spite of the fact that the sodium and chloride levels in sea water are approximately 509 and 561 mmol respectively (Giammona and Modell, 1967). The serum potassium level may rise because of the metabolic acidosis, intravascular haemolysis, or the onset of acute renal failure. Haemoglobinaemia is most commonly seen with fresh water drowning and may necessitate transfusion with fresh blood. An exchange transfusion with fresh blood may be indicated where intravascular haemolysis is severe and urine output poor.

Acute renal failure is a well recognised complication of near-drowning in fresh water (Kvittingen and Naes, 1963) and is thought to be related to acute intravascular haemolysis, hypoxia and hypotension. Grausz and co-workers (1971) reported two cases of near-drowning in sea water who developed acute renal failure. It was thought to result from a combination of hypoxia and hypotension.

Urine output should therefore be monitored and a urine plasma osmolality ratio taken to assess renal tubular function. Should renal failure be present, intravascular volume and serum potassium must be carefully observed. Dialysis may be indicated (see Part 1, ch. IV).

Treatment of hypothermia

The treatment of hypothermia is discussed in detail on p. 127. A near-drowned victim whose core temperature is 28°C or below may develop ventricular fibrillation spontaneously or more usually following mechanical irritation (Ross, 1957). Active rewarming should be established in patients with core temperatures of 32°C or below, since poor results have been obtained in patients with temperatures below this figure (Tolman and Cohen, 1970). Under hypothermic conditions there is a heat transfer gradient from the surface 'shell' to the centre 'core'. Core temperature may therefore continue to fall after the loss from the skin has been stopped. By the time the victim reaches hospital, the heat transfer has probably stopped and the core temperature steady (Freeman and Pugh, 1969). These patients should not have active surface rewarming since with peripheral vasodilation, cold blood will be transferred to the core and may precipitate ventricular fibrillation. Active surface rewarming should not be employed if the core temperature is 33°C or less since during the first phase of rewarming, the core temperature may fall by 3–4°C (Freeman and Pugh, 1969). Active rewarming should therefore be done from within outwards by heating the humidified gas being supplied to the airway so that the temperature at the mouth is approximately 40°C. Intravenous fluids should be warmed to 37°C and should the situation be critical, the core temperature can be even more rapidly raised by peritoneal dialysis (Lash et al., 1967).

In patients with ventricular fibrillation, external cardiac massage should be continued until the core temperature has reached 30°C. Metabolic acidosis should be corrected with sodium bicarbonate and d.c. cardioversion performed. In patients with severe bradycardia – external cardiac massage should be performed until the femoral pulse volume is good and the pupils are reacting to light. Deeply hypothermic patients may suffer little anoxic damage during periods of up to 15–20 min of circulatory arrest (Blair, 1964; Swann et al., 1955). Passive rewarming should be used for patients with temperatures of 32°C or above.

SECONDARY DROWNING

Even if the victim survives the immediate effects and appears to have recovered, there is a great danger of developing acute pulmonary oedema 15 min to 72 h after the drowning incident (Fuller, 1963a;

Rivers *et al.*, 1970). The symptoms range from rapid shallow breathing to inability to take a deep breath, laryngospasm, burning retrosternal discomfort, pleuritic pain and expectoration of pink frothy sputum. Radiological changes may not be present. Biochemical findings are similar to those found immediately following severe drowning and treatment is similar.

Additional findings include a high temperature (which may necessitate body cooling) and a neutrophil leucocytosis. The most severely ill patients may also have transient neurological symptoms and signs such as trismus, motor hyperactivity, convulsions, anxiety and headaches. Return of coma is a serious sign (Fuller, 1963b) and is generally fatal.

Many of the symptoms and signs can be attributed to hypoxia; the high fever may be related to the onset of a secondary respiratory infection.

DELAYED EFFECTS

Delayed effects involving the treatment of drowning include a condition resembling the respiratory distress syndrome – which may be related to oxygen toxicity (Nash *et al.*, 1967), permanent cerebral damage subsequent to cerebral hypoxia, and secondary pulmonary infection (Redding *et al.*, 1970).

REFERENCES

Alexander, I. G. S. (1968). The ultrastructure of the pulmonary alveolar vessels in Mendelson's (acid pulmonary aspiration) syndrome. *Brit. J. Anaesth.* **40**, 408.

Blair, E. (1964). 'Clinical Hypothermia', p. 33. McGraw-Hill, New York.

Editorial (1972). Drowning. *Lancet* **2**, 691.

Freeman, J. and Pugh, L. G. C. E. (1969). Hypothermia in mountain accidents. *Int. Anaesthesiol. Clin.* **7**, 997.

Fuller, R. H. (1963a). Drowning and the post immersion syndrome: a clinicopathologic study. *Military Medicine* **128**, 22.

Fuller, R. H. (1963b). The clinical pathology of human near drowning. *Proc. Roy. Soc. Med.* **56**, 33.

Giammona, S. T. and Modell, J. H. (1967). Drowning by total immersion. Effects on pulmonary surfactant of distilled water, isotonic saline and sea-water. *Amer. J. Dis. Child.* **114**, 612.

Glasser, K. L., Civetta, J. M. and Flor, R. J. (1975). The use of spontaneous ventilation with constant-positive airway pressure in the treatment of salt water near drowning. *Chest* **67** (3), 355.

Glauser, F. L. and Smith, W. R. (1975). Pulmonary interstitial fibrosis following near-drowning and exposure to short-term high oxygen concentrations. *Chest* **68**, 873.

Golden, F. St. C. and Rivers, J. F. (1975). Thoughts on immediate care. The immersion incident. *Anaesthesia* **30**, 364.

Gooden, B. A. (1972). Drowning and the diving reflex in man. *Med. J. Aust.* **2**, 583.

Grausz, H., Amend, W. J. C. Jr. and Earley, L. E. (1971). Acute renal failure complicating submersion in sea-water. *JAMA* **217**, 207.

Keatinge, W. R., Prys-Roberts, C., Cooper, K. E., Honour, A. J. and Haight, J. (1969). Sudden failure of swimming in cold water. *Brit. Med. J.* **1**, 480.

Kvittingen, T. D. and Naes, A. (1963). Recovery from drowning in fresh water. *Brit. Med. J.* **1**, 1315.

Lash, R. F., Burdette, J. A. and Ozdil, T. (1967). Accidental profound hypothermia and barbiturate intoxication. *J. Amer. Med. Ass.* **201**, 123.

Miles, S. (1968). Drowning. *Brit. Med. J.* **3**, 597.

Modell, J. H., Davis, J. H., Giammona, S. T., Maya, F. and Mann, J. B. (1968). Blood gas and electrolyte changes in human near-drowning victims. *JAMA* **203**, 99.

Modell, J. H. (1971). 'The Pathophysiology and Treatment of Drowning and Near-drowning.' Thomas, Springfield, Ill.

Modell, J. H., Calderwood, H. N., Ruiz, B. C., Downs, J. B. and Chapman, R. (1974). Effects of ventilatory patterns on arterial oxygenation after near-drowning in sea-water. *Anaesthesiology* **40**, 376.

Nash, G., Blennerhessett, J. B. and Pontopiddan, H. (1967). Pulmonary lesions associated with oxygen therapy and artificial ventilation. *New Engl. J. Med.* **276**, 368.

Plueckhahn. V. D. (1972). The aetiology of 134 deaths due to 'drowning' in Geelong during the years 1957 to 1971. *Med. J. Aus.* **21**, 849.

Redding, J. S., Voight, G. C. and Sapar, P. (1960). Drowning treated with intermittent positive pressure ventilation. *J. Appl. Physiol.* **15**, 849.

Redding, J. S., Yakaitis, R. W. and Herschel-King, C. (1970). Problems in the management of drowning victims. *Maryland State Med. J.* **19**, 58.

Ritchie, B. C. (1972). The physiology of drowning. *Med. J. Aust.* **2**, 1187.

Rivers, J. F., Orr, G. and Lee, H. A. (1970). Drowning: its clinical sequelae and management. *Brit. Med. J.* **2**, 157.

Rosenthal, S. L., Zuger, J. H. and Apollo, E. (1975). Respiratory colonisation with Pseudomonas putrefaciens after near-drowning in salt water. *Am. J. Clin. Pathol.* **64**, 382.

Ross, D. N. (1957). Problems associated with the use of hypothermia in cardiac surgery. *Proc. Roy. Coll. Med.* **50**, 76.

Rutledge, R. R. and Flor, R. J. (1973). The use of mechanical ventilation with positive end-expiratory pressure in the treatment of near-drowning. *Anaesthesiology* **38**, 194.

Sladen, A. and Zauder, H. L. (1971). Methylprednisolone therapy for pulmonary oedema following near-drowning. *JAMA* **215**, 1793.

Swann, H. G. and Spafford, N. R. (1951). Body salt and water changes during fresh and sea-water drowning. *Texas. Rep. biol. Med.* **9**, 356.

Swann, H., Virtue, R. W., Blount, S. G. and Kircher, L. T. (1955). Hypothermia in surgery: analysis of 100 clinical cases. *Ann. of Surgery* **142**, 382.

Tolman, K. G. and Cohen, A. (1970). Accidental hypothermia. *Cent. Afr. J. Med.* **11**, 151.

Section 5: Acute Massive Pulmonary Embolism

M. PANETH

HISTORICAL

Trendelenburg in 1908 first advocated a rational surgical approach to the treatment of this condition. He supported these views by conclusions drawn from animal experiments; although he undertook a number of emergency embolectomies he never had a long-term survivor. His pupil Kirschner in 1924 performed the first successful emergency pulmonary embolectomy.

During the next 37 years only a relatively small number of patients were saved by the operation as advocated by Trendelenburg (Cooley et al., 1961) although the literature does not indicate the number of unsuccessful attempts. But Sharp in 1962 reported the first case successfully treated with the aid of extra-corporeal circulation. Since then the advent of improved diagnostic and operative techniques, i.e. emergency pulmonary angiography and cardiopulmonary bypass respectively, has resulted in an increasing number of patients being submitted to pulmonary embolectomy. Naturally the question has been asked whether the operation has really been necessary in all cases. The use of thrombolytic agents has become increasingly widespread and there are therefore now three alternative treatment regimes available for critically ill patients with acute massive pulmonary embolism.

These are: 1. Pulmonary embolectomy; 2. Thrombolytic therapy; 3. Anti-coagulation. Which of these lines of treatment should be employed will depend on the clinical state of the patient, the effectiveness of resuscitation and the response to pharmacological support.

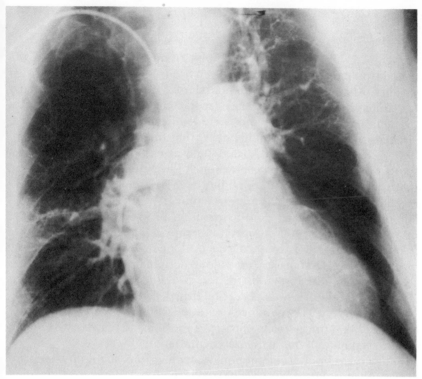

Fig. 1. Pulmonary arteriogram in massive pulmonary embolism. Effective perfusion is confined to the left upper lobe.

PATHOPHYSIOLOGY

To be life threatening the embolus must occlude at least 75% of the available pulmonary arterial tree (Fig. 1). Faced by a sudden and extreme rise in resistance to emptying, the right ventricle rapidly fails. The clinical picture therefore is one of sudden circulatory collapse with an elevated systemic (central) venous pressure. Since these patients are surviving on a very low and fixed cardiac output, the obstruction being proximal to the left-sided circulation, there will be no evidence of left-sided failure such as orthopnoea or signs of pulmonary venous congestion. The peripheries will therefore be constricted and cold in an attempt to maintain cerebral, coronary and renal blood flow. It follows that any agent or manoeuvre which encourages peripheral vasodilatation such as morphia, isoprenaline or the injudicious administration of a general anaesthetic will result in a precipitous fall in the blood pressure followed by bradycardia and circulatory arrest.

TREATMENT

Resuscitation

Gorham in 1961 analysed the survival time of patients with acute massive pulmonary embolism and reported that some two-thirds died within the first two hours, the remainder up to 14 days later. His study was undertaken before external cardiac massage became a routine resuscitative measure for any sudden and unexplained case of circulatory collapse. It is highly likely that the proportion who cannot be resuscitated by modern means such as external cardiac massage, intubation and ventilation is now much lower; but it must be stressed that pharmacological support by intravenous infusion of alpha-receptor stimulants such as noradrenaline in a concentration of 4 mg/l and infused at a rate sufficient to maintain a recordable blood pressure may be necessary until appropriate therapy has been instituted. Quite frequently external cardiac massage alone will have propelled the massive embolus a short distance along both main pulmonary arteries, so that the initial total obstruction is reduced and a critical but adequate circulatory state is re-established.

These modern means of resuscitation are frequently sufficiently effective so that the majority of patients regain consciousness and do not require intubation and artificial ventilation at this stage.

Following resuscitation pulmonary angiography should be performed if at all possible in order to confirm the diagnosis. The procedure may cause momentary cardiac arrest – full resuscitation facilities should therefore be available.

Immediate assessment

Immediately following angiography or after resuscitation (should the patient be too shocked for angiography), the patient should be transferred to an intensive therapy unit. For complete control a central venous pressure line, radial artery cannula for frequent blood gas analysis and pressure monitoring, and a urinary catheter should be inserted. Invariably a considerable metabolic acidosis will have developed from – (a) the antecedent episode of circulatory arrest, and (b) the persistent low output state. This acidosis should be corrected by the intravenous administration of appropriate quantities of sodium bicarbonate solution. If the systemic blood pressure tends to fall an intravenous drip of noradrenaline should be given at a rate sufficient to keep the systolic blood pressure at or above 80 mm Hg. Adrenaline itself

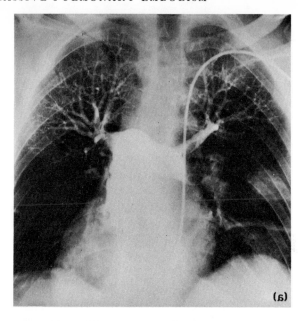

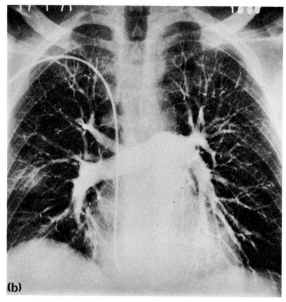

Fig. 2. Pulmonary arteriogram in massive pulmonary embolism. (a) before treatment with streptokinase, and (b) on completion of thrombolytic treatment. Restoration to normality has been achieved.

should be kept in reserve if emergency embolectomy becomes necessary. Urine production should be measured and if – (i) the blood pressure has to be maintained by increasing doses of vasopressors, (ii) urine production falls below 20 ml/h, (iii) the peripheral temperature fails to rise, then emergency embolectomy should be advised. If the clinical state as judged by these three parameters remains stable, thrombolytic therapy is the treatment of choice.

Thrombolytic therapy or 'medical embolectomy'

In most 'non-shock' patients, i.e. those with a blood pressure above 80 mm Hg systolic and urine flow maintained at or above 20 ml/h without the need for increasing doses of vasopressors, thrombolytic therapy will be effective. Streptokinase is used in the U.K. although urokinase has become increasingly popular in the U.S.A. because of its higher purity with resultant fewer unpleasant side-effects.

Usually a large catheter has been left in the main pulmonary trunk following pulmonary angiography and this route is used for the infusion at a dosage of 600 000 in 30 min followed by 100 000 units/h for 72 h. In addition 100 mg of hydrocortisone is administered intravenously 6 hourly as steroid cover. Provided the clinical state remains stable over

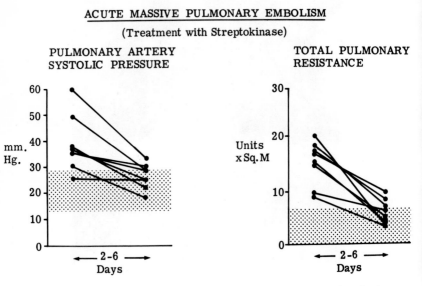

Fig. 3. Effect of thrombolytic therapy on pulmonary artery systolic pressure and total pulmonary vascular resistance.

the next 12 h, streptokinase in this dosage will produce complete resolution in three days or at any rate accelerate resolution sufficiently so that the patients own thrombolytic system will complete the process and a normal pulmonary arterial tree will eventually be restored (Fig. 2a and b). During the first 12 h of streptokinase administration one will notice a clinical improvement in the patient, such as increased pulse volume and hourly urine flow, and serial estimations of pulmonary artery pressure and pulmonary vascular resistance have shown restoration to normality by the end of three to four days (Fig. 3) (Miller *et al.*, 1971; Hall *et al.*, 1975).

Analysing the experience at the Brompton Hospital of 68 patients with acute massive pulmonary embolism without associated cardio-respiratory disease treated by pulmonary embolectomy, streptokinase and heparin, Miller *et al.* (in press) conclude unequivocally that streptokinase is the treatment of choice in the 'non-shock' group as defined above. Heparin treatment, being anticoagulant only and not thrombolytic, has an unacceptable failure rate even in this group of patients.

The contraindications to streptokinase therapy are:

(*i*) An operation within the preceding 72 h.
(*ii*) Severe systemic hypertension or previous cerebro-vascular accident.
(*iii*) Coagulation defect.
(*iv*) Recent history of gastro-intestinal ulceration or haemorrhage.

The precautions which should be taken are:

Frequent estimation of euglobulinlysis time (which should be maintained at 15–20 minutes on streptokinase therapy).
Frequent estimation of haemoglobin and P.C.V. and observation for hidden bleeding, i.e. retroperitoneal, intestinal or renal.
Blood transfusion for a falling haemoglobin concentration.

Pulmonary embolectomy

This emergency procedure is now reserved for patients whose circulatory state continues to deteriorate in spite of maximal medical support and in whom clinical experience suggests that there will not be enough time for thrombolytic therapy to be effective. That is to say, even with maximal medical support, they are not expected to survive another twelve hours. The operation should be performed also if there are contra-indications to 'medical embolectomy' as outlined in the previous section. The position has been clearly defined by Sasahara and Barsamian (1973).

Optimum operating conditions are obtained by the use of total cardiopulmonary bypass and the immediate availability of sterile, disposable oxygenators of various types has made any other technique (Pisko-Dubienski, 1968) obsolete and only necessary where an 'open heart team' is not available on a standby basis.

Contrary to a number of other reports, the experience at the Brompton Hospital with patients from a distance of up to 60 miles suggests that, after successful initial resuscitation and in spite of progressive deterioration, they can still be transported to a suitable centre equipped for modern pulmonary embolectomy.

Trendelenburg (1908) was the first to point out the dangers of conventional general anaesthesia in these patients when he advocated that one should wait until the patient had lost consciousness.

General anaesthesia should be delayed until the surgical team is scrubbed-up, the bypass equipment is fully primed, the patient is connected in the operating room to the E.C.G. with the arterial and central venous pressures continuously displayed. Intermittent estimations of the blood pressure by cuff techniques are unsuitable in these severely vasoconstricted patients. Intravenous thiopentone sodium and scoline anaesthesia at a minimal dosage is used to permit intubation. The inevitable fall in blood pressure, which accompanies this, is anticipated and counteracted by adding a small dose of metaraminol (Aramine) to the thiopentone sodium syringe. Further small doses of this vasopressor or even adrenaline may require to be administered to maintain a recordable blood pressure up to the moment of instituting cardiopulmonary bypass.

The incision. A vertical median sternotomy with longitudinal incision of the pericardium affords immediate access to the ascending aorta and right atrium (Fig. 4). Heparin in a dose of 2 mg/kg body weight* is administered as soon as adequate haemostasis has been achieved and due allowance must be made for the grossly retarded circulation time. If time allows a purse-string suture is placed at the aortic cannulation site, but if the blood pressure is critically depressed, immediate cannulation of the aorta for arterial return and single right atrial cannulation, via its appendage, for venous drainage is performed and these two cannulae

---

* Sodium heparin mucous 1 mg = 130 International Units.

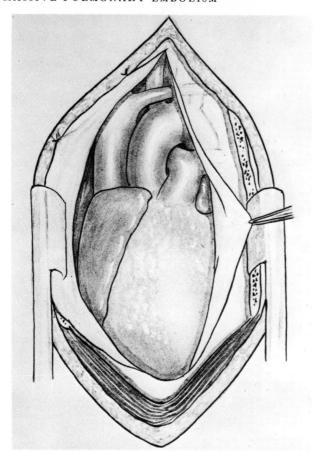

Fig. 4. Pulmonary embolectomy: exposure of the heart by vertical median sternotomy.

are rapidly connected to the arterial and venous limbs of the 'sash' of the bypass circuit in the usual way (Fig. 5). Bypass is commenced and continued with the heart beating for a suitable period to allow correction of the severe acid base imbalance and readjustment of the high arterio-venous oxygen difference. The institution of cardiopulmonary bypass in itself is beneficial for the following reasons:

(*i*) The right ventricle is relieved of its 'overload'.

(*ii*) The 'systemic output' and blood pressure (perfusion pressure) are improved.

(*iii*) Arterial oxygen tension is raised improving cerebral, coronary and renal oxygen supply.

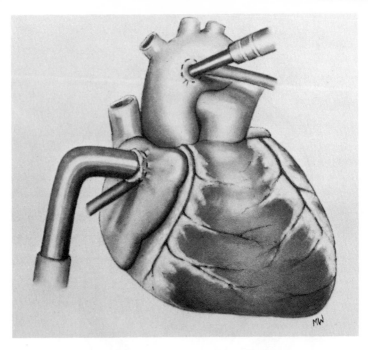

Fig. 5. Pulmonary embolectomy: cannulation of ascending aorta and right atrium.

(*iv*) General tissue oxygen tension is improved by the reduction in arterio venous difference.

After a suitable interval of total body perfusion the heart is electively fibrillated and the pulmonary trunk is opened by a longitudinal incision extending from just distal to the pulmonary valve almost to its bifurcation (Fig. 6).

By careful use of the cardiotomy sucker the pulmonary trunk is emptied and thrombus invariably present in the main pulmonary arteries is slowly and gently extracted with Desjardine forceps until each pulmonary arterial tree has been inspected to its basal divisions (Fig. 7). The strong sucker is next passed down each pulmonary artery in turn to remove impacted embolic fragments and finally the anaesthetist inflates both lungs (Valsalva manoeuvre) to demonstrate reflux of red blood from the pulmonary capillaries into each pulmonary artery in turn thereby proving that the pulmonary arterial tree has been completely cleared on both sides.

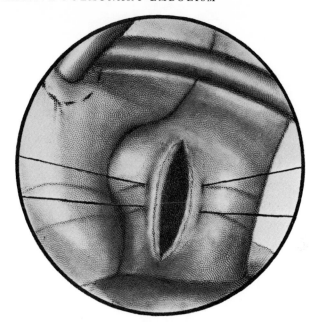

Fig. 6. Pulmonary embolectomy: the pulmonary trunk is opened to its bifurcation.

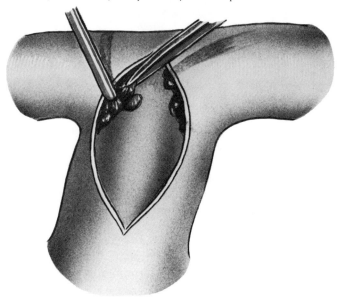

Fig. 7. Pulmonary embolectomy: the emboli are extracted from each pulmonary arterial tree in turn.

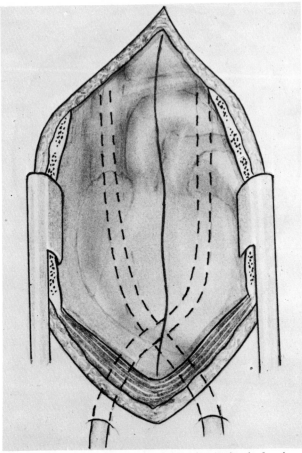

Fig. 8. Pulmonary embolectomy: the sternotomy incision is closed after decannulation with substernal and retrocardiac drainage tubes.

Following repair of the incision of the pulmonary trunk in two layers by continuous monofilament suture, the heart is defibrillated.

A period of supportive perfusion may be necessary in cases of severe right ventricular failure and at this stage isoprenaline may be required by continuous intravenous infusion. After 'weaning off', decannulation and the administration of protamine sulphate in suitable dosage, the pericardium is loosely closed and the sternum approximated over two drainage tubes (Fig. 8).

Artificial ventilation may be necessary for a few hours on return to the intensive therapy unit.

MANAGEMENT FOLLOWING TREATMENT OF PULMONARY EMBOLISM

Inferior caval ligation has been advocated by some (Crane *et al.*, 1969) and Little *et al.* (1968) have claimed that this procedure significantly lowers the recurrent embolic rate which in some series is estimated to be as high as 30%. The author has never interrupted the inferior vena cava or interfered in any way with the venous system. Virchow's statement (1856) that stasis and trauma are the main factors in venous thrombosis is still true.

We advocate instead that all patients after successful medical or surgical embolectomy should be maintained on conventional oral anticoagulants for a minimum period of three months unless there are overt signs of venous obstruction when anti-coagulants should be continued until these have completely resolved or for a minimum period of six months whichever is the longer. The prothrombin ratio should be maintained at 2 to 2.5:1.

When this regime has been properly carried out there has been no significant incidence of recurrent embolism in our series.

SUMMARY

Patients with suspected acute massive pulmonary embolism should be resuscitated by external cardiac massage and transferred to the Intensive Therapy Unit. The diagnosis may then be confirmed by pulmonary arteriography and their treatment will depend on the clinical state.

(*i*) *'Non-shock group'*. Blood pressure 80 or above, urine production 20 cc/hour or more, increasing doses of vasopressors not required.
– Thrombolytic therapy with streptokinase.

(*ii*) *'Shock group'*. Blood pressure 80 or below, requiring increasing doses of vasopressors, urine production below 20 ml/h, failure of rise of peripheral skin temperature.
– Emergency pulmonary embolectomy, preferably with cardio-pulmonary bypass.

At the Brompton Hospital the emergency embolectomy rate has fallen since this treatment protocol based on a clinical trial, has been established.

REFERENCES

Cooley, D. A., Beall, A. C. and Alexander, J. K. (1961). Acute massive pulmonary embolism. *J. Amer. Med. Ass.* **177**, 283.

Crane, C., Hartsuck, J., Birtch, A., Couch, N. P., Zollinger, R., Matloff, R., Dalen, J. and Dexter, L. (1969). Management of major pulmonary embolism. *Surg. Gynec. Obstet.* **128**, 27.

Gorham, L. W. (1961). Study of pulmonary embolism. *Arch. intern. Med.* **108**, 8.

Hall, R., Sutton, G. C. and Kerr, I. H. (1975). Resolution of pulmonary embolism. *Circulation* **52** (Supp. 2 – abstract no. 515), 131.

Kirschner, M. (1924). Ein durch die Trendelenburgsche Operation geheilter Fall von Embolie der Art. pulmonalis. *Arch. klin. Chir.* **133**, 312.

Little, J. M. and Lowenthal, J. (1968). Pertrochanteric venography in the study of human renal transplant recipients. *Surg. Gynec. Obstet.* **127**, 777.

Miller, G. A. H., Sutton, G. C., Kerr, I. H., Gibson, R. V. and Honey, M. (1971). Comparison of streptokinase and heparin in treatment of isolated acute massive pulmonary embolism. *Brit. Med. J.* **2**, 681.

Miller, G. A. H., Hall, R. and Paneth, M. *Amer. Heart J.* In press.

Pisko-Dubienski, Z. A. (1968). A new approach to pulmonary embolism. *Brit. J. Surg.* **55**, 138.

Sasahara, A. A. and Barsamian, E. M. (1973). Another look at pulmonary embolism. *Ann. thorac. Surg.* **16**, 317.

Sharp, E. H. (1962). Pulmonary embolectomy. *Ann. Surg.* **156**, 1.

Trendelenburg, F. (1908). Über die Operative Behandlung der Embolie der Lungenarterie. *Arch. klin. Chir.* **86**, 686.

Virchow, R. (1856). Thrombose und Emboli. Gefässentzündung und septische Infektion. *In* 'Gesammelte Abhandlungen zur wissenschaftlichen Medizin', p. 219. Meidinger, Frankfurt-am-Main.

Section 6: Decompression Sickness and Air Embolism

GILLIAN C. HANSON

AETIOLOGY

Vascular gas embolism results when gases (particularly inert) enter the circulation and lodge in organs, thereby affecting their function. Since air embolism is relatively rare, early diagnosis and appropriate treatment is essential. The condition should be avoided if at all possible by being aware of the aetiology. Hart (1974) categorised the causes of air embolism into accidental, criminal and iatrogenic.

Rapid decompression

Accidental air embolism may follow rapid decompression during flying or diving. The majority of the affected individuals will be treated by the Navy or Air Force at the site nearest to the accident. However, decompression sickness may develop in compressed air construction workers, in water sports and industrial diving. Decompression injury can occur from diving in relatively shallow water and has a nationwide distribution since scuba diving has become a popular sport. The other added problem is that there is commonly a latent period before the onset of symptoms – the victim during this period may have travelled some distance from the site of compression. Industrial and naval divers and aviators generally are aware of the symptoms and will contact the nearest recompression site as soon as symptoms arise – unless symptoms are too severe for them to do so. Amateur divers may not diagnose the symptoms and may on rare occasions attend the nearest accident centre.

603

Trauma

Accidental air embolism may follow trauma to the great vessels where the heart is gravitationally below the injured vein and blast injury where the alveolar membrane may be torn and respiration pumps air through the torn surface (Mason *et al.*, 1971).

Air embolism has been reported following oral genital sexplay – air being forced into the vagina by the sex partner. The pregnant female appears most susceptible – deaths have been reported (Aronson and Nelson, 1967).

Criminal causes of air embolism including the introduction of a septic abortion by injection of air into the cervical os, intravascular injection of air to terminate life and stab or gunshot wounds involving the great vessels situated above the heart.

Iatrogenic. Iatrogenic air embolism may arise in surgery performed on the head or neck in the upright position, during vascular surgery and during open heart surgery. Ericsson and co-workers (1964) collected 93 cases of iatrogenic air embolism from the world literature with an overall mortality rate of 73%; in their own series of 7 cases the mortality rate was 28%. Heller and co-workers (1970) reported that 9% of patients following cardiopulmonary bypass developed an organic brain syndrome and that 2% of these had permanent neurological deficits – they attributed this in part to inert gas microembolism.

Other iatrogenic causes may arise during the management of patients in the intensive therapy unit. Air embolism has been reported as occurring during haemodialysis (Ward *et al.*, 1971). It may arise following catheterisation of the internal jugular, external jugular or subclavian vein or during intravenous therapy via a central vein when performed in the head-up position (Gottlieb *et al.*, 1965). It may also follow diagnostic procedures such as angiography (Bergeron and Rumbaugh, 1971) and on rare occasions air may be forced during hand ventilation through the alveolar membrane (Hart, 1974).

PREVENTION

It is clear that certain basic measures should be taken in order to reduce the iatrogenic incidence of air embolism. These include, cannulation of any vein above the heart in the head down position (this is even more important in the patient suspected to be hypovolaemic), ensuring that all connectors leading to lines centred in the thorax are airtight and that all intravenous injections given into such lines are given if at all possible with the patient in the horizontal plane. Air may be pumped into the circulation with a fluid pump which does not switch off when the fluid being infused from a solid container has finished – this is a particular danger when blood is being pumped rapidly into the circulation to replace massive blood loss. Plastic intravenous fluid containers have been shown to be a source of air embolism, particularly when the infusion rate is increased by pumping (Yeakel, 1968). Air may also enter the circulation when the air inflow to the infusion bottle is too close to the infusion outflow, this in particular applies where fluid is being infused rapidly.

DIAGNOSIS AND TREATMENT OF DECOMPRESSION SICKNESS

Diagnosis of decompression sickness

The diagnosis has been discussed in detail by Elliott *et al.* (1974). Classically decompression sickness has been divided into Type 1, the limb-bends and Type 2, the more serious features. Any symptom however should be taken seriously since minor symptoms may proceed to more serious manifestations. The inexperienced practitioner may also misclassify the patient, the patient thus not receiving adequate treatment. At least 70% of divers develop symptoms within one hour of surfacing, whereas in compressed air workers, limb-bends develop on an average three hours after decompression – more serious manifestations however occur earlier (Golding *et al.*, 1960).

Pain in the region of a large joint is the commonest manifestation of acute decompression sickness in man. In conventional diving with compressed air, the upper limbs are affected approximately three times as often as the lower limbs, whereas in aviators and compressed air workers and deep oxyhelium diving, the lower limbs are most commonly affected (Elliott *et al.*, 1974). More than one site is affected but the distribution is rarely symmetrical, the knees and shoulders being involved most commonly.

The pain is usually near a joint but may be described as deep seated and the severity is extremely variable. The pain may move from one joint to another, or persist in one site. Generally local physical signs are absent, occasionally there is diminished voluntary movement and oedema over the joint site. Cutaneous involvement occasionally occurs, transient pruritis, localised itching followed by vasodilatation and central cyanotic areas and patches of oedema have been described.

Fatigue and anorexia may precede more serious symptoms. Respiratory decompression sickness generally occurs immediately after the dive but may be delayed several hours. The patient is generally pale and sweating and gets pleuritic pain on inspiration; dyspnoea may be present.

Nervous system involvement occurs in 8–35% of victims (Elliott *et al.*, 1974). Neurological manifestations may be bizarre and a patient presenting with a history consistent with recent decompression must be observed carefully. The first symptom may be mild weakness, paraesthesiae or epigastric or girdle pain. The disturbance may be predominantly cerebral migrainous-like headache, visual disturbances with nystagmus and papillary abnormalities, or disturbances of vestibular function 'the staggers'.

Haemoconcentration associated with loss of intravascular volume may occur in severe decompression sickness, this may be complicated by hypotension, inadequate organ perfusion and pulmonary oedema.

Differential diagnosis

Pulmonary barotrauma may be difficult to distinguish from decompression sickness. The symptoms are apparent almost immediately after surfacing from a dive. The symptoms are predominantly cerebral. There may be evidence of pulmonary trauma in the form of a pneumothorax, or mediastinal emphysema. The patient requires recompression as in decompression sickness.

Treatment of decompression sickness

The most important treatment is recompression. It is important however when severe decompression sickness is present or suspected, that an Hct and chest X-ray are taken beforehand. A high Hct may justify the insertion of a central venous pressure line and infusion of fluid. Cockett and Nakamura (1964) have demonstrated that low molecular weight dextran or plasma is the best treatment for this syndrome but this must be combined with appropriate recompression. Delay in recompression is detrimental, the probability of residual symptoms varies from 1% of patients treated within 30 min of onset, to 13% if the delay exceeds 6 h (Elliott *et al.*, 1974). The longer the delay in applying recompression treatment, the greater the pressure likely to be required for complete relief from symptoms (Doll and Berghage, 1967). Should a patient with severe decompression sickness be admitted to the intensive therapy unit – pure oxygen should be delivered via a tightly fitting face mask and advice should be sought regarding emergency recompression (see Table 1). The officer on call holds up-dated lists of available compression chambers and can also provide the telephone number of a specialist medical officer should advice be required. Should a single person oxygen chamber be available in the hospital – recompression may be considered in this chamber but should not be undertaken without expert advice. Hart (1974) advises that recompression in oxygen is preferable to that of air, since the best gas partition coefficient would be reached to excrete inert gas emboli in a delivery system where the patient is compressed in an atmosphere of oxygen and breathing oxygen. A patient compressed in air and breathing oxygen by mask cannot excrete all the nitrogen as absorption across the cutaneous boundary occurs. Statistically, in severe cases the failure rate using the American decompression tables, has been 47% (Goodman and Workman, 1965).

Table 1. Decompression sickness. Emergency recompression and advice regarding management

Telephone:	Portsmouth Dockyard Telephone Exchange
	Portsmouth 22351
State that you have a patient suffering from decompression sickness	
Call transferred during	
working hours to – Superintendent of Diving	
other hours to – Duty Lieutenant-Commander H.M.S. *Vernon*	

Advice extracted from the Royal Naval Diving Manual

Severe decompression sickness may require artificial ventilation for neurological failure or for severe pulmonary oedema. Should I.P.P.V. or C.P.P.V. be required, the patient must be carefully observed for the onset of a pneumothorax. Shock and hypovolaemia may be complicated by a metabolic acidosis which should be corrected with sodium bicarbonate (Kindwall and Margolis, 1975).

Agitated patients may require diazepam for sedation. Philp (1964) has demonstrated that heparin may be valuable largely for its anti-lipaemic rather than anti-coagulant properties. The doses should be small (approximately 2000 units 6 hourly) because of the danger of haemorrhage subsequent to vestibular gas bubble damage (Elliott *et al.*, 1974).

Associated pulmonary barotrauma may require drainage of a pneumothorax.

DETECTION AND TREATMENT OF AIR EMBOLISM

In venous air embolism, air enters the venous system and in sufficient quantity can obstruct the right heart (Durant *et al.*, 1949). Generally air continues onto the lungs producing acute pulmonary hypertension followed by pulmonary oedema.

Twenty-four per cent of the population (Hart, 1974) have a probe-patent foramen ovale. Air may therefore pass in venous air embolism from the right to the left side of the heart. Left heart embolism or arterial air embolism may produce myocardial infarction through air entering a coronary artery, may enter the cerebral vessels producing neurological deficits as in decompression sickness and may also enter other tissues such as the kidney, liver and bone, producing silent infarcts. A cardiac arrest or dysrhythmia may occur on the table during an operative procedure where arterial air embolus is a possibility (Donato *et al.*, 1975), or air may be seen entering the venous or arterial circulation. The presence of air in the right heart can be detected with the use of a Doppler probe (Tinker *et al.*, 1975) and Breckner and Bethune (1968) describe an early warning system by monitoring exhaled carbon dioxide. A sudden drop in exhaled carbon dioxide is consistent with air embolism but may also occur when the cardiac output falls (the drop then generally being gradual) and during ventricular tachycardia (Lippmann, 1972). The sudden appearance of a cardiac murmur, especially if mill-wheel in character, should be considered to be confirmatory evidence of air embolism until proven otherwise. The immediate treatment is directed to the venous or arterial side of the circulation depending upon the site of involvement.

If the diagnosis is suspected, the surgeon should be notified immediately so that the source of air is eliminated if at all possible. In venous air embolism the venous pressure should be raised by intubation and hand ventilation with 100% oxygen. Discontinuance of nitrous oxide administration is essential since nitrous oxide is 34 times more soluble in blood than nitrogen. Consequently when a bubble of air appears in venous blood containing a high concentration of nitrous oxide there is a rapid transfer of many molecules of nitrous oxide into the bubble with an exit of only a few molecules of nitrogen.

The patient should be placed in the left lateral head-down position 'Durant' Manoeuvre (Lippmann, 1972). This prevents air from passing through a patent foramen ovale or into the pulmonary circulation. External cardiac massage should be commenced if air obstructs right ventricular output or if Durant's manoeuvre cannot be carried out.

Massive venous air embolism should be treated with placement of a right atrial catheter and evacuation of the air using a 250 ml vacuum container. Angelis (1975) has demonstrated a very neat system whereby the right atrial catheter is attached to a three-way tap – one to an intravenous fluid source, the other to a 250 ml empty container (Haemo-Vac Blood Container, McGaw). The catheter is positioned with the line connected to the intravenous infusion bottle and switched over to the vacuum bottle once the position is confirmed. Since the evacuated container described contains A.C.D. solution, should only blood be evacuated, this can be returned to the patient. Following evacuation of the air – the patient should be compressed if at all possible in hyperbaric oxygen. Oxygen delivered at 3 A.T.A. will afford the greatest displacement of the inert gas to obtain the best quality of survival (Hart, 1974).

In severe arterial air embolism compression in a hyperbaric oxygen chamber or compressed air chamber is essential (Hart, 1974). The authorities mentioned in Table 1 should be consulted.

EMBOLISM FROM CARBON DIOXIDE

Pulmonary embolism during insufflation of the fallopian tubes with carbon dioxide is rarely observed because of the high solubility of carbon dioxide in blood and tissues. With massive embolisation the gas may be trapped in the pulmonary artery producing obstruction to right ventricular outflow. Gas may also occupy the pulmonary capillary bed producing failure of gas exchange and death from hypoxia. The gas may be displaced by Durant's manoeuvre (see p. 608). External cardiac massage may be necessary if Durant's manoeuvre does not improve right ventricular output.

REFERENCES

Angelis, J. de (1975). A simple and rapid method for evacuation of embolised air. *Anaesthesiology* **43**, 110.

Aronson, M. E. and Nelson, P. K. (1967). Fatal air embolism in pregnancy resulting from an unusual sex act. *Obstet. Gynec.* **30**, 127.

Bergeron, R. T. and Rumbaugh, C. L. (1971). Air embolism associated with the use of malfitting plastic connectors in angiography. *Radiology* **98**, 689.

Breckner, V. L. and Bethune, R. W. (1968). Retention of venous air embolism by carbon dioxide monitoring. *Anaesthesiology* **29**, 178.

Cockett, A. T. K. and Nakamura, R. M. (1964). A new concept in the treatment of decompression sickness (dysbarism). *Lancet* **1**, 1102.

Doll, R. E. and Berghage, T. E. (1967). U.S. Navy Experimental Diving Unit Research report, p. 7.

Donato, A. T., Arciniegus, E. and Lam, C. R. (1975). Fatal air embolism during thoracotomy for gunshot injury to the lung. Report of a case. *J. Thorac. and Cardiovasc. Surg.* **69**, 827.

Durant, T. M., Oppenheimer, M. J., Webster, M. R. and Long, J. (1949). Arterial air embolism. *Am. Heart J.* **38**, 481.

Elliott, D. H., Hallenbeck, J. M. and Bove, A. A. (1974). Acute decompression sickness. *Lancet* **2**, 1193.

Ericsson, J. A., Gottlieb, J. D. and Sweet, R. B. (1964). Closed chest cardiac massage in treatment of venous air embolism. *New Engl. J. Med.* **270**, 1356.

Golding, F. C., Griffiths, P., Hempleman, H. V., Paton, W. D. M. and Walder, D. N. (1960). Decompression sickness during construction of the Dartford tunnel. *Brit. J. Ind. Med.* **17**, 167.

Goodman, M. W. and Workman, R. D. (1965). Minimal Decompression, Oxygen Breathing Approach of Treatment. Decompression Sickness in Divers and Aviators. BUSHIPS Proj. SF0110605 Task 11 513 – 2. Research rep. p. 5. Bureau of Med. and Surg. Washington, D.C.

Gottlieb, J. D., Ericsson, J. A. and Sweet, R. B. (1965). Venous air embolism. A review. *Anesth. Analg.* **44**, 773.

Hart, G. B. (1974). Treatment of decompression illness and air embolism with hyperbaric oxygen. *Aerospace Med.* **45**, 1190.

Heller, S. S., Frank, K. A., Malm, J. R., Bowman, F. O. Jr., Harris, P. D., Charlton, M. H. and Kornfield, D. S. (1970). Psychiatric complications of open-heart surgery. *New Engl. J. Med.* **283**, 1015.

Kindwall, E. P. and Margolis, I. (1975). Management of severe decompression sickness with treatment ancillary to decompression: Case Report. *Aviation, Space and Environ. Med.* **46**, 1065.

Lippmann, M. (1972). Air embolism. *Int. Anaesthesiol. Clin.* **10**, 93.

Mason, W. Van. H., Damm, E. G., Dickinson, A. R. and Nevison, T. O. Jr. (1971). Arterial gas emboli after blast injury. *Proc. Soc. Exp. Biol. Med.* **136**, 1253.

Philp, R. B. (1964). The ameliorative effects of heparin and depolymerised hyaluranate on decompression sickness in rats. *Cana. J. Physiol and Pharmacol.* **42**, 819.

Tinker, J. H., Gronert, G. A., Messick, J. M. and Michenfelder, J. D. (1975). Detection of air embolism, a test for positioning of right atrial catheter and doppler probe. *Anaesthesiology* **43**, 104.

Ward, M. K., Shadforth, M., Hill, A. V. L. and Kerr, D. N. S. (1971). Air embolism during haemodialysis. *Brit. Med. J.* **3**, 74.

Yeakel, A. E. (1968). Lethal air embolism from plastic blood-storage container. *JAMA* **204**, 267.

VI

The Management of Poisoning

PATRICIA STONE AND P. L. WRIGHT

INTRODUCTION

Drug overdose continues to be a major cause of admission to medical wards. It is estimated that more than 100 000 admissions annually take place in the United Kingdom. In many units it may represent the commonest single cause of admission, especially those units serving depressed urban areas. The overall mortality is of the order of 1%, Matthew and Lawson (1966). It is very important to recognise this in the planning of treatment for a poisoned individual. *Primum non nocere*. It is especially necessary to remember this dictum as new suggestions are made for treatment. Older physicians will remember the now outmoded analeptic therapy given to patients poisoned with barbiturates which, being found wanting, led to the 'Scandinavian Method' of elective supportive therapy depending on the maintenance of respiratory function and the treatment of circulatory failure.

Patients with drug overdose in this country are usually referred to casualty departments. A history is often obtainable since most patients are conscious at the time of admission. There will remain a number of patients who refuse to co-operate or are unconscious on admission. Diagnosis in such cases may be difficult even if overdose is suspected.

PRODUCTS PRODUCING INTOXICATION. INFORMATION SERVICES

Medicinal products

In theory, identification of dispensed medicines should now be easy as the names appear on the labels. Doctors should remember the

611

extraordinary propensity patients have for putting tablets in different bottles. Many tablets and capsules bear an identification, and any pharmacist can easily identify many products by experience and from the manufacturers' literature. When no pharmacist is available, a tablet identification guide may prove helpful, although accurate colour reproduction is difficult and slight alterations in shade may cause errors. It is advisable to compare the unknown with an authentic specimen, colours and tablet weights should exactly coincide. A guide appears in the 'Chemist and Druggist Directory and Tablet and Capsule Identification Guide'. This book is published annually by Benn Brothers Limited.

Industrial and household products

The constituents of products available may be unknown. Information about all types of poisons and the management of the patient may be obtained from one of the national network of Poisons Information Centres. Their telephone numbers are:

Belfast	0232	40503
Cardiff	0222	33101
Edinburgh	031229	2477
Leeds	0532	32799
London	01–407	7600
Manchester	061 740	2254
Newcastle	0632	25131

A second source of information about drugs and poisons is the network of Drug Information Centres set up by the hospital pharmaceutical service (Table 1). These are able, usually at short notice, to provide detailed information.

Plants and animals

There are many poisonous plants in the wild and cultivated flora. Among these a number may cause serious poisoning. A useful book in which the major poisonous plants are illustrated in colour and the type of poison is described in that published by North (1967).

The only native poisonous snake is the Adder or Northern Viper, *Vipera bera*. The antiserum suitable for treating cases is commercially available in the United Kingdom.

For foreign snakes, information about treatment and a supply of serum for emergency treatment of bites can be obtained from either The

Table 1. Regional drug information centres

Region	Telephone number	Extension
East Anglian	0473 72233	–
Mersey	051–236 8464	347
Northern	0632 25131	–
North East Thames	01–247 5454	62 and 147
North West Thames	01–373 2316	35
North Western	061–224 9633	270
Oxford	0865–49891	483
South East Thames	01–407 7600	2548
South West Thames	0483 71122	536
South Western	0272 22041	2867
Trent	0533 541414	491
Wessex	0703 777222	3751
West Midlands	021–355 6161	3314
Yorkshire	0532 32799 and	547
	0532 30715	49
Wales	0222 755944	2979
Greater Glasgow	041–552 3535	486
Lothian	031–229 2477	–
Tayside	0382 26975	2351
Northern Ireland	0232 40503	–

National Poisons Information Centre at New Cross Hospital, Avonley Road, London, SE14 5ER (telephone number 01–407 7600), or the Pharmacy Department of the University Hospital of Wales, Heath Park, Cardiff, CF4 4XW (telephone number 0222 755944).

Hazardous freight

Arrangements exist for obtaining advice and assistance in the cases of any incident involving hazardous freight. Three publications, primarily intended for the Fire and Ambulance Services, may provide useful information.

1. The Chemical Industries Association publishes Transport Emergency Cards (*Tremcards*) which are intended to be carried in the cabs of vehicles carrying dangerous substances. They give details of action to be taken by emergency services. Complete sets can be obtained from the C.I.A., Alembic House, 93 Albert Embankment, London, SE1 7TU.

2. The C.I.A. publishes a manual '*Chemsafe*' detailing the procedure recommended to manufacturers and traders who handle dangerous

substances for establishing emergency arrangements in advance for providing advice and assistance should a mishap occur.

3. I.C.I. publish a book, 'A Guide for Public Authorities' describing the I.C.I. emergency scheme for providing expert advice when an incident involving hazardous freight occurs. Centres all over the country are listed, some of which can provide technical advice day or night, and others which can also provide emergency equipment.

THE NON-SPECIFIC MANAGEMENT OF POISONING

A summary of the emergency treatment of poisoning is shown in Table 2.

Initial management

A full medical history should be taken and the patient examined carefully. The quantity and type of ingested drug should be noted. Special attention should be given to factors which might alter the patient's responsiveness to drugs or to his ability to detoxicate or excrete them, e.g. respiratory depression from barbiturates will be more serious in patients with chronic chest disease; opiates may precipitate hepatic encephalopathy in the cirrhotic patient.

The level of consciousness and the time of examination should be recorded in order that future observers will be able to gauge the progress of the patient.

It is the author's policy to continue to recommend what has been called a 'punitive policy' to conscious patients. An overdose being suspected, a stomach washout is performed using a wide bore lubricated tube. Plain tap water is used for this purpose. Washouts should not be performed if the patient is thought to have swallowed a corrosive poison. Removal of the drug from the stomach or its destruction chemically is occasionally possible *viz*:

Salicylate	Sodium bicarbonate 1 teaspoonful of powder in 500 ml lavage water (approx. isotonic).
Yellow phosphorus	Potassium permanganate solution 1 to 5000 dilution.
Iron	Sodium bicarbonate 1% followed by 5000 mg desferrioxamine in 10 ml of water to be left in the stomach.

Table 2. Summary of emergency treatment of poisoning

1. Check airway. Tongue, dentures, food, vomit. Bronchial secretions. If unconscious, insert airway.
2. Nurse in coma position. Vomiting is common.
3. Confirm the heart is beating. If not, intubate, ventilate and start external cardiac massage.
4. Assess adequacy of ventilation by measurement if possible. Treat if inadequate. Give 100% oxygen if patient in coma.
5. Assess circulatory state. Treat.
6. Arterial blood for acid base status, PaO_2, $PaCO_2$, drug identification, haemoglobin, blood urea, electrolytes if required.
7. Measure core temperature.
8. Check if there is a specific antidote (unlikely).
9. Consider gastric lavage. ? any specific method of removal. (See p. 614)
10. Give adequate intravenous fluids. Treat acid base disturbances, cardiac dysrhythmia, hyper/hypotension or convulsions, should they be present.
11. Promote excretion if needed. Forced acid/alkaline diuresis. Renal dialysis. Haemoperfusion.
12. If in doubt consult the poisons reference service (Table 1)

In children it may be preferable to induce vomiting instead of performing gastric lavage, provided the child has not taken an antiemetic drug, corrosive poison or petroleum product. The preparation used is ipecacuanha paediatric emetic draught B.P.C. The dosages are: child 6 months to 18 months, 10 ml; child 18 months to 5 years, 15 ml, followed by 200 ml of water. The dose may be repeated once if no vomiting occurs after 20–25 minutes.

The unconscious patient should be nursed in the coma position. Careful attention should be paid to the patient's respiratory function. Foreign matter should be carefully removed from the mouth and pharynx. A sucker should be to hand in case of vomiting. If ventilation appears inadequate or the cough and gag reflex absent, it is safer to insert an endotracheal tube under direct vision in order to prevent the aspiration of stomach contents. With a tube inserted and the cuff of the endotracheal tube inflated, a wide bore stomach tube may be passed and a washout performed. Samples of the fluid may be saved for forensic analysis should this be considered necessary. The amount of drug removed, especially from this type of patient, may be small but important. Highly soluble compounds are unlikely to be present many hours after drug ingestion. The authors are themselves impressed by the quantity of material which is present in the stomachs of patients found dead. Gastric lavage is certainly useless if performed in a perfunctory manner, with too small a volume of fluid or through a narrow tube.

After attending to the airway blood should be taken for estimation of drug levels if needed for the management or confirmation of the diagnosis, e.g. salicylate, paracetamol and barbiturate. Except in mild cases, an arterial blood gas analysis should be performed to give a baseline indication of respiratory performance. Analysis of blood urea, electrolytes, haemoglobin etc. are occasionally useful. A chest X-ray should be obtained if possible to assist in the early diagnosis of pulmonary aspiration or atelectasis.

As stated, the majority of patients will recover from their drug overdose, no special treatment being required to antagonise or remove the offending material from their circulatory system. The patient should be kept under observation until full recovery occurs. Should respiratory depression develop the patient should be intubated in order to protect the airway, mechanical ventilation should be commenced if serial estimations of minute volume and blood gases indicate respiratory failure. Where aspiration is suspected, ventilation should be instituted on admission because of the complications which may arise in this condition if the patient is allowed to breathe spontaneously (Part 2, ch. V, p. 563). In the semiconscious patient with drug overdose complicated by pulmonary aspiration, intubation may necessitate the use of a muscle relaxant.

The blood pressure and pulse should be monitored; a cardiac monitor should be used in tricyclic anti-depressant overdosage to detect the onset of dysrhythmias. If shock is present an intravenous infusion line should be inserted and a central venous catheter used to assess right atrial filling pressure and the patient infused with normal saline to restore the pressure to +5 cm water. Pressor amines do not appear to have any useful role here. Isoprenaline or dopamine (see Part 2, ch. II, p. 372) may occasionally be valuable in counteracting the myocardial suppressant effect of drugs (e.g. barbiturates).

The elimination of drugs from the patient may be enhanced by the following techniques:

Forced diuresis
Peritoneal dialysis
Haemodialysis
Haemoperfusion using an activated charcoal column
Exchange transfusion.

These techniques are complex, carry their own risks and complications and should only be considered in the management of severe poisoning where there is good evidence that their use may save life. Their use is not advocated to shorten a period of unconsciousness.

Forced acid and alkaline diuresis

This treatment increases the urinary excretion of those drugs which are weak electrolytes; two principles are involved. Firstly by increasing urinary flow larger amounts of certain drugs are excreted since reabsorption in the proximal and distal renal tubules is reduced. This has been applied particularly to the treatment of barbiturate overdosage. Secondly, tubular reabsorption is influenced by the amount of ionisation of the drug: a greater degree of ionisation by reducing the lipid-solubility would favour reabsorption. For example, at an alkaline pH, salicylates, which are weak acids, are highly ionised and so are eliminated at an enhanced rate. Conversely, the excretion of a weak base such as pethidine is increased by an acidic urinary pH.

A detailed account of these principles may be found in the book by Smith and Rawlins (1973). In addition, the authors list many drugs with chemical and pharmacological characteristics which can be used to predict whether their elimination may be enhanced by either a forced acid or alkaline diuresis.

Table 3. The use of forced diuresis in drug intoxication (in decreasing order of effective drug removal)

Forced alkaline diuresis	Forced acid diuresis
Diodone	Amphetamine
Salicylic acid	Ephedrine
Probenecid	Nicotine
Acetylsalicylic acid	Pethidine
Phenylbutazone	Quinine
Tolbutamide	Chlorpromazine
Phenobarbitone	Morphine
Nitrofurantoin	
Cyclobarbitone	

Forced alkaline diuresis (Cumming et al., 1964)

A catheter is inserted into the bladder and released hourly. Isotonic sodium chloride, 5% dextrose and 2% sodium bicarbonate are infused in sequence at a flow rate initially of 500 ml every 30 min. The rate of infusion can be maintained for several hours, care being taken that the patient is not overloaded. In the older patient right atrial pressure monitoring is advisable. After 2–3 h the infusion should be slowed to match the urinary output. Intravenous frusemide 40 mg at the onset will help to initiate diuresis. Supplemental potassium will be necessary; after one hour the serum potassium should be measured and replaced at the rate of 10 mmol/h. Most easily and safely a prepared solution of sodium chloride 0.9% and potassium chloride can be substituted for the plain saline after the first hour. A continual watch is necessary despite this precaution for some patients will excrete very high levels of potassium in their urine. The author has himself caused a fall in potassium level to 1.1 mmol/l in this way.

A forced alkaline diuresis should be continued until the patient has regained consciousness or in the case of salicylate intoxication, the serum salicylate level has fallen to 60 mg/100 ml or less.

Forced acid diuresis

Forced acid diuresis is rarely indicated and hence rarely instituted. Rapid acidification of the urine is difficult to achieve and is probably best done using arginine monohydrochloride. It should occasionally be considered in severe chlorpromazine overdose. Senior medical advice should be obtained before starting this form of treatment.

1. L-Arginine hydrochloride (30 g* in 50 ml) to be added to 500 ml 5% dextrose and infused over one hour.
2. 500 ml normal saline and 100 ml 10% mannitol over one hour.
3. Keep drip open with normal saline.
4. Repeat (1) after 2 h if diuresis < 150 ml.
5. If diuresis > 150 ml give one litre normal saline + 500 ml 5% dextrose in one hour. Repeat in next hour, give frusemide 20 mg i.v.
6. Continue infusion at 500 ml/h using normal saline alternating with 5% dextrose. Potassium chloride should be added at 10 mmol/l. Output should be 12 l/day.

If serum K falls below 3.5 mmol/l, increase the potassium in the infusate. Check T-waves on monitor.
7. Calcium gluconate should be given 10 ml of 10% 8-hourly.
8. The patient should be catheterised.

Peritoneal dialysis and haemodialysis

The former is simpler and requires less complex apparatus and can usually be managed by a nurse. The costs involved are similar. Dialysis should be considered:

In renal failure.
When deterioration occurs despite adequate supportive treatment in the presence of a dialysable poison.
Uncorrectable acid base imbalance, e.g. salicylate poisoning.

* L-Arginine hydrochloride 30 g/500 ml containing 142 mmol H^+.

It is essential to monitor right atrial pressure when dialysing a patient with drug overdose.

Peritoneal dialysis is performed with continuous recycling of 1 litre of isotonic solution every 20 min. If serum potassium is normal, potassium 5 mmol is added to alternate litres. The serum potassium should be checked after 2 hours and the potassium in the dialysate adjusted accordingly.

Lipid peritoneal dialysis

Glutethemide poisoning may be severe and since it is highly lipid soluble is rapidly distributed into the liver and body fat after ingestion. Because of the lipid solubility, haemodialysis with lipid dialysate has been used with reports of enhanced clearance of glutethemide, this however has been subsequently disproved (Leitzell *et al.*, 1971).

We have found a minimal increase in clearance rate in one case using lipid peritoneal dialysis. The method used involved continuous recycling of a combination of 100 ml 10% Intralipid with 500 ml isotonic dialysis solution every 30 min. Potassium monitoring is essential. This form of treatment has not been investigated extensively because of the rare incidence of severe glutethemide intoxication.

Haemodialysis

Haemodialysis is known to be more efficient in removing dialysable poisons from the blood stream. We have not found it necessary, however, to institute haemodialysis in any patient admitted with drug overdose over the last 7 years. Over this period there has been no death directly attributable to the effect of a dialysable poison, death being due to complications which would be unaffected by dialysis, e.g. massive pulmonary aspiration. An excellent survey on the effect of dialysis in removal of various drugs and poisons has been made by Schreiner and Teehan (1972).

Charcoal haemoperfusion

The technique and its attendant complications are described by Trewby and Williams (p. 984). It's use in the management of drug overdose is highly controversial but there is evidence to suggest that it may be of value in the treatment of patients severely poisoned with all types of barbiturate and glutethemide (Vale *et al.*, 1975). The technique is simpler and more effective than haemodialysis but until its value has been proven, should be preferably performed by medical personnel experienced in its use.

Exchange transfusion

May be life saving in babies and small infants.

THE MANAGEMENT OF SPECIFIC INTOXICATIONS

Salicylates

Aspirin and other salicylate compounds produce complex effects on the poisoned patient. The effects stem from the ability of salicylate to uncouple oxidative phosphorylation and thus markedly increase the metabolism of glucose and then fats. This results in a marked increase in oxygen consumption and carbon dioxide production. Respiration is stimulated both by the increase in carbon dioxide and also by the direct effect of salicylate on the respiratory centre. Higher levels of salicylate ultimately cause respiratory depression. The metabolic effect on the patient is therefore complicated. Levels of pyruvate lactate and ketone bodies rise; aspirin is itself an organic acid and thus a metabolic acidosis supervenes and a mixed picture is often seen. In advanced cases respiratory acidosis is present. Encephalopathy may be present and the patient may develop hyperthermia. Salicylate levels are useful in the assessment of severity of poisoning; at levels below 50 mg/100 ml no specific therapy is usually required. Levels of 80–110 mg/100 ml or more constitute a serious risk to the patient and require additional therapy in the form of forced alkaline diuresis or more rarely renal dialysis.

In view of the metabolic and respiratory changes which may occur in moderate to severe salicylate intoxication (salicylate blood level >80 mg/100 ml), serial acid base and blood gas analyses are essential. The quantity of sodium bicarbonate infused in the forced alkaline diuresis regime (see p. 617) may have to be altered in the light of these changes. Associated changes in salicylate intoxication include gastric haemorrhage, gastric perforation, a haemorrhagic diathesis (usually due to hypoprothrombinaemia and correctable by vitamin K, but sometimes due to thrombocytopenia) and occasionally acute renal failure. Vitamin K_1 should be given routinely on admission and urine output must be observed carefully during forced alkaline diuresis.

Opiate drugs

Note that the patient may be a drug addict and be suffering from the consequences of his addiction. Frequent complications include hepatitis and septicaemia. Not all patients with hepatic encephalopathy are jaundiced, thus an addict admitted in coma may not necessarily be suffering from opiate poisoning. Expected signs of poisoning include pin-point pupils and slow, deep respiration. Improvement may rapidly be expected with nalorphine 10 mg intravenously, repeated as necessary. Nalorphine itself is a respiratory depressant and overdose must be avoided. Alternatively, naloxone hydrochloride 0.4 mg in one ml is given by intravenous injection. The injection may be repeated at 2–3 min intervals. Failure to obtain improvement suggests an alternative diagnosis to opiate poisoning.

Paracetamol

In overdose, the normal metabolic pathways of paracetamol are overwhelmed, and unusual conjugates are formed. It is the reactive precursors of these conjugates which may combine with hepatocyte proteins, with resultant hepatic necrosis. Work describing this process is reviewed by Davis *et al.* (1976) in a paper in which they also describe their own work on paracetamol conjugates in the urine.

Paracetamol sulphate is the major metabolite formed in the liver after therapeutic doses. However, this metabolic route is soon saturated even with therapeutic doses, and alternative conjugative pathways come into action. The most important of these is glucuronide conjugation. When potentially hepatotoxic doses have been taken, this route also becomes saturated. At this stage, a related transient unconjugated hyperbilirubinaemia may develop – insufficient glucuronic acid being available for conjugation with bilirubin. Other available metabolic pathways involve conjugation with cysteine and mercapturic acid. The paracetamol forms chemically unstable precursors which combine with reduced glutathione in the liver cell. These then break down to form the cysteine and mercapturic acid conjugates which are excreted in the urine. In therapeutic use, this pathway accounts for a very small proportion of the dose, so that the very small amounts of the unstable precursors are soon combined with reduced glutathione. In overdose the reduced glutathione levels soon fall and the excess precursor combines with the sulphydryl (-SH) groups of the liver cell protein.

Individuals may vary in their susceptibility to this form of liver damage, and various predisposing factors have been identified such as consumption of alcohol and enzyme inducing drugs, diet and genetic factors.

Treatment has been based theoretically on the assumption that -SH donor groups will displace unstable precursors from their combination with glutathione or -SH groups of the liver cell, reviewed by Penn (1976). One approach is to use the glutathione precursors L-cysteine and L-methionine since glutathione is not taken up by liver cells. L-Methionine tablets are available commercially. Alternatively cysteamine has been shown to reduce paracetamol toxicity when given up to 10 h from ingestion. Prescott *et al.* (1974, 1976a and 1976b). Its mode of action may be as above or by the inhibition of microsomal oxidation of paracetamol.

The admission plasma paracetamol concentration estimated as an emergency and related to the time ingestion is used as a guide to the need for treatment (Fig. 1).

Cysteamine is given by intravenous infusion, 1–2 g initially, 800 mg in the next 4 h, 400 mg in the subsequent 8 h, followed by 400 mg in the final 12 h. Cysteamine is not commercially available as a sterile solution for intravenous use and must be prepared by the hospital pharmacist and sterilised, or injected through a Millipore filter.

The treatment of paracetamol poisoning can alternatively be attempted by haemoperfusion through a charcoal column, the efficacy of this technique remains to be proven.

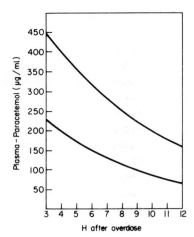

Fig. 1. Plasma-paracetamol concentrations in relation to time after overdosage. (Reproduced by kind permission of Prescott *et al.*, 1976.)

The treatment therefore of paracetamol overdosage remains controversial and was reviewed in 'Drug and Therapeutics Bulletin' (1976). A paracetamol estimation kit is commercially available from Winthrop Laboratories. It is suggested that guidance be sought from one of the Poisons Information Centres since the position regarding therapy is likely to be clarified in the near future.

Iron

Serious poisoning can occur in a child following ingestion of as few as 5 tablets of ferrous sulphate. Early symptoms are of nausea, vomiting and metallic taste in the mouth. Sudden death from cardiac toxicity may occur up to 24 h after iron ingestion. Gastric lavage is essential (p. 614).

On admission the patient is given 2000 mg desferrioxamine intramuscularly each 500 mg vial being dissolved in 2 ml water for injection. Desferrioxamine should then be infused intravenously at a rate of not more than 15 mg/kg/h to a maximum dose in 24 h of 80 mg/kg. The drug may be added to normal saline, dextrose or dextrose saline. It should be dissolved first in 2–3 ml water per injection. The intramuscular injection can be repeated 12 hourly. Desferrioxamine, 100 mg, will chelate 8.5 mg iron or 5 g will inactivate the iron in 10 tablets of ferrous sulphate.

Tricyclic anti-depressants

In overdosage anti-cholinergic side effects are seen such as dryness of the mouth, pupillary dilatation, urinary retention, failure of sweating complicated by hyperthermia and ileus. Hyperreflexia, convulsions and respiratory depression are common. Signs of both pyramidal and extrapyramidal disturbance are seen. Hypotension and hypertension are common. Treatment with physostigmine may be considered but is often unnecessary (Noble and Matthew, 1969). Convulsions and/or extreme agitation may require the use of intravenous diazepam. A period of mechanical ventilation is invariably required if diazepam is used to control convulsions – respiratory depression commonly arising not only as a result of the use of the drug but also subsequent to the seizures. Benztropine mesylate 1–2 mg intramuscularly or intravenously is valuable in controlling severe extrapyramidal symptoms.

The major problem with tricyclic poisoning is the late onset of ventricular fibrillation, this may occur up to 48 h after drug ingestion and is generally but not always preceded by ventricular extrasystoles.

These patients should therefore be constantly monitored in an area where prompt resuscitation is available. No difficulty was experienced by the author in defibrillating four such cases who were subsequently given lignocaine for 48 h. If extrasystoles are noted, it seems wise to attempt to prevent ventricular fibrillation by the prophylactic administration of lignocaine 50 mg intravenously as a loading dose and then as a continuous infusion of 1–2 mg/min. Myocardial suppressant drugs, in particular β-adrenergic blockers should be used with extreme care, since their use may be complicated by a radical fall in pulse rate and cardiac output and even asystolic arrest. Phenytoin sodium has proven to be valuable in not only controlling convulsions but also in suppressing any cardiac dysrhythmia and is one of the drugs of choice when both occur simultaneously.

Cyanide

Cyanides are used in several industrial processes such as electro-plating and have also been used in domestic products such as metal polishes. There are a number of plants which contain cyanogenetic glycosides in the seeds which break down to form hydrocyanic acid. All are members of the Rosaceae and include the kernels and pips of apricot, bird cherry, apple, pear, plum and bitter almond.

The metabolic processes described below are described in greater detail by Goodman and Gilman (1975). The symptoms of cyanide poisoning are due to cytotoxic hypoxia, the cyanide ion reacting with cytochrome oxidase in the cell mitochondria to form a cytochrome oxidase-cyanide complex. Formation of this complex inhibits cellular respiration. The cytochrome oxidase-cyanide complex is dissociable; the mitochondrial enzyme sulphur transferase mediates the transfer of sulphur from thiosulphate to the cyanide ion, with the formation of thiocyanate. This releases the cytochrome oxidase which is now available for cell respiration. Endogenous thiosulphate is only available in limited amount and once used up the cytochrome oxidase-cyanide complex is no longer dissociable. An alternative metabolic pathway is that in which cyanide combines with methaemoglobin to form cyanmethaemoglobin. In the presence of high concentrations of methaemoglobin, this metabolic route is utilised preferentially to the one involving cytochrome oxidase. Administration of nitrites converts haemoglobin to methaemoglobin, thereby diminishing the production of cytochrome oxidase-cyanide complex.

The emergency treatment of cyanide poisoning must be started immediately. Poisoning is usually accidental and in laboratories etc. where cyanide is used, a treatment kit is kept. Such a kit must be kept in the casualty department. Cyanide poisoning is usually with potassium or sodium cyanide; free hydrocyanic acid (prussic acid) is almost instantaneously fatal. A patient who has swallowed cyanide may be slow to liberate hydrocyanic acid from the stomach if the stomach acid concentration is low or the patient has recently taken food. Two forms of treatment are available. The first to be described is traditional and effective. The second has theoretical advantages and fewer side effects.

1. An ampoule of amyl nitrite is broken and the patient inhales it from a fibre swab. Ten ml of 3% sodium nitrite is injected as soon as possible at the rate of 2.5–5 ml/min. Using the same needle, sodium thiosulphate 12.5 g (50 ml of 25% solution) should be injected over a period of 10 min. The injections may be repeated at half the initial doses. Severe and paroxysmal headache is the main side effect, marked hypotension invariably occurs.

2. Cobalt edetate/tetracemate: 'Kelocyanor' Rona Laboratories Ltd. (0.3 g in 20 ml for intravenous injection). This acts by forming a stable complex with cyanides, in which form it will be excreted from the body. Cobalt itself is normally toxic and a reciprocal antidote effect occurs in that the formation of the complex with the cyanide reduces the potential toxicity of the cobalt. It is important therefore to establish the diagnosis of cyanide poisoning before it is given. Forty ml (0.6 g) should be given intravenously followed immediately by 50 ml of 50% dextrose. Should there be no response, a further 0.3 g of cobalt edetate tetracemate should be given followed by another dose of 50 ml 50% dextrose. Side effects are likely to last for one minute and include a fall in blood pressure, a rise in pulse rate and retching.

Organo-phosphorus compounds

These compounds are powerful anti-cholinesterase agents. The inhibition of this enzyme leads to the accumulation of acetyl choline and consequently provides continuous stimulation of the cholinergic fibres of the central and peripheral nervous systems. In some cases the organo-phosphorus compounds bind irreversibly to the enzyme, and the return of anticholinergic activity is dependent on the formation of new enzyme, which may take days or months. A detailed account may be found in Goodman and Gilman (1975).

Most of the organo-phosphorus compounds are highly lipid soluble, so they are well absorbed by all routes, including through the skin. In acute poisoning, muscarinic and nicotinic signs are present in addition to the effects on the nervous system. Peripheral muscle fasciculation and paralysis occur. Death is from respiratory failure due to laryngospasm and bronchoconstriction, complicated by increased tracheobronchial and salivary secretion. Cardiovascular effects may also occur.

Treatment

1. Atropine in large doses should be used; it reverses the effects at the muscarinic receptor sites.

2. Pralidoxime mesylate (P2S) acts by displacing the organophosphorus compound from its complex with the cholinesterase enzyme, thus reactivating it. An intravenous injection of 5 ml of the 20% solution restores the response to stimulation of motor nerves within a few minutes. The effect of pralidoxine mesylate on the autonomic receptors is less and it has an insignificant effect on the central nervous system.

A list of designated centres which hold stocks of pralidoxime mesylate injection will be found in the circular 'Supply of Certain Prophylactic and Therapeutic Agents' D.H.S.S. (1964). This circular is currently under review (1977) and a new edition may be expected.

Amanita phalloides

Over 90% of human deaths from fungus poisoning are caused by *Amanita phalloides* (Death cap), which is fairly common in deciduous woods in autumn. Less commonly occurring species which contain the same toxins are *A. verna* (Gill, Fool's mushroom) and *A. virosa* (Destroying angel). The effects of eating the fungus are reviewed in an editorial *Lancet* (1972). The toxins present fall into two groups: one group known as the phallotoxins are heptapeptides and these are responsible for the violent nausea, vomiting and diarrhoea which characteristically develop after a delay of some hours. The other group, amatoxins, are octapeptides. The principal one which has been identified is alpha-amanitin. It is the amatoxins which cause the fatal hepatorenal symptoms. In small doses, the epithelial cells of the proximal convoluted tubules of the kidney are damaged, a high concentration being present at this site because the toxins are reabsorbed from the glomerular filtrate. In higher doses, alpha-amanitin irreversibly damages the hepatocyte nuclei by binding to ribonucleic acid polymerase in eukaryotic cells.

Treatment

There is no specific antidote. The only agents which have shown promise are those which displace alpha-amanitin from its plasma protein binding sites, thus facilitating its excretion. Skrabal and Dittrich (1973) report that haemodialysis has been effective, particularly in combination with drugs which displace alpha-amanitin from plasma binding sites. Such drugs which have been used are penicillin, chloramphenicol and phenylbutazone. Experimental work has also tried cytochrome C – its mode of action is not clear, but it has been used to increase intracellular respiration in anoxaemic states.

Paraquat

This is a dipyridylium weedkiller or herbicide marketed by I.C.I. in a range of products. Trade names likely to be met in the U.K. are listed below:

U.K. products containing paraquat	
Dextrone X*	Gramoxone S*
Dexuron*	Pathclear
Esgram*	Terraklene*
Gramonol*	Tota-Col*
Gramoxone*	Weedol

An oral dose of 3 g of paraquat (15 ml of a 200 g/l liquid concentrate) is likely to be fatal for an adult.

The concentrate is corrosive so that immediate effects are by irritation and ulceration in the gastro-intestinal tract. Splashes in the eyes cause inflammation of the conjunctivae and cornea. A *Lancet* editorial (1976) summarised the symptoms of poisoning.

Large doses. Ingestion leads to death by pulmonary oedema and haemorrhage within a few days. Many organs, including the kidneys, liver, heart and adrenal glands are damaged.

Smaller doses. (10–20 ml of concentrate.) The symptoms develop more slowly. Excretion via the urine declines after the first day as renal damage occurs. Progressive pulmonary fibrosis develops and death

* Most fatalities are caused by these concentrated liquid preparations.

from respiratory failure ensues. This process, outlined below, is described by Copland *et al.* (1974):

Paraquat destroys the epithelial lining of ventilated pulmonary alveoli. This then leads to extensive intra-alveolar avascular fibrosis. Its destructive effect on the epithelium appears to be due to the liberation of hydrogen peroxide during its metabolic cyclic reduction and subsequent re-oxygenation. Lung tissue is particularly vulnerable because of its close contact with atmospheric oxygen and well perfused capillary network. In addition, paraquat is preferentially accumulated by lung tissue for which it has a particular affinity.

The makers of paraquat, Imperial Chemical Industries, publish a handbook for doctors giving details of the diagnosis and treatment of paraquat poisoning, I.C.I. (1977), which should be available in the intensive therapy unit.

Treatment of paraquat poisoning

Unabsorbed paraquat still present in the gut acts as a reservoir for further absorption. The prime object of treatment is to remove this from the gut. Fuller's Earth and similar fine clays have the ability to absorb paraquat – after washing out the stomach, 1 litre of a 30% suspension of Fuller's Earth Surrey Finest Grade (obtainable in sterilised one-treatment packs from I.C.I. Plant Protection Division, Fernhurst, Haslemere, Surrey) be given orally, followed by a sodium or magnesium sulphate cathartic. Alternatively, the same amount of a 7% Bentonite suspension may be given. A repeat dose of 200–500 ml of Fuller's Earth suspension should be given every two hours for the first 24 h and then every four hours for the second 24 h. Further doses of cathartic should also be given during this period to speed up elimination.

Haemoperfusion through a charcoal column or haemodialysis should be considered.

REFERENCES

Blood Paracetamol Kit, Winthrop Laboratories, Surbiton-upon-Thames, Surrey.

Copland, G. M., Kolin, A. and Shulman, H. S. (1974). Fatal pulmonary intra-alveolar fibrosis after paraquat ingestion. *New Engl. J. Med.* **291**, 290.

Cumming, G., Dukes, D. C. and Widdowson, G. (1964). Alkaline diuresis in treatment of aspirin poisoning. *Brit. Med. J.* **2**, 1033.

Davis, M., Labadarios, D. and Williams, R. S. (1976). Metabolism of paracetamol after therapeutic and toxic doses in man. *J. Int. Med. Res.* **4** (Suppl. 4) 40.

Department of Health and Social Security (1964). Supply of certain prophylactic and therapeutic agents. *H.M.* **71**, 64.

Drug and Therapeutics Bulletin, 1976, Paracetamol overdosage **14** Nos 2, 5–6.

Editorial (1972). Death cap poisoning. *Lancet* **1**, 1320.

Editorial (1976). Paraquat poisoning. *Lancet* **1**, 1057.

Goodman, L. S. and Gilman, A. (1975). 'The Pharmacological Basis of Therapeutics', Fifth Edition. Macmillan Publishing Company Inc.

Imperial Chemical Industries, Plant Protection Division (1977). Treatment of Paraquat Poisoning.

Leitzell, B. J., Barton, L. J., Wilcox, H. G. and Bloomer, H. A. (1971). Comparison of lipid and aqueous dialysis for removing glutethemide from plasma. *Clin. Res.* **19**, 152.

Matthew, H. and Lawson, A. A. (1966). Acute barbiturate poisoning – A review of two years experience. *Quart. J. Med. New Series* **35** (No. 140) 539.

Noble, J. and Matthew, H. (1969). Acute poisoning by tricyclic antidepressants: clinical features and management of 100 patients. *Clinical Toxicology* **2** (4), 403.

North, P. (1967). 'Poisonous Plants and Fungi in Colour'. Blandford Press Ltd.

Penn, R. G. (1976). A theoretical approach to the management of paracetamol overdosage. *J. Int. Med. Res.* **4** (Suppl. 4) 98.

Prescott, L. F., Newton, R. W., Swainson, C. P., Wright, N., Forrest, A. R. W. and Matthew, H. (1974). Successful treatment of severe paracetamol overdosage with cysteamine. *Lancet* **1**, 588.

Prescott, L. F., Park, J. and Proudfoot, A. T. (1976a). Cysteamine, L-methionine and D-penicillamine in paracetamol poisoning. *J. Int. Med. Res.* **4** (Suppl. 4) 112.

Prescott, L. F., Park, J., Sutherland, G. R., Smith, I. J. and Proudfoot, A. T. (1976b). Cysteamine, methionine and penicillamine in the treatment of paracetamol poisoning. *Lancet* **2**, 109.

Skrabal, F. and Dittrich, P. (1973). Death Cap poisoning. *Lancet* **1**, 767.

Schreiner, G. A. and Teehan, B. P. (1972). Dialysis of poisons and drugs. *Am. Soc. Artif. Inter. Org.* **18**, 503.

Smith, S. E. and Rawlins, M. D. (1973). 'Variability in Human Drug Response'. Butterworths.

Vale, J. A., Rees, A. J., Widdop, B. and Goulding, R. (1975). Use of charcoal haemoperfusion in the management of severely poisoned patients. *Brit. Med. J.* **1**, 5.

VII

The Management of Endocrine Emergencies

P. L. WRIGHT

THE THYROID

Hyperthyroidism

Presentation and diagnosis

It is important to note the tendency for thyrotoxicosis to present with severe congestive heart failure or digitalis resistent atrial fibrillation, especially in the elderly. Associated clinical features of thyrotoxicosis may not be present (Table 1). The thyrotoxic patient requiring intensive therapy is either suffering from severe disease, presents with a predominant facet of the disease, or is coincidentally diagnosed as suffering from hyperthyroidism during the treatment of another illness. In the latter case, a persistent tachycardia, a restless sweating patient who may be pyrexial, should make one consider hyperthyroidism since disease of minor degree may increase in severity under conditions of stress.

The diagnosis may be confirmed by estimation of the serum thyroxine (T_4), normal limits being 60–150 mmol/1. Serum T_4 is affected by the level of the thyroid binding protein and when there is doubt about this level, the free thyroxine index should be calculated. On the rare occasions when the clinical features are consistent with thyrotoxicosis and serum T_4 is normal, serum T_3 must be estimated in order to exclude T_3 toxicosis.

Table 1. Clinical features of
thyrotoxicosis

General
Weight loss
Polyphagia
Fatigue and muscular weakness
Intolerance to heat and sweating
Chorea
Anxiety
Fine tremor

Neurological
Proximal muscle wasting and
weakness

Cardiac
Tachycardia
Atrial fibrillation
Congestive cardiac failure

Ophthalmic
Proptosis and staring
Lidlag
Chemosis
External ophthalmoplegia

Thyroid
Goitre ± Bruit

Treatment

In an obvious case of thyrotoxicosis, treatment should not be delayed until biochemical confirmation is obtained – the latter is more necessary when a patient is seen with an anxiety state or obscure symptoms which might be referable to the thyroid gland. Treatment is always in the first place medical. In less severe cases (rarely seen in the intensive therapy unit) treatment is initially with carbimazole 60 mg or propylthiouracil 300 mg in divided doses thrice daily.

Acute severe hyperthyroidism (thyroid crisis) is rare and may be precipitated by some other form of stress or follow thyroidectomy on an inadequately prepared patient. Treatment in such cases can be directed towards control of body temperature, reduction of oxygen demands, correction of salt and water depletion and treatment of any cardiac dysrhythmia or failure that may be present.

Body temperature control. These patients commonly have a high core temperature which may, if uncontrolled, lead to death. The core temperature should be lowered to 39°C by the methods described in Part 1, ch. VI, p. 147. The patient should be cooled on a cold water blanket, ice-cold water be dripped into the stomach via a Ryles tube, intravenous fluids should be cooled by placing the blood warming coil in iced water and sheets soaked in methylated spirits may be placed on the patient and the patient fanned. Core temperature monitoring is essential and active cooling (other than leaving the patient on a cooling blanket) should be stopped once the core temperature is 39°C or less.

Reduction of oxygen demands. Because of the greatly increased catabolism, hyperpyrexia, a high $PaCO_2$ and a lactic acidosis is common. A hyperventilating, hyperdynamic sweating patient with a PaO_2 of 8.7 kPa (65 mm Hg) or less is an indication for mechanical ventilation. Prior to intubation the tachycardia should be controlled with propranolol 5–15 mg titrated intravenously, and once intubated, muscle activity should be suppressed with a muscle relaxant such as pancuronium. The onset of congestive cardiac failure invariably necessitates ventilation since the increased oxygen demands following the increased work of breathing together with the decreased oxygen transfer capacity, leads to dangerous hypoxia.

Correction of salt and water depletion. Severe water depletion is common and may be complicated by sodium loss from vomiting – a right atrial pressure line is essential in order to assess the dynamic circulating blood volume. Fluid and metabolic balance should be restored according to the advice given in Part 1, ch. VII.

Treatment of cardiac complications. A rapid supraventricular tachycardia if not controlled will inevitably lead to congestive cardiac failure. The drug of preference in order to control the tachycardia is propranolol 5–15 mg titrated intravenously followed by a continuous infusion of 5–15 mg 4 hourly. Rapid atrial fibrillation is an indication for digitalisation and pulmonary oedema should be treated with thiazide diuretics. Should the patient have severe bronchospasm – propranolol is contra-indicated, a small dose of oxprenolol should be titrated slowly intravenously – and should the airway pressure not increase, be continued as a continuous intravenous infusion.

Anti-thyroid drugs in severe hyperthyroidism. Anti-thyroid drugs in large doses should be given orally, or crushed and put down the Ryles tube. Prophylthiouracil is preferred in this situation since it has an additional extrathyroidal action of reducing conversion of thyroxine to the metabolically more active triiodothyronine. Thyroid secretion is more rapidly suppressed by giving oral potassium iodide (60 mg daily in divided doses). Should the iodide not be absorbed orally, sodium iodide may be given intravenously.

By these measures the severe hyperthyroid state can generally be sufficiently well controlled to wean the patient off the ventilator within one week of onset. The mortality in a thyrotoxic crisis is high especially in the elderly where death from myocardial failure is common. Infection frequently complicates severe hyperthyroidism and should be treated appropriately.

Further discussion of the management of thyrotoxicosis is beyond the scope of this chapter – *viz.* – continued medical treatment, surgery or radiotherapy.

Complications following thyroidectomy for hyperthyroidism
Post-operatively important immediate complications may ensue, specific to thyroid surgery. These are: haemorrhage at the operative site, thyroid crisis and hypocalaemic tetany.

Haemorrhage. The thyroid is an extremely vascular gland and there is always a risk of bleeding especially after sub-total thyroidectomy. It is more likely after a difficult operation and is less frequent with increasing surgical experience. The result of haemorrhage is dramatic, in that the haematoma compresses the trachea and causes asphyxia. When it happens it usually occurs shortly after the operation is finished and realisation of the cause of sudden cyanosis may be difficult with a bulky dressing in place. For this reason only an experienced person should be permitted to observe or escort these patients back to the ward. Careful observation of the patient for the 24 h postoperatively is essential in order to detect early haemorrhage around the operation site. On observing severe respiratory difficulty or cyanosis, the nurse should immediately take down the dressing and open the wound herself to allow decompression. Fortunately this is not often necessary but it can be life saving.

Thyroid crisis. The management of thyroid crisis has already been discussed (p. 682).

Hypocalcaemic tetany. This results from the removal of or damage to the parathyroid glands. Its treatment is referred to in Part 1, ch. VII, p. 191.

Hypothyroidism

Presentation and diagnosis

Hypothyroidism is likely to be encountered in the intensive therapy unit causing in the main two problems, hypothermic coma and cardiac tamponade. The physical appearances of hypothyroidism are characteristic but may mimic hypothermic coma.

Table 2. Physical appearance of hypothyroidism

Puffy pale facies
Low skin and core temperature
Ice cold extremities
Extreme bradycardia
Reptilian reflexes
Absence of shivering
J-waves on electrocardiogram

A history of previous thyroid treatment or a family history of thyroid disease is useful in suspecting the diagnosis. Tests of thyroid function may not be available for a week or more so that treatment of the severe hypothermia should include thyroxine or triiodothyronine when hypothyroidism is suspected. The most useful confirmatory laboratory investigations are the serum cholesterol and the level of thyroid stimulating hormone.

Treatment

Treatment of severe hypothyroidism should be directed towards restoration of normal body temperature, control of respiration and maintenance of blood gases, control of electrolyte and fluid balance and correction of hypoglycaemia, treatment of any cardiac complication, hormone replacement therapy and treatment of any underlying infection. The mortality from myxoedema coma is high and the basis of treatment is gradual correction to normality. A high percentage of these patients sustain irreversible residual cerebral damage, or die during treatment or some weeks later from refractory congestive cardiac failure, intercurrent infection or cerebral haemorrhage.

Restoration of normal body temperature

Temperature should be restored to normal by slow rewarming (p. 133). Rewarming by simple insulation is generally adequate. The clinical management of the hypothermic hypothyroid patient should be conducted on similar lines to that of pure hypothermia; Part 1, ch. VI, p. 133.

Control of respiration and maintenance of blood gases
Caution should be exercised in interpreting blood samples and arterial sampling is essential even for electrolyte analysis. Corrections must be made for pH, $PaCO_2$ in relation to body temperature (Part 1, ch. VI, p. 134, Fig. 1).

Ventilatory failure associated with hypercapnoea is common and frequently necessitates mechanical ventilation. Ventilation should not be started before inserting a right atrial pressure line and measuring right atrial pressure. A high right atrial pressure with no respiratory swing in the presence of a low pulse volume, would suggest cardiac tamponade; on rare occasions careful fluid replacement is necessary in order to restore circulating blood volume. Ventilation has to be adjusted in order to maintain cardiac output at the optimum. Gross pulmonary oedema associated with hypoxia and commonly hypercapnoea is also an indication for mechanical ventilation. Sedation during ventilation should be kept to the minimum. A tracheostomy is frequently indicated since weaning from the ventilator may take many weeks. Tracheostomy should not be considered for at least a week after commencing treatment since the extra stress may precipitate a myocardial infarction.

Control of electrolyte and fluid balance and correction of hypoglycaemia
Fluid balance should be regulated according to the right atrial pressure – water overload is common, but once thyroid replacement therapy is started, a water diuresis generally occurs which may be complicated by hypokalaemia. An indwelling urinary catheter is essential in order to monitor urine output and electrolyte content.

Hypoglycaemia or hyperglycaemia may occur – the blood glucose should be maintained between 6 and 9 mmol/l by careful glucose monitoring and an appropriate dextrose regime with or without added insulin. These patients are frequently very sensitive to insulin which must be introduced in low dosage – e.g. 16 units intravenously as a start dose followed by 4 units intravenously hourly for the treatment of hyperglycaemia. Dextrose and insulin (if necessary) is the most appropriate source of calories, since the regime is known to produce a sodium diuresis and also may have a myocardial inotropic effect.

Treatment of cardiac complications

An extreme bradycardia is frequently present and provided peripheral perfusion, urine output and blood gases are adequate, should not be treated. On occasions cardiac output is totally inadequate, urine output very poor and there develops an increasing lactic acidosis. Under such circumstances isoprenaline should be titrated intravenously in a dosage sufficient to restore the blood pressure systolic to 60 mm Hg or more and a urine output of 40 ml/h or more. The drug must be used with extreme caution since it may precipitate a cardiac dysrhythmia or a myocardial infarction if the dose is too high.

An inotropic agent must not be used if cardiac tamponade is suspected. The diagnosis and management of cardiac tamponade is described in Part 1, ch. III. The signs of tamponade may be due to a tense pericardial effusion but may also be due to an accumulation of pseudomucinous fluid in the myocardium thus reducing its contractility as in an infiltrative cardiomyopathy. Diagnosis depends firstly on the recognition of the physical signs which are very easy to miss and secondly on the chest X-ray which may show a marked increase in the transverse cardiac diameter. On rare occasions pericardiocentesis is necessary.

Thiazide diuretics may be indicated for the treatment of gross pulmonary oedema – but must be used with caution since hypokalaemia is common.

Hormone replacement therapy

Thyroid hormone should be given very gradually and in a ventilated patient should be given intravenously since oral absorption is unpredictable. Serum T_3 should be given initially as 5 μg intravenously twice daily for 3 days gradually increasing over the subsequent week to 40 μg daily. Oral therapy with L-thyroxine should be started as soon as possible as 0.025 mg daily increasing to 0.05 mg daily after the first week. Intravenous T_3 should be discontinued once oral absorption is assured. The dose of T_3 or thyroxine should not be increased if there is E.C.G. evidence of increasing myocardial ischaemia.

Treatment of infection

These patients may be admitted with infection (in particular bronchopneumonia) and are very susceptible to superinfection during treatment. Creatinine clearance levels are often low at the onset of patient management and therefore nephrotoxic antibiotics must be used with care – antibiotic blood levels being estimated whenever necessary.

THE ADRENAL GLANDS

Cushing's syndrome

The general features of Cushing's syndrome are well-known and will not be discussed. It is important to recognise however that severe biochemical disturbances of Cushing's syndrome may present to an intensive therapy unit, *viz.* hypernatraemia and hypokalaemia, occasionally resulting in paralysis without loss of consciousness. Normally in Cushing's syndrome, whether due to adrenal hyperplasia or adenoma formation the potassium level is rarely less than 3 mmol/l. When the fall in potassium is profound, to 2 mmol/l or less, the cause is likely to be an adrenal carcinoma or an ectopic A.C.T.H. producing tumour – usually an oat cell carcinoma of the lung. Both are associated with very high plasma cortisol levels. Patients with ectopic A.C.T.H. production are often pigmented and suffer severe psychiatric complications. Suicidal attempts are common. Chest radiograph, sputum examination for malignant cells, and even bronchoscopy are often negative until a late stage. Treatment of patients with ectopic A.C.T.H. producing tumours is unfortunately rarely curative because of the nature of the primary tumour. The severity oi the hypercorticism may be reduced with metapyrone up to 750 mg/day with aminoglutethemide 250 mg 4 times daily. Such patients may suffer an acute Addisonian crisis which may be prevented by giving the patient maintenance therapy with cortisone 25 mg twice daily.

Operative steroid management of Cushing's syndrome
When surgery is planned for the treatment of ordinary Cushing's syndrome, it is necessary to remember that the patient has become tolerant to high levels of plasma cortisol. In order therefore to prevent a hypoadrenal crisis it is necessary to plan the supplemental steroid therapy given at the time of surgery. A suitable regime is given (Table 3). It should be modified in the light of the actual plasma cortisol levels and urinary outputs measured for the individual patient. Little harm will be done if an excess is given; it can always be tapered off. An adrenal crisis however is a very serious postoperative complication with a substantial mortality.

Occasionally it may be many weeks before the residual suppressed adrenal tissue becomes active. It is an error to stimulate this with ACTH for this does nothing to increase the activity of the suppressed hypothalamic/pituitary axis. Occasionally it may be necessary to continue treatment with exogenous steroids indefinitely, e.g. for an

Table 3. Operative steroid management of Cushing's syndrome

Pre-operative day	100 mg cortisone acetate i.m.
Operative day	6.00 a.m. – 100 mg cortisone acetate i.m. pre-med. – 100 mg hydrocortisone semi-succinate i.v. + 100 mg cortisone acetate i.m.
During operation	Continuous infusion of hydrocortisone 100 mg in 500 ml N saline repeated after 2 h.
Immediate post-operation	100 mg hydrocortisone by continuous infusion 6 hourly for rest of that 24 hour period. 8.00 p.m. – cortisone 100 mg i.m.
Postoperative 1st day	Cortisone 100 mg i.m. thrice daily. Hydrocortisone 150 mg in 500 ml n saline by continuous infusion during 24 h.
Postoperative 2nd day	Cortisone 100 mg i.m. thrice daily.
Postoperative 3rd day	Cortisone 75 mg i.m. thrice daily.
Postoperative 4th day	Cortisone 75 mg i.m. or oral thrice daily and then slow reduction over two weeks to nil if possible.

average patient, cortisone 37.5 mg daily with fludrohydrocortisone 0.1 mg daily.

Addison's disease

Presentation

Hypoadrenalism may present in a variety of ways: with sudden prostration and circulatory collapse, asthenia, weakness, pigmentation, general inanition, diarrhoea, etc. Now that tuberculosis is less commonly seen in the United Kingdom, it will often be the result of adrenal atrophy, possibly associated with other deficiencies, e.g. hypothyroidism, idiopathic thrombocytopenia and hypoparathyroidism. It may also be the result of surgical removal of tissue in the treatment of Cushing's or Conn's syndrome or be due to infiltration of the gland by sarcoid or amyloid. Carcinomatous infiltration though common, rarely gives rise to hypoadrenalism.

Clinical features of hypoadrenalism include: brown pigmentation of mucous membranes, diffuse brown pigmentation of skin, especially wound scars, skin creases and pressure points, muscular weakness, hyporeflexia, hypotension and marked postural hypotension.

Metabolic changes include: sodium depletion and dehydration, a low plasma sodium and chloride, a high plasma potassium and hypoglycaemia.

Hypotension and marked postural hypotension are the most reliable signs in the author's experience. Hypoadrenalism is unlikely if the blood pressure exceeds 100 mm Hg and a fall of > 20 mm Hg is likely on standing.

Diagnosis may be confirmed by measurement of the plasma cortisol level and failure of response to A.C.T.H., but in a critical situation results of these tests should not be awaited.

A low plasma sodium has little discriminating value in critically ill patients but a raised potassium and blood urea level (in the absence of renal failure) and frequently hypoglycaemia and hypercalcaemia are all suggestive findings.

Treatment

Before starting treatment a precipitating factor must be looked for, blood cultures should be taken routinely. Treatment consists of restoration of blood volume, correction of the metabolic deficits, hormonal replacement therapy and treatment of any precipitating factor such as sepsis or a haemorrhagic diathesis (e.g. following anti-coagulant therapy).

Restoration of blood volume and correction of metabolic imbalance

Restoration of blood volume should be done under right atrial pressure monitoring control since it is easy to swing from hypovolaemia to fluid overload. Fluid should be initially replaced with N saline changing to dextrose saline once the right atrial pressure has been restored to normal. The serum potassium rarely requires specific treatment returning to normal with volume and hormonal replacement. Urine output should be observed carefully since, following a period of severe hypotension, there may ensue an oliguric phase or a period of acute intrinsic renal failure.

Hypoglycaemia may be initially corrected by intravenous dextrose at a rate of 40 g/h for the first 2 h and subsequently titrated intravenously according to the blood glucose. The blood glucose generally returns to normal following cortisol therapy. Some of these patients have associated diabetes mellitus, serial blood glucose levels are therefore important and insulin (in low dosage) given if necessary. These patients are very sensitive to insulin and excess dosage may lead to fatal hypoglycaemia.

Hormonal replacement therapy

Cortisol should be initially given as 100 mg intravenously 4 hourly slowly reducing over the subsequent 3 days. Salt retaining steroid in the form of oral 9-α-fluorohydrocortisone or intramuscular aldosterone is generally required once the dosage of cortisol has been reduced to 50 mg 8 hourly or less.

Treatment of any precipitating factor
Intercurrent infection must be excluded and any haemorrhagic diathesis corrected.

Finally after investigation and treatment of the primary disorder, if possible the patient should be stabilised on the minimum possible replacement dose of steroids which is usually 25–37.5 mg of cortisone with 0.1 mg fludrohydrocortisone daily. The patient should be warned that in the event of illness or injury, the cortisone should be increased pending medical advice, which should be sought rapidly in the event of vomiting.

PHAEOCHROMOCYTOMA

Presentation and diagnosis
Phaeochromocytoma is occasionally discovered to be the cause of sustained hypertension as a result of routine investigation. More frequently it will be suspected as the possible cause of paroxysmal attacks which may be of considerable variety. The patient may complain of episodic but transient intense headaches at the vertex, syncopal attacks, palpitation, sweating, flushing, central chest pain, blanching of the extremities, abdominal pain and diarrhoea. Paroxysmal hypertension may be recorded intermittently only and high blood pressure readings taken by a junior nurse in casualty on admission may occasionally be the only clue to the diagnosis as in one of the author's personal cases; the patient being found to be in acute pulmonary oedema and treated appropriately, hypertension not being recorded again during the first admission. The history in patients with paroxysmal attacks may include a number of the symptoms listed above. Not surprisingly a number of such patients have been classified as neurotic.

Phaeochromocytomata are seen more frequently in association with other disorders, some familial, of tissue derived from the neural crest. These include:

Neurofibromata
Café au lait pigmentation
Meningiomata
Medullary carcinoma of the thyroid
Hyperparathyroidism

Carcinoid tumour
Multiple phaeochromocytoma

Phaeochromocytomata are usually benign in the strict neoplastic sense (90%) but represent an extremely hazardous condition. In the untreated patient sudden death may occur at any time from heart failure, ventricular fibrillation or stroke. Death may occur as a result of examination of the patient, especially from deep palpation of the kidneys to cause a pressor response, venepuncture, intravenous pyelography, angiography and especially from presacral air insufflation. It is therefore of considerable importance to establish an early diagnosis and if on clinical grounds the condition seems likely, to admit the patient to an intensive therapy unit for full α- and β-blockade while investigations are being performed.

Obsolete and dangerous investigations include the pressor response to abdominal palpation and the pressor tyramine or histamine provocation tests. All are safe in the absence of the disease but potentially fatal if positive. Details of their performance will not be given. The intravenous phentolamine test is still too widely used (Belchetz, 1976). The principle looked for is a fall in diastolic blood pressure greater than 20 mm Hg but false positives are frequent and sudden complete adrenergic blockade may cause acute hypovolaemic shock due to loss of fluid through a hypoxic post-arteriolar capillary bed.

Definite diagnosis is usually made by the assay of breakdown products of adrenaline and noradrenaline in the urine. Substances commonly measured include 4-hydroxy-3-methoxymandelic acid (V.M.A.) the normal range being up to 9 mg/24 h. False positives may be obtained in patients eating vanilla as in ice cream or bananas. The metabolites metadrenaline and normetadrenaline may be measured, 24 h outputs in the urine being less than 1.3 mg. (Direct measurement of plasma adrenaline and noradrenaline is difficult and rarely useful outside a research centre.) Urine is collected in 24-h aliquots into a plastic container with 15 ml 6 N hydrochloric acid to maintain the pH below 3. Drugs should not be given during collections if possible; monamine oxidase inhibitors and catecholamine releasing drugs may give false positive reactions; though theoretically methyldopa may interfere by causing the formation of methylnoradrenaline etc. it does not seem to invalidate the assay either of normetadrenaline or V.M.A.

Occasionally it may not be possible to prove the diagnosis from a study of 24-hour specimens; it may be useful to collect smaller aliquots of urine from 4–6 h after a paroxysm of hypertension.

Treatment

Pre-operative preparation. On making the diagnosis, treatment should be immediately begun with partial α- and β-blockade. These are best started together, for full α-blockade may cause hypovolaemic shock and full β-blockade may provoke paroxysmal hypertension. Treatment is best started with oral phenoxybenzamine 10 mg thrice daily and oral propranolol 10 mg thrice daily titrating the doses in order to provide control of both tachycardia and hypertension. Paroxysms of hypertension despite the above may be most rapidly controlled with intravenous phentolamine mesylate 10 mg by rapid injection.

Patients with extreme blood pressure swings should have the blood pressure monitored at regular intervals by the Doppler technique (Part 2, ch. II, p. 305) and the right atrial pressure recorded in order to ensure an adequate circulating blood volume. Some patients with phaeochromocytoma are known to have a low circulating blood volume from prolonged excessive secretion of vasoconstrictor substances (Brock, 1975). In such patients shock may be precipitated with the use of peripheral vasodilators unless circulating blood volume is restored simultaneously.

Once blockade has been established, the right atrial line may be removed and the patient may then safely be investigated by intravenous pyelography selective arteriography and/or presacral carbon dioxide insufflation. It is important to try to establish the site of a phaeochromocytoma as excessive handling of tissues during a prolonged search for the tumour at operation may provoke paroxysms of hypertension despite adequate blockade. The tumours are usually found in the adrenal glands but 10–30% are extra-adrenal and may be found in the para-aortic region down to the bladder base.

Management of the patient immediately pre-operatively and during surgery

Pre-operative preparation. A right atrial pressure line must be inserted and an adequate circulating blood volume ensured. Continuous monitoring of the arterial pressure during operation is essential (see p. 304) since paroxysmal episodes of hypertension may occur despite blockade. These are particularly likely to occur during intubation and during handling of the tumour. Because of these pressure swings, a physician should be present who in co-operation with the anaesthetist, is responsible for blood volume control and drug administration. Hypovolaemia may complicate haemorrhage or follow clamping of the adrenal veins and removal of the tumour. A sudden fall in blood pressure should not follow catecholamine depletion providing the vascular compartment is full (Ross, 1967). Two peripheral infusion lines should be set up, the right atrial line being used for monitoring purposes only and (provided the solution is warmed) for volume replacement.

One infusion line should contain a Y connection for infusion of phentolamine or noradrenaline. The phentolamine should be prepared in a concentration of 1 mg/ml of N saline and be infused via a 100 ml burette. Noradrenaline should be prepared in a concentration 8 mg/500 ml N saline and infused via a 100 ml burette. The other infusion should be similarly prepared with isoprenaline 4 mg in 500 ml N saline and propranolol 0.08 mg/ml in N saline (see Table 1). A cardiac monitor and defibrillating apparatus are essential.

Preparation for theatres therefore includes the continuation of full blockade. Premedication with hyoscine 0.4 mg or papaveretum 20 mg will not cause release of excess catecholamine. If the blood pressure is above 160/100, phenoxybenzamine is given 50 mg intravenously. Induction will usually be with thiopentone which does not cause catecholamine release though this may produce some hypotension from myocardial depression. This however is transient. Great care is necessary to avoid a profound fall which may occur with as little as 125 mg of thiopentone. Halothane as an anaesthetic gas appears to be safe.

Intra-operative and postoperative management (see Table 4). During the operation as noted the plasma volume must be maintained by transfusion in order to maintain the right atrial pressure (R.A.P.) level. Phentolamine should be infused according to the observed blood pressure responses and propranolol also infused according to the heart rate.

Paroxysmal rises in blood pressure should be treated with bolus IV injections of phentolamine 2.5–5 mg and paroxysmal rises in heart rate with an injection of propranolol 5–10 mg given over a period of 3–5 min.

As mentioned above if the circulatory plasma volume is maintained, hypotension is not to be expected after removal of the tumour and will normally respond to blood transfusion. Noradrenaline infusion has not in my experience been required. Treatment with α- and β-blocking drugs is discontinued pre-operatively. The patient should be returned to the intensive therapy unit for post-operative monitoring. Blood pressure monitoring can be changed to the Doppler technique (Part 2, ch. II, p. 305). Hypotension is generally related to hypovolaemia; cardiac dysrhythmias may arise over the subsequent 24 h requiring appropriate therapy. Continuation of paroxysms of hypertension or tachycardia obviously lead to suspicion of the tumour being multiple.

Table 4. Pre-operative and intra-operative management of a patient with phaeochromocytoma

Observations
Continuous intra-arterial blood pressure. Continuous E.C.G. recording and pulse rate. Right atrial pressure (R.A.P.) monitoring. Skin/core temperature differential. Urine output/hour

BLOOD PRESSURE
Hypertension
Blood pressure > 100 D.P. preoperatively give phenoxybenzamine 50 mg i.v. (observe
 R.A.P. fluid top-up may be necessary).
B.P. > 110 D.P. on induction or during operation, phentolamine mesylate 2.5–5.0 mg
 as a bolus. Lasts 5–10 min and then if B.P. starts to rise, commence continuous
 infusion 0.5–2.0 mg/min (phentolamine 1 mg/ml N saline infused via a 100 ml
 burette).

Hypotension
Generally associated with a low R.A.P. – restore circulating volume.
Occasionally R.A.P. high normal, skin temperature normal. Then use noradrenaline
 (8 mg/500 ml N saline and infused via 100 ml burette) as a continuous infusion
 0.002–0.004 mg/min. R.A.P. high normal, skin temperature low, use isoprenaline
 (4 mg/500 ml N saline) as a continuous infusion 0.001–0.004 mg/min.

Supraventricular tachycardia
Propranolol 1–5 mg intravenously titrated under E.C.G. monitoring control over
 3 min.
Should tachycardia persist give 8 mg of propranolol as a continuous infusion at a rate of
 80 mg/4 h.

Ventricular extrasystoles
Lignocaine hydrochloride given as a bolus 60–120 mg intravenously.

REFERENCES

Belchetz, P. E. (1976). Management of acute endocrine emergencies. *Update* **2**, 371.
Brock, Lord (1975). Hypovolaemia and phaeochromocytoma. *Ann. roy. Coll. Surg. Engl.*
 56, 218.
Ross, E. J., Prichard, B. N. C., Kaufman, L., Robertson, A. I. G. and Harries, B. J.
 (1967). Preoperative and operative management of patients with phaeochromocytoma. *Brit. Med. J.* **1**, 191.

VIII

The Management of Haematological Problems Related to Intensive Therapy

P. JONES

The particular aspects of haematology discussed in this chapter concern three topics that frequently arise in the care of the critically ill – haemolysis, haemostasis and blood component transfusion. When assessing a patient's haematological status it should be remembered that history, clinical signs and laboratory features are dependent on the demand, supply, destruction and removal of blood components, and that bone marrow, lymph nodes, bowel, liver, spleen and kidney are all partners in the dynamic picture apparent in health or disease.

HAEMOLYSIS

Haemolysis, the premature destruction of erythrocytes, may result from a primary defect of the red cell or from the secondary action of an extrinsic agent.

Primary red cell defects

These may be hereditary or acquired. Among the former are hereditary spherocytosis, inherited enzymopathies, haemoglobinopathies, and thalassaemia. Acquired defects include those in which alterations in plasma lipids affect the shape of red cells (severe hepatocellular disease and alcoholic cirrhosis) (Zieve, 1958; Dacie, 1967a, b).

647

Table 1. Drugs contra-indicated in G-6-PD deficient patients. (Adapted from Table II.' Grimes and de Gruchy, 1974)

Aminoquinolines	*Sulphonamides*	*Miscellaneous*
Chloroquine	Co-trimoxazole	Acetylphenylhydrazine
Mepacrine	Sulphonamide	Ascorbic acid (massive dosage)
Primaquine	Sulphacetamide	Dimercaprol (BAL)
Pamaquine	Sulphafurazole	Methylene blue
	Sulphamethoxy-	Para-aminosalicylic acid
Analgesics	pyridazine	Phenylhydrazine
Acetylsalicylic acid	Sulphisoxazole	Probenecid
Acetophenacetin		Vitamin K water soluble analogue
Acetanilide	*Sulphones*	Chloramphenicol ⎫
	Dapsone	Quinidine ⎬ Not in negroes
Nitrofurans	Sulphoxone	Quinine ⎭
Furazolidone	Thiazosulphone	
Nitrofurantoin		
Nitrofurazone		

Recognition of the *enzymopathies* is important because of the contra-indication to certain drugs. The commonest of these disorders is glucose-6-phosphate dehydrogenase (G-6-PD) deficiency, present in an estimated 100 million people (Carson and Frischer, 1966). Variants of G-6-PD deficiency are found principally in Mediterranean, Negro and Oriental races, the defect being X-linked with intermediate dominance. Haemolysis results from exposure to infection and to oxidant drugs (Fraser and Vessell, 1968) (Table 1) which cause glutathione depletion with denaturation of haemoglobin in old red cells, resulting in Heinz body formation. In the Mediterranean variant acute haemolysis which may be life threatening and necessitates exchange transfusion may follow exposure to fava or broad beans (favism). Apart from the avoidance of oxidant drugs and the prompt treatment of infections, treatment consists of transfusion after haemolytic episodes (Grimes and de Gruchy, 1974).

The *haemoglobinopathies* include a wide range of disorders character-ised by the presence of structurally abnormal haemoglobins. Among these sickle cell disease and sickle cell trait are of particular importance in the critical care situation because of the need to avoid hypoxia, hypotension, acidosis and dehydration. In the homozygote severe haemolytic and embolic disease, and painful crises due to infarction, are precipitated by these variables, and by infection and cold (Serjeant, 1974). Crises are unusual in the heterozygote with sickle cell trait but do occur (Huehns, 1974), and it is therefore wise to screen all patients with

Negroid ancestry for haemoglobin S prior to anaesthesia, in pregnancy, or in states predisposing to general or localised anoxia.

Management of sickle cell disease consists of the prompt treatment of infections, the avoidance of the variables mentioned above, and transfusion with normal red cells in the event of crises. Partial exchange transfusion may be indicated prior to major surgery in the homozygote, and is of especial importance before by-pass surgery for heart valve replacement, and when crises occur in pregnancy (Huehns, 1974). Tourniquets should be used with caution.

Indiscriminate transfusion and treatment with iron preparations should be avoided in sickle cell disease, and the thalassaemias, because of the dangers of haemosiderosis.

Apart from transfusion, and the use of iron chelating agents, there is no specific treatment in the thalassaemias, which are inherited disorders of haemoglobin synthesis. Mixed syndromes, in which a structural defect is combined with thalassaemia, are not uncommon.

Secondary defects

The broad classification here is of immune and non-immune haemolytic anaemias (Delamore, 1976).

(*a*) The immune haemolytic anaemias are characterised by a positive antiglobin (Coombs') test. Haemolytic anaemia with warm auto-antibodies is associated with hepatic and collagen disorders, and that with cold auto-antibodies with infections, classically atypical pneumonia. Both types are found in lymphoma. Drug causes are listed in Table 2.

Table 2. Drugs and chemicals that may cause haemolysis

Arsine	Melphalan	Quinidine
Cephaloridine	Methyldopa	Quinine
Chlorpromazine	Nitrobenzene	Rifampicin
Hydantoins	Para-amino salicylic	Salazopyrin
Insulin	acid	Sodium chlorate
Isoniazid	Paracetamol	Sulphonamides
Lead	Penicillin	Sulphones
Levodopa	Phenacetin	Sulphonureas
Mefenamic	Phenothiazine	Vitamin K water soluble
acid	Potassium	analogues

(*b*) The non-immune haemolytic anaemias are associated with infection, the mechanical destruction of red cells ('cardiac haemolysis') (Marsh and Lewis, 1969), micro-angiopathic haemolysis (Brain *et al.*, 1962), and certain drugs and chemicals (see Table 2).

The clinical signs of haemolytic anaemia depend on the rate of haemolysis, the capability of bone marrow to compensate for cellular loss, the binding capacity of plasma haptoglobins, and hepatic and renal function. Suspicion of a haemolytic process should be aroused whenever a falling haemoglobin level cannot be explained by bleeding. (See also Part 3, ch. I, p. 811.)

Management of haemolytic anaemia rests on the treatment of identified underlying disorders and the avoidance of known predisposing agents. Steroid therapy is indicated in the immune diseases, and blood transfusion may of course be necessary in severe haemolysis. *Folate deficiency*, which may accompany any chronic haemolytic state, should be treated.

HAEMOSTASIS

Normal haemostasis depends on the intimate interaction of at least three mechanisms – contraction of blood vessels and consequent alteration in blood flow, aggregation of platelets, and formation of fibrin polymer as the end-point of the coagulation cascade.

A classification of the causes of disordered haemostasis is shown in Table 3. In practice, although localised haemorrhage strongly suggests

Table 3. Causes of disordered haemostasis

Localised bleeding
Medical cause
    (i.e. nasal polyp, peptic ulcer, Meckel's diverticulum, glomerulonephritis etc.)

Surgical cause
    (i.e. unsecured haemostasis at operation, wound infection etc.)

Systemic bleeding
Thrombocytopenia
Qualitative platelet defect
Anti-coagulant effect
Vitamin K deficiency
Hepatic failure
Disseminated intravascular coagulation
'Haemophilic' disorder

Table 4. Haemostatic enquiry

Present or past history or physical signs of:
Bruising
Telangiectasia
Purpura
Haemarthrosis or arthropathy
Epistaxes
Gastro-intestinal bleeding
Haematuria
Menorrhagia
Response to injury: prolonged or secondary haemorrhage following lacerations, intra-
    muscular injections, dental extractions, operations, childbirth
Blood product transfusion
Drug ingestion, especially aspirin and anticoagulants
Family history of bleeding
Evidence of other disease, especially hepatic dysfunction

---

either a medical or surgical cause, and systemic bleeding a breakdown in either platelet or coagulation function, unexplained haemorrhage from any site warrants laboratory investigation. The tests chosen for laboratory diagnosis depend on information from the history and physical signs, and assessment of these should always be the first step in a 'haemostatic screen' (Table 4).

Whenever unexpected bleeding occurs laboratory help should be sought early, and certainly before replacement therapy or drugs are given. Blood for haemostatic studies should, if possible, always be obtained by 'clean' venepuncture.

Separate aliquots are required for blood and platelet counts, coagulation studies, and fibrin degradation product estimation. All samples should be sent directly to the laboratory. Artefacts may be introduced by:

1. Collection from indwelling catheters (platelet aggregation at catheter tip may give low count in sample).
2. Slow or difficult withdrawal of sample with haemolysis.
3. Multiple attempts at one site (admixture of sample with tissue fluid will trigger coagulation).
4. Contamination with heparin or dextran.
5. Inaccurate dilution with the 3.8 sodium citrate required for coagulation studies (dilution factor is 9 parts blood: 1 part citrate; i.e. 4.5 ml blood to 0.5 ml citrate, or equivalent).

Thrombocytopenia and qualitative platelet defects

A simplified classification of the causes of thrombocytopenia and platelet

Table 5. Some causes of thrombocytopenia and platelet dysfunction

---

Thrombocytopenia
1. Failure in platelet supply—
   Marrow aplasia
   Acute marrow failure (viral infection especially in childhood, aplastic crises in
      chronic haemolytic anaemias)
   Marrow infiltration (leukaemia, carcinomatosis, myelofibrosis etc.)
   Defective maturation (vitamin B_{12} or folate deficiency)

2. Premature destruction—
   Idiopathic (auto-immune) thrombocytopenic purpura
   Drug sensitivity
   Infections (viral, especially in childhood)
   Disseminated lupus erythematosus
   Disseminated intravascular coagulation
   'Hypersplenism'
   Massive blood transfusion

Platelet dysfunction
Uraemia
Drug induced—aspirin, phenylbutazone, oxyphenbutazone, indomethacin and
   sulphinpyrazone
von Willebrand's disease
Thrombasthenia
Thrombocythaemia in myeloproliferative disease

---

dysfunction is shown in Table 5. Those that should be particularly borne in mind in the critically ill patient are thrombocytopenia secondary to massive blood transfusion, infection, disseminated intravascular coagulation (D.I.C.), and drugs.

The list of drugs implicated as causes of thrombocytopenia continues to grow. It is clearly impossible either to remember them all, or to identify easily a culprit when multiple drug therapy is employed. Those most commonly reported in the United Kingdom are: ampicillin, aspirin, co-trimoxazole, frusemide, indomethacin, oxyphenbutazone, paracetamol and phenylbutazone (Girdwood, 1976). It is sometimes forgotten that drugs used for the treatment of malignant disease will also cause marrow depression and thrombocytopenia. Rarely, transient thrombocytopenia occurs seven days after a blood transfusion, platelet antibodies destroying transfused incompatible platelets (Morrison and Mollison, 1966).

Management depends on the underlying cause. The patient's present and immediate past therapy should be reviewed. Steroid therapy is

COAGULATION

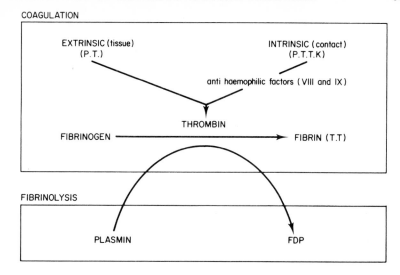

Fig. 1. The diagram shows, in a very simplified form, the relationship between coagulation and fibrinolysis. The two coagulation pathways, *extrinsic* triggered by admixture of blood and tissue enzymes and *intrinsic* triggered by contact between blood and foreign surfaces, activate prothrombin to the enzyme *thrombin*. Thrombin cleaves the fibrinogen molecule to form *fibrin*. The fibrinolytic enzyme *plasmin* breaks down fibrin to form *fibrin degradation products*.

Platelets and ionised calcium are required at several stages of coagulation.

A simple clotting screen includes the P.T., which measures the extrinsic and final common pathway, the P.T.T.K., which measures the intrinsic (including factor VIII and IX) and final common pathway, and the T.T. which measures the conversion of fibrinogen to fibrin. The level of F.D.P. may be assessed rapidly using a latex slide test.

P.T., prothrombin time; P.T.T.K., partial thromboplastin time with kaolin; T.T., thrombin time; F.D.P., Fibrin degradation products.

sometimes indicated in thrombocytopenic purpura due to an immunological mechanism. Platelet transfusion is rarely indicated, severe spontaneous haemorrhage being unlikely with platelet counts of over 40 000/mm³. Platelet transfusion will boost immunity in cases of immune thrombocytopenia, but the results of transfusion are disappointing because of shortened platelet survival time.

Coagulation

Coagulation depends on the presence within the circulation of adequate levels of functionally normal platelets and coagulation *factors*. There are 12 recognised coagulation factors (Table 6), and two coagulation pathways – extrinsic and intrinsic (Fig. 1).

The majority of clotting factors are proteins manufactured in the

Table 6. The coagulation factors

Factor I	Fibrinogen	Factor VIII	Anti-haemophilic factor (A.H.F.), Anti-haemophilic globulin (A.H.G.)
Factor II[1]	Prothrombin		
Factor III	Tissue factor	Factor IX[1]	Christmas factor
Factor IV	Ca^{++}	Factor X[1]	
Factor V		Factor XI	
Factor VII[1]		Factor XII	
		Factor XIII	Fibrin stabilising factor

[1] Dependent on normal vitamin K absorption and metabolism.

liver and therefore dependent on adequate hepatic function. Four of them (II, VII, IX and X; the 'prothrombin complex') are also dependent on fat-soluble vitamin K, and will become deficient in conditions of malabsorption of this vitamin, for instance in biliary tract disease causing obstructive jaundice, in gastrocolic fistula, and in steatorrhoea. Vitamin K deficiency may occur in patients on prolonged intravenous nutrition as the usual vitamin supplements prescribed (i.e. Parentrovite) do not contain vitamin K. Factors II, VII, IX and X are also the factors affected by oral anticoagulation.

The fibrinolytic system removes fibrin through the proteolytic action of the enzyme plasmin. The breakdown products (Fibrin Degradation Products, F.D.P.s) are normally removed by the reticulo-endothelial system.

Disseminated intravascular coagulation

Disseminated intravascular coagulation (consumption coagulopathy, defibrination syndrome) is an increasingly recognised complication of a wide range of different disorders (Table 7). Its recognition is important because not only does it sometimes signal unsuspected underlying disease, but also because successful early management buys time for the clinician faced with a critically ill patient. D.I.C. is triggered either by the release of thromboplastins into the bloodstream, or by endothelial damage as a result of blood vessel disruption. The clinical and laboratory effects depend on the nature and persistence of the triggering agent, the general health of the host (and in particular hepatic function), fibrinolytic activity, and the integrity of reticulo-endothelial system. The paradoxical picture of both bleeding and intravascular clotting gives rise to a wide spectrum of clinical signs ranging from the classical picture of persistent oozing from body orifices and venepuncture sites to widespread thrombosis. A simple explanation of this paradox is shown in Fig. 2.

Table 7. Clinical conditions associated with disseminated intravascular coagulation. (Reproduced with kind permission from Mersky, 1976)

Acute variety
1. Shock
   Haemorrhage, post-traumatic, cardiogenic, anaphylactic shock, acute allergic reaction to drugs, e.g. meprobamate; or other causes
   Septicaemia (with shock) due to meningococci, pneumococci, streptococci, pseudomonas or other gram negative bacteria (see also Part 2, ch. II, p. 364)
2. Acute intravascular haemolysis
   Incompatible blood transfusion
   Severe haemoglobinaemia due to other causes, e.g. malaria, drowning, ingestion of strong acids
3. Purpura fulminans
4. Acute viral infections
5. Obstetrical causes (see also Part 2, ch. XI, p. 723)
   Abruptio placentae, amniotic fluid embolism, septic abortion
6. Acute pulmonary embolism; dissecting aneurysm
7. Burns
8. Surgical operations especially involving thoracic viscera
9. Acute anoxia, e.g., in cardiac arrest with resuscitation
10. Heat stroke
11. Bites of certain poisonous snakes
12. Following extracorporeal circulation
13. Renal disease – glomerulonephritis, haemolytic-uraemic syndrome, transplant rejection
14. Thrombotic thrombocytopenic purpura (?), diabetic ketoacidosis
15. Other causes

Subacute variety
1. Malignant disease
   Disseminated carcinoma
   Acute promyelocytic leukaemia and other types of acute leukaemia, disseminated rhabdomyosarcoma
2. Obstetrical causes
   Retained dead foetus syndrome
3. Thrombosis at local site, e.g. aortic aneurysm

Chronic variety
1. Giant haemangioma (Kasabach–Merritt syndrome) and haemangioendothelioma
2. Massive cavernomatous transformation of blood vessels, e.g. in the splenoportal venous system

The laboratory results may, depending on the severity of the process and time of sampling, show:

Thrombocytopenia.

Decreased coagulation factors reflected in abnormally prolonged clotting times and low assay results, particularly that of fibrinogen.

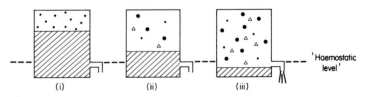

Fig. 2. In (*i*) the normal state is shown with plentiful coagulation factors and platelets. As a result of the triggering process intravascular coagulation begins, consuming both some of the coagulation factors and platelets. Demand for these components eventually exceeds supply and their level in the blood stream falls. Meanwhile fibrin deposition begins in the small blood vessels, particularly affecting kidney, lung and cerebral vasculature. A concurrent rise in fibrinolytic activity breaks down fibrinogen and fibrin, and fibrin degradation products increase in the circulation swamping the normal removal mechanism of the reticulo-endothelial system (*ii*).

Eventually (*iii*) consumption of clotting factors is so great that their 'haemostatic level' is passed and bleeding results. Bleeding may also occur because of associated thrombocytopenia, although this is not invariable.

Key: •, Platelets; ////, Clotting factors; ●, Microemboli; △, F.D.P.

High fibrin degradation products and other evidence of abnormal fibrinolytic activity.

Fragmented red cells on the blood film. These are one of the features of micro-angiopathic haemolytic anaemia, red cells being damaged by fibrin strands laid down in the microvasculature (Brain *et al.*, 1967).

Management of D.I.C. As D.I.C. is potentiated by *hypovolemia, hypoxia,* and *acidosis* initial treatment should be directed at the correction of these abnormalities, and at the *primary cause of the syndrome.* In the majority of cases once the trigger is removed D.I.C. will cease and no further treatment will be necessary.

The importance of early recognition cannot be overstressed, and patients with conditions which predispose to D.I.C. should be carefully monitored by regular physical examination and laboratory investigation. Physical signs suggesting the onset of D.I.C. include easy bruising, purpura, oozing from vein or artery puncture sites and mucous membranes, aspiration of blood from the naso-gastric tube and suction catheters, acrocyanosis, thrombosis, and evidence of renal impairment. A regular laboratory assessment should include haemoglobin and haematocrit, platelet count, and thrombin time. Death directly attributable to D.I.C. occurs either because of haemorrhage, commonly intracerebral or pulmonary, or because of the effects of micro-embolisation, commonly of the kidney. Both are preventable with early treatment, although the mode of presentation of some of the diseases associated with D.I.C., for instance haemolytic uraemic syndrome, make this extremely difficult. Apart from the removal of the trigger and the application of general supportive measures to the patient, further care rests on the judicious use of blood products and heparin.

Blood products in D.I.C. If D.I.C. can be brought under control, either by the removal of the trigger or by the use of heparin, replacement of coagulation factors or platelets is usually unnecessary unless urgent surgery or organ biopsy is contemplated. However there are certain clear indications for their use and these are the presence of serious or potentially serious haemorrhage, particularly when this involves the central nervous system, and in those patients who are unlikely to correct quickly their own defect. The latter group includes patients with hepatic insufficiency, and the newborn.

There is still a place for replacement therapy even in those situations where D.I.C. cannot be controlled. In the presence of life threatening haemorrhage it obviously takes precedence over concern about 'adding fuel to the fire' by increasing the likelihood of micro-embolisation. Similarly in those patients with malignant disease and chronic D.I.C. replacement therapy should be used to control distressing haemorrhagic symptoms.

Heparin in D.I.C. The decision to use heparin must be based on both the clinical and laboratory signs. It should never be used without clear laboratory evidence of D.I.C. and is usually contra-indicated in the presence of recent major injury, whether accidental or surgical. Heparin short-circuits the consumption of coagulation factors and platelets (Fig. 3) and therefore prevents further micro-embolisation. *It has no effect on fibrin already laid down in the micro-vasculature*, and this is probably why it is so ineffective in conditions like the haemolytic uraemic syndrome, in which the damage has already been done by the time the patient presents in renal failure.

In conditions in which the triggering agent can definitely be removed there may still be a case for heparin in management. A particular

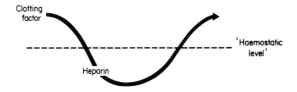

Fig. 3. Heparin blockage in D.I.C.

example here is in meningococcal septicaemia when the patient presents with early clinical signs suggesting the Waterhouse–Friderichsen syndrome. In this condition a bolus of heparin should be given before the administration of steroids, blocking further fibrin deposition in the adrenal glands and subsequent haemorrhagic necrosis. Obstetric cases will normally recover without the need for heparinisation, provided that the uterus has been evacuated and that measures have been taken to ensure adequate uterine contraction.

In states of continuing D.I.C. both bleeding and micro-embolisation may be controlled by heparinisation, with or without blood product replacement. The dosage regime employed by the author is that suggested by Mersky (1972), 50 to 100 units of heparin/kg body weight being given as an initial dose with 10–15 units/kg body weight hourly thereafter. In severe thrombocytopenia the smaller dose should be used because of lowered platelet-linked heparin resistance (Conley et al., 1948). Heparin should be given by continuous infusion by pump rather than as intermittent intravenous injections (Salzman et al., 1975).

Laboratory monitoring of the patient's progress should include measurement of platelet count, fibrogen and F.D.P.s. The platelet count is often the last variable to return to normal (Colman et al., 1972).

In general, *antifibrinolytic therapy is contra-indicated in D.I.C.* Fibrinolytic blockade with E.A.C.A. ('Epsikapron') or similar drugs, predisposes to further micro-embolism. D.I.C. is discussed further in relation to severe infection and obstetric practice in Part 2, ch. II, p. 364 and ch. XI, p. 723, respectively.

Management of other coagulopathies

Treatment is summarised in Table 8. Patients with a bleeding tendency *should not receive intramuscular injections or aspirin-containing drugs.* Occasionally haemorrhage for which there is no clinical or laboratory explanation is encountered. These patients should be transfused with fresh frozen plasma (2–3 packs in the adult) the dose being repeated at 12 h. Patients with unexplained and persistent haemorrhage and those with haemophilia or a similar disorder should be referred to a special centre for further treatment as soon as possible. A list of Haemophilia Reference Centres is given at the end of the chapter.

BLOOD COMPONENT TRANSFUSION

With the increasing use of whole blood fractionation, plasmapheresis, and the introduction of the cell separator a whole range of components

Table 8. Management of haemorrhage caused by coagulopathy other than D.I.C.

Cause	Treatment
Heparin	Reversal with i.v. protamine sulphate. Approximate dose: 1 mg protamine sulphate neutralises 1 mg (100 units) heparin. Adjust according to time last dose heparin. Acts immediately.
Oral anti-coagulants	1. Reversal with vitamin K_1. Dose: 5 mg i.v. if oral anti-coagulation to continue. 25–50 mg i.v. if oral anti-coagulation discontinued (patient resistant to further therapy for 2 weeks). Rate of infusion: 10 mg/min. Acts in 6–8 h. 2. Immediate action with prothrombin complex (II, VII, IX, X concentrate), or F.F.P. Give vitamin K_1 simultaneously.
Liver failure	Fresh frozen plasma; dosage and frequency according to laboratory results.
Haemophilic disorder	See text.
'Unexplained' haemorrhage	Fresh frozen plasma (see text).

designed to meet the needs of particular patients is becoming available to clinicians. Blood is an expensive human resource, and in spite of increasingly sensitive methods of testing, its use is still not without risk. The basic rules of safety in blood transfusion should be known and understood by all medical and nursing staff employed in clinical care. In particular it should be appreciated that the major cause of severe transfusion reaction remains that of human error in checking a patient's particulars with those of the blood pack provided for transfusion.

Table 9 summarises the blood products available for transfusion in the United Kingdom. Whole blood is only indicated after acute blood loss when the indication is to restore blood volume and the oxygen carrying capacity in the patient. It should not be necessary in patients who have lost less than 20% of their blood volume, either plasma protein fraction or dextran being substituted (Tovey and Bird, 1974). Fresh whole blood is very rarely indicated; multiple deficiencies can be made up by choosing the specific blood components necessary to correct the deficit in the patient. Whole blood should be less than five days old when indicated for the newborn or for open heart surgery because of the dangers of hyperkalaemia.

Bank blood (over 48 h old) will be deficient in leucocytes, platelets, and factors V and VIII. Patients requiring massive transfusion should therefore have factor V and VIII replaced using fresh frozen plasma. A good rule of thumb is to transfuse one pack of fresh frozen plasma for

Table 9. Summary of blood components available for transfusion (U.K.)

Product	Indication	Comment
Whole blood	Restoration blood volume and oxygen carrying capacity after acute loss of more than 20% patient's blood volume	Cross match essential. Use blood less than 5 days old for newborn and open heart surgery
Red cells	Correction of anaemia. Haemoglobin rises by approximately 1 g/dl/pack in adult	Cross match essential. Caution in severe anaemia
Dried plasma	Volume expander	Deficient in clotting factors V and VIII
Fresh frozen plasma (F.F.P.)	Correction of coagulation factor defects and complement deficiency in angioneurotic oedema	Preferably ABO/Rh specific. Always use Rh negative F.F.P. for Rh negative females
Plasma protein fraction Albumin	Volume expander. Contains 5 g/protein/dl, mostly albumin Volume expander, 25 g/bottle. Replacement therapy in hypo-albuminaemia	Salt poor
Fibrinogen	Replacement therapy, 4 g/bottle	
Cryoprecipitate	Replacement therapy in haemophilia A and von Willebrand's disease. Contains VIII and fibrinogen	Preferably ABO/Rh specific. Should be Rh specific in females
AHG lyophilised concentrates	Treatment haemophilia A	No correction platelet defect in von Willebrand's disease
Prothrombin complex concentrates	Contain either II, VII, IX, X or II, IX, X. Replacement therapy haemophilia B (Christmas disease), and pro-thrombin complex deficiency	Risk of thrombo-embolic phenomena – do not use in newborn
Platelet concentrates	Either platelet rich plasma (P.R.P.) or concentrates for replacement therapy in thrombocytopenia	Preferably HL-A typed when frequent transfusions necessary
Granulocytes	Granulocytopenia in leukaemia and marrow aplasia	HL-A compatibility preferable. Obtained by cell separator

every six packs of blood transfused. Rarely platelet transfusion will also be necessary.

Red cells are indicated for the correction of anaemia, with due caution in cases of severe anaemia.

Dried plasma, which is rapidly going out of production, plasma protein fraction (P.P.F.), and albumin are all volume expanders, P.P.F. and albumin being hepatitis free in the United Kingdom. These three products are of no value in coagulation defects although dried plasma does contain some fibrinogen.

Fresh frozen plasma contains all the coagulation factors and is the material of choice for replacement therapy in D.I.C. as there is less risk of hepatitis from its use than with fibrinogen concentrate. Problems of circulatory overload restrict its use for the treatment of haemophilia A (factor VIII deficiency), but it is sometimes of value in the treatment of haemophilia B (Christmas disease, factor IX deficiency) in *minor* bleeding episodes.

Cryoprecipitate contains factor VIII and is used for the treatment of both haemophilia A and von Willebrand's disease. It also contains a significant amount of fibrinogen and may be used for replacement therapy in hypofibrinogenaemia.

Mild allergic reactions are common with both F.F.P. and cryoprecipitate, and it is the author's practice to prescribe intravenous chlorpheniramine routinely prior to transfusion with these products. A rare but potentially lethal complication is acute allergic pulmonary oedema (Kernoff *et al.*, 1972), presenting with dyspnoea and acute praecordial or epigastric pain, chest radiology revealing multiple fluffy opacities. Treatment is with intravenous hydrocortisone and diuretics.

The A.H.G. (factor VIII) lyophilised concentrates are used for replacement therapy in haemophilia A. They do not correct the platelet defect in von Willebrand's disease. Prothrombin complex concentrates at present carry an indeterminate risk of thrombo-embolism (Menache, 1975) and should be used with caution, particularly in the newborn and in patients with hepatic failure. They are indicated for replacement therapy in haemophilia B.

Platelet concentrates are now available from most major transfusion centres. Unfortunately they cannot be stored for more than two to three days. Similarly white cells cannot be stored but with the increasing use of the cell separator should become more freely available for use in patients with granulocytopenia.

With the exception of plasma protein fraction and albumin all the products mentioned carry the risk of serum hepatitis transmission.

Those products prepared from pooled plasma (fibrinogen, A.H.G. and prothrombin concentrates) carry a greater risk than products from individual blood donation.

United Kingdom Haemophilia Reference Centres

St. Thomas' Hospital	01-928 9292	London, the South East
The Royal Free Hospital	01-794 0500	and East Anglia
The Churchill Hospital, Oxford	0865 64841	Oxford, Wessex, the South West, the Midlands and Northern Ireland
The Royal Infirmary, Manchester	061 273 3300	The North West, North Wales, Trent and Yorkshire
The Royal Infirmary with the Children's Hospital, Sheffield	0742 20977	
The Royal Victoria Infirmary, Newcastle	0632 25131	The North of England
University Hospital of Cardiff	0222 755944	South Wales

In Scotland, Haemophilia Centres are situated in:

Aberdeen	0224 23423
Dundee	8382 60111
Edinburgh	031 229 2477
Glasgow	041 552 3535
Inverness	0463 34151

ACKNOWLEDGEMENTS

The author is grateful to Dr W. Walker of the Department of Haematology, Royal Victoria Infirmary for his help in the preparation of this chapter.

REFERENCES

Brain, M. C., Dacie, I. V. and Hourihane, D. O'B. (1962) Micro-agiopathic haemolytic anaemia: the possible role of vascular lesions in pathogenesis. *Brit. J. Haemat.* **8**, 358.

Brain, M. C., Easterly, J. R. and Beck, E. A. (1967). Intravascular haemolysis with experimentally produced vascular thrombi. *Brit. J. Haemat.* **13**, 868.

Carson, P. E. and Frischer, H. (1966). Glucose-6-phosphate dehydrogenase deficiency and related disorders of the pentose phosphate pathway. *Am. J. Med.* **41**, 744.

Colman, R. W., Robboy, S. J. and Minna, J. D. (1972). Disseminated intravascular coagulation (D.I.C.): An approach. *Am. J. Med.* **52**, 679.

Conley, C. L., Hartmann, R. C. and Lalley, J. S. (1948). The relationship of heparin activity to platelet concentration. *Proc. Soc. Exp. Biol. Med.* **69**, 284.

Dacie, J. V. (1967a). 'The Haemolytic Anaemias'. Part III, Secondary or symptomatic haemolytic anaemias. Churchill, London.

Dacie, J. V. (1967b). 'The Haemolytic Anaemias'. Part IV, Section on Paroxysmal nocturnal haemoglobinuria. Churchill, London.

Delamore, I. W. (1976). Haematological clues in systemic disease *Practitioner* **216**, 27.

Fraser, I. M. and Vessell, E. S. (1968). Effects of drugs and drug metabolites on erythrocytes from normal and glucose-6-phosphate dehydrogenase – deficient individuals. *Ann. N.Y. Acad. Sci.* **151**, 777.

Girdwood, R. H. (1976). Haematological side effects of drugs. *Practitioner* **216**, 37.

Grimes, A. J. and de Gruchy, G. C. (1974). Red cell metabolism: hereditary enzymopathies. *In* 'Blood and its Disorders' (Ed. R. M. Hardisty and D. J. Weatherall) p. 473. Blackwell, Oxford.

Huehns, E. R. (1974). The structure and function of haemoglobin: clinical disorders due to abnormal haemoglobin structure. *In* 'Blood and its Disorders' (Ed. R. M. Hardisty and D. J. Weatherall) p. 526.

Kernoff, P. B. A., Durrant, I. J., Rizza, C. R. and Wright, F. W. (1972). Severe allergic pulmonary oedema after plasma transfusion. *Brit. J. Haemat.* **23**, 777.

Marsh, G. W. and Lewis, S. M. (1969). Cardiac haemolytic anaemia. *Seminars in Haematology* **6**, 133.

Menache, D. (1975). 'The use of factor IX concentrates in conditions other than congenital clotting factor deficiencies'. Proceedings of the X Congress of the World Federation of Hemophilia, Helsinki.

Mersky, C. (1972). The defibrination syndrome. *In* 'Human Blood Coagulation, Haemostasis and Thrombosis' (Ed. R. Biggs) p. 1444. Blackwell, Oxford.

Morrison, F. S. and Mollison, P. L. (1966). Post-transfusion purpura. *New Engl. J. Med.* **275**, 243.

Salzman, E. W., Deykin, D., Shapiro, R. M. and Rosenberg, R. (1975). Management of heparin therapy *New Engl. J. Med.* **292**, 1046.

Serjeant, G. R. (1974). The clinical features of sickle cell disease. North-Holland Publishing Company, Amsterdam.

Tovey, G. H. and Bird, G. W. G. (1974). Blood transfusion and the use of blood products. *In* 'Blood and its Disorders' (Ed. R. M. Hardisty and D. J. Weatherall) p. 1481. Blackwell, Oxford.

Zieve, L. (1958). Jaundice, hyperlipemia and haemolytic anaemia: a heretofore unrecognised syndrome associated with alcoholic fatty liver and cirrhosis. *Ann. Intern. Med.* **48**, 471.

IX

The Management of Severe Gastrointestinal Disorders

Section 1: The Management of Severe Gastrointestinal Haemorrhage

P. L. WRIGHT

INTRODUCTION. CLINICAL ASSESSMENT

Gastrointestinal haemorrhage is a common medical emergency causing sudden prostration often not associated with pain. An assessment of the amount lost is seldom helpful as the patient is unable to estimate accurately the volume lost in vomit or faeces. Generally speaking the more massive the haemorrhage the more likely it is that vomitus will be bright or dark red and the melaena will be frankly bloody rather than showing the more characteristic shiny tarry colour. A history of recurrent melaena suggests that bleeding has been occurring over several days. The time of haemorrhage may be indicated by a syncopal attack. Coffee ground vomit may be associated with massive bleeding; it may represent a small quantity of blood from the duodenum refluxing into the stomach while the majority is passing downward.

A detailed history should be taken with specific enquiry into past history of indigestion, known hiatus hernia, gastric and duodenal ulcer etc. The drug history is important; specific reference should be made to alcohol, aspirin, antirheumatic drugs and steroids. The patient should be asked if he has taken 'pain killers' and if a woman, medication for period pains as these may contain salicylates. A meticulous physical examination may reveal signs of associated disease. The skin should be

665

searched carefully for spider naevi, striae and telangiectases; the latter especially if there is a recurrent history of haemorrhage. A clinical estimate of the degree of blood loss is made and the patient started on a pulse and blood pressure chart. In an acute bleed the relationship of the volume of blood lost (as a percentage of the estimated total blood volume) to the clinical findings is shown in Table 2, p. 336, and is discussed in greater detail on p. 335. It should be noted that recurrent concealed haemorrhage is not always associated with a rising pulse and falling blood pressure especially in the younger patient when paradoxically intense vaso-spasm may put up the blood pressure before total circulatory collapse occurs.

MANAGEMENT

Blood should be sent for immediate grouping and cross-match in all but trivial cases. If significant haemorrhage has taken place a minimum of 4 units should be requested; if transfusion is deemed necessary at the start 8 units are ordered so that there will be a reserve available after the immediate resuscitation of the patient. Blood should also be sent for urea measurement, haemoglobin and packed cell volume. A moderately raised urea is common in association with intestinal haemorrhage, e.g. 10–12 mmol/l. A high urea may indicate renal failure, suggesting uraemic gastritis or colitis as the cause; however in severe blood loss over several days the fall in renal blood flow may permit the urea to rise

Table 1. The management of severe gastrointestinal haemorrhage

---

1. Early admission.
2. Clinical assessment of severity of shock (see Part 2, ch. II, p. 336, Table 2).
3. Intravenous infusion with saline. Sedation. Avoid opiates.
4. (a) Blood for haemoglobin, urea and electrolytes, coagulation studies, liver function. Tests for Australia antigen if required.
   (b) Blood for group and cross match – 4 units of reserve; 8 units if transfusion indicated.
5. Insert a right atrial pressure line and monitor. On rare occasions other monitoring systems may be required.
6. Gastric aspiration and continuous drainage.
7. Blood transfusion should massive volumes of blood be required; refer to Part 2, ch. II, p. 349.
8. Diagnosis by endoscopy or emergency barium meal.
9. Early consultation with surgeons.
10. Cimetadine.
11. Early surgery in persisting or massive haemorrhage.

---

to levels of 25–35 mmol/l. The haemoglobin will be normal in acute haemorrhage and if low suggests chronic blood loss or a previous haemorrhage.

An intravenous infusion should be set up even when minor haemorrhage is suspected and the patient infused with normal saline/plasma/dextran, as seems indicated by the clinical state of the patient. Solutions suitable for volume expansion, their properties and most appropriate solution to select under different clinical circumstances are described in detail in Part 2, ch. II, p. 341.

The resuscitation of a patient suffering from shock related to a severe gastrointestinal bleed is similar to that described in the patient with severe blood loss following trauma (see Part 2, ch. II, p. 335) and is summarised in Table 6, p. 350. Patient monitoring is essential especially in the elderly or when the bleeding is moderate to profound.

Any patient may bleed again, sometimes catastrophically, and the insertion of a needle in a collapsed patient may be extremely difficult. A right atrial pressure line should be inserted and the pressure recorded in order to facilitate the rapid resuscitation of the patient and to recognise early further haemorrhage; a sudden fall in the central venous pressure (C.V.P.) being often the first sign. With a C.V.P. line in place, rapid transfusion to a pressure of 10–12 cm H_2O allows effective volume replacement. More elaborate monitoring systems are rarely required in the patient suffering from gastrointestinal bleed except in profound shock where vital organ function may fail. Monitoring indices which may be needed under such circumstances are described in Part 2, ch. II, p. 316.

A nasogastric tube is inserted to aspirate residual fluid or blood from the stomach and again to detect early further bleeding. The tube can be left to drain continuously into a reservoir bag; ritual hourly aspiration and plugging of the tube is not recommended.

At this point, with the patient resuscitated and in a safe state, consideration is given to the diagnosis and subsequent management should further bleeding occur. It is well established that bleeding need not necessarily come from known lesions. At least 40% of patients with known varices bleed from acute or chronic peptic ulcers or oesophago/gastritis. Similar figures are obtained in the study of ulcer patients. For this reason, in recent years great effort has been made to establish the diagnosis actively and early, by emergency barium meal and/or endoscopy. Both methods have their advocates, the latter having a higher success rate in establishing diagnosis though requiring the services of an experienced endoscopist: not available on call at all hospitals. It has not however been shown to date that early diagnosis reduces the overall mortality of this group of patients.

Special procedures for the investigation of gastrointestinal haemorrhage

Emergency endoscopy

This procedure may be performed on the patient's bed. The patient is placed in the left lateral position, the pharynx is sprayed with 1% lignocaine. A lubricated wide stomach tube with multiple apertures is passed and aspiration begun. Lavage is performed with ice cold tap water using enough to clear the stomach and get a clear return. Usually if bleeding has stopped this takes 30–45 min as a maximum but if bleeding is active the effluent remains bright red. The important thing is that clots should be removed and the procedure should be continued until clots cease to appear.

Endoscopy may then be performed; most operators prefer to do this under intravenous diazepam, 10–15 mg being injected till the patient is drowsy. A forward looking endoscope is passed and an attempt at full oesophago-gastro-duodenoscopy performed. Mallory Weiss lesions, gastric and duodenal ulcers, acute gastric erosions, acute gastric ulcers, diffuse oesophago-gastritis and varices are systematically sought. Rarer lesions may be found, gastric carcinoma, telangiectasia, leiomyomata and lymphosarcoma of the stomach. Biopsy is performed if indicated and the instrument withdrawn. Considerable difficulty occurs in the presence of clot or severe sustained haemorrhage where it may be impossible to do more than indicate the probable site of haemorrhage. Some work is being done to develop endoscopic techniques for arresting haemorrhages with argon laser coagulation and diathermy (Cottom, 1976) – this is highly experimental.

Arteriography

Selective coeliac axis angiography is increasingly used to diagnose the site of haemorrhage in patients who continue to bleed. Again the main requirement is for highly skilled personnel, and it may well be argued that if operation seems inevitable it should not be delayed excessively by these techniques.

In my own practice I do not believe in an aggressive approach to diagnosis in all patients with haemorrhage, even though it may have been severe. I rarely endoscope as an emergency patients with a history of aspirin ingestion or who give a good account of a Mallory Weiss lesion (retching, vomiting on one or more occasions, followed by bright red blood especially after a heavy meal plus or minus alcohol). I prefer to investigate the majority of patients who stop bleeding by barium meal and endoscopy (if required) as a cold procedure and reserve endoscopy as an emergency for patients who are elderly. The elderly patient is more likely to have a perforating ulcer eroding a major artery or persisting bleeding related to possible or known varices. I believe in the value here of an early consultation with surgical colleagues and working out an agreed programme for the individual patient.

In coming to a decision risks of endoscopy should be discounted, *viz.* oesophageal and gastric perforation and aspiration pneumonia since, in experienced hands, they are very rare.

Continuing care
The vital functions of the patient are monitored during transfusion, great care being taken not to overload the patient and precipitate acute pulmonary oedema. When massive blood replacement is necessary, the routine summarised in Table 6, p. 350, should be followed. Nothing should be given by mouth other than crushed ice to suck if desired by the patient. Instillation of alkalis or acid adsorbants does not affect the likelihood of further haemorrhage but may be given if the patient complains of pain. The patient should be sedated if required with diazepam intramuscularly 5–10 mg. Opiates should be avoided especially in patients with liver disease because of the risk of precipitation of hepatic encephalopathy. A high proportion of patients thus treated stop bleeding and may resume feeding and await definitive diagnostic procedures or continue with indicated medical treatment for their primary disease.

Recurrent or persistent haemorrhage from peptic ulcer, oesophago-gastritis and gastric erosions may be controlled with the new H_2-receptor antagonist cimetadine. This may be given orally 200 mg thrice daily and 400 mg at night. An intravenous preparation is available, the recommended dose being 200 mg repeated at 2–4 hourly intervals up to a maximum of 2 g/day. It may be given by continuous infusion, the average rate should not exceed 75 mg/h. This compound has been found to increase the rate of healing of both duodenal and gastric ulcer, oesophagitis etc. and has been used in the treatment of acute haemorrhage. It appears useful but sufficient controlled trials are not yet available to assess its true worth in this acute situation.

Surgery
Active surgical intervention may be necessary if bleeding is prolonged. Factors which should be considered include:

(*a*) *Age.* The older the patient the higher is the mortality from gastrointesinal haemorrhage. The difficulty of maintaining such a patient in a good clinical state is greater.

(*b*) *Acute gastric erosions, diffuse gastritis, Mallory Weiss syndrome.* Bleeding may be severe and continuous. Surgery should be avoided if at all possible especially in the latter two conditions because the surgeon may have to perform total gastrectomy to obtain haemostasis.

(*c*) *Gastric ulcer.* The history may be of several small/intermediate bleeds before catastrophic haemorrhage occurs. This is particularly likely in the elderly and therefore early surgery is advisable.

(*d*) *Duodenal ulcer.* It should be noted that such patients are more likely to bleed postoperatively from the gastric suture line or from acute gastric erosions. Continued vigilance is therefore necessary post-operatively. A very difficult patient is the young adult with bleeding and no previous history of indigestion. Such patients frequently develop chronic postoperative complications such as dumping. Surgery should therefore be avoided if possible.

(*e*) *Hereditary telangiectasia.* The diagnosis may be made in the absence of family history or signs by gastroscopy. Bleeding is usually self limiting and moderate though it is frequently recurrent.

(*f*) *Benign or malignant tumour.* Surgery is best delayed if possible to allow a cold planned extirpation of the disease.

In bleeding from oesophageal varices the initial management of the bleeding patient is similar, but investigations should include bilirubin, the serum albumin and clotting factors. Blood should be taken for Australia antigen. The specimens should be labelled 'High Risk' and sent separately to the laboratory in a leak-proof plastic bag. The laboratory should be warned of the arrival of the specimens so that due care can be taken to avoid infection of laboratory staff. Further investigations should be minimised should the patient be found to be Australia antigen positive.

Gastrointestinal haemorrhage associated with liver failure

The management of this condition is described in detail in Part I, ch. V, p. 101.

REFERENCE

Cottom, P. B. (1976). Upper gastrointestinal endoscopy. *Brit. J. Hosp. Med.* **16**, 7.

Section 2: The Management of acute ulcerative colitis, pseudomembranous colitis and Crohn's disease.

P. L. WRIGHT

ACUTE ULCERATIVE COLITIS

Introduction

Patients may be admitted in their first attack of colitis or less commonly as an acute relapse in a patient with previous or chronic ulcerative colitis. The history will include diarrhoea with loss of blood and mucus. In a severe case frequent watery diarrhoea is associated with severe prostration, abdominal pain and circulatory collapse. After a careful history and physical examination, sigmoidoscopy should be performed as soon as possible to verify the likely diagnosis.

Investigation and differential diagnosis

Sigmoidoscopy

The patient is placed in the left lateral position. A well lubricated wide bore sigmoidoscope is gently inserted, directed towards the sacrum, and the obturator removed. Gentle air insufflation allows inspection of the mucosal lining and the instrument advanced with great care. It can usually be easily inserted to 12–15 cm in an adult. Above this level reverse rotation of the instrument handle is necessary to negotiate the sacral curve and permit inspection of the upper rectum. The typical appearance of acute ulcerative colitis is of friable ulcerated mucosa with an excess of mucus, pus and bright red blood. The mucosa bleeds to touch. A biopsy should be taken in the lower rectum, care being taken that the bite is superficial to avoid perforation. Specimens of mucus should be taken for bacteriological examination on a warm microscope

671

stage if amoebic colitis is suspected from the history, recent residence abroad or the sigmoidoscopic appearance is suggestive of amoebic ulcers.

It cannot be stressed too highly that if this procedure is not performed with great care and gentleness, local perforation is the likely consequence. If insufflation is excessive, perforation may occur in the bowel higher up and this may ultimately prove to be fatal in the critically ill toxic patient.

Differential diagnosis

The differential diagnosis is from acute Crohn's disease; ischaemic colitis (even in young adults, Clark *et al.*, 1972); diverticulitis, pseudomembranous colitis, radiation colitis, etc.

Management

The treatment of ulcerative colitis consists of supportive and definitive therapy. Initial studies after sigmoidoscopy include a plain abdominal X-ray to assess possible colonic distension and to check that no perforation has occurred. Blood should be taken for haemoglobin, urea and electrolyte measurement and in a severe case blood should be cross-matched. Stool should be sent for culture and the abdominal girth measured and charted. Severe ulcerative colitis is associated with severe diarrhoea, gross rectal bleeding, abdominal pain and distension, fever, salt and water depletion and circulatory collapse.

Assessment of the extent and severity of the ulcerative colitis by barium enema should not be performed in a seriously ill patient because of the risk of perforation. It should be performed later when the acute process is coming under control. Colonoscopy may also be used at this juncture to make visual assessment and biopsy of suspicious looking polyps (pseudopolyps) above the reach of the sigmoidoscope.

The management of abnormalities in metabolic and fluid balance have been described in detail in Part 1, ch. VII. Classically the patient with fulminating ulcerative colitis develops predominant water depletion, potassium depletion and a gradually increasing metabolic acidosis. Potassium and magnesium depletion may be severe in patients with explosive diarrhoea.

In severe cases the modified intravenous regime of Truelove and Jewel (1974) should be used.

1. No fluid is allowed orally except ice to suck or sips of water.

2. After transfusion and correction of electrolyte imbalance, the patient should be fed intravenously. Daily weighing is essential in order to assess fluid balance. Right atrial pressure monitoring is important during the acute phase – thus ensuring an adequate dynamic fluid volume. The central line can also be used for feeding – these patients are particularly susceptible to infection – the line should therefore be changed at least once every 10 days (earlier if there is evidence of sepsis). The long-term metabolic and nutritional management should be based upon that described in Part 1, ch. IX, p. 247.

In the absence of overt hepatic or renal failure, Aminosol 10% is the protein solution of choice – 1500 ml should be given daily in an adult in the first instance.

Fluid and potassium requirements are high – at least 6 litres of fluid being generally needed to maintain fluid balance. The average potassium requirement during intravenous feeding and in the presence of severe diarrhoea, is 140–200 mmol daily. Magnesium requirements are generally 12–15 mmol daily. Sequential observations as enumerated in Part 1, ch. IX, Table 1, p. 248, are essential, additives (Part 1, ch. IX, p. 252) are invariably required and vitamins and haematinics (Part 1, ch. IX, p. 253) should be replaced from the onset.

Blood transfusion is generally required once every 3–5 days during the acute toxic phase of the illness and 40–60 mg of prednisolone phosphate should be given intravenously daily.

Truelove and Jewel (1974) recommended the administration of tetracycline intravenously daily but because of its potential nephrotoxic and hepatotoxic effects, it is probably wise to use intravenous co-trimoxazole as an alternative – keeping in mind that this may precipitate folate depletion.

3. The patient is given a rectal drip of 100 mg hydrocortisone hydrochloride in 120 ml warm normal saline twice daily.

4. After 5 days' intravenous feeding, oral feeding is recommended with 20 mg oral prednisolone daily and prednisolone retention enemata twice daily, being continued as required.

Daily observation of abdominal girth should be made, the frequency and type of stool recorded and frequent checks of haemoglobin and electrolyte status made according to the progress of the patient. Repeat abdominal films should be taken if deterioration occurs in order to detect early the onset of toxic megacolon. In such cases gross increase in the transcolonic diameter occurs (greater than 6.5 cm).

Less severely ill colitic patients may be allowed a normal diet from the start with 60 mg of oral prednisolone and twice daily prednisolone retention enemata. The patient should be given also salazopyrine 1 g thrice daily. The same observations should be made. I do not consider that antidiarrhoeal agents such as codeine phosphate and dephenoxylate with atropine (Lomotil) are useful and I believe they mask the severity of the disease process.

Early consultation with surgical colleagues should take place. Indications for surgical intervention by defunctioning ileostomy or total colectomy include –

1. Progressive deterioration despite adequate medical treatment.
2. Failure to improve.
3. Increasing abdominal distension especially with ileus.
4. Perforation.
5. Toxic megacolon.
6. Pyoderma gangrenosa.

The management of ulcerative colitis in pregnancy is described in Part 2, ch. XI, p. 717.

PSEUDOMEMBRANOUS COLITIS

Introduction

This disease is increasingly recognised as a complication of antibiotic therapy, particularly lincomycin and broad spectrum antibiotics. It should be differentiated from fulminating staphylococcal enterocolitis, also usually a consequence of antibiotic therapy (Editorial, 1975).

The mechanism of development of pseudomembranous colitis is not understood. Patients have diarrhoea of all grades of severity and death may occur from this condition.

Management

The offending antibiotic should be stopped and the patient treated as per ulcerative colitis. The intensive intravenous regime described above is effective (Goodman and Truelove, 1976). Intravenous feeding should not be started until fluid and metabolic balance has been corrected. Explosive diarrhoea may be complicated by hypovolaemic shock and tetany (which may be due to hypokalaemia and/or hypomagnesaemia). Because of the rapid fall in serum albumin, volume replacement should be preferably with a protein-containing solution such as plasma, P.P.F. or blood (if the haemoglobin is low).

Surgery should be avoided if at all possible because of the good long-term prognosis.

CROHN'S DISEASE

Introduction

Crohn's disease remains an illness of unknown aetiology and presents diverse and complex problems in management. Originally recognised as a non-tuberculous cause of terminal ileitis it has become increasingly recognised as a cause of single or multiple granulomatous inflammation from the mouth to the anus. It is being increasingly recognised as a cause of colitis. The disease may present at all ages with a tendency for it to occur in young women. The condition is not predictable, recurrences of disease at the original site or others occurring without reason.

Clinical manifestations. Investigations

The clinical manifestations of Crohn's disease are listed in Table 1.

Table 1. The clinical manifestations of Crohn's disease

Fever
Weight loss
Diarrhoea – with blood and mucus if the colon is involved
Perianal fissures and fistula
Abdominal pain
Subacute and acute intestinal obstruction
Perforation. Local abscess formation. Perforation into bladder or vagina
Erythema nodosum
Arthritis
Facial pigmentation and finger clubbing
Sacro-ileitis and aortic incompetence

In this section we will be considering in the main the management of an acute attack or recurrence. Diagnosis may have been made by follow-through barium examination in the investigation of abdominal pain, or by laparotomy in patients admitted with an 'acute abdomen', or presenting with a mass in the right iliac fossa etc.

A full clinical assessment of the patient is made, particular note being taken of his state of nutrition. Investigations should include haemo-globin, white cell count, E.S.R., urea and electrolytes, fasting calcium and magnesium, plasma albumin, stool culture x 3 for acid-fast bacilli, blood for Yersinnia antibodies, folic acid, iron and vitamin B_{12} levels.

A full survey of the gastrointestinal tract should be made radiologically (if the condition of the patient permits) by follow-through barium meal and barium enema. The latter should be done without previous washout. Sigmoidoscopy and biopsy should be performed even if the rectal mucosa looks normal; the specimens should be examined for acid-fast bacilli. Colonoscopy, though offering an accurate assessment of the extent of the disease process, does not especially improve understanding or management of the disease.

Management

The patient should be managed by medical treatment so far as is possible. Unless vomiting occurs, the patient should be allowed a normal diet. Elemental diets have shown no advantage in the management of these patients, many of whom find these diets nauseating when taken over a long period. Severely ill patients may require feeding by the intravenous route. The same principles apply as in feeding the ulcerative colitic and are described in greater detail in Part 1, ch. IX. Many of these patients develop multiple fistula and chronic intra-abdominal sepsis – this is particularly likely to occur following laparotomy for an 'acute abdomen'. The management of severe chronic intra-abdominal sepsis is described in Part 2, ch. IV, p. 511. Treatment of the patient with Crohn's disease is similar to that described in this chapter. Surgery for closure of a fistula resistant to medical management should be delayed if at all possible until the serum albumin and body weight has returned to the lower limits of normal.

Corticosteroids

In severely ill patients prednisolone 60 mg/day should be given orally or hydrocortisone 100 mg 4–6 hourly by continuous infusion. This has a dramatic effect on the condition with rapid resolution of diarrhoea, a sense of well being, loss of fever, weight gain and loss of abdominal pain etc. The corticosteroids should then be tailed off over 1–2 weeks to maintenance therapy of 15 mg prednisolone per day in divided doses. The prednisolone should then be gradually decreased and discontinued providing the patient remains well.

Azathioprine

Though there was a number of encouraging reports of improvement in patients with Crohn's disease treated with azathioprine controlled trials have failed to show objective benefit (Rhodes *et al.*, 1971).

At the present time I would reserve it for patients who fail to improve on corticosteroids alone. When used it is given in a dosage of 2 mg/kg body weight orally. Checks of haemoglobin, white blood count and platelets should be done twice weekly initially.

Metronidazole
Ursing and Kamme (1975) introduced metronidazole in the treatment of Crohn's disease with an encouraging report of improvement in 5 cases. Extensive controlled trials to assess its usefulness are not yet available but dramatic responses do seem to occur. It is given on a continuous basis in a dosage of 400 mg three times daily for up to 1 year. It is likely to be useful in patients with suspected abscesses because of its effectiveness in suppressing anaerobes.

Other Agents
Sulphasalazine is often used in patients with Crohn's colitis. No controlled trials exist to demonstrate its effectiveness. The dosage is as in ulcerative colitis.

Surgery
Indications for surgery in Crohn's disease are: the relief of obstruction, drainage of abscess, persistent fistula, obstruction to ileostomy stoma, correction of blind loop syndrome, toxic megacolon and development of carcinoma (rare).

It is tempting to advise resection in patients with apparently localised disease. Experience shows however that the condition tends to flare up after surgery, other normal part of the bowel becoming affected. I have been impressed by this process occurring in a number of patients with apparent 'burned out' Crohn's disease who had surgery for mild chronic pain attributable to a minor degree of obstruction. In my own experience the longest case of this type recurred severely after 15 years of apparent inactivity.

REFERENCES

Clark, A. W., Lloyd-Mostyn, R. H. and de C. Sadler, M. R. (1972). 'Ischaemic colitis' in young adults. *Brit. Med. J.* **4**, 70.

Conn, H. O. and Ramsby, G. R. *et al.* (1975). Intra arterial vasopressin in the treatment of upper gastrointestinal haemorrhage. A prospective controlled trial. *Gastroenterology* **68**, 211.

Editorial (1975). Antibiotic diarrhoea. *Brit. Med. J.* **4**, 243.

Goodman, M. J. and Truelove, S. C. (1976). Intensive intravenous regimen for membranous colitis. *Brit. Med. J.* **2**, 354.

Rhodes, J., Beck, P., Bainton, D. and Campbell, H. (1971). Controlled trial of azathioprine in Crohn's disease. *Lancet* **2**, 1273.

Truelove, S. C. and Jewel, D. P. (1974). Intensive intravenous regimen for severe attacks of ulcerative colitis. *Lancet* **1**, 1067.

Ursing, B. and Kamme, C. (1975). Metronidazole for Crohn's disease. *Lancet* **1**, 775.

Section 3: The Management of Acute Pancreatitis

J. E. TRAPNELL

PATHOPHYSIOLOGY

The actual cause of acute pancreatitis is still not known and its treatment is therefore to some extent empirical, but there is now a much better understanding of the changes which occur in the gland once the auto-digestive process has commenced. Originally all that was available was a macroscopic description of oedema progressing to haemorrhage and sometimes to necrosis, but a more sophisticated view can now be presented and this has had a double impact. First of all, it has become apparent that acute pancreatitis is a multi-organ disease and, secondly, this better understanding of the pathophysiology has allowed a more scientific approach to treatment.

With the development of an episode of acute pancreatitis, there is

Table 1. Acute pancreatitis – pathophysiology

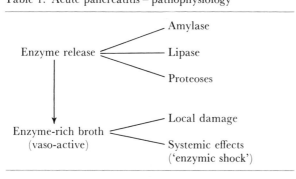

within the gland an explosive release of enzymes. This may be contained locally or may leak into the general circulation (Table 1). Of the three main components of pancreatic juice, amylase is in one respect the most important, for it is vital in the biochemical confirmation of a clinical diagnosis. However, this particular enzyme, even at high levels in the serum, is apparently quite harmless to the patient. Lipase is also released and is involved in some complicated mechanism not fully understood in the development of fat necrosis. It is, however, the proteolytic enzymes which cause the main tissue damage and which make acute pancreatitis so dangerous. In the past, there has been a tendency to concentrate on a particular named enzyme or enzyme systems – for instance trypsin or elastase, lysolecithin or kallikrein – but it is now quite clear that within the 'broth' which is produced in this condition, it is not so much the individual constituent which is important, but the overall effect of the 'witches brew'. This is vaso-active and highly tissue-destructive.

The local effect of this proteolytic enzyme release is, first of all, an increased tissue permeability. This leads to a leakage of very large amounts of fluid into the pancreas, the peripancreatic tissues and the peritoneal cavity. Clinically this is seen as oedema in and around the gland, increased lymphatic flow and a peritoneal exudate, all resulting in loss of extra-cellular fluid volume. In severe cases of pancreatitis as much as five to six litres of fluid may be lost from the circulation. A further local action of release of the enzyme-rich fluid is irritation and disorganisation of the coeliac plexus. It is this which causes the severe pain which is such a marked clinical feature in the majority of cases. In addition, because of a slowing in the micro-circulation and also because of a direct enzymic effect on the blood, there is small vessel thrombosis and extravasation leading to haemorrhage and subsequently to ischaemic necrosis.

When the proteolytic enzymes fail to be contained in the vicinity of the pancreas by the body's own defence mechanisms, the syndrome of enzymic shock is produced and this results in much more widespread and more serious effects. All the major organs and systems are affected directly or indirectly. In the circulation, there is alteration in the coagulation mechanism, probably as a result of kinin release (Kwaan et al., 1971), which takes the form of a consumptive coagulopathy. There is a direct effect on the heart (Lefer et al., 1971) with depression of the central pump mechanism and it is this which accounts for the E.C.G. changes which have been well recognised in acute pancreatitis for a long time. Finally, there is an *increase* in the general peripheral resistance (Sankaran *et al.*, 1974) which results initially in a rise in systemic blood pressure, before hypovolaemia and myocardial depression take over to produce hypotensive shock.

Alteration in liver function is present in nearly all cases of acute pancreatitis (Kitamura *et al.*, 1973). This is reflected in a disturbance of liver enzyme patterns and in certain clinical aspects (Trapnell, 1972), but these do not have any impact on treatment in the critical early stage of the illness. Enzymic release does, however, affect the lungs immediately and insidiously. The mechanism is not at all clear but it would appear that there is a primary effect on the alveoli themselves with an alteration in pulmonary compliance and resistance and an increase in total pulmonary water content (Ranson *et al.*, 1974). There is also an element of pulmonary hypertension (Halmagyi *et al.*, 1974). In clinical terms these changes are very important for it is now recognised that in many patients with acute pancreatitis, there is a marked, and at the same time often a totally unexpected, fall in the arterial oxygen tension in the first 12 to 24 hours of the illness. The degree of fall does not correlate fully with the patient's clinical condition and these changes occur in the absence of any radiological alteration of the chest film. Certainly PO_2 levels should be measured in all cases of acute pancreatitis on admission, for urgent corrective action may be required even in a patient whose breathing is *apparently* quite normal.

The syndrome of 'enzymic shock' also produces a direct effect on the kidneys. Renal failure is a well recognised complication of acute pancreatitis (Gordon and Calne, 1972). Originally it was thought that this resulted purely from hypovolaemia. It then began to be apparent that there was a renal as well as a pre-renal element and quite recently Werner and his colleagues (1974) in a well designed clinical study have demonstrated a local pressor mechanism which produces an alteration in renal blood flow and glomerular filtration rate.

A small percentage of patients with acute pancreatitis develop an acute confusional state usually within 24–48 h of the onset of their illness. This lasts for two to three days and then subsides, the patients usually being fully reorientated within five days of the onset of the illness. A clinical study of a group of such cases did not reveal any evidence of any previous or subsequent psychiatric illness (Trapnell, 1972) and it has therefore been concluded that this confusion may be regarded as a form of toxic psychosis. Much more rarely the condition of 'pancreatic encephalopathy' may develop (Sharf and Bental, 1969). This complication has only been diagnosed at autopsy and is apparently due to a lipolytic demyelinisation of the central nervous system. It has been postulated that lipase may be combining with the proteolytic enzymes to produce the central nervous system damage.

In summary then, it is clear that acute pancreatitis can produce a multi-systems failure and the disease should no longer be regarded as one simply localised to a gland in the retro-peritoneum.

TREATMENT

An understanding of this concept of 'enzymic shock' in acute pancreatitis and the pathophysiological changes which result from it have led to a number of advances in the routine management of this condition. These will now be considered under three headings.

1. Supportive treatment

The general principles of the conservative management of acute pancreatitis are now well recognised. The first and most important step which should be undertaken is the massive replacement of lost fluid. An intravenous infusion should be set up and large amounts of saline, plasma and, in the later stages of the illness, blood will be required. In order that this fluid can be given rapidly, the rate of infusion should be monitored by the measurement of central venous pressure (C.V.P.) and it is now mandatory to insert a C.V.P. line in all patients with acute pancreatitis. In the mildest cases, there will be a deficit of 2 litres while in a severe episode as much as 6 to 8 litres or more may be lost from the extracellular compartment.

In addition to the replacement of fluid, minerals are also required and these may be given intravenously. The need for sodium, potassium and chloride is well recognised. The importance of magnesium is less certain. A deficiency has been described in acute pancreatitis (Feller *et al.*, 1974) but the symptoms of this syndrome are not at all clear. However, with a severe or long standing attack of pancreatitis, magnesium supplements should perhaps be administered later in the illness. In contrast, to this rather uncertain area of our knowledge, the need for calcium supplements is clear cut. It is well recognised that a fall in the calcium level occurs in all cases of acute pancreatitis – and at times this may be profound and of grave prognostic significance. This loss is due to some extent to colloid leakage from the intravascular compartment but a much greater proportion is 'mopped up' by fatty acids which have been released following lipolysis. This trend must be monitored by daily estimations of the serum levels because it is clinically important and tetany can occur. Calcium gluconate is generally required in a dosage of 20–40 ml 10% calcium gluconate (5.0–10.0 mmol/Ca^{++}) given intravenously daily until the serum level is 2.0 mmol/l or above.

Some patients may also require intravenous nutrition. This is particularly important either when ileus persists for more than five to seven days, or in the patient who is already malnourished before an episode of acute pancreatitis. This is typically the case in the chronic alcoholic. It cannot be stressed too strongly that in acute pancreatitis there is not only loss of fluid, but also of protein and it is for this reason that this condition has aptly been described as a 'pancreatic burn'.

On theoretical grounds it is rational to advocate not only an intensive management of fluid loss in all its aspects but also some attempt to support the 'pump' too. 'Enzymic shock' produces myocardial depression and for this reason patients should be digitalised, especially if they are in the older age group.

A naso-gastric tube is also passed. It has been stated that the main value of this form of treatment is that by keeping the stomach empty the passage of gastric contents into the duodenum is prevented and so the duodenal release of secretin is inhibited. In fact, this is probably not important because, from all experimental evidence, the pancreas is fully 'shut down' during the acute stage of the illness (Dreiling, 1961). The main benefit from regular gastric aspiration accrues from relief of the vomiting and retching which can be so very distressing to the patient.

The relief of pain is also of critical importance. The amount of analgesia which will be required depends more on the patient's pain threshold than on the severity of the disease. Severe pain is a cardinal feature of the illness and it is now our practice to control this with small doses of intravenous heroin in a fashion similar to that used in the management of ischaemic cardiac pain. It has been suggested that epidural anaesthesia may have a place in this particular aspect of treatment. We have no experience of this ourselves but the method has been used in certain centres, particularly in North America (Feller et al., 1974).

The use of steroids has also been fashionable in the treatment of acute pancreatitis but there is no evidence that they convey any benefit and it is our view that these drugs are absolutely contraindicated for they may be dangerous. Steroids may mask the clinical signs of hypovolaemia. The attending physician is therefore lulled into a false sense of security for he is not able to appreciate the patient's real need, which is for fluid.

2. Preventive treatment

It has been traditional in the treatment of acute pancreatitis to give a full course of antibiotics and anti-cholinergics in all cases. However, neither of these forms of treatment has ever been subjected to any form of proper assessment and there is no evidence that either is beneficial. The regular use of anti-cholinergics is being discontinued in many centres. Antibiotics are indicated in the patient with chest complications or if an acute cholecystitis is suspected; if they are given it should be remembered that they will not prevent retroperitoneal abscess formation later in the course of the acute illness in a severe case where there has been wide-spread tissue destruction.

Oxygen via a humidifier at the appropriate oxygen percentage will be required in approximately one third of patients with acute pancreatitis. Studies by Imrie in Glasgow (1976) have shown that a PO_2 below 8.0 kPa (60 mm Hg) is critical and that if this cannot be raised to above 10–10.7 kPa (75–80 mm Hg) then intubation and positive pressure respiration should be considered. It should again be stressed that these low arterial oxygen tensions may be present with a normal chest X-ray and are often seen in patients without any respiratory embarrassment who are apparently in good general condition.

In spite of the fact that patients with acute pancreatitis are hypovolaemic, it is now the practice in a number of centres to administer a diuretic. The theoretical rationale for this is based on the specific alterations in renal blood flow and glomerular filtration rate already discussed. Frusemide is particularly indicated, not only because of its direct effect on the kidney, but also because there is some evidence that it is beneficial in reducing pulmonary water content in the shock lung state. It is our practice to give 80 mg frusemide twice daily until the patient's condition is fully stable and clearly improving. It is, however, clearly important if this drug is to be given in this way that hypovolaemia must be fully corrected, and therefore the C.V.P. must be maintained within the normal range. The combination of adequate fluid replacement plus a diuretic should go far to prevent the development of renal failure in these patients.

Finally, it has been suggested that glucagon may be beneficial in cases of acute pancreatitis. The inhibitory effect of glucagon on the pancreas has been recognised for some time and it has been suggested that this inhibition of pancreatic secretion will rest the gland. Condon *et al.* (1973) reported a dramatic clinical improvement in a series of 30 patients with only two deaths. As this mortality was 7% as compared with a prevalent figure of 20% in other much larger series, they concluded that the difference was important and that this was due to the treatment given. Their report is certainly most interesting and stimulating but unfortunately there was no control group in their study and in addition the authors did not say how many of their patients were suffering from recurrent acute or chronic relapsing pancreatitis with its very different and much reduced mortality. Certainly glucagon does have a physiological effect on pancreatic secretion but there are some theoretical objections to this very simple explanation of its effectiveness in acute pancreatitis. Not only has it been well shown that the pancreas shuts down at the onset of an attack of acute pancreatitis but there is also a considerable release of endogenous glucagon at this time (Paloyan *et al.*, 1967), which forms part of the general response to shock. However, glucagon in addition to suppressing pancreatic secretion also increases coeliac blood flow and this could be highly beneficial in acute pancreatitis as will be discussed in the next section. The use of glucagon in the treatment of acute pancreatitis has been taken up enthusiastically in Great Britain but with very conflicting results. Its role is currently being assessed on a double blind basis by the Medical Research Council (Welbourne and Cox, 1974) and the findings of this study are awaited with interest. The dosage recommended is 2 mg initially followed by 2 mg given as a continuous infusion 6 hourly for five days. Glucagon may cause a depression of the blood glucose which should therefore be monitored daily.

3. Specific treatment

When we return to consider the specific treatment of enzymic shock there are four main ways in which the problem may be tackled. In general terms an antidote to the 'witches brew' may be given – an anti-enzyme: the pancreatic collection may be diluted and dissipated so that the body's own defence mechanisms may have a chance to prevent a local build-up: the poison may be artificially washed away or finally the factory making it may be removed. Each of these approaches will now be discussed.

Anti-enzymes

The kallikrein and trypsin inhibitor Trasylol which is derived from the bovine parotid gland was first introduced into clinical practice in 1958. In the early 1960s there were many enthusiastic reports of its effectiveness, mainly in the German literature. However, during the latter half of the 1960s serious doubts about the effectiveness of this form of treatment were raised and it began to fall into disuse, so that by 1972 Trapnell, among others, had concluded that this form of treatment was 'of little proven value in the treatment of acute pancreatitis'. However, a full trial of the use of this drug was commenced in 1967 on a strict protocol. It was completed in 1973 and the results were published recently (Trapnell et al., 1974). In a double blind study of 105 patients there was a significant improvement in the mortality when Trasylol was used. This difference was even more marked in the sub-group of patients over the age of 50. The findings of this trial are at variance with many other reports but in a critical review of the literature Trapnell and co-workers have concluded that these other studies did not provide sufficient data to support some of the conclusions which had been drawn. Certainly no drug should be finally accepted on the basis of just one report, and their findings (Trapnell et al., 1974) is being re-checked by the Medical Research Council (Welbourne and Cox, 1974). In the light of this new evidence it would seem that Trasylol should now be used for the treatment of acute pancreatitis until it is proved to be ineffective. The drug is given intravenously by a continuous infusion. The present recommended dose is 300 000 units as a bolus statim and then 300 000 units 6 hourly for five days (total dose 6 300 000 units). The Trasylol may be added to the general infusion fluid and need not be divided so that the concentration is constant in each vacuolitre but it is advised that there should be some enzyme inhibitor in each bottle.

As Trasylol is a protein, sensitivity reactions can occur with repeated courses of treatment and therefore a skin test should be performed on every patient who has received the drug on a previous occasion. However, this situation should not arise very often for the prognosis of recurrent acute pancreatitis is quite different from the first attack. The mortality is very low – around 1% (Trapnell and Duncan, 1975) – and therefore the use of Trasylol is rarely indicated, in this situation.

Maintenance of the micro-circulation
It has already been suggested that if a build-up of concentration of the enzymic broth can be prevented by dissipation, then the damage that it produces will be diminished. One of the first effects of enzymic release in acute pancreatitis is on the local micro-circulation. There is first stasis and then the formation of micro-thrombi resulting in ischaemia and local tissue necrosis. The importance of the maintenance of the micro-circulation in this condition has been stressed by Goodhead (1969). He suggested that low molecular weight dextran might be beneficial

because of its anti-sludging effect. However, it is now recognised that this particular form of treatment is not only ineffective but may be harmful. In acute pancreatitis, because there is an increase in tissue permeability, the low molecular weight dextran while it may prevent sludging is readily extravasated from the intravascular compartment into the tissue spaces taking fluid with it and so increasing the oedema which is a feature of this condition. An alternative approach is to attempt to increase pancreatic blood flow. Glucagon has just this effect and if studies currently in progress show that this drug is beneficial in the treatment of acute pancreatitis, then it may be that it is this action which conveys the benefit rather than an inhibition of pancreatic secretion.

Peritoneal dialysis

Peritoneal dialysis is certainly theoretically attractive because it allows removal of the enzyme rich broth from the vicinity of the gland. A number of reports of the use of this treatment in a small series of cases have appeared in the literature recently (Rosato *et al.*, 1973) and Slavotinek (1975) has recommended that the dialysis catheters should be placed in the lesser sac to allow perfusion of the surface of the gland. In studies performed in Adelaide and Seattle, free active trypsin has been demonstrated in the dialysate (Slavotinek, 1975). Clearly placement of catheters in this exact fashion will only be possible if a laparotomy has been performed. Otherwise general peritoneal dialysis may be set up in the usual fashion; it is now recommended that Trasylol should be added to the dialysing fluid in a dose of 200 000 units per litre.

Pancreatectomy

Finally, if the enzymes cannot be counteracted or washed away then the gland which is producing them should theoretically be excised. On this basis immediate sub-total pancreatectomy has been recommended and indeed it is being practised in a few centres (Hollander *et al.*, 1971; Rives and Laudennois, 1974). Once again experience of this form of treatment is very limited and it will be a number of years before any firm assessment of this major undertaking can be made.

CONCLUSION

A summary of the management of acute pancreatitis is shown in Table 2. In deciding which of these various forms of treatment should be instituted the clinician is faced with the real difficulty that there is at

Table 2. Summary of management of acute pancreatitis

All cases	Additional treatment	Indications
I.v. fluids according to the central venous pressure	Oxygen	$PaO_2 < 9.3$ kPa (70 mm Hg)
	Digitalis	Patient >65 years
Analgesics	Antibiotics	Chest infection and/or cholecystitis
Continuous naso-gastric suction	Intravenous calcium gluconate	Serum Ca^{++} <2.0 mmol/l
Trasylol	Intravenous nutrition	Ileus >5 days
	Peritoneal dialysis	Failure to respond to resuscitation within 24 h
	Frusemide (observe central venous pressure and serum potassium levels)	$PaO_2 < 9.3$ kPa (70 mm Hg) P.C.V. $>40\%$

present no reliable method of establishing a prognosis at the outset of an attack of acute pancreatitis. It is therefore impossible to decide which patient merely requires adequate fluid replacement and little else, and which one is doomed unless immediate pancreatectomy is performed. In the last instance, the decision is particularly critical for a major resection is a major undertaking, not only with a short-term risk but with a considerable long-term morbidity as well, and in the majority of cases it will be clearly unnecessary for full recovery will take place without resort to such a drastic measure.

Striking a balance in this unsatisfactory situation is always difficult but clearly it is right that all patients should have the benefit of the general supportive and preventive measures which have been outlined. Trasylol should also be given, while the value of glucagon should be clarified shortly. While surgical resection may indeed be life-saving in a few cases, it does not seem right that it should come into general use in the treatment of this condition until the patients who actually need it can be identified more clearly. On the other hand, peritoneal dialysis is less invasive and could well be employed much more frequently than at present.

REFERENCES

Condon, J. R., Knight, M. and Day, J. L. (1973). Glucagon therapy in acute pancreatitis. Brit. J. Surg. **60**, 509.

Dreiling, D. A. (1961). The pathological physiology of pancreatic inflammation. *J. Amer. Med. Ass.* **175**, 183.

Feller, J. H., Brown, R. A., Toussenit, G. P. M. and Thompson, A. G. (1974). Changing methods in the treatment of severe acute pancreatitis. *Am. J. Surg.* **127**, 196.

Goodhead, B. (1969). Vascular factors in the pathogenesis of acute haemorrhagic pancreatitis. *Ann. roy. Coll. Surg. Eng.* **45**, 80.

Gordon, D. and Calne, R. Y. (1972). Renal failure in acute pancreatitis. *Brit. Med. J.* **3**, 801.

Halmagyi, D. F. U., Karis, J. H., Stenning, F. G. and Varga, D. (1974). Pulmonary hypertension in acute haemorrhagic pancreatitis. *Surgery* **76**, 637.

Hollander, L. F., Gillet, M. and Kohler, J. J. (1971). Urgent pancreatectomy in acute pancreatitis. *Langenbecks Arch. Chir.* **328**, 314.

Imrie, C. W. (1976). Personal communication.

Kitamura, O., Ozawa, K. and Honjo, I. (1973). Alterations of liver metabolism associated with experimental acute pancreatitis. *Am. J. Surg.* **126**, 379.

Kwaan, H. C., Anderson, M. C. and Gramatica, L. (1971). A study of pancreatic enzymes as a factor in the pathogenesis of disseminated intravascular coagulation during acute pancreatitis. *Surgery* **69**, 663.

Lefer, A. M., Glenn, T. M., O'Neill, T. J., Lovett, W. M., Geissinger, W. T. and Wangensteen, S. L. (1971). Inotropic influences of endogenous peptides in experimental haemorrhagic pancreatitis. *Surgery* **69**, 220.

Paloyan, E., Paloyan, D. and Haper, P. V. (1967). The role of glucagon hypersecretion in the relationship of pancreatitis and hyperparathyroidism. *Surgery* **62**, 167.

Ranson, J. H. C., Turner, J. W., Roses, D. F., Rifkind, K. A. and Spencer, F. C. (1974). Respiratory complications of acute pancreatitis. *Ann. Surg.* **179**, 557.

Rives, J. and Lardennois, B. (1974). La therapeutique d'assechement dans le traitement des pancreatites argues necroticohemorrhagiques, *J. Chir.* (Paris) **107**, 249.

Rosato, E. F., Mullis, W. F. and Rosato, F. E. (1973). Peritoneal lavage therapy in haemorrhagic pancreatitis. *Surgery* **74**, 106.

Sankaran, S., Lucas, C. E. and Walt, A. J. (1974). Transient hypertension with acute pancreatitis. *Surg. Gynec. Obstet.* **138**, 235.

Sharf, B. and Bental, E. (1971). Pancreatic encephalopathy. *J. Neural. Neurosurg. Psychiat.* **34**, 357.

Slavotinek, A. (1975). Communication to European Pancreatic Club.

Trapnell, J. E. (1972). Natural history and management of acute pancreatitis. *Clin. Gastroent.* **1**, 127.

Trapnell, J. E., Rigby, C. C., Talbot, C. H. and Duncan, E. H. L. (1974). A controlled trial of trasylol in the treatment of acute pancreatitis. *Brit. J. Surg.* **61**, 177.

Trapnell, J. E. and Duncan, E. H. L. (1975). Incidence patterns in acute pancreatitis. *Brit. Med. J.* **2**, 179.

Welbourne, R. B. and Cox, A. G. (1974). Glucagon therapy in acute pancreatitis. *Brit. Med. J.* **1**, 244.

Werner, M. H., Hayes, D. F., Lucas, C. E. and Rosenberg, K. K. (1974). Renal vasoconstriction in association with acute pancreatitis. *Amer. J. Surg.* **127**, 185.

X

The Management of Some Neurological Problems

J. M. K. Spalding

Many neurological problems are dealt with elsewhere, including head injuries (p. 398), spinal cord injuries (p. 412), meningitis, encephalitis and raised intracranial pressure (p. 484), and tetanus (p. 491). The present chapter is mainly concerned with life-threatening effects of paralysis, and in particular with the management of patients who have respiratory difficulties due to paralysing diseases.

Paralysis may threaten the life of the patient because it affects either respiratory muscles or those of swallowing. The cause of the paralysis may be important as it may affect ethical decisions. It is hardly ever ethical to ventilate a patient with a progressive paralysing disease such as motor neurone disease, but often the diagnosis may not be certain at the time when action has to be taken and the patient should then be given the benefit of the doubt.

RESPIRATORY MUSCLE WEAKNESS

Recognition and treatment

If a patient with progressive paralysing disease is allowed to develop so much respiratory paralysis that he is unable to ventilate adequately, the effects of asphyxia rapidly combine with the original disease to cause increasing weakness and the patient may die before artificial ventilation is instituted. It is vital therefore to assess the strength of the respiratory muscles regularly so that progressive weakness can be detected and

691

precautions taken before underventilation occurs. The vital capacity is the important measurement. In a rapidly progressing disease such as acute idiopathic polyneuritis artificial respiration should be instituted if the vital capacity falls below one third to one quarter of normal. In respiratory failure from lung disease, blood gases are an important monitor, but they are not useful in paralysing disease as such, for they do not become abnormal until the weakness has already progressed to a dangerous stage. Their value in paralysing disease is to detect early complicating lung disease such as aspiration.

Muscle disease

Patients with *polymyositis* occasionally require artificial ventilation (Hewer *et al.*, 1968). In the younger age groups the prognosis is reasonably good, though in the elderly there is an increasing possibility that the polymyositis is a symptom of underlying carcinoma. Treatment with corticoids is important, and adequate dosage is essential, prednisolone 100 mg daily reducing to 5–15 mg daily over two to three months may be suitable (DeVere and Bradley, 1975). A.C.T.H. may also be used for immediate relief but is unsuitable in the long term, for treatment will probably be required for two or three years. In resistant cases intravenous methotrexate and oral cyclophosphamide have been used, but the advice of someone experienced in these muscle diseases should be sought for such patients. Before treatment is begun every effort should be made to establish the diagnosis firmly, including muscle biopsy, for treatment may make subsequent diagnosis very difficult. Ventilation of patients with muscular dystrophy is rarely ethically justified except where the condition is complicated by reversible pulmonary disease such as bronchopneumonia.

Disease of neuromuscular junction

Patients with *myasthenia gravis* may require extensive artificial ventilation. The ultimate prognosis is usually good but severe cases may need ventilating on several occasions over a number of years but may ultimately make a good recovery. When a myasthenic patient is admitted to hospital as an emergency he usually cannot swallow, so that the normal medication may need to be given parenterally. The anticholinesterase neostigmine is very imperfectly absorbed from the gastrointestinal trace and therefore the parenteral dose is much smaller than the oral dose. The factor varies from person to person but a working rule is that the parenteral dose should be one twentieth of the oral. For these purposes an oral dose of neostigmine 15 mg (prostigmine, 1 tablet) is regarded as equivalent to an oral dose of pyridostigmine 60 mg (Mestinon, 1 tablet). If there is doubt whether the patient is in a myasthenic or cholinergic crisis edrophonium chloride (Tensilon), a short-acting anticholinesterase, should be given intravenously, 2 mg followed if there is no reaction in 30 s by 8 mg. If there is an obvious response more neostigmine should be given, but if there is no response, or a doubtful one, it should not. Unless the crisis is fairly modest and the vital capacity over 1 litre, it may be safer to establish artificial ventilation first and then to adjust the anticholinesterase dosage and consider other forms of treatment. For the long-term management of anticholinesterases, and the possible use of atropine, corticoids and thymectomy advice should be sought from someone with experience in these problems.

If the thymus is to be removed it is useful to determine whether artificial respiration will be needed postoperatively so that the need for tracheostomy can be assessed. Indications that this is likely are a pre-operative vital capacity, with the patient on optimum anticholinesterase treatment, of less than two litres. In borderline patients, the presence of a thymoma, bulbar symptoms especially dysphagia, and age over 50 years may be indications for artificial ventilation. Usually the effect of thymectomy on anticholinesterase requirements is extremely gradual and therefore the pre-operative anticholinesterases, or their parenteral equivalent, should be continued postoperatively (Loach et al., 1975). Occasionally the patient becomes more sensitive to these drugs and if there is uncertainty about this an edrophonium test should be done.

Abnormalities of neuromuscular conduction also occur in the *myasthenic* syndrome (Lambert et al., 1956; Lambert et al., 1965). In this condition a myasthenic (fatigueable) type of weakness occurs usually in the proximal limb muscles, rather than the eyes, masseters and mouth as in myasthenia gravis, and there are characteristic electromyographic abnormalities. The weakness may respond for a time to anticholinesterases, but is almost always associated with an underlying neoplasm usually of the bronchus. Disorders of neuromuscular conduction can also occur in systemic lupus erythematosis. Artificial respiration is justified as a holding measure since steroid therapy may produce remarkable improvement.

Peripheral nerve disease
The commonest form of peripheral neuritis for which artificial respiration is required is *acute idiopathic polyneuritis* (Guillain-Barré

syndrome). It occurs at all ages, including young adults. Paralysis of voluntary movement may be complete but recovery is usually excellent. Paralysis may spread rapidly so that artificial respiration is required within a few days of the first symptom. Respiratory muscle power (vital capacity) and patency of the airway (swallowing) must therefore be assessed frequently. Most patients who require artificial respiration do so within three weeks of the first symptoms (Hewer *et al.*, 1968). Steroid treatment has been suggested on the basis that this form of polyneuritis is an autoimmune condition which may be suppressed by steroids. Occasionally there seems to be a good response, but comparison between treated and untreated groups has shown to the disadvantage of the treated group, either due to slower recovery or to complications of treatment (Hewer *et al.*, 1968; Eisen and Humphreys, 1974; Goodall *et al.*, 1974; Sliman, 1978). I do not use them routinely. The baroreceptor reflexes controlling blood pressure are dependent on the glosso-pharyngeal nerve as the afferent limb of the reflex arc and on the sympathetic nerves and the vagi as the efferent limb. Either limb may be affected in polyneuritis. There may be hypotension, irregular blood pressure or more rarely hypertension (Spalding and Smith, 1963). Orthostatic hypotension may occur so that when the patient is tilted head-up for physiotherapy to the chest the blood pressure may fall dangerously. In a badly paralysed patient this may go unnoticed if not looked for. Usually treatment by slight head-down tilt is satisfactory but plasma expanders are sometimes required. Nasogastric feeding is normally satisfactory and may have to be continued for some weeks; a small tube should be used to avoid the tendency to pull the nostril away from the upper lip. Dehydration should be avoided as it exacerbates any difficulties with circulatory control.

Polyneuropathy other than acute idiopathic polyneuritis may occur and require treatment with artificial ventilation. Peripheral nerves have so great a power of recovery that unless the cause of the neuropathy is known to be progressive as in malignant polyneuropathy, artificial ventilation should be given until the cause is found. This is sometimes a protracted process. Advice should be sought from someone with special knowledge of these diseases both on the diagnosis and the treatment. The polyneuropathy of acute porphyria should be suspected if there have been previous attacks, abdominal pain often severe enough to cause one or more negative laparotomies, hypertension and tachycardia, or discoloured urine – classically port wine in colour but often browner 'Bristol Milk' in appearance. If it is suspected, no drugs should be given until the position is clarified.

Spinal cord disease (for further details of the injuries see p. 413).

Acute life-threatening disturbances due to spinal cord lesions are usually the result of injuries to the cervical or upper thoracic spinal cord and occasionally to rapidly progressive myelitis. Life may be threatened by respiratory or circulatory problems. Lesions at this level of the spinal cord paralyse all or most of the intercostal muscles so that respiration has to be maintained by the diaphragm innervated by the phrenic nerve from about the C4 segment. Such a patient with healthy lungs ultimately develops a good respiratory reserve, being able voluntarily to hyperventilate until the arterial PCO_2 falls to about 2.9 kPa (22 mm Hg). In the acute stage however, and especially if the lungs have been damaged (either in the original injury or by inhalation of vomit or secretions), artificial ventilation may be required until the lungs are restored to health. If the level of the lesion is near the C4 segment, respiratory function (vital capacity and blood gases) should be carefully assessed. Sensory loss over the shoulders and weakness of the deltoids and biceps indicate C5 loss and raise doubts about C4. Partial involvement of C4 in the acute stage may be compatible with recovery of satisfactory respiratory function, due to recovery of function in the cord and to hypertrophy of the diaphragmatic muscle whose innervation has survived.

High spinal cord lesions cut off the sympathetic outflow (T1 to L2) from control by the brain. In the acute stage a patient with such a lesion is extremely liable to orthostatic hypotension. Even a few degrees of head-up tilt may be enough to drop the blood pressure to unacceptable levels, and it may be best to nurse the patient in a slightly head-down position. These patients are also liable to reflex bradycardia particularly in response to stimuli to the airway such as aspirating from the pharynx or through a tracheostomy (Dollfus and Frankel, 1965). Fatal bradycardia may occur in such patients receiving artificial respiration. Immediate treatment is cardiac massage and intravenous atropine (0.6 mg). Prophylactic treatment consists of prevention of hypoxia and if this is not possible, or successful, continuous atropinization (0.6 mg intramuscularly four hourly) (Frankel *et al.*, 1975).

Brain diseases and respiratory depressants

In vascular disease and in head injury affecting the brain stem, if spontaneous respiration ceases (and the airway is clear) the brain stem is commonly beyond recovery, and artificial ventilation is contraindicated unless there is some substantial form of immediate treatment available, such as removing an intracranial haematoma. In *encephalitis* it is often impossible to be sure what the prognosis will be and the patient should be artificially ventilated if spontaneous breathing ceases. Occasionally excellent results follow when the acute state was very unpromising. Encephalitis and its management is discussed in greater detail in Part 2, ch. IV, p. 489.

In *poisoning* with barbiturates and other respiratory depressants, the respiratory centre may be paralysed and artificial ventilation is indicated as soon as there is doubt about the adequacy of breathing. Cardiovascular control will also be paralysed and the blood pressure sometimes falls precipitously, especially when the patient is moved. The management of poisoning is discussed in greater detail in Part 2, ch. VI, p. 611.

In *status epilepticus* (recurrent fits without recovery of consciousness between them) respiratory function, though not paralysed, is disordered and its failure may be the cause of death. The best treatment is prompt control of the fits by continuing any previous anticonvulsant regime, parenterally if necessary, and adding the agent with whose use the doctor is most familiar, such as paraldehyde, diazepam (Valium), chlormethiazole (Heminevrin) or thiopentone (Pentothal) (Table 1). I prefer paraldehyde used as described. If control has not been achieved and the patient's ventilation or circulation is deteriorating artificial ventilation should be given. This will probably be through an endotracheal tube and special care must be taken to see that the tube is not bitten if a fit occurs. Often the restoration of a good oxygen supply to the brain arrests the fits. If not, they can be brought under control with one of the drugs mentioned, but while this is occurring it may be advisable to give the patient enough curare to weaken the fits though not enough to make them undetectable.

THE AIRWAY

In a patient with a paralysing disease the airway may become blocked because of paralysis affecting the upper airway, either because the patient may be unable to hold his tongue forward or because *difficulty in swallowing* leads to the contents of the mouth, whether saliva, food or vomit, entering the airway. If the possibility is not foreseen the obstruction may be sudden and disastrous. A patient with a paralysing disease who coughs when given water to drink is unable to protect his airway adequately. In such a case if the patient can breathe satisfactorily (as in occlusion of the posterior inferior cerebellar artery), he can often be treated by being nursed prone or semi-prone. Should

Table 1. Anticonvulsants in *status epilepticus* (doses for an average adult)

Drug and reference	Regime	Special problems
Paraldehyde (Whitty and Taylor, 1949)	1. Paraldehyde 10 ml injected into glutaei. 2. If fits continue, intravenous paraldehyde solution, graded according to fit frequency.[1] Dissolve paraldehyde 1 in 10 in physiological saline and give 25 ml solution (2.5 ml paraldehyde) each time the patient has a generalised fit, up to once every 20 min. Focal twitching alone, without interference with respiration, does not require a further dose.	Test plastic apparatus with neat paraldehyde to ensure that the apparatus is not dissolved.
Diazepam (Valium)	1. 10–15 mg by slow intravenous injection. 2. If fits continue, intravenous diazepam graded according to fit frequency.[1] 5.0 mg each time the patient has a generalised fit up to a maximum of about 200 mg daily.	Control not always maintained.
Chlormethiazole (Heminevrin) (Harvey *et al.*, 1975)	Constant intravenous infusion of 0.8% solution 60–90 ml solution per hour (480–720 mg/h).	Biological half-life only 46 min. Needs an infusion pump to maintain infusion rate constant.
Thiopentone (Pentothal)	1. Thiopentone as for induction of anaesthesia until the fit stops. 2. Intravenous infusion of thiopentone 1 g in 500 ml physiological saline run in as slowly as possible. Run it in fast if a fit occurs until the fit stops.	Short acting. Anaesthesia and toxicity (respiratory and circulatory) may occur with heavy dosage. Facilities to deal with it must be immediately available.

[1] Graded doses may be given conveniently with two drip sets connected to a common intravenous canula. One is an ordinary set to keep the canula patent with a slow infusion of, say, 'dextrose-saline'. The other is a paediatric set which includes a calibrated portion. This portion is filled to the required level to give the necessary dose which is run in each time a fit occurs.

this not keep the airway clear or should there be substantial weakness of the respiratory muscles, endotracheal intubation or a tracheostomy is indicated.

THE TANK RESPIRATOR

Occasionally artificial ventilation should be given with a tank respirator not with intermittent positive pressure ventilation. This is true mainly in people with chronic weakness of respiratory muscles from poliomyelitis, chronic polyneuritis or occasionally muscular dystrophy. Such a patient may have a vital capacity just enough to enable him to achieve a limited but satisfying range of activities. If he gets a lung infection he does not have the reserve of respiratory strength to breathe adequately. If an endotracheal tube or tracheostomy is used it may be difficult and perhaps dangerous to take it out when no longer required. In these circumstances a tank respirator is useful to keep the patient breathing so that he can get some rest and save his strength for coughing. With increasing age such a patient may find that he needs some respiratory help every day and a cuirass, pneumobelt or rocking bed may be the solution (Spalding and Smith, 1963; Goodfield and Spalding, 1976).

REFERENCES

DeVere, R. and Bradley, W. G. (1975). Polymyositis. Its presentation, morbidity and mortality. *Brain* **98**, 637.
Dollfus, P. and Frankel, H. L. (1965). Cardiovascular reflexes in tracheostomised tetraplegics. *Paraplegia* **2**, 227.
Eisen, A. and Humphreys, P. (1974). Guillain-Barré syndrome: a clinical and electrodiagnostic study of 25 cases. *Arch. Neurol.* **30**, 438.
Frankel, H. L., Mathias, C. J. and Spalding, J. M. K. (1975). Mechanisms of reflex cardiac arrest in tetraplegic patients. *Lancet* **2**, 1183.
Goodall, J. A. D., Kosmidis, J. C. and Geddes, A. M. (1974). Effect of corticosteroids on course of Guillain-Barré syndrome. *Lancet* **1**, 524.
Goodfield, R. N. and Spalding, J. M. K. (1976). 'A Nurse's Guide to Artificial Ventilation'. Edward Arnold, London.
Harvey, P. K. P., Higenbottam, T. W. and Loh, L. (1975). Chlormethiazole in treatment of *status epilepticus*. *Brit. Med. J.* **2**, 603.
Hewer, R. L., Hilton, P. J., Crampton Smith, A. and Spalding, J. M. K. (1968). Acute polyneuritis requiring artificial respiration. *Q.J.M.* **37**, 479.
Lambert, E. H., Eaton, L. M. and Rooke, E. D. (1956). Defect of neuromuscular conduction associated with malignant neoplasm. *Am. J. Physiol.* **187**, 612.
Lambert, E. H., Okihiro, M. and Rooke, E. D. (1965). 'Clinical Physiology of Neuromuscular Junction in Muscle' (Ed. W. M. Paul, E. E. Daniel, C. M. Kay and G. Moukton) p. 487. Pergamon Press, New York.

Loach, A. B., Young, A. C., Crampton Smith, A. and Spalding, J. M. K. (1975). Post operative management for thymectomy. *Brit. Med. J.* **1**, 309.

Sliman, N. A. (1978). Outbreak of Guillain-Barré syndrome associated with water pollution. *Brit. Med. J.* **1**, 751.

Spalding, J. M. K. and Crampton Smith, A. (1963). 'Clinical Practice and Physiology of Artificial Respiration'. Blackwells Scientific Publications, Oxford.

Whitty, C. W. M. and Taylor, Margaret (1949). Treatment of status epilepticus. *Lancet* **2**, 591.

XI

Obstetric Problems which may require Intensive Therapy

GILLIAN C. HANSON AND DAPHNE KAYTON

INTRODUCTION

The majority of obstetric emergencies are treated on the obstetric unit, the services of an intensive therapy unit being only required when either the problem is not immediately solved by appropriate therapy because of complications arising as a result of treatment, or when organ failure is sufficiently severe that support systems are indicated. No attempt is made here to deal with obstetric emergencies which can be safely treated in the obstetric unit, but with the present shortage of nursing personnel it is anticipated that a greater number of obstetric patients will be treated in the intensive therapy unit. An attempt will be made to stress the physiological changes which occur in pregnancy and hence the possible effects it may have in patient management. Various physiological changes take place during pregnancy which if not recognised may lead to misinterpretation of pathological and physio-logical indices. The physiological changes and alterations in bio-chemical and haematological data which occur during pregnancy are summarised by Barnes (1970a) and this is also an excellent reference for the management of medical disorders which may arise in obstetric practice.

The management of an obstetric crisis requires close co-operation between the obstetrician in charge of the case, the consultant in charge of the intensive therapy unit, and with any other consultant with particular expertise relating to the problem present. A severe obstetric crisis is rare and without adequate consultation and co-operation the mortality is likely to be high.

CARDIOVASCULAR EMERGENCIES IN OBSTETRIC PRACTICE

Introduction

In the normal patient cardiac output rises by up to 40 per cent in pregnancy – this increase starts early and most of this increase has occurred by the end of the first trimester. The rise in cardiac output is not due to extra blood to the uterus alone since there is simultaneous increase in flow to other organs, e.g. the kidneys (Sims and Krantz 1958). The rise in cardiac output is maintained until the end of labour and the risk of dying from cardiac failure increases as gestation continues after 36 weeks (D.H.S.S., 1975). Patients with cardiac disease are therefore very susceptible to the development of cardiac failure during pregnancy. In addition to the rise in cardiac output, other factors may increase this susceptibility. These factors include anaemia, hypertension, obesity, multiple pregnancy, thyroid disease and cardiac arrhythmias.

The changes in blood pressure that occur during pregnancy are reviewed by MacGillivray and workers (1969). The systolic and diastolic pressures fall to their lowest between the 16th and 24th weeks – the systolic falling by approximately 5 mm Hg and the diastolic pressure by 15–20 mm Hg. After 30 weeks, hypotension may develop in a certain number of patients in the supine position.

The aetiology of hypertension developing during pregnancy is uncertain. Homeostasis is undoubtedly affected. In normal pregnancy there is a progressive increase in plasma volume (700–1700 ml) and an increase in total exchangeable sodium (> 500 mmol towards term). A mild fall in serum sodium develops towards term because of haemodilution. In spite of the increase in total exchangeable sodium, pregnant women are much less able to withstand depletion of sodium (as with indiscriminate thiazide diuretic therapy). The hypertensive pregnant patient has smaller increases in total exchangeable sodium and plasma volume than normal (Chesley, 1972) except when there is a rapid rise in blood pressure when sodium and water retention may be marked. It is possible that widespread fibrin deposition in the capillaries of the kidneys, lungs and placenta may be an important factor in the aetiology of pre-eclampsia and eclampsia.

Superimposed on the haemodynamic alterations of pregnancy are those encountered during labour and delivery. Maternal posture has a significant effect, and from the data of Ueland and Hansen (1969a) cardiac output and stroke volume are maintained at higher levels between contractions when the patient is in the lateral recumbent position. Values during contraction are found to be similar whether the patient is in the lateral recumbent or supine position. Uterine contractions are also associated with other changes in haemodynamics. With each contraction as cardiac output increases, arterial blood pressure rises and there is reflex bradycardia, while simultaneously blood is redistributed to the upper half of the body at the expense of the lower part (Bieniarz et al., 1968). These changes are less marked in lateral recumbency than in the supine position.

Different methods of anaesthesia and delivery also produce haemodynamic changes which should be taken into account when deciding upon the method of delivery in a critically ill patient. Cardiac output between contractions increases progressively during labour in patients receiving local anaesthesia (paracervical or pudendal block), whereas those receiving a caudal anaesthetic show less increase during the second stage (Ueland et al., 1969b). The increase in cardiac output in patients delivered under local anaesthesia is thought to be due to pain and is associated with an increase in the pulse rate.

Delivery by Caesarean section at term before the onset of labour avoids the haemodynamic changes associated with labour but a major abdominal procedure with postoperative pain produces in itself increased demands on the circulation. A general anaesthetic in itself increases maternal morbidity. The rise in cardiac output during general anaesthesia can be obviated by the use of an epidural anaesthetic without adrenaline in the anaesthetic solution (Ueland, et al., 1972).

Epidural anaesthesia should not be used in the management of labour in a patient with cardiac disease without knowledge of the right atrial pressure prior to its use. Patients with severe mitral valve disease may benefit from an epidural anaesthetic if pulmonary oedema is imminent, venous return being decreased. Certain patients however, because of lack of cardiac compensation, may develop severe hypotension following its use. Not only may the mother suffer as a result but since maternal placental flow depends upon an adequate perfusion pressure, the foetus may suffer from hypoxia.

The cardiac output during general anaesthesia remains fairly stable except during intubation and extubation and in skilled hands many of these changes can be prevented (Ueland and Metcalfe, 1975). It is therefore clear that anaesthesia for an obstetric patient with cardiac disease requires the services of a skilled anaesthetist. During the second stage of labour central venous pressure and blood pressure rise during contractions and following delivery the pulse volume systolic pressure and central venous pressure rise almost immediately because of the increase in venous return.

Hendricks and Brenner (1970) reviewed the cardiovascular effects of uterine stimulants commonly used postpartum, and showed that ergometrine when given parenterally may produce transient hypertension which is clearly hazardous in a patient who is susceptible to the development of cardiac failure. Browning (1974) analysed the serious side effects which may arise during the use of ergometrine and recommended that it should not be used in hypertensive patients, particularly those with pre-eclampsia. The writer went so far as to suggest that because the drug may precipitate eclamptic convulsions (he also reported a cardiac arrest following its use) it should no longer be used in obstetrics. Clearly, ergometrine should not be used in any patient with cardiac disease or severe hypertension (blood pressure D.P. > 110 mm Hg) and should be used with extreme caution in patients with any degree of hypertension.

Syntocinon is known to exert an anti-diuretic effect and may produce water intoxication when infused in high concentrations for a prolonged period. Most of the cases reported have occurred in connection with its administration during saline-induced abortion, missed abortion and postpartum haemorrhage. This condition may be prevented by early recognition, serial observations of serum electrolytes and urine output and administration of syntocinon in an electrolyte solution as opposed to 5% dextrose (Laverson and Birnbaum, 1975). The commonest manifestation of water intoxication in these patients was a convulsive seizure. The diagnosis and management of water intoxication is discussed on p. 169. During induction of labour water intoxication is unlikely to occur, but clearly the anti-diuretic effect may be dangerous in a cardiac or toxaemic patient and can be prevented by the simultaneous use of a thiazide diuretic.

Oxytocic drugs when used at the time of delivery produce uterine contraction following which 300–500 ml of blood is returned to the circulation. This may precipitate acute pulmonary oedema in a patient with imminent cardiac failure. Sytocinon, however, should not be denied to a patient with mild valvular disease where the risks of a post-partum haemorrhage are greater than their use. The risk can be offset by intravenous frusemide 80 mg which should be given approximately 30 minutes beforehand. Thiazide diuretics should not be used if the serum potassium is less than 3.5 mmol/l.

Cardiac failure

Introduction

Heart disease is the principal non-obstetric cause of maternal death; the largest number of patients dying will have had pre-existing rheumatic heart disease and the immediate cause of death is acute congestive cardiac failure (Pack *et al.*, 1965). Other more rare causes of acute congestive cardiac failure include patients suffering from congenital heart disease (who may have undergone cardiac surgery), puerperal cardiomyopathy, myocardial infarction, constrictive or infective peri-carditis, hypertensive heart failure, or the onset of an acute cardiac dysrhythmia.

Acute pulmonary oedema may develop during pregnancy in a patient with preceding asymptomatic mitral stenosis. Precipitating factors include pulmonary embolism, acute onset of atrial fibrillation or flutter in a patient previously in sinus rhythm, infection (in particular pulmonary), excessive weight gain and the recurrence of rheumatic fever. Bacterial endocarditis affecting an abnormal valve whether congenital or acquired may also precipitate heart failure.

The management of heart failure before term

Chronic congestive cardiac failure in pregnancy has a much lower mortality than the onset of acute pulmonary oedema. Management should be similar to the treatment of cardiac failure in the non-pregnant patient and can generally be quite safely conducted on the wards. Delivery is planned to coincide with optimum improvement in the haemodynamic state.

Acute congestive cardiac failure developing in pregnancy is of serious import and is preferably treated in an I.T.U. Treatment should be similar to the routine management of acute cardiac failure, keeping in mind that the foetal outcome is closely related to the adequacy of placental oxygenation. It is therefore important to correct the precipitating factor as quickly as possible. The acute onset of atrial fibrillation or flutter can generally be brought under control with rapid digitalisation. Should the cardiac output and peripheral perfusion be poor in a patient with a cardiac dysrhythmia unrelated to rheumatic or congenital heart disease (e.g. myocardial infarction, cardiomyopathy, severe infection), d.c. cardioversion should be considered. It is wise before cardioversion to correct any acid base or potassium abnormalities (Part 1, ch. VII) and provided the clotting screen (prothrombin time, fibrinogen titre and platelets) is normal, to give heparin 10 000 units intravenously. Sodium citrate 15 ml (0.3 molar) should be given orally to neutralise the stomach contents (Lahiri *et al.*, 1973). Drainage of the stomach in a patient with a rapid cardiac dysrhythmia may produce a further deterioration in the cardiac output and is preferably avoided. Cardioversion should be performed 30 minutes after giving the intravenous heparin and oral sodium citrate, using intravenous diazepam as a sedative (provided delivery is not imminent), the anaesthetist preoxygenating the patient and carefully observing the airway prior to cardioversion. The patient should be premedicated on a bed or operating table (which can be tipped head-down) and facilities for suction and intubation must be available. The minimum number of Joules should be used starting at 20 and increasing by increments of 50. Should cardioversion not be successful at 120 J, the use of an antidysrhythmiac drug followed by d.c. shock should be considered. The foetal effects of these drugs is poorly documented but clearly in a desperate situation their use outweighs the possible dangers to the foetus which is greater from hypoxia than from the drug used. A β-adrenergic blocker should be avoided in patients with suspected myocardial damage, e.g. cardiomyopathy – the drug selected can be according to p. 41. Digitalis and quinidine can probably be used safely throughout pregnancy (Cabaniss, 1971) although digitoxin has been known to produce digitalis intoxication in the foetus (Blinick *et al.*, 1973). Phenytoin may be teratogenic if used during the first trimester (Yaffe, 1975) and if used long term the serum concentrations should be monitored and folic acid prescribed. β-Adrenergic blockers are known to cross the placenta and are definitely contraindicated towards term since the foetal heart rate and cardiac output may be impaired (Stirrat *et al.*, 1973).

The onset of acute heart failure prior to labour with no definite precipitating factor is a serious occurrence and generally requires oxygenation, intravenous opiates, diuretics, digitalisation, reduction of the venous return with rotating cuffs and/or venesection, hypotensive agents (should there be diastolic hypertension) and rarely cardiac surgery. Intravenous papaveretum must be titrated slowly intravenously, overdosage may lead to respiratory depression. Bradycardia is particularly likely to occur in the patient with a recent myocardial infarction and the dosage inducing adequate sedation can frequently be reduced by using intravenous haloperidol (2.5 mg). Diuretics can be given with safety during pregnancy – the pregnant patient appears particularly susceptible to hypokalaemia, and potassium monitoring is therefore important. It must be remembered that the serum sodium concentration decreases by 2–3 mmol/l and the serum potassium by 0.3 mmol/l during pregnancy.

Rotating cuffs are invaluable during the management of severe left ventricular failure, may prevent the necessity for venesection and should be continued until oxygenation has improved either through digitalisation, reversal of a rhythm abnormality or a diuresis. Venesection should not be deferred if response is poor following cuff rotation. Urgent haemoglobin and haematocrit estimation is essential if a high output failure due to anaemia is suspected. When the haemoglobin is 5.0 g/dl or less, venesection of 500–1000 ml should be performed replacing simultaneously with 2 units of packed cells. Packed cells should be given gradually over the subsequent 48 h in conjunction with diuretic therapy until the haemoglobin is restored to 7.0 g/dl.

Acute hypertensive cardiac failure requires exclusion of severe thyrotoxicosis, phaeochromocytoma, underlying renal disease or coarctation of the aorta. In severe thyrotoxicosis or phaeochromocytoma the blood pressure may be satisfactorily dropped with α and β-blockade (p. 714) whereas underlying renal disease or coarctation is best treated with intramuscular hydrallazine followed by oral hypotensive therapy (see p. 53). Severe hypertension related to essential hypertensive disease is most unusual in the mid-trimester. The foetus rarely survives if hypertension with left ventricular failure occurs during the first trimester.

Cardiac surgery is rarely considered during pregnancy and is associated with a high foetal mortality. A relative indication is the failure to maintain cardiac compensation under therapeutic conditions in a patient with valvular disease after the 16th–20th week. Foetal mortality in open heart surgery is about 33% (Zitnik et al., 1969) and, because of the possible detrimental effects on the foetus of open heart surgery during the first trimester, therapeutic abortion should be considered if open heart surgery is considered essential for maternal survival.

The management of congenital coarctation of the aorta during pregnancy is well reviewed by Goodwin (1961). A patient with simple coarctation associated with a high diastolic pressure and large gradient with poor perfusion below the narrowed segment should undergo surgery during the first seven months of pregnancy. When coarctation is accompanied by other cardiac lesions such as aortic valve disease, the prognosis is more serious and the incidence of congestive cardiac failure is increased. Congestive cardiac failure should be treated as mentioned previously remembering that left ventricular failure may be complicated by ischaemic disease; surgical referral is essential.

The management of acute heart failure near term

Severe heart failure near term often precipitates labour. The effects of uterine contraction and the consequences of delivery on cardiovascular function have been discussed on p. 703. These effects have to be taken into account when treating the patient with severe pulmonary oedema during labour and the mode of delivery should be decided by discussion between an anaesthetist, physician and obstetrician. Venous return during labour can be decreased by maintaining the patient on her back with the bed tilted foot-down. The utilisation of epidural anaesthesia for labour and delivery should be considered, vasodilatation in the lower limbs decreasing the circulating blood volume. The patient should receive 100% oxygen before and during epidural blockade and right atrial pressure should be monitored. Following epidural blockade the systolic blood pressure should not be allowed to fall below 90 mm Hg and any fall in the right atrial pressure associated with a rising pulse rate, falling pulse volume and falling systolic pressure is an indication to infuse 200 ml alliquots of P.P.F. until the systolic pressure is 90 mm or above.

Ancillary measures include oxygen via a face mask, adequate sedation, digitalis and/or antidysrhythmics (avoiding β-blockers because of the dangers to the baby), diuretics and occasionally positive pressure ventilation. Should the patient be orthopnoeic and centrally cyanosed (in spite of oxygen via a face mask), rotating cuffs should be introduced, followed by phlebotomy. At least 500 ml of blood should be removed prior to delivery and a wide bore cannula should be left *in situ* in preparation for a further phlebotomy after delivery of the placenta. Deterioration is common after delivery of the placenta – a P.P.H. of approximately 500 ml is therefore beneficial. Ergometrine must not be used but should the P.P.H. be excessive Syntocinon 2.5–5 units intramuscularly may be given. Recrudescence of pulmonary oedema following delivery may necessitate a further venesection of 500 ml and rotation of cuffs around all four limbs. The critical period is the first hour following delivery of the placenta – when intubation and ventilation may be necessary if the PaO_2 is low.

It is essential to have a paediatric team available to resuscitate the baby at the time of delivery, should the baby be small or premature.

Patients with underlying valvular disease should receive prophylactic antibiotics prior to delivery and for three days following delivery. The most satisfactory combination available (unless resistant organisms are suspected) is clindamycin and cephalosporin.

Following delivery, urinary output and renal function must be carefully observed.

Other rarer forms of acute biventricular failure developing during pregnancy are maternal cardiomyopathy (Rand *et al.*, 1975) and peripartum heart failure most commonly found in Nigerian women. The latter is probably hypertensive in origin – the blood pressure rising after resolution of the cardiac failure (Brockington, 1971).

Myocardial infarction developing during pregnancy is rare but may be precipitated by the efforts of labour and be complicated by left ventricular failure. It must be recalled that aortic valve disease or cardiac disease associated with a fixed low left ventricular output may be complicated by poor coronary perfusion, in particular during stress – such as labour (Hughes, 1975).

The diagnosis of bacterial endocarditis during pregnancy and the puerperium may be difficult – the initial manifestation may be cardiac failure in the presence of cardiac murmurs which were not detected at the beginning of pregnancy. The antibiotics to be used must be related to the organism isolated and the possible effects of long-term parenteral antibiotics on the foetus. Tetracyclines, chloramphenicol, sulphonamides, trimethoprim and amino glycosides, should not be used before delivery (Ashton, 1971). The penicillins appear to be safe in pregnancy but sensitisation to these and other drugs may occur *in utero* (Kelsey, 1965).

The management of severe hypertension, pre-eclampsia and eclampsia

The normal changes in blood pressure and homeostasis during pregnancy have already been discussed. Factors relating to the development of hypertension in pregnancy are described in a Lancet

Editorial (1975) and its management is discussed by Finnerty (1975). A phaeochromocytoma must be excluded (see p. 641). A rapid and profound rise in blood pressure with associated vascular complications should not often occur provided careful monitoring of the blood pressure and appropriate drug therapy is used (Finnerty, 1975). Eclampsia is one of the most dangerous conditions in obstetrics and carries with it a maternal mortality of 4 to 5% and a perinatal mortality of 15–20% (Editorial, 1974).

Michael (1973) has reported no case of eclampsia in 4100 consecutive booked deliveries in Western Australia since the introduction of diazoxide for the control of hypertensive crises in pregnancy.

Suggested methods of treatment of acute hypertension, pre-eclampsia and eclampsia are summarised in Table 1.

Table 1. Suggested methods of treatment for acute severe hypertension, pre-eclampsia and eclampsia
(For the management of hypertension related to phaeochromocytoma see p. 643)

A. *Rapid blood pressure reduction*
Method 1

Promethazine hydrochloride 12.5 mg
Chlorpromazine 12.5 mg $\Big\}$ i.v. stat.

then infusion of the 'lytic' cocktail at a rate adequate to produce sedation and control blood pressure *without* respiratory depression.

'Lytic' cocktail – Pethidine 100 mg
Chlorpromazine 50 mg $\Big\}$ added to 500 ml
Phenergan 50 mg $\;$ 5% dextrose

Method 2
Hydrallazine hydrochloride 20–40 mg given by slow intravenous injection, subsequent dosage can be given intramuscularly.
Do *not* use if pulse greater than 120/min.
Should pulse rate rise greater than 130/min after its use, titrate IV oxyprenolol 1–2 mg until pulse rate 120/min or less.
Right atrial pressure monitoring recommended.

Method 3
Method possibly preferable to 1 or 2 in patients with severe hypertension B.P. D.P. >110 mm.
Diazoxide 300 mg i.v. over 10 s (should the patient weigh over 90 kg give 5 mg/kg B.W.).
Monitor blood pressure initially until maximal fall has occurred (generally within 3 min) and until the blood pressure is steady (generally within 10 min).
Should the blood pressure not fall within 15 min, give diazoxide as a bolus in a dosage of 5 mg/kg B.W.
B.G. monitoring essential.

Table 1.—*Continued*

Sedation. No sedation achieved with Methods 2 and 3. Should sedation be required, give haloperidol 2.5 mg i.v. followed by papaveretum 10–20 mg titrated intravenously to produce adequate sedation without respiratory depression.

B. *Management of severe pre-eclampsia or eclampsia*

Method 1

Haloperidol and papaveretum i.v. (see above) followed by rectal Bromethol 0.075 m/kg B.W.
Bromethol must be freshly prepared.

Method 2

'Lytic' cocktail (see A, Method 1) in conjunction with intravenous diazoxide A, Method 3).

Method 3

The combination of intravenous diazoxide (A, Method 3) and intravenous chlormethiazole is probably the preferable combination in an extremely ill eclamptic where complications may arise and where rapid lightning of sedation for examination may be required.

Chlormethiazole. Initially 30–50 ml of 0.8% solution i.v. then infuse continuously so that the patient remains drowsy but rousable with a good cough reflex and adequate ventilation. Pulse rate may rise by approx. 10/min during its use but should remain at the same rate or fall during continuous infusion.

Should convulsions recur in spite of adequate sedation, use diazepam 5–10 mg, or clonazepam 1 mg i.v. slowly (observe the airway and adequacy of ventilation) and/or phenytoin sodium 125 mg intravenously. Diazepam or clonazepam *must not* be used as a continuous infusion because of the insidious onset of respiratory depression and danger of pulmonary aspiration.

In non-delivered patients once blood pressure under control for A.R.M. or Caesarean section.

Observations

Pulse rate.
Blood pressure and pulse pressure (see text).
Right atrial pressure.
Cerebral state.
Urine output – if <40 ml/h for a thiazide diuretic provided serum potassium normal.
U/P osmolality ratio (prior to diuretic therapy).
B.U. electrolytes.
Acid base status and blood gases.
B.G. >12 mmol/l for insulin.
Abdominal girth.

Artificial ventilation may be indicated if:

Multiple convulsions.
Convulsions following G.A. reversal after Caesarean section.
Acute left ventricular failure PaO_2 < 9 kPa (67.5 mm Hg) on oxygen via a face mask.

Table 1.—*Continued*

A thiazide diuretic should be considered if:
The patient is oedematous.
Syntocinon is going to be used.
The right atrial pressure is raised.

An acute hypertensive crisis in early pregnancy may, if rapidly controlled, be treated conservatively until the foetus is viable and thereby the foetal survival rate may be improved. If not treated, cerebral haemorrhage, dissecting aneurysm, myocardial infarction, acute cardiac failure, subcapsular rupture of the liver or renal failure may occur.

In late pregnancy the aims of treatment in the severe hypertensive crisis, severe pre-eclampsia and eclampsia are to reduce the blood pressure, prevent or control convulsions and to deliver a live infant if possible. The latter is achieved either by A.R.M. and Syntocinon infusion if a rapid labour is anticipated, or by Caesarean section which is becoming more extensively used. The treatment of these cases is generally conducted in an obstetric unit but if complications arise, the patient is probably more safely treated in an I.T.U. and should be transferred there following delivery.

The management of the acute hypertensive crisis in early pregnancy differs little from that in the non-pregnant patient. Treatment should aim at reducing the diastolic to 90 mm Hg or less and the systolic below 160 mm if possible (see Table 1A). A useful combination of drugs is intravenous diazoxide followed by intravenous haloperidol and papaveretum or the 'lytic' cocktail, in order to achieve adequate sedation. This method is, in our experience, the one of choice, since hydrallazine tends to produce a tachycardia and the lytic cocktail alone may not lower the blood pressure adequately unless given in a high dosage with the attendant risk of respiratory depression. Once the blood pressure has been controlled, and it has been decided to treat the patient conservatively, control may be continued with a hypotensive agent of the clinician's choice (e.g. debrisoquine or methyl dopa).

In the severe pre-eclamptic or eclamptic where early delivery is anticipated a variety of drugs or combination of drugs have been used (Table 1B). Rectal Bromethol is extremely efficacious in that blood pressure levels fall and excellent sedation is rapidly achieved, but suffers from the difficulty that it is not easily and quickly available. Should this not be available, a hypotensive such as intravenous diazoxide with a sedative such as continuous intravenous chlormethiazole, or the 'lytic' cocktail, may be used. The patient must be very carefully monitored, in view of the risk of respiratory depression. When using the 'lytic' cocktail in combination with diazoxide, lower doses than those required to induce hypotension are required because of the hypotensive effect of diazoxide.

The continuous infusion of diazepam, in our opinion, should be avoided unless the patient is in an intensive therapy unit – the onset of respiratory depression is insidious and pulmonary aspiration may occur (personal experience). Moreover, although the mother is the primary concern, the depressant effect of diazepam on the foetus should be remembered.

It is advisable, when using an intravenous hypotensive agent, to insert a central venous pressure line. A hypertensive crisis may be complicated by haemorrhage (e.g. rupture of an aneurysm along the coeliac axis, subcapsular rupture of the liver) and peripheral vasodilation in the presence of haemorrhage may produce fatal hypotension. Right atrial pressure monitoring should be commenced if at all possible prior to delivery so that appropriate volume replacement can be given. A thiazide diuretic should be used if the patient is oedematous, Syntocinon is to be used, or the right atrial pressure is raised. Epigastric pain is generally associated with haemorrhage beneath the liver capsule – serial observation of the abdominal girth is therefore important because of the danger of intraperitoneal haemorrhage. Pulse rate and blood pressure may be misleading should an intraperitoneal haemorrhage occur, since the pulse volume may fall but the diastolic pressure remain high (Browne *et al.*, 1975) – this may be further confused by the use of hypotensive agents. Chlormethiazole may increase the pulse rate (Wilson *et al.*, 1969). Right atrial pressure monitoring is therefore essential in the severe eclamptic, a sudden fall in the absence of overt blood loss suggests an intraperitoneal bleed – peritoneal tap may be diagnostic. A suspected intraperitoneal bleed is an absolute indication for laparotomy and appropriate surgery (Beecham *et al.*, 1974; Browne *et al.*, 1975). Continuous convulsions may be an indication for ventilation especially if complicating recovery from the anaesthetic for Caesarean section.

Eclampsia and pre-eclampsia may be complicated by disseminated intravascular coagulation; indeed, it has been suggested but not proven that this may be an important aetiological factor in toxaemia of pregnancy (Beecham *et al.*, 1974). Haematuria may be the first clinical sign of D.I.C. Heparin therapy should be considered but generally replacement of clotting factors is sufficient, D.I.C. resolving once the hypertension is controlled and the baby delivered. The changes in clotting factors during pregnancy are described on p. 722 and the treatment of D.I.C. is described on p. 723.

Congestive cardiac failure associated with prolonged coma may follow eclampsia and is associated with a poor prognosis.

Urine output and renal function must be observed carefully and should there be evidence of deterioration, renal dialysis may have to be considered. The indications for dialysis are similar to those in the non-pregnant patient – the baby preferably should be delivered prior to commencement. Insulin and dextrose may be required in order to prevent a dangerous rise in serum potassium during labour and the development of a respiratory acidosis must be avoided. The management of renal failure is described in Part 1, ch. IV.

The management of hypertension related to a phaeochromocytoma

All patients with hypertension in pregnancy should be screened for a phaeochromocytoma. This condition is characterised by an acute and severe rise in blood pressure during the first trimester of pregnancy. Phaeochromocytoma and pregnancy has been reviewed by Scheneker and Chowers (1971) and its emergency management is discussed on p. 643. In the total of 112 pregnancies associated with phaeochromocytoma, foetal wastage was 55% (Scheneker and Chowers, 1971). It has been shown that the blood levels of catecholamines are much lower in the cord than in the mother (Thiery *et al.*, 1967) but the foetus may be affected during a crisis. The maternal mortality of undiagnosed phaeochromocytoma is 58% and 17.3% if diagnosed and appropriately treated (Scheneker and Chowers, 1971).

The crisis should be treated with intravenous phentolamine and β-blockade – monitoring of right atrial pressure is essential in order to ensure an adequate circulating blood volume. It is recommended that even during pregnancy the tumour should be localised and removed. Should the foetus be considered viable, Caesarean section should be performed before X-rays are performed to confirm the site of the tumour. The mother should be prepared for operation with an appropriate dose of β-adrenergic blocker (propranolol) and blood pressure should be controlled with a phentolamine infusion (because of the prolonged effect of phenoxybenzamine and possible foetal effects). β-Blockade may produce bradycardia in the foetus but where the maternal mortality is so high, control of maternal pulse rate is essential.

ENDOCRINE CRISES AND PREGNANCY

Thyroid and adrenal disorders during pregnancy

The incidence of hyperthyroidism during pregnancy is about 0.75 per 1000 (Javert, 1940) and the incidence of hypothyroidism even less. The annual incidence of Addison's disease is 39 per million population and is therefore rarely encountered during pregnancy.

The chance of encountering an acute thyrotoxic or Addisonian crisis during pregnancy is extremely rare. The manifestations of hypopituitarism following postpartum pituitary necrosis are insidious and its management is unlikely to be the responsibility of an intensive therapy unit team.

Thyroid function tests are radically affected during pregnancy since thyroid-binding globulin (T.B.G.) is doubled and any test that measures binding (e.g. T_3 resin uptake) gives a result in the hyperthyroid range because of the increase in vacant binding sites. Multiplying the total T_4 by the resin uptake measurement gives the free thyroxine index (FT_4I) which remains normal throughout pregnancy (Goolden et al., 1967) and is therefore valuable in the diagnosis of thyrotoxicosis.

The adrenal cortex hypertrophies during pregnancy and increased amounts of free cortisol are found particularly in the last three months of pregnancy. The plasma cortisol level begins to rise in the third month of pregnancy and increases steadily until term. Cope and Black (1959) have shown that the mean cortisol production in the last month of production is 25 mg/day compared with 11 mg/day in non-pregnant women.

Thyrotoxic crisis in pregnancy

The authors have had no experience in treating this condition in pregnancy and no report has been found in the literature. Since the mortality is high it is likely that abortion would be precipitated and therefore treatment should be orientated towards saving the mother (see p. 632). Should the foetus survive the crisis, congenital goitre and hypothyroidism may develop subsequent to treatment of the mother with iodides (Bongiovanni et al., 1959). The use of β-adrenergic blockade to control maternal tachycardia in the mother may produce bradycardia in the foetus – but since T_3 and T_4 are known to cross the placenta (Dussault *et al.*, 1969), it is probable that the effect would be beneficial. Langer *et al.* (1974) have treated 4 pregnant thyrotoxic patients long term with propranolol – they found no adverse effect on the foetus or on labour. They suggested that this may be the treatment of choice when the patient's symptoms are sufficiently severe to warrant therapy. Following control of maternal thyrotoxicosis, serial observations of FT_4I are essential; should this fall, full doses of T_4 must be used in order to prevent hypothyroidism developing in the infant. At the time of delivery T_4 and FT_4I of the cord blood should be estimated so that foetal abnormalities may be quickly recognised. Neonatal thyrotoxicosis may be caused by the transplacental passage of thyroid-stimulating immunoglobulins (Ramsay, 1976).

Acute adrenal failure due to haemorrhage or thrombosis of the glands occasionally occurs during pregnancy. It can be a complication of pre-eclampsia or of shock following accidental or postpartum haemorrhage and may follow endotoxin shock, acute pyelonephritis or amniotic fluid embolism. Brudenell (1972) reported one case occurring in association with toxaemia of pregnancy. Abdominal pain and rigidity with absent foetal heart sounds and low blood pressure were the presenting symptoms. Massive adrenal haemorrhage was found at post-mortem.

Treatment should be similar to the non-pregnant patient, p. 640. Once the crisis has been appropriately treated, should the foetus be still alive, steroids should be reduced to a minimum because of the increased risk of congenital abnormalities in children whose mothers receive high doses of steroids during pregnancy (Popert, 1962).

Mothers suffering from adrenal insufficiency may require parenteral replacement therapy during the first trimester because of vomiting. Maintenance dosage is generally 25 mg cortisone daily with 9-α fluorohydrocortisone 0.05–0.1 mg daily. An adrenal crisis may be precipitated by failing to increase the steroid dosage during stress (e.g. labour or infection) in a known Addisonian patient, or in a patient who has been on high doses of steroids for some other condition (e.g. asthma, collagen disease). The management of the crisis due to phaeochromocytoma are described on p. 714 and Part 2, ch. VII, p. 643).

Diabetic ketoacidosis in Pregnancy

Diabetic ketoacidosis, sufficiently severe to warrant intensive therapy, should rarely arise unless the patient is an undiagnosed diabetic or is poorly controlled because of irregular clinic attendances and failure to adhere to advice.

Diabetic ketoacidosis may be precipitated in the first trimester because of poor dietary intake associated with increasing insulin demands secondary to pregnancy. Should serum sodium levels be raised because of dehydration from vomiting, it is important to use hypotonic solutions (1/5 normal saline) if the serum sodium is 145 mmol/l or greater. During the second and third trimesters the renal threshold for glucose may fall – urine glucose thus being an unreliable reflection of blood glucose. Patients with heavy glycosuria may lose up to 100 g of glucose per day in the urine (Essex, 1976); extra glucose should be added to the diet otherwise starvation ketoacidosis may develop.

The management of acute diabetic ketoacidosis during pregnancy is similar to the non-pregnant patient (p. 233), rapid restoration of the blood volume is important, the blood glucose should be lowered gradually by a constant insulin infusion. Glucose should be given once the blood glucose is 9 mmol/l or less. Because of the danger of hypocalcaemia in the infant, should the baby be delivered during or following a period of ketoacidosis, maternal monitoring of serum calcium is essential.

Severe diabetic ketoacidosis may induce abortion or precipitate labour. A paediatrician and anaesthetist must be present at delivery because of the increased incidence of respiratory distress, hypo-glycaemia and hypocalcaemia in the infant. The foetal mortality is very high.

GASTROINTESTINAL CRISES AND PREGNANCY

Ulcerative colitis and Crohn's disease

Fielding (1976) described the management of inflammatory bowel disease in pregnancy.

Patients who develop acute ulcerative colitis for the first time during pregnancy appear to be most at risk. The attack is generally in the first trimester and approximately 68% of patients (Crohn et al., 1956) are likely to have a severe attack. It would appear that the maternal mortality of 15% (Crohn et al., 1956) is little different from the mortality in a non-pregnant patient of 19% (Rice-Oxley and Truelove, 1950) in the first attack. Patients who develop ulcerative colitis for the first time in the puerperium are also at significant risk (Banks et al., 1957) since these attacks are generally severe.

Should the disease become active during pregnancy it should be treated similarly to the non-pregnant patient (see Part 2, ch. IX,

p. 671). Surgery should not be denied if there is an indication in spite of the risks of an increased foetal mortality. Georgy (1974) advises that should a fulminating attack of ulcerative colitis develop during the first trimester of pregnancy and continuation of pregnancy is highly desired, immediate subtotal colectomy and ileostomy should be performed. Should the pregnancy be unwanted, or there be evidence of emotional instability, therapeutic abortion should be considered.

Patients with quiescent Crohn's disease may go through pregnancy uneventfully. Martimbeau and co-workers (1975) reported two cases who developed Crohn's disease during pregnancy and reviewed 8 others reported in the English-language literature. The 10 pregnancies yielded 11 infants, six of whom died. They found that deterioration during pregnancy may require emergency surgery. A severe attack of Crohn's disease should therefore be treated as in the non-pregnant (Part 2, ch. IX, p. 676).

Acute pancreatitis

The management of acute pancreatitis is described on page 682. The mortality rate from acute pancreatitis during pregnancy is higher than in the non-pregnant, the overall maternal mortality being 37% (Wilkinson, 1973) compared to 3.1–6.6% in the non-pregnant patient under 50 years (Becker, 1954; Romer and Carey, 1966). Other factors of note is that maternal mortality is 9% higher in the primigravida than in the multigravida and perinatal mortality is 13.5% higher in the primigravida, the average foetal mortality being 34.6% (Wilkinson, 1973). Wilkinson (1973) showed a high maternal mortality when acute fatty liver of pregnancy was associated with pancreatitis. A high percentage of these patients had received tetracycline and it is possible that tetracycline is not only toxic to the liver but also to the pancreas. Tetracycline must never be used during pregnancy. Certain other features were associated with a high maternal mortality; these included pulmonary involvement, a white blood cell count above 22 000/mm³, anaemia, hypoglycaemia and hyperglycaemia (Wilkinson, 1973). A severe attack of acute pancreatitis in the third trimester in conjunction with these poor prognostic features, would suggest that termination of the pregnancy should be seriously considered. The foetal mortality is so high in such cases, that continued development *in utero* is unlikely. The management of acute pancreatitis is similar to the management in the non-pregnant patient. Laparotomy should be performed if the diagnosis is in doubt; this does not appear to increase maternal or foetal mortality (Wilkinson, 1973). Unfortunately peritoneal lavage, a valuable aspect of therapy, cannot be performed after 16 weeks and when conducted at less than 16 weeks may precipitate an abortion. Fluid volume and metabolic control and adequate oxygenation is essential in order to maintain adequate placental function. Trasylol may be used during pregnancy. A cholecystogram should be performed approximately 8 weeks after an acute attack of pancreatitis, in pregnancy this should be deferred until postpartum.

Acute surgical crisis during obstetrics

The diagnosis of an acute surgical emergency during obstetrics may be difficult – but when suspected and diagnosis uncertain, laparotomy should be performed early rather than late. Acute perforation due to peptic ulcer is rare in pregnancy. Acute gastric erosion with haematemesis may develop as a complication of eclampsia or pre-eclampsia (Langmade, 1956). The incidence of acute appendicitis in pregnancy is about one in 2500. The overall maternal mortality rate is about 9% the high mortality being related to delay in surgery because of an incorrect diagnosis and unwillingness to operate for fear of disturbing the pregnancy (Barnes, 1970b). Appendicitis developing after the seventh month increases the risk of peritonitis, probably because of upward displacement of the uterus and intermittent uterine contractions preventing localisation. Should an acute intra-abdominal surgical catastrophe develop near term, it may be necessary to deliver the baby by Caesarean section before proceeding to intra-abdominal surgery.

HAEMATOLOGICAL CRISES AND PREGNANCY

Introduction

Erythropoiesis is accelerated during pregnancy resulting in an increased number of circulating red blood cells, the red cell volume increasing gradually so that at term the volume is 20–33% above the non-pregnant value. Erythrocytes behave essentially the same as in the non-pregnant state. The markedly increased plasma volume and a definite but less increase in red cell volume, results in a slight drop in haematocrit and haemoglobin during the second trimester with a slight increase in the last month. A haemoglobin of less than 11.0 g/dl, or a haematocrit of less than 33% should be considered pathological until proven otherwise.

Anaemias and pregnancy

Iron deficiency anaemia is rarely encountered in pregnancy sufficiently severe to warrant intensive therapy. It must be remembered that these patients tolerate transfusion very poorly and it may precipitate left heart failure, in particular towards term.

An anaemia related to protein malnutrition and described in pregnant Nigerian women but occurring elsewhere (Woodruff, 1955) may deteriorate and present in late pregnancy. The condition characterised by hepatosplenomegaly, is refractory to haematinics and improves *pari passu* with the increase in serum albumin. The services of an I.T.U. are unlikely to be required unless the patient develops left ventricular failure from over enthusiastic blood transfusion.

Folate deficiency in pregnancy rarely requires intensive therapy. The patient may present with a pyrexia, severe anaemia and leucopenia complicated by thrombocytopenic purpura and sepsis, and such patients may be admitted to an intensive therapy unit.

Aplastic anaemia in pregnancy is rare and may be present before the pregnancy starts, or the pregnancy *per se* may produce bone marrow depression. The mother is particularly at risk from haemorrhage due to thrombocytopenia. The management of these patients is lucidly described by Messer (1974).

The haemolytic anaemias most commonly seen in pregnancy are those related to the haemoglobinopathies, see also Part 2, ch. VIII, p. 648. Inherited haemoglobinopathies may be classified into two types, (1) defective rate of synthesis of one or more of the polypeptide chains and (2) structural alterations in the haemoglobin molecule. The presence of the abnormal haemoglobin S results in the sickling phenomenon, and those persons homozygous for S are far more likely to manifest *in vivo* sickling and clinical symptoms than the heterozygotes where blood contains both HbS and HbA. While lowered oxygen tension is most directly responsible for sickling, other variables such as acidaemia and dehydration are known to play an important role. Erythrocytes with 100% HbS will sickle at oxygen tensions that can be found within the body tissues, while cells that contain both HbS and HbA will rarely sickle under physiological conditions. Other haemoglobin variants may produce sickling under physiological oxygen tensions, e.g. HbS with HbC or HbD. A high concentration of HbF within the red cell seems to protect against sickling. Intravascular sickling results in stasis of blood flow and increased erythrocyte destruction, the abnormal morphology of the sickled cells producing increased blood viscosity and microthrombosis. The stasis is further augmented by the onset of hypoxia and acidosis at the site of thrombosis.

Pregnancy in a patient with S/S disease is associated with a high perinatal mortality rate and increased incidence of maternal morbidity and mortality. The maternal mortality in S/S disease varies from 0–25% (Perkins, 1971) and is commonly complicated by a medical illness which may require admission to an intensive therapy unit. These include, pneumonia, urinary tract infection, pulmonary embolism, anaemia (which may be due to folate deficiency) and congestive cardiac failure. An emergency general anaesthetic for an obstetric complication may also warrant post-operative admission to an I.T.U.

The painful sickle cell crisis occurs in most patients during pregnancy, the frequency increasing as the pregnancy proceeds, and is particularly common during labour and in the puerperium.

Murdoch and Nathanson (1969) have reported the use of a partial exchange program in sickle cell disease. This necessitates the exchange of 1 to 2 units of blood at six week intervals starting at the third month of pregnancy. Work so far suggests that this technique may lower the foetal and maternal mortality rate.

The management of the sickle cell crisis is described on p. 649 and consists of rest, oxygen, hydration (if necessary) and analgesics. Sodium bicarbonate should be given (50 mmol HCO_3^-) if the base deficit is greater than 8. It is wise to use heparin during the last month of pregnancy should a crisis arise in order to prevent microthrombosis. Some authors have advised prophylactic antibiotics during a painful crisis, during labour and the puerperium (Hendrickse et al., 1972).

It is particularly important during management of a crisis to observe the serum uric acid, renal function, and the coagulation factors. The condition may be complicated by the onset of D.I.C., or in particular with haemoglobin S/C disease, the fat embolism syndrome. The use of oxytocin should be questioned in these patients since it may precipitate a crisis. The fat embolism syndrome has been successfully treated with exchange transfusion (Chmel and Bertles, 1975).

Caesarean section should be considered in a patient with S/S or S/C disease if labour is prolonged. Anaesthesia should be given with care, hypoxia should be avoided and blood loss kept to a minimum. The haematocrit should be maintained around 28% prior to delivery.

The thalassaemia syndromes are hereditary haemoglobinopathies caused by reduction in the rate of synthesis of one or more of the polypeptide chains of the globin portion of the haemoglobin molecule. These abnormalities affect the quantity produced rather than the structural quality of haemoglobin. These patients rarely require intensive therapy, generally presenting with severe anaemia, increasing during the second and third trimester, and frequently folate depletion.

Intravascular haemolysis has been reported following intra-amniotic mid-trimester abortion with hypertonic saline (Adachi *et al.*, 1975). Intravascular haemolysis (which may occur up to 46 h after instillation) may be associated with haemoglobinuria, hypotension and disseminated intravascular coagulation. The hypotension is generally related to volume depletion following blood loss and if prevented, renal failure and D.I.C. is unlikely to occur. The technique is now rarely used in this country.

HAEMORRHAGIC DISORDERS AND PREGNANCY

The investigation of a haemorrhagic disorder is described in detail in Part 2, ch. VIII, p. 650. The haemorrhagic disorders in pregnancy which may produce severe haemorrhage or be precipitated by some other disease include: idiopathic thrombocytopenic purpura, thrombocytopenia due to other causes (see Part 2, ch. VIII, p. 652, Table 5), hereditary deficiency of coagulation factors and disseminated intravascular coagulation.

Introduction

There are a variety of coagulation factors that increase during pregnancy: fibrinogen and factors II, VII, VIII, IX and X. only factor XIII seems to be slightly reduced (Coopland *et al.*, 1969) and platelets are normal. Fibrinogen begins to increase in the 20th–25th week of pregnancy and reaches its highest values at term. The fibrinolytic enzyme system is reduced. There have been a variety of coagulation studies during labour and delivery, and these have shown only minor fluctuations (Bonnar *et al.*, 1970). Fibrinolytic activity is decreased by lower activator activity and higher concentrations of plasma inhibitors and the clotting time is shortened. Fibrin degradation products are not present during normal gestation or delivery. It has been proposed that pregnancy is a condition where chronic D.I.C. exists, the placenta being the site for the consumptive process, and that D.I.C. may be one of the pathophysiological factors in pregnancy toxaemia (Page, 1972).

Idiopathic thrombocytopenic purpura (I.T.P.)

The incidence of I.T.P. is approximately three times greater in females than in males and since it is most frequently seen before the age of 20, I.T.P. and pregnancy may coexist. Untreated, the symptoms tend to worsen during pregnancy (Zilliacus, 1964) and it is possible that severe bleeding related to I.T.P. may necessitate I.T.U. care. Should the bleeding not be controlled with steroids (prednisone 40, 80 mg daily) and platelet infusions, splenectomy should be performed (Laros and Sweet, 1975). Platelet infusions should be given prior, during and after the splenectomy and adequate surgical homeostasis is essential. P.P.H. from the placental site is rarely a problem but severe haemorrhage can arise from vaginal or cervical lacerations. It is essential to prepare the patient for any operative intervention with platelets.

Thrombotic thrombocytopenic purpura (T.T.P.)

Although T.T.P. is rare, it may occur in women of child-bearing years. Anaemia, thrombocytopenia, neurological abnormalities, renal failure and fever are the classic manifestations. The peripheral film shows distortion and fragmentation of the red cells. The disease is invariably acute and is generally fatal. No patient during pregnancy has been known to survive without splenectomy (Barrett and Marshall, 1975) and this treatment should be combined with steroids and heparin (see Part 2, ch. VIII, p. 658).

Hereditary deficiency of coagulation factors

Patients with Von Willebrand's disease should be monitored carefully during pregnancy and if factor VIII levels are low at term, cryoprecipitate infusions are recommended and continued for several days postpartum (Flessa, 1974). Because of the rise in factor VIII during pregnancy, the patient with the haemophilia carrier state is unlikely to bleed, except postpartum when cryoprecipitate may be required. Aspirin should not be used in either of these bleeding diatheses since the inhibition effect on platelets may accentuate the bleeding tendency.

Disseminated intravascular coagulation (D.I.C.) and severe haemorrhage

Disseminated intravascular coagulation has been discussed in Part 2, ch. VIII, p. 654 and its management in relation to septicaemia is described in Part 2, ch. II, p. 364. The obstetrician is concerned with the acute forms of this phenomenon, which may arise in abruptio placentae, amniotic fluid embolism, saline termination of pregnancy, endotoxin and septic shock (see p. 735) and, rarely in a more chronic form, the dead foetus syndrome.

Coagulation defects in obstetrics most frequently follow premature separation of the placenta, usually normally sited. Pregnancy toxaemia is generally present. Severe haemorrhage from a placenta praevia may also be complicated by D.I.C. and in these cases there is frequently a history of bleeding in previous pregnancies. Blood replacement is imperative and should be preceded by taking blood for baseline clotting factors (see Part 2, ch. II, p. 365, Table 3). Severe ante-partum haemorrhage necessitates right atrial pressure monitoring, monitoring of urine output, pulse rate and blood pressure; and volume replacement as recommended in Part 2, ch. II, p. 341. Blood pressure is not a reliable indicator of hypovolaemia at term, falling late because of the physiological increase in blood volume. The blood pressure may also be high before bleeding occurs, falling to the normal range after haemorrhage. It is essential to replace labile clotting factors with F.F.P. Blood is unlikely to clot if the fibrinogen value is less than 100 mg/100 ml or the fibrinogen titre less than 1/64 – this should also be replaced with F.F.P. The platelet count is commonly low either from D.I.C. or old blood transfusion and rarely causes a clotting defect until 40 000/mm^2 or less. A haemorrhagic diathesis related to replacement with old blood is common in obstetric practice and can be differentiated from D.I.C. by the table illustrated in Part 2, ch. II, p. 365. Heparin is rarely required, labile clotting factors being replaced with F.F.P. and the haemoglobin defect with blood. Should the fibrinogen titre repeatedly fall after the use of F.F.P. and the thrombin time and P.T. remain prolonged with continued haemorrhage, heparin should be considered. Under such circumstances heparin should be given in a dosage of 50–100 units/kg B.W. intravenously stat then 10–15 units/kg B.W. hourly as a continuous infusion (lower dosage if the platelets less than 100 000/mm^2) and clotting factors replaced with fresh blood. Hysterectomy may be necessary if bleeding continues. The timing for hysterectomy is critical, a platelet count of less than 40 000/mm^3 necessitating preoperative preparation with fresh blood, platelet-enriched plasma or platelet packs, and fresh blood should be available for the operation. Operation should proceed once the fibrinogen titre has returned to 1/64 or more, and the thrombin time is less than 5 times normal. Blood volume if at all possible should be replaced pre-operatively and a urine output of greater than 40 ml/h established. Severe blood loss with massive replacement may be associated with a tachycardia unrelated to volume depletion. The cause for this is unknown and may be related to pyrogens or serotonins in the transfused blood. The tachycardia may be reduced (if greater than 140/min and therefore likely to compromise cardiac output) with cautious administration of a β-blocker.

The management of severe obstetric haemorrhage should be conducted along the lines suggested in Table 6, Part 2, ch. II, p. 350. Frequently these patients benefit from elective sedation, intubation and ventilation in order to reduce the oxygen demand for breathing, anxiety and pain.

Provided blood volume is replaced sufficiently rapidly and adequate oxygenation is maintained, metabolic problems and renal failure rarely arise. Rapid volume replacement in obstetric haemorrhage generally requires two peripheral vein drips – the central venous pressure line being used for clear fluids and right atrial pressure monitoring.

Dead foetus syndrome

This condition is less likely to be encountered since the syndrome is now well recognised and the uterus evacuated early. There appears to be a lapse of approximately 5 to 6 weeks between the intra-uterine death and the onset of the syndrome (Pritchard and Ratnoff, 1955). The mechanisms involved are still not clear but seem to be related to chronic activation of the coagulation system. The coagulation defect consists mainly of a decrease in plasma fibrinogen with an increase in degradation products and a decrease in factors V and VIII. The platelet count may remain normal.

Prevention by emptying the uterus is clearly the most important aspect of management. Should an intra-uterine death have occurred three or more weeks before the condition is diagnosed, it is wise to check the coagulation factors and should there be evidence of D.I.C. to use intravenous heparin for 24 hours prior to inducing labour or evacuating the uterus. Should the fibrinogen titre be 1/64 or less, then four packs of F.F.P. should be given whilst starting heparin therapy.

Frank haemorrhage in the presence of a dead foetus necessitates the use of intravenous heparin and F.F.P. as suggested in Part 2, ch. II, p. 366, Table 4. Platelets are rarely required.

Amniotic fluid embolism

This may be associated with D.I.C. This syndrome has been the topic for a number of review articles (Anderson, 1967; Sicuranza and Tisdall, 1975). Predisposing factors include strong uterine contractions, uterine stimulants, uterine trauma, multiparity and premature placental

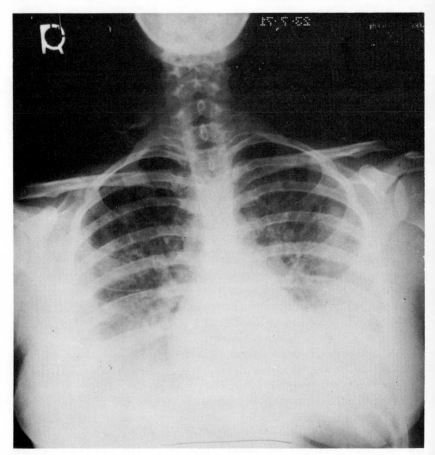

Fig. 1. Chest X-ray of a patient presumed to be suffering from amniotic fluid embolism. Admitted as an emergency following a septic abortion. Patient shocked, orthopnoeic and cyanosed on admission. No coagulation abnormality detected. Spontaneous resolution and steady clinical improvement over a period of 5 days. Treatment included volume replacement and antibiotics. *E. coli* isolated from the blood stream.

separation. The mortality is around 80%. The diagnosis is confirmed by the presence of foetal debris or meconium in the blood aspirated from the right side of the heart.

The clinical manifestations include the sudden onset of shock associated with respiratory distress, cyanosis and evidence of a bleeding tendency. The chest X-ray shows evidence of pulmonary oedema (Fig. 1) in the absence of any clinical evidence of left ventricular failure. The

Table 2. Summary of the management of the patient with suspected amniotic fluid embolism

---

Investigations
Astrup analysis
B.U. Electrolytes. B.G.
Blood culture
Culture of $\begin{cases} \text{placenta} \\ \text{H.V.S.} \\ \text{urine} \end{cases}$
Chest X-ray
Clotting factors (P.T. thrombin time. Fibrinogen titre)
Hb. W.B.C. and diff. Platelets.

Treatment
Insert central venous pressure line and record right atrial pressure (R.A.P.).
R.A.P. > 12 cm H_2O insert thermodilution catheter to measure cardiac output (see Part 2, ch. II, p. 322).
R.A.P. < 10 cm H_2O increase blood volume with appropriate fluid (fresh blood if patient bleeding and P.C.V. < 30%).

Do not use blood <3 days old without filtration

Fibrinogen titre < 1/64 or T.T. or P.T. prolonged give F.F.P.
Intubate and ventilate if PaO_2 < 9.3 kPa (70 mm Hg) on high flow oxygen via a face mask. *Avoid pulmonary aspiration if at all possible.*
Achieve optimum ventilation as recommended in Part 2, ch. V, p. 552.

Drugs
Heparin 50–100 units/kg B.W. i.v. stat then 10–15 units/kg B.W. hourly as continuous infusion (lower dosage if platelet count < 100 000/mm²) Trasylol.
Antibiotics – cephalothin or cephaloridine i.v. and clindamycin i.v.

---

management of a patient suffering from amniotic fluid embolism is summarised in Table 2.

The pathophysiology is considered to be related to the mechanical blockage of the pulmonary circulation, activation of D.I.C. and possible activation of the kinin system and release of serotonin and other vasoactive peptides.

Should the condition be suspected, blood should be taken for clotting factors, acid base and blood gas studies, urea, electrolytes, blood glucose and blood cultures. A right atrial line should be inserted as soon as possible and if severe shock is present, insertion of a thermodilution Swann Ganz catheter should be considered for measurement of cardiac output. Cardiac output monitoring is certainly indicated if the systolic blood pressure is 90 mm or less in the presence of a high right atrial pressure and deteriorating lung function necessitating pulmonary ventilation. Ventilatory management should be based on the management of the shock lung syndrome described in Part 2, ch. V, p. 552. Evidence of a low platelet count less than 100 000³ and a fibrinogen titre 1/64 or less, is an indication to start heparin therapy. Heparin therapy should be started early since it is probable that D.I.C. has an important part to play in pulmonary failure. Trasylol, a proteose inhibitor, should be given in addition to heparin. We found no literature to suggest that this drug was of benefit in this condition, but since the syndrome is so rapidly fatal, time cannot be wasted in trying out drugs sequentially. Zimmermann and co-workers (1972) suggested that the combination of Trasylol and heparin in the traumatic lung syndrome (presumably largely related to fat embolism since many of his patients were not shocked at the time of the accident) is of greater therapeutic benefit than heparin alone.

A haemorrhagic diathesis is an indication for the use of fresh frozen plasma, blood for haemoglobin replacement and fresh blood or platelets if haemorrhage continues in spite of clotting factor replacement and the platelet count is less than 60 000/mm³.

Antibiotics should be given routinely since the condition may follow a septic abortion. The combination of a cephalosporin and clindamycin (given intravenously initially) seems a reasonable combination unless there is evidence to suggest that an organism resistance to cephalosporin is present. High vaginal swabs, catheter specimen of urine and blood cultures must be taken before starting antibiotics.

Postpartum haemorrhage and coagulation abnormalities

Haemorrhage in the third stage of labour and postpartum is either from the placental site in a uterus which fails to contract adequately, or from trauma to the birth canal. Treatment should be directed towards appropriate obstetric methods to stop the bleeding and replace blood loss as recommended in Part 2, ch. II, p. 349. Blood for coagulation studies should be taken if the bleeding is not controlled. Bleeding may continue if labile coagulation factors are not replaced during massive transfusion. Rarely it could be related to a haemorrhagic disorder unrelated to the pregnancy or to the defibrination syndrome.

Although it has been suggested that development of haemorrhage in patients 30–240 min after an apparently uneventful delivery may be due to primary fibrinolysis (Beller and co-workers, 1961; Phillips *et al.*, 1962), our limited experience suggests that if all obvious obstetric or medical causes are excluded and dealt with the condition is invariably associated with D.I.C. and that antifibrinolytic therapy (e.g. E.A.C.A.)

is contraindicated (Jones, 1977). Replacement of clotting factors with F.F.P. or fibrinogen concentrate, appropriate red cell and volume replacement coupled with the necessary obstetric measures is generally adequate. On the rare occasion when haemorrhage continues in spite of evacuation of the uterus and appropriate surgical haemostasis – heparin should be considered. The diagnosis of D.I.C. based on simple clotting indices and the dosage of heparin recommended are described in Part 2, ch. II, p. 365, Table 3 and p. 366, Table 4 respectively.

Generally clotting occurs with component therapy (F.F.P., red cells, and platelet concentrates) and intravenous heparin, but should bleeding continue, fresh blood should be considered. We have had experience with two cases where bleeding slowed down only after the use of fresh blood. Under such desperate circumstances – where blood volume replacement and bleeding has been profound, hysterectomy should be considered as soon as the extent of bleeding has decreased and before further blood loss occurs.

Jones (1977) states that a definitive laboratory diagnosis of primary fibrinolysis might very rarely suggest the use of antifibrinolytics. The use of E.A.C.A. should be prescribed in the knowledge that the patient primed to clot by the physiological changes of pregnancy will be exposed to an increased danger of systemic thrombosis.

THE MANAGEMENT OF MASSIVE PULMONARY EMBOLISM IN OBSTETRIC PRACTICE

The presentation and diagnosis have been described in Part 2, ch. V, p. 590. Pulmonary embolectomy is not contraindicated at any time during pregnancy should it be considered that the mother will die without an operation. The use of anti-coagulants has been excellently reviewed by Flessa and co-workers (1974). Heparin only should be used, streptokinase and oral anti-coagulants are contraindicated. Oral anti-coagulants may increase the tendency to a retroplacental haemorrhage and increase the risk of foetal haemorrhage especially when the foetus is born prematurely (and therefore the anti-coagulant not stopped for 3 days prior to delivery), or when anti-coagulant control has been poor (Flessa et al., 1965). The dosage of intravenous heparin should be based on anti-coagulant studies. Flessa and co-workers (1974) recommend that intravenous heparin should be continued for approximately 10 days, the administration then being changed to the subcutaneous route.

OVERDOSE AND PREGNANCY

The management of drug overdose in pregnancy is generally similar to that described in Part 2, ch. VI. It is imperative that in the presence of respiratory failure the airway and adequate oxygenation is maintained. There is a great danger of pulmonary aspiration towards term and therefore the airway should be secured (by intubation) as soon as the cough reflex has been lost. Gastric lavage should not be attempted (without prior endotracheal intubation) unless the patient has a good cough reflex and objects to the tube being inserted. Maintenance of an adequate cardiac output is also important and therefore any dysrhythmia should be treated as soon as it arises (by d.c. cardioversion if necessary). Thermodilution cardiac output monitoring should be considered if the blood pressure systolic falls to 80 mm Hg or below and the urine output less than 40 ml/h. Cardiac output should be maintained by volume replacement (under right atrial pressure monitoring control) or more frequently by the use of a drug such as dopamine (Part 2, ch. II, p. 371, Table 5). The drug should be titrated intravenously as recommended in Part 2, ch. II, p. 373. Monitoring of the foetal heart rate is imperative.

Barbituate overdose during pregnancy has been well documented – we have experience with one case who had ingested a barbiturate of medium duration of activity at 36 weeks gestation. This patient was treated conservatively with intubation and ventilation for four days, nutrition via a Ryles tube and a high fluid turnover rate. The blood pressure fell to 80 mm Hg and remained around this level for the first 24 h – the urine output and skin perfusion remained good, the foetal heart rate fell to 80/min for approximately 12 h then slowly returned to a normal rate. Delivery of an active normal infant occurred 12 hours after the mother had started to breathe spontaneously.

It is therefore felt that conservative management of barbiturate overdose on the lines advised on p. 614 is wise, since clearly delivery of the infant with a slow pulse rate and presumably respiratory depression would be hazardous. Barbiturates are known to cross the placenta and pass rapidly into the foetal tissues (Crawford, 1965). Most authors consider that the difference between the maximal concentrations of drugs in the maternal and foetal blood is 15–30%. There is no evidence to suggest that barbiturates cause abortion (Fouts, 1965) and it is probable that a fall in foetal heart rate is not dangerous provided the maternal oxygenation and cardiac output is maintained, since barbiturates are known to reduce the oxygen requirements of the brain (Secher and Wilhjelm, 1968).

SHOCK IN OBSTETRICS

The pathophysiology and management of various forms of shock have been discussed in detail in Part 2, ch. II. It is therefore proposed to mention particular forms of shock which may occur in obstetric practice and to stress aspects of management which differ from the non-pregnant individual.

The monitoring of the shocked patient is described in ch. II, p. 301 and a similar approach to patient assessment applies during obstetric shock. It is important to be aware of certain physiological adaptations which take place during pregnancy – changes in blood volume, cardiac output, and haematological alterations have already been mentioned (pp. 702 and 722 respectively). The venous pressure in the arm remains unchanged in pregnancy but there is a progressive increase in the femoral venous pressure due to the increasing pressure of the uterus and the relatively high pressure of the blood discharged from the uterine veins. Pressures on the right side of the heart are unaffected by pregnancy – an average right atrial pressure of 10 cm H_2O in the third trimester has been reported by O'Driscoll and McCarthy (1966). In pregnancy the peripheral blood flow is increased and the finger skin temperature rises from 34.2°C in the non-pregnant to 35.9°C at 36 weeks (Herbert *et al.*, 1958). The normal reaction to stress is peripheral vasoconstriction but in pregnancy a vasodilator response may occur (Lloyd and Pickford, 1961). Awareness of this response is of great importance since the pregnant woman particularly at term is less likely to compensate for a fall in dynamic blood volume than the non-pregnant patient. It is our impression that the pregnant septic patient remains peripherally vasodilated for longer, a fall in dynamic blood volume is therefore more likely to occur than in the non-pregnant patient where peripheral vasoconstriction occurs at a relatively early stage of the shock state.

The pregnant or postpartum shocked patient is particularly vulnerable to the development of D.I.C. and therefore baseline coagulation factors are particularly important. The changes in clotting indices and the management of D.I.C. have been discussed in detail in Part 2, ch. II, p. 364 and in relation to pregnancy on p. 723.

In normal pregnancy a small but consistent fall occurs in the concentration of serum electrolytes. In early pregnancy the serum sodium falls by 2–3 mmol/l and the potassium by 0.2–0.3 mmol/l and then remain constant. The bicarbonate concentration falls early and is related to a fall in $PaCO_2$ so that the $PaCO_2$ has fallen from 5.2 kPa (38.8 mm Hg) to 4.1 kPa (30.6 mm Hg) by the end of the second trimester (Lyons and Antonio, 1959).

It is proposed to discuss particular aspects of management under the following headings – certain of these topics have already been discussed and it is not proposed to discuss them further.

Predominantly hypovolaemic
Water and electrolyte losses:
    gastrointestinal, p. 671
    pancreatic, p. 679
    lightning injury, p. 467
    burns, p. 443
    aspiration syndrome, p. 563
    endocrine, p. 631
Blood loss:
    gastrointestinal, p. 665
    trauma following an accident or due to an obstetric complication e.g. ruptured uterus, pp. 733–734
    postpartum haemorrhage, p. 728
    ante-partum haemorrhage, p. 724
Emboli:
    thromboembolism, p. 590
    amniotic fluid embolism, p. 725
    air embolism, p. 603

Septic
Predominantly cardiac:
    myocardial infarction ⎫
    myocardial failure   ⎬ Part 1, ch. III
    dysrhythmias   ⎭
    cardiac arrest, Part 2, ch. I

Shock in obstetrics predominantly related to hypovolaemia

Most of these conditions have been discussed elsewhere (see above). It is not proposed to discuss hypovolaemic shock complicating obstetric practice.

Non-obstetric trauma
Trauma from non-obstetric causes has been recently reviewed by London (1974) and Crosby (1974).

Lightning accidents

Lightning injury has been discussed in detail in Part 2, ch. III, p. 467. Lightning stroke during pregnancy has been reported (Chan and Sivasamboo, 1972). It is probable that the gravid uterus serves as a preferential conducting pathway – labour is frequently induced at term but this may not occur if the pregnancy is not very advanced (Rees, 1965). Lightning has been reported to induce violent uterine contractions and rupture of the uterus (Samsoenarjo, 1959). General management is similar to that of the non-pregnant patient – ventilation may be required if there is severe lung contusion; maintenance of blood volume and metabolic balance is an essential part of therapy. The pregnant woman is particularly susceptible to pulmonary aspiration; early gastric drainage with neutralisation of its contents is important. In a semiconscious patient with an impaired cough reflex – intubation may be indicated prior to drainage.

Burns

The experience by Schmitz (1971) suggests that the incidence of burns in pregnancy is approximately 1 in every 250 women. The pregnancy is not affected unless more than one third of the total body surface is involved when there is an increased incidence of premature labour. The management of burns is described in Part 2, ch. III, p. 443, particular attention must be paid to volume replacement and adequate oxygenation during resuscitation. Blood glucose monitoring is particularly important if glucose infusions are used. Antibiotics must be chosen with care because of the possible effects on the foetus.

Trauma

Woodhall (1942) reviewed the literature concerning rupture of the uterus. Uterine rupture is rare in belted victims but may occur with lap-belt restraint (Rubovits, 1964). The presence of a lap-belt may focus some of the force of deceleration on the pelvic structures. Previous uterine surgery also increases the risk of rupture during sudden increases of intra-uterine pressure. The pregnant uterus may provide protection for the other organs during an automobile accident, the greater the size of the uterus the greater the protection provided. Elliott (1966) reported 39 pregnant women seriously injured in vehicle accidents – the cause of death in all 8 patients who died was uncontrollable haemorrhage: 5 of the 8 had retroperitoneal haemorrhage, 3 had placental separation and 3 intraperitoneal haemorrhage.

Pregnancy itself appears to predispose the patient to splenic rupture (Sparkman, 1958) and this may occur after trivial injury.

Fracture of the pelvic ring during pregnancy increases the risk of retroperitoneal haemorrhage and foetal injury. With increased vascularity of the pelvic region in pregnancy, retroperitoneal haemorrhage around the fracture site may be exceptionally severe (Crosby, 1974). Deformity of the pelvis following displacement of the fractured bones may necessitate Caesarean section (Delaney, 1973).

A severe automobile accident involving a pregnant woman may be complicated by premature separation of the placenta. Beyond 12 weeks' gestation an incidence of 5.7% has been reported (Crosby and Costiloe, 1971). Premature placental separation may be the only complication of injury, the injury may not necessarily be serious. The severity of clinical symptoms and foetal outcome both depend upon the area of the placental surface separated. When less than 23% of the placenta is involved, clinical symptoms are external bleeding and premature labour. Larger areas of separation are generally associated with hypovolaemic shock, uterine tenderness and occasionally D.I.C.

Management of the severely ill traumatised pregnant woman

The management of traumatic haemorrhagic shock is discussed in detail in Part 2, ch. II, p. 333. The mother can survive shock for a considerably longer period than the foetus, indeed during maternal shock constriction of the uterine arteries helps salvage the mother at the expense of the foetus. In acute blood loss, uterine blood flow is reduced, foetal PaO_2 is reduced and foetal bradycardia is usually present (Romney *et al.*, 1963). Vasopressors must never be used in maternal shock because of the dangers in decreasing uterine blood flow which may be reduced below that produced by hypotension alone (Boba *et al.*, 1965).

The relationship between clinical symptoms and volume of blood lost is shown in Table 1, p. 334. In the pregnant patient clinical symptoms may not develop until 30–35% of the blood volume has been lost (Marx, 1965); right atrial pressure monitoring is therefore essential whenever there has been a history of trauma and the pulse rate is greater than 100/min. Blood volume should be replaced along the lines described in ch. II, p. 341, uncrossmatched blood should not be given unless considered absolutely essential. Clotting factors must be monitored, F.F.P. being used according to Table 6, p. 350. In late pregnancy venal caval compression may occur when the patient lies supine. The resultant reduction in venous return may decrease cardiac output and simultaneously increase the venous pressure in the lower part of the body, thereby increasing the volume of blood lost from any traumatised site. The patient should be nursed on her side and should remain in this position preoperatively until induction of anaesthesia. It must be recalled that the pregnant traumatised victim is particularly susceptible to pulmonary aspiration. Internal abdominal injuries should be suspected in any seriously ill accident victim – splenic and hepatic rupture are more common during pregnancy. Diagnostic paracentesis is often not helpful in the second half of pregnancy and periodic diagnostic peritoneal washouts are not possible.

Although the diagnosis of internal bleeding and/or bowel rupture is more difficult in the pregnant patient, absent bowel sounds, tenderness and increasing distension are indications for laparotomy. Should a ruptured uterus be suspected – laparotomy should be performed as soon as sufficient infusion cannulae and a right atrial pressure monitoring line have been inserted.

In late pregnancy, surgical exposure may be compromised by the bulk of the uterus, in such cases the uterus may have to be emptied first. Caesarean section should also be considered near term when there is extensive intraperitoneal faecal contamination.

If premature separation of the placenta should be suspected following trauma and the foetus is alive and viable, delivery must be considered urgent and Caesarean section probably necessary.

Shock associated with sepsis

The pregnant patient may suffer from non-obstetric severe sepsis such as pyelonephritis, bowel perforation or meningococcal septicaemia. It is proposed to devote this section mainly to sepsis related to obstetric and gynaecological practice.

In obstetric-gynaecological practice, situations most likely to predispose the patient to severe sepsis are abortion, the presence of a dead foetus in association with membrane rupture, prolonged labour followed by an instrumental delivery, Caesarean section after prolonged labour and, rarely, the presence of an intra-uterine device in association with pregnancy (Zuckerman and Stubblefield, 1974). The mortality rate among obstetric-gynaecological patients is much lower than other patients developing septic shock. Explanations for this include, the source of sepsis (generally the pelvis) which is amenable to surgical drainage, the age of the patient and the decreasing incidence of illegal abortion.

The range of bacteria isolated in a series of obstetric-gynaecological patients with bacteraemia gives a guide to the most suitable antibiotic combination. Ledger and co-workers (1974) isolated anaerobic organisms in 29.2% of their patients. The three most frequently recovered aerobes were *E. coli*, enterococci and beta haemolytic streptococci, while the most commonly isolated anaerobes were streptococci and Bacteroides. They found that patients with a gynaecological malignancy were the most difficult patients to treat, Candida and Pseudomonas species being common. Occasionally two organisms were isolated from the blood culture, *Cl. welchii* being rarely found since the incidence of illegal abortion has decreased. An unfamiliar organism recovered in this study was *Salmonella typhi*. The isolation of staphylococci was rare except in patients with gynaecological malignancy.

Because of this limited range of organism, it seems reasonable to use a combination of cephaloridine and clindamycin in the management of the obstetric patient with shock associated with sepsis, gentamicin being confined to the gynaecological patient with malignancy. In pregnant patients suffering from non-obstetric sepsis, should the foetus be considered viable, antibiotics must be selected with care. Tetracycline, chloramphenicol, sulphonamides and combinations of sulphonamides with antifolate agents should be avoided. Aminoglycoside antibiotics should only be used in very severe infection where there is no suitable alternative. Monitoring of antibiotic blood levels is essential since aminoglycosides may cause damage to the eighth cranial nerve in the foetus.

The management of septic shock should be conducted along the lines suggested for the non-obstetric patient (Part 2, ch. II, p. 361, Table 2). Respiratory distress is more likely to arise in the pregnant septic patient towards term than in the non-pregnant – exhaustion, basal atelectasis and pulmonary aspiration is more likely to occur. Intubation and ventilation should be considered early on in patient management. The obstetric patient with associated sepsis invariably has a low circulating blood volume and compensatory vasoconstriction does not occur until late. Right atrial pressure monitoring and adequate volume replacement is therefore essential in order to maintain adequate placental flow. The septic obstetric patient appears to be particularly vulnerable to the development of pulmonary oedema secondary to fluid overload in the presence of acute oliguric renal failure. Right atrial pressure monitoring is therefore essential.

Blood cultures are essential; cultures should also be taken of the urine, vaginal secretions and in the obsetric patient from the cervix and, when available, the products of conception.

In severe septic shock, non-responsive to these measures, a massive dose of prednisolone should be given. Dopamine hydrochloride is probably safe in the pregnant patient provided only a low dose is used, 1–4 µg/kg B.W./min. Drug therapy in septic shock is described in greater detail in Part 2, ch. II, p. 367.

The incidence of acute renal failure in septic abortion is high and early diagnosis prior to surgery is essential. The pre-operative preparation of such a patient should be on the lines described in Part 2, ch. II, p. 377. The obstetric patient is particularly predisposed to D.I.C. Baseline clotting factors are therefore important, any evidence of D.I.C. (Part 2, ch. II, p. 365, Table 3) is an indication for blood replacement with fresh blood; the operation should be preceded by an infusion of 4 packets of F.F.P. Platelets are rarely required.

The surgical management of severe obstetric sepsis deserves special mention since it forms an essential part of treatment. In septic abortion the uterus should be evacuated as soon as the patient has been resuscitated and covered by antibiotics. If sepsis has spread to the pelvis and an abscess has developed it must be drained, either by colpotomy or abdominally depending on its site and extent. Hysterectomy may have to be considered if there is evidence of severe myometrial infection such as uterine gangrene or microabscess formation. In cases of known clostridial septic abortion, evacuation or any other operation should be preceded and followed by a course of hyperbaric oxygen (Hanson *et al.*, 1966 and Part 2, ch. IV, p. 504).

Should intravenous feeding be required in the pregnant patient – amino acid and glucose solutions should be infused as advised in Part 1, ch. IX. The amino acid preparation should be the crystalline laevorotatory amino acid Vamin N or Vamin Glucose. Towards term, it is advisable to restrict the intake of fat (as Intralipid) to 10% of the total calorie supply until the possibility of fatty infiltration of the placenta with attendant decreased placental function has been excluded (Heller, 1972). Vitamin supplementation is important, the mother being particularly susceptible to folate deficiency; adequate supplies of calcium and Vitamin D are essential for foetal maturation. Vitamins should preferably be supplied as Vitlipid and Solivito (Part 1, ch. IX, p. 254).

THE MANAGEMENT OF ORGAN FAILURE IN PREGNANCY

Renal failure

By the third month of pregnancy, renal plasma flow begins to increase and by the end of the fourth month is 30–40% more than in the non-pregnant patient. At the seventh month renal plasma flow begins to subside and at term is only slightly above the non-pregnant patient. Glomerular filtration-rate also increases and by the fourth month is over 50% normal, it subsequently decreases but does not return to the non-pregnant mean. The blood urea during pregnancy is 2–3.3 mmol/l and the creatinine clearance may be as high as 150% of normal renal function.

Patients with severe renal failure do not become pregnant. A recent survey on patients who became pregnant with pre-existing renal disease suggest that the incidence of complications is small provided renal insufficiency and severe hypertension is absent before conception (Strauch and Hayslett, 1974). Pregnancy is therefore most likely to be complicated by acute renal failure than acute on chronic renal failure. Successful pregnancy has now been reported in patients on regular dialysis but severe complications arising in these patients are most likely to be handled in a specialist unit and will therefore not be discussed.

Management of acute renal failure in pregnancy

The treatment of acute renal failure has been discussed in detail in Part 1, ch. IV. Acute renal failure most commonly complicates shock associated with sepsis (e.g. after abortion), severe haemorrhage or pregnancy toxaemia, and is therefore most likely to arise postpartum. Cortical necrosis is nearly always a complication of concealed accidental haemorrhage in the last trimester and is uncommon in acute renal failure after septic abortion (Barnes, 1970c).

The indications for dialysis are similar to the non-pregnant patient – the majority (because of the underlying pathology) being extremely catabolic. Should these patients require emergency surgery – this should be performed under insulin dextrose cover in order to prevent a dangerous rise in serum potassium and the patient should be hyperventilated throughout the operation. Care must be taken not to overload the patient – we have the impression that these patients have a greater tendency towards the development of acute pulmonary oedema than the non-pregnant patient. Dialysis is generally indicated immediately postoperatively.

Acute renal failure complicating septic abortion is commonly associated with severe hypotension and an unstable circulation for several days postoperatively. During this period it has been found preferable to 'hold' the patient with peritoneal dialysis (the catheter being inserted high in the abdomen either during operation or under direct vision) and subsequently changing to haemodialysis once the blood pressure and cardiovascular state has stabilised. Trauma to the pelvic floor or uterine rupture generally necessitates haemodialysis from the onset because of leakage of peritoneal dialysis fluid.

Dialysis is unlikely to be required as an acute measure in the presence of a viable foetus but has been used for limited periods to prolong pregnancy in severe pre-eclamptic toxaemia (Goldsmith *et al.*, 1971), acute nephritis due to systemic lupus (Mitra *et al.*, 1972) and chronic renal disease not requiring dialysis prior to pregnancy (Herwig *et al.*, 1965). Under such circumstances, careful control of hypertension and uraemia, adequate nutrition and transfusion to maintain a haemoglobin value of around 7.0 g/dl, seem to be important factors in allowing adequate foetal growth. Clearly the management of such patients requires close co-operation with a nephrologist and the foetal outcome is gloomy if the mother is sufficiently sick to warrant intensive therapy in addition to haemodialysis.

Hepatic failure

The management of acute hepatic failure has been described in Part 1, ch. V. In normal pregnancy, biochemical tests of hepatic function show a slight rise in the alkaline phosphatase in the last eight weeks of gestation; the increase is in the heat-stable moiety and is derived from the placenta. Turbidity tests, transaminases and bilirubin remain normal. The level of serum albumin falls steadily until the seventh or eighth month of pregnancy when it may have fallen by as much as 10 g/l. The serum globulin is slightly raised, electrophoresis showing a fall in γ-globulin but a rise in the γ- and β-globulins – this pattern may not revert to normal until several months after delivery (Owen, 1958). Spider naevi and vascular spiders are common in pregnancy. Acute hepatocellular failure may be due to disorders not directly related to pregnancy or less commonly to a condition which develops during pregnancy – acute fatty liver of pregnancy.

Idiopathic acute fatty liver of pregnancy
An uncommon clinical entity characterised by the development of jaundice in the third trimester in association with nausea, vomiting, abdominal pain, rapidly progressive hepatic failure and a mortality of approximately 85%. The condition is similar to acute fulminant hepatitis, the histology however is different, there being little or no hepatocellular necrosis. This condition has been related to protein malnutrition and to depression of protein synthesis by drugs, in

particular tetracycline. Laboratory findings include a leucocytosis, hyperbilirubinaemia, moderately elevated alkaline phosphatase and transaminase and an increase in blood urea. Severe renal involvement associated with anuria or oliguria is common. Disseminated intravascular coagulation has been recently documented (Cano *et al.*, 1975) and gastrointestinal bleeding is common.

Treatment is similar to that described in Part 1, ch. V. The patient generally delivers spontaneously a stillborn infant. Following delivery a high fever commonly develops, the mother dying several days later of hepato-renal failure.

Toxaemia, eclampsia and subcapsular rupture of the liver

Pre-eclamptic toxaemia and eclampsia may be complicated by bleeding beneath the liver capsule which if severe may rupture into the peritoneal cavity. Bis and Waxman (1976) reviewed 89 cases – toxaemia was present in all but 4 cases and convulsions occurred in 24. The onset may be insidious with nausea, vomiting and epigastric pain. The diagnosis may be difficult, the diastolic pressure remaining high in spite of bleeding (Browne *et al.*, 1975), the pulse volume however being low and the rate rapid. Diagnosis is frequently based on sudden collapse following a convulsion, associated with increasing abdominal distension, liver tenderness and free blood on tapping the peritoneal cavity. The mortality is high unless laparotomy and haemostasis is carried out. Adequate volume replacement is essential, diazoxide (see p. 710) may be necessary to control the blood pressure postoperatively. Replacement of labile clotting factors during transfusion is important; D.I.C. and acute renal failure may be complications which require appropriate treatment.

Pulmonary failure

Cugell *et al.* (1953) carried out a detailed analysis of respiratory function during pregnancy and found that the vital capacity remained unchanged although the total lung capacity and residual volume diminished. The diaphragm rises during the course of pregnancy, thus increasing the tendency towards basal atelectasis in the seriously ill pregnant patient towards term.

The management of severe respiratory failure in the pregnant patient is similar to that of the non-pregnant – and has been described in Part 2, ch. V.

Bronchial asthma is generally little affected by pregnancy (Shaefer and Silverman, 1961).

Bronchopneumonia developing during pregnancy may produce intra-uterine death, this being most likely to occur between the 25th and 36th week of pregnancy. Blood gas monitoring when a pregnant patient develops severe bronchopneumonia is imperative, the PaO_2 should not be allowed to fall below 8.7 kPa (65 mm Hg) – a PaO_2 below this level on oxygen via a face mask is an indication for artificial ventilation. It is essential during ventilation of a pregnant patient to ensure an adequate venous return – the patient may have to be nursed on her side, right atrial pressure monitoring is important since ventilation should not be commenced in the presence of a decreased circulating blood volume.

Viral pneumonia may be particularly lethal when contracted during pregnancy. Respiratory failure may be rapid, is often complicated by intravascular haemolysis; D.I.C. and renal failure may also be present. Recovery of a pregnant patient with viral pneumonia complicated by D.I.C. (treated with fresh blood and intravenous heparin) and renal failure (treated by dialysis) has been reported by Griffith (1974). Spontaneous labour occurred whilst she was on the ventilator, the baby weighed 1.2 kg and died 50 hours after delivery.

Pulmonary aspiration and pregnancy (Mendelson's syndrome)
The management of pulmonary aspiration has been described in detail in Part 2, ch. V, p. 563. The obstetric patient is particularly likely to develop the aspiration syndrome, because of the frequent presence of gastric contents of high acidity, and the increased intra-abdominal pressure related to the enlarged uterus which is further increased during labour. The obstetric patient most commonly aspirates during induction or recovery from anaesthesia, following an eclamptic fit, or following excessive sedation during the management of eclampsia or pre-eclampsia. Any suspicion of aspiration is an absolute indication for intubation and ventilation (with a positive end expiratory pressure) for at least 24 hours after the incident. Further management should be conducted on the lines described in Part 2, ch. V, p. 573.

Pneumomediastinum
Pneumomediastinum is a well recognised complication of oesophageal rupture (Gray and Hanson, 1966), bronchopneumonia and chest injury. Occasionally the condition is spontaneous and is known to be a rare complication of parturition. It generally occurs during the second

stage of labour, principally in primigravidas and although the prognosis is excellent, death from cardiopulmonary failure has been reported (Gordon, 1927).

Sudden onset of dyspnoea, chest pain and cyanosis should alert the physician to the possible diagnosis. Should the air remain trapped in the mediastinum, venous return and cardiac output may be impaired leading to severe hypotension. The diagnosis may be suspected by detecting emphysema in the neck or the presence of a crunching sound just medial to the apex beat (Hamman's sign). The chest X-ray appearance is diagnostic (Fig. 2). Should the patient's condition be critical, air can be removed by needling the neck just above the sternum and aspirating the air which has tracked up from the mediastinum. Oxygen should be given by face mask and should the patient remain cyanosed (due to splinting of the lungs with air), the patient should be intubated and hand-ventilated with oxygen. It has been our limited experience that by this method a pneumothorax is frequently created – air then being removed via a pleural drain. The efforts of labour should be reduced, if necessary with a general anaesthetic, and delivery expedited by a forceps delivery or Caesarean section. Once the increased intrathoracic pressure created by labour is reduced, the amount of air diverted into the mediastinum from a ruptured alveolus decreases.

NEUROLOGICAL CRISES AND PREGNANCY

The management of various neurological disorders has been described in Part 2, ch. V, p. 485 and ch. X. The majority of neurological crises arising in the pregnant patient are treated similarly to the non-pregnant – three disorders deserve special mention: epilepsy, the Guillain-Barré Syndrome and myasthenia gravis.

Epilepsy and pregnancy

It has been found that epileptics who experience more than one fit a month are very likely to deteriorate further during pregnancy, while only 25% of those with rare convulsions (intervals greater than 9 months) will do so (Knight and Rhind, 1975). For patients receiving anti-convulsants, the slight teratogenic properties must be accepted in order to prevent *status epilepticus*. Folic acid supplementation is essential when the patient is receiving a folate antagonist – this may reduce the anti-convulsant property of the drug.

Status epilepticus demands the rapid deployment of an anti-convulsant regime sufficient to abolish fits as quickly as possible. The management

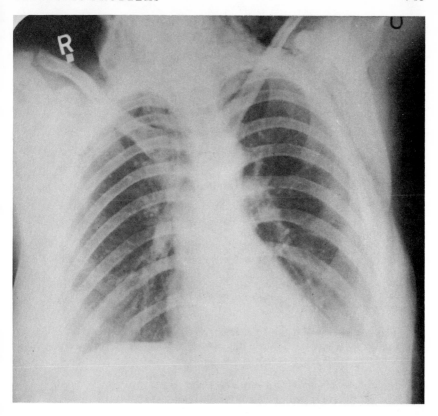

Fig. 2. Chest X-ray appearance of spontaneous pneumomediastinum. Sudden onset of retrosternal chest pain, dyspnoea and transient cyanosis during the second stage of labour. Crepitus noted in the neck. Note air dissecting along the right side of the trachea and its presence in the neck and down the left chest wall.

of the non-pregnant patient with status epilepticus is described in Part 2, ch. X, p. 696.

Intravenous diazepam and intramuscular paraldehyde are generally the drugs of choice. Clonazepam like diazepam, a member of the benzodiazepine group of compounds, may prove to be more effective in the control of *status epilepticus* than diazepam. Experimentally its anti-convulsant activity is more marked and faster than diazepam. Gastaut *et al.* (1971) found that clonazepam was effective when diazepam had failed and concluded that it was the most effective agent available at present for treatment of *status epilepticus*. Monitoring of blood gases and acid base state are essential in a patient whose convulsions are not

Table 3. Summary of the management of the obstetric patient with *status epilepticus*

Drugs   refer to Part 2, ch. X, p. 697, Table 1.

Author's preference: i.m. paraldehyde, i.v. diazepam plus previous anti-convulsant drugs (phenytoin sodium should be given via the Ryles tube).

In a known severe epileptic consider clonazepam 1 mg i.v. given over 30 seconds, then as a continuous infusion (concentration 3 mg in 250 ml 5% dextrose) given at a rate sufficient to control convulsions.

Investigations   Astrup analysis.
Observations   B.G.   B.U.   electrolytes.
                Hb.   P.C.V.
                Hourly urine output.
                ½-hourly skin core temperature.
                ½-hourly pulse and blood pressure.

Intubate and ventilate under the following circumstances:
1. Evidence of respiratory depression $PaCO_2 > 6$ kPa (45 mm Hg) or presence of hypostatic pneumonia or pulmonary aspiration or
2. Pulse rate > 120/min for more than 1 h with a core temperature $> 38°C$ (in the absence of sepsis) or
3. $PaO_2 < 9.3$ kPa (70 mm Hg) on highest possible inspiratory oxygen percentage via face mask or
4. pH < 7.3

Ventilation

Avoid pulmonary aspiration during intubation if at all possible.

Use pancuronium to ensure muscle relaxation (allow relaxant to wear off 2 hourly to assess irritability).

Use regular doses of   i.m. paraldehyde.
                      i.v. diazepam or clonazepam.

Continue preceding anti-convulsant therapy.

Check the blood levels of these drugs and maintain in the therapeutic range.

Do not stop ventilation until:
    Temperature normal   ⎫ for at
    Pulse rate < 100/min   ⎬ least
    No evidence of twitching after lightening ⎭ 12 h

---

controlled within 5 min. A falling pH, rising pulse rate (> 120/min) and rising temperature are indications for muscle relaxation, intubation and artificial ventilation. Ventilation should be continued until the pulse rate has fallen to 100/min or less and the temperature and pH returned to normal. During ventilation, the patient's usual anti-convulsant drugs should be used with the addition of regular doses of clonazepam or diazepam given intravenously and paraldehyde intramuscularly.

The patient should be lightened periodically to assess whether muscle irritability is present. Adequate airway control and oxygenation is an essential aspect of management – deterioration in the mother (increasing metabolic acidosis, rising pulse rate and temperature) is likely to be complicated by intra-uterine death or the onset of premature labour. A suggested plan for the management of *status epilepticus* in pregnancy is shown in Table 3. Once the convulsions are controlled, pregnancy should be allowed to continue. It is essential to ensure adequate anticonvulsant control by maintaining therapeutic blood levels of the anticonvulsant drugs being used.

Management of the Guillain-Barré syndrome in pregnancy

Approximately twenty-seven cases of Guillain-Barré syndrome in pregnancy have been reported in the world literature. Sudo and Weingold (1974) reported on two further cases and reviewed the literature. The management of the non-pregnant patient is discussed in Part 2, ch. X, p. 693. Maternal mortality is largely related to pulmonary aspiration, bronchopneumonia, cardiac arrest, circulatory failure and complications of tracheostomy (Sudo and Weingold, 1974). The pregnant woman requires meticulous observation of ventilatory function; intubation and early tracheostomy is indicated should there be an inadequate cough reflex, difficulty in swallowing, or a rising $PaCO_2$.

It is generally accepted that efficient uterine contractions can occur in spite of severe neurological disease. The onset of labour in the presence of minimal respiratory failure is an indication for a tracheostomy in order to control the airway. Caesarean section is not necessary unless there are obstetric indications. The infants born to mothers with this disease are normal and there is no indication for pregnancy termination.

Myasthenia gravis

The effect of pregnancy on myasthenia gravis is variable, it is usual for exacerbations to occur in the first trimester and remissions in the second and third. About 20% of the babies of myasthenic mothers develop transient neonatal myasthenia. There is a tendency for an exacerbation of the disease to occur in the puerperum (Fraser and Aldren Turner, 1963).

The management of a myasthenic or cholinergic crisis is described in Part 2, ch. X, p. 692. Should the patient go into labour during a myasthenic crisis, delivery should be assisted by low forceps under local blockade or general anaesthesia. All muscle relaxants and drugs related to the belladonna group, including scopolamine, must be avoided. The baby must be observed and if necessary treated for myasthenia.

REFERENCES

Adachi, A., Spivak, M. and Wilson, L. (1974). Intravascular haemolysis: a complication of midtrimester abortion. *Obstet. Gynec.* **45**, 467.

Anderson, D. G. (1967). Amniotic fluid embolism: a re-evaluation. *Am. J. Obstet. Gynec.* **96**, 336.

Ashton, H. (1971). Drugs and the foetus and neonate. *Adverse Drug Reaction Bull.* **28**, 80.

Banks, B. M., Korelitz, B. I., Zetzel, L. (1957). The course of non-specific ulcerative colitis: review of twenty years' experience and late results. *Gastroenterology* **32**, 983.

Barnes, C. G. (1970a). 'Medical Disorders in Obstetric Practice' (Ed. C. G. Barnes) Third Edition. Blackwell Scientific Publications, Oxford and Edinburgh.

Barnes, C. G. (1970b). Disorders of the Alimentary Tract. *In* 'Medical Disorders in Obstetric Practice' (Ed. C. G. Barnes) p. 140. Blackwell Scientific Publications, Oxford and Edinburgh.

Barnes, C. G. (1970c). Non-toxaemic Hypertension. *In* 'Medical Disorders in Obstetric Practice' (Ed. C. G. Barnes) Third Edition, p. 93. Blackwell Scientific Publications, Oxford and Edinburgh.

Barrett, C. and Marshall, J. R. (1974). Thrombotic brombocytopenic purpura. *Obstet. Gynec.* **46**, 231.

Becker, W. F. (1954). Acute pancreatitis, clinical study of one hundred cases. *J. Louisiana M. Soc.* **106**, 166.

Beecham, J. B., Watson, W. J. and Clapp, J. F. (1974). Eclampsia, pre-eclampsia and disseminated intravascular coagulation. *Obstet. Gynec.* **43**, 576.

Beller, F. K., Glas, H. and Roemer, H. (1961). Fibrinolysis as the cause of obstetrical haemorrhage. *Am. J. Obstet Gynec.* **82**, 620.

Bieniarz, J., Crottogini, J. J., Curuchet, E., Romero-Salinas, G., Yoshida, T., Poseiro, J. J. and Caldeyro-Barcio, R. (1968). Aortocaval compression by the uterus in late human pregnancy. An arteriographic study. *Am. J. Obstet. Gynec.* **100**, 203.

Bis, K. A. and Waxman, B. (1976). Rupture of the Liver associated with pregnancy: a review of the literature and report of 2 cases. *Obstet. Gynec. Survey* **31**, 763.

Blinick, G., Jerez, E. and Wallach, R. C. (1973). Methadone maintenance, pregnancy and progeny. *J. Amer. Med. Assoc.* **225**, 477.

Boba, A., Plotz, E. J. and Linkie, D. M. (1965). Effect of atropine on fetal bradycardia and arterial oxygenation. Experimental study in the dog during graded haemorrhage and following vasopressor administration. *Surgery* **58**, 267.

Bongiovanni, A. M., Di George, A. M. and Grumbach, M. M. (1959). Masculinisation of the female infant associated with oestrogen therapy alone during gestation: four cases. *J. Clin. Endocr.* **19**, 1004.

Bonnar, J., Prentice, C. R. M., McNichol, G. P. and Douglas, A. S. (1970). Haemostatic mechanism in the uterine circulation during placental separation. *Brit. Med. J.* **1**, 564.

Brockington, I. F. (1971). Post-partum hypertensive heart failure. *Am. J. Cardiol.* **27**, 650.

Browne, C. H., Hanson, G. C., De Jode, L. R. and Roberts, P. A. (1975). Rupture of subcapsular haematoma of the liver in a case of eclampsia. *Brit. J. Surg.* **62**, 237.

Browning, D. J. (1974). Serious side effects of ergometrine and its use in routine obstetric practice. *Med. J. Aust.* **1**, 857.

Brudenell, J. M. (1972). *In* 'Integrated Obstetrics and Gynaecology for Post-graduates' (Ed. C. J. Dewhurst) p. 332.

Cabaniss, C. D. (1971). Management of heart disease in pregnancy. *Southern Med. J.* **64**, 293.

Cano, R. I., Delman, M. R., Pitchummi, C. S., Lev, R. and Rosenthal, W. S. (1975). Acute fatty liver of pregnancy. Complication by disseminated intravascular coagulation. *JAMA* **231**, 159.

Chan Yew-Foon and Sivasamboo, R. (1972). Lightning accidents in pregnancy. *J. Obstet. Gynaec. Brit. Cwlth.* **79**, 761.

Chesley, L. C. (1972). Plasma and red cell volumes during pregnancy. *Amer. J. Obstet. Gynec.* **112**, 440.

Chmel, H. and Bertles, J. F. (1975). Haemoglobin S/C disease in a pregnant woman with crisis and fat embolisation syndrome. *Am. J. Med.* **58**, 563.

Coopland, A. T., Alkjaersig, N. and Fletcher, A. P. (1969). Reduction in plasma factor XIII (fibrin stabilising factor) concentration during pregnancy. *J. Lab. Clin. Med.* **73**, 144.

Cope, C. L. and Black, E. G. (1959). The hydrocortisone production in late pregnancy. *J. Obstet. Gynaec. Brit. Empire* **66**, 404.

Crawford, J. S. (1965). 'The Placenta, Drugs and the Foetus in Principles and Practice of Obstetric Anaesthesia', Second Edition, p. 811. Blackwell Scientific Publications, Oxford.

Crohn, B. B., Yarnis, H., Crohn, E. B., Walter, R. I. and Gabalove, L. J. (1956). Ulcerative colitis and pregnancy. *Gastroenterology* **30**, 391.

Crosby, W. M. and Costiloe, J. P. (1971). Safety of lap belt restraint for pregnant victims of automobile collisions. *N. Engl. J. Med.* **284**, 632.

Crosby, W. M. (1974). Trauma during pregnancy: maternal and fetal injury. *Obstet. Gynec. Survey* **29**, 683.

Cugell, D. W., Frank, N. R., Gaensler, E. A. and Badger, T. L. (1953). Pulmonary function in pregnancy. *Amer. Rev. Tuberc.* **67**, 568.

Delancy, J. J. (1973). 'Obstetrical and Gynecological Injuries in the Management of Trauma.' (Ed. W. P. Ballinger, R. B. Rutherford and G. D. Zuidema) p. 479. W. B. Saunders, Philadelphia, London and Toronto.

D.H.S.S. (1975). Reports on confidential enquiries into maternal deaths in England and Wales. 1970–72, H.M.S.O., London.

Dussault, J., Row, V. V. Lickrish, G. and Volpé, R. (1969). Studies of serum triiodothyronine concentration in maternal and cord blood; transfer of tri-iodothyronine across the human placenta. *J. Clin. Endocrinol. Metab.* **29**, 595.

Editorial (1974). Hypertensive crises in pregnancy. *Med. J. Aust.* **2**, 233.

Editorial (1975). Hypertension in pregnancy. *Lancet* **2**, 487.

Elliott, M. (1966). Vehicular accidents and pregnancy. *Aust. N.Z. J. Obstet. Gynec.* **6**, 279.

Essex, N. (1976). Diabetes and pregnancy. *Brit. J. Hosp. Med.* **15**, 333.

Fielding, J. F. (1976). Inflammatory bowel disease and pregnancy. *Brit. J. Hosp. Med.* **15**, 345.

Finnerty. F. A. (1975). Hypertension in pregnancy. *Clin. Obstet. Gynec.* **18**, 145.

Flessa, H. C., Glueck, H. I. and Dritschilo, A. (1974). Thromboembolic disorders in pregnancy; pathophysiology, diagnosis and treatment, with emphasis on heparin. *Clin. Obstet. Gynec.* **17**, 195.

Flessa, H. C., Kapstrom, A. B., Glueck, H. I. and Will, J. J. (1965). Placental transport of heparin. *Am. J. Obstet. Gynec.* **93**, 570.

Flessa, H. C. (1974). Haemorrhagic disorders and pregnancy. *Clin. Obstet. Gynec.* **17**, 236.

Fouts, J. R. (1965). Metabolism of drugs by the foetus in embryopathic activity of drugs. Smith, Churchill, London.

Fraser, D. and Aldren Turner, J. W. (1963). Myasthenia gravis and pregnancy. *Proc. roy. Soc. Med.* **56**, 379.

Gastaut, H., Courjon, J., Poiré, R. and Weber, M. (1971). Treatment of *status epilepticus* with a new benzodiazepine more active than diazepam. *Epilepsia* (Amst.) **12**, 197.

Georgy, F. M. (1974). Fulminating ulcerative colitis in pregnancy. *Obstet. Gynec.* **66**, 603.

Goldsmith, H. J., Menzies, D. N., De Boer, C. H., Caplan, W. and McCandless, A. (1971). Delivery of healthy infant after five weeks dialysis treatment for fulminating toxaemia of pregnancy. *Lancet* **2**, 738.

Goodwin, J. F. (1961). Pregnancy and congenital coarctation of the aorta. *Clin. Obstet. Gynec.* **4**, 645.

Goolden, A. W. G., Gartside, J. M. and Sanderson, C. (1967). Thyroid status in pregnancy and in women taking oral contraceptives. *Lancet* **1**, 12.

Gordon, C. A. (1927). Respiratory emphysema in labour. Two new cases and review of 130 cases in the literature. *Amer. J. Obstet. Gynec.* **14**, 633.

Gray, J. M. and Hanson, G. C. (1966). Mediastinal emphysema: etiology, diagnosis and treatment. *Thorax* **21**, 325.

Griffith, E. R. (1974). Viral pneumonia in pregnancy: report of a case complicated by disseminated intravascular coagulation and acute renal failure. *Am. J. Obstet. Gynec.* **120,** 201.

Hanson, G. C., Slack, W. K., Chew, H. E. R. and Thomas, D. A. (1966). Clostridial infection of the uterus – a review. Treatment with hyperbaric oxygen. *Post. Grad. Med. J.* **42**, 499.

Heller, L. (1972). Problems of parenteral nutrition in pregnancy. *In* 'Parenteral Nutrition' (Ed. A. W. Wilkinson) p. 180. Churchill-Livingstone, Edinburgh and London.

Hendricks, C. H. and Bennner, W. E. (1970). Cardiovascular effects of oxytocic drugs used post-partum. *Am. J. Obstet. Gynec.* **108**, 751.

Hendrickse, J. P. de V., Harrison, K. A., Watson-Williams, E. J., Luzzatto, L. and Ajabor, L. N. (1972). Pregnancy in homozygous sickle-cell anaemia. *J. Obstet. Gynaec. Brit. Commonw.* **79**, 396.

Herbert, C. M., Banner, E. A. and Wakim, K. G. (1958). Variations in the peripheral circulation during pregnancy. *Amer. J. Obstet. Gynec.* **76**, 742.

Herwig, K. R., Merrill, J. P., Jackson, R. L. and Oken, D. E. (1965). Chronic renal disease and pregnancy. Case report of haemodialysis and delivery of viable infant. *Amer. J. Obstet. Gynec.* **92**, 1117.

Hughes, T. B. J. (1975). Myocardial infarction and rheumatic heart disease in pregnancy. *Brit. J. Obstet. Gynaec.* **82**, 505.

Javert, C. T. (1940). Hyperthyroidism and pregnancy. *Amer. J. Obstet. Gynec.* **39**, 954.

Jones, P. (1977). Personal communication.

Kelsey, F. O. (1965). *In* 'Drug Induced Diseases' (Ed. L. Meyler and H. M. Peck) p. 13. Excerpta Medical Foundation.

Knight, A. H. and Rhind, E. G. (1975). Epilepsy and pregnancy: a study of 153 pregnancies in 59 patients. *Epilepsia* **16**, 99.

Lahiri, S. K., Thomas, T. A. and Hodgson, R. M. H. (1973). Single-dose antacid therapy for the prevention of Mendelson's syndrome. *Brit. J. Anaesth.* **45**, 1143.

Langer, A., Hung, C. T., McA'Nalty, J. A., Harrigan, J. T. and Washington, E. (1974). Adrenergic blockade. A new approach to hyperthyroidism during pregnancy. *Obstet. Gynec.* **44**, 181.

Langmade, C. F. (1956). Epigastric pain in pregnancy toxaemias. *West. J. Surg. Obstet. Gynec.* **64**, 540.

Laros, R. K. and Sweet, R. L. (1975). Management of idiopathic thrombocytopenic purpura during pregnancy. *Am. J. Obstet Gynec.* **122**, 182.

Laverson, N. H. and Birnbaum, S. J. (1975). Water intoxication associated with oxytocin administration during saline induced abortion. *Am. J. Obstet. Gynec.* **121**, 2.

Ledger, W. J., Norman, M., Gee, C. and Lewis, W. (1975). Bacteremia in an obstetric-gynecologic service. *Am. J. Obstet. Gynec.* **121**, 205.

Lloyd, S. and Pickford, M. (1961). The action of posterior pituitary hormones and oestrogens on the vascular system of the rat. *J. Physiol.* (Lond.) **155**, 161.

London, P. S. (1974). Injury and pregnancy. *Injury* **6**, 129.

Lyons, H. A. and Antonio, R. (1959). The sensitivity of the respiratory centre in pregnancy and after the administration of progesterone. *Trans. Ass. Amer. Phys.* **72**, 173.

MacGillivray, L., Rose, G. B. and Rowe, B. (1969). Blood pressure survey in pregnancy. *Clin. Sci.* **37**, 395.

Martimbeau, P. W., Welch, J. S. and Weiland, L. H. (1975). Crohn's disease and pregnancy. *Am. J. Obstet. Gynec.* **122**, 746.

Marx, G. F. (1965). Shock in the obstetric patient. *Anaesthesiology* **26**, 423.

Messer, R. H. (1974). Pregnancy anaemias. *Clin. Obstet. Gynec.* **17**, 163.

Michael, C. A. (1973). Intravenous diazoxide in the treatment of severe pre-eclamptic toxaemia and eclampsia. *Aust. N.Z. J. Obstet. Gynec.* **13**, 143.

Mitra, S., Vertes, V., Roza, O. and Berman, L. E. (1970). Hemodialysis in pregnancy. *Am. J. Med. Sci.* **259**, 333.

Murdock, D. E. and Nathanson, B. N. (1969). Partial exchange transfusion in pregnant women with sickle cell disease. *New York State J. Med.* **69**, 2686.

O'Driscoll, K. and McCarthy, J. R. (1966). Abruptio placentae and central venous pressure. *J. Obstet. Gynae. Brit. Cwlth.* **73**, 923.

Owen, J. A. (1958). *In* 'Advances in Clinical Chemistry', p. 237. Academic Press, New York and London.

Pack, S., Bader, M. E., Bader, R. A. and Gelb, I. J. (1965). 'Heart Disease, Medical, Surgical and Gynecological Complications.' Williams and Wilkins, Baltimore.

Page, E. W. (1972). On the pathogenesis of pre-eclampsia and eclampsia. *J. Obstet. Gynaec. Brit. Commonw.* **70**, 883.

Perkins, R. P. (1971). Inherited disorders of haemoglobin synthesis and pregnancy. *Am. J. Obstet. Gynec.* **111**, 120.

Phillips, L. L., Skrodelis, V. and Taylor, H. C. (1962). Haemorrhage due to fibrinolysis in abruptio placentae. *Am. J. Obstet. Gynec.* **88**, 1447.

Popert, A. J. (1962). Pregnancy and adrenocortical hormones. Some aspects of their interaction in rheumatic diseases. *Brit. Med. J.* **1**, 967.

Pritchard, J. A. and Ratnoff, O. D. (1955). Studies of fibrinogen and other hemostatic factors in women with intrauterine death and delayed delivery. *Surg. Gynec. Obstet.* **101**, 467.

Ramsay, I. (1976). Thyroid and adrenal disease in pregnancy. *Brit. J. Hosp. Med.* **15**, 373.

Rand, R. J., Jenkins, D. M. and Scott, D. G. (1975). Maternal cardiomyopathy of pregnancy causing stillbirth. *Brit. J. Obstet. Gynec.* **82**, 172.

Rees, W. D. (1965). Pregnant women struck by lightning. *Brit. Med. J.* **1**, 103.

Rice-Oxley, J. M. and Truelove, S. (1950). Ulcerative colitis. Course and prognosis. *Lancet* **1**, 663.

Romer, J. F. and Carey, L. C. (1966). Pancreatitis, a clinical review. *Am. J. Surg.* **111**, 795.

Romney, S. L., Gabel, P. V. and Takada, Y. (1963). Experimental haemorrhage in late pregnancy. *Am. J. Obstet. Gynec.* **87**, 636.

Rubovits, F. E. (1964). Traumatic rupture of the pregnant uterus from 'seat belt' injury. *Am. J. Obstet. Gynec.* **90**, 828.

Samsoenarjo (1959). Rupture of a pregnant uterus by lightning. *J. Indonesian Med. Assoc.* **9**, 420.

Schaefer, G. and Silverman, F. (1961). Pregnancy complicated by asthma. *Am. J. Obstet. Gynec.* **82**, 182.

Scheneker, J. G. and Chowers, I. (1971). Phaeochromocytoma and pregnancy. *Obstet. Gynec. Survey* **26**, 739.

Schmitz, J. T. (1971). Pregnancy patients with burns. *Am. J. Obstet. Gynec.* **110**, 57.

Secher, O. and Wilhjelm, B. (1968). The protective action of anaesthetics against hypoxia. *Can. Anaesth. Soc. J.* **15**, 423.

Sicuranza, B. J. and Tisdall, L. H. (1975). Amniotic fluid embolism. Respiratory problem. *New York State J. Med.* **75**, 1517.

Sims, E. A. H. and Krantz, K. E. (1958). Serial studies of renal function during pregnancy and the puerperium in normal women. *J. Clin. Invest.* **37**, 1764.

Sparkman, R. S. (1958). Rupture of the spleen in pregnancy. *Am. J. Obstet. Gynec.* **76**, 587.

Stirrat, G. M. and Beard, R. W. (1973). Drugs to be avoided or given with caution in the second and third trimesters of pregnancy. *Prescribers' Journal* **13**, 135.

Strauch, B. S. and Hayslett, B. S. (1974). Kidney disease and pregnancy. *Brit. Med. J.* **4**, 578.

Sudo, N. and Weingold, A. B. (1974). Obstetric aspects of the Guillain-Barré syndrome. *Obstet. Gynec.* **45**, 39.

Thiery, M., Deron, R. J., Van Ketz, H. E., de Schacpehyver, A. F., Bernard, P. J., Berkaert, S. A., Hooft, C. M., Derum, F., Roley, G. and Roels, H. J. (1967). Phaeochromocytoma in pregnancy. *Am. J. Obstet. Gynec.* **98**, 21.

Ueland, K. and Hansen, J. M. (1969a). Maternal cardiovascular dynamics II. Posture and uterine contractions. *Am. J. Obstet. Gynecol.* **103**, 1.

Ueland, K., Hansen, J. M. (1969b). Maternal cardiovascular dynamics III. Labour and delivery under local and caudal anaesthesia. *Am. J. Obstet. Gynec.* **103**, 8.

Ueland, K., Akamatsu, T. J., Eng, M. and Bonica, J. J. (1972). Maternal cardiovascular dynamics VI. Caesarean section under epidural anaesthesia without epinephrine. *Am. J. Obstet. Gynec.* **114**, 775.

Ueland, K. and Metcalfe, J. (1975). Circulatory changes in pregnancy. *Clin. Obstet. Gynec.* **18** (3), 41.

Wilkinson, E. J. (1973). Acute pancreatitis in pregnancy. A review of 98 cases and a report of 8 new cases. *Obstet. Gynec. Survey* **28** (5), 281.

Wilson, J., Stephen, G. W. and Scott, D. B. (1969). A study of the cardiovascular effects of chloramethiazole. *Brit. J. Anaesth.* **41**, 840.

Woodhall, R. B. (1942). Traumatic rupture of the pregnant uterus resulting from an automobile accident. *Surgery* **12**, 615.

Woodruff, A. W. (1955). The natural history of anaemia associated with protein malnutrition. *Brit. Med. J.* **1**, 1297.

Yaffe, S. J. (1975). A clinical look at the problem of drugs in pregnancy and their effect on the foetus. *C.M.A. J.* **112**, 728.

Zilliacus, H. (1964). Thrombocytopenia in pregnancy. *Clin. Obstet. Gynec.* **2**, 404.

Zimmermann, W. E., Vogel, W., Mittermeyer, C. H., Walker, F., Kuner, E., Shäfer, H., Birzle, H., Netenjacob, J. and Hirschauer, M. (1972). Gas exchange and metabolic disorders in traumatic-haemorrhagic and septic shock and their treatment. Paper read at a symposium on shock, Buenos Aires, S. America. October 1972, p. 141.

Zitnik, R. S., Brandenberg, R. O., Sheldon, R. and Wallace, R. B. (1969). Pregnancy and open-heart surgery. *Circulation* **39** and **40** (Suppl. 1), 1.

Zuckerman, J. E. and Stubblefield, P. G. (1974). *E. coli* septicaemia in pregnancy associated with the shield intra-uterine contraceptive device. *Am. J. Obstet. Gynec.* **120**, 951.

XII

The Management of Auto-Allergic Diseases

A. J. Rees

Patients critically ill with an auto-allergic disease represent a particular problem for the intensive care physician. Diagnosis may be difficult and necessitate procedures requiring special expertise and it needs great confidence to give the appropriate emergency treatment of steroids and immunosuppressives to a patient in whom the alternative diagnosis is one of infection. These difficulties are compounded by the rarity of severe auto-allergic diseases in general medical practice. This denies most clinicians the opportunity to acquire adequate experience.

INTRODUCTION. PATHOPHYSIOLOGY

Development of auto-allergy

Although the first intimations of auto-allergic disease mechanisms were voiced in the early 1900s (Erlich and Morgenroth, 1901; Donath and Landsteiner, 1904) it is not until the last twenty years that the subject has developed. During this time the concepts governing the origin of auto-allergy have changed. The original supposition which provided the rationale for immunosuppressive therapy, namely that the primary defect was over-activity of the antibody producing cells, has been replaced by a suspicion that these cells are over-active only because of the failure of another population of cells that normally control them.

753

This change of emphasis forces us to reconsider whether the quest for more and more powerful immunosuppressive regimes is appropriate and suggests that future therapy may include stimulation of some immune cells with suppression of others. The whole subject of the control of the immune response, tolerance of self antigens and loss of this tolerance with the development of auto-allergy has been well reviewed recently (Gershon, 1974; Weigle, 1973; British Medical Bulletin, 1976; Lachmann, 1975).

The allergic reaction

For convenience Gell and Coombs (1962) have divided allergic reactions into four classes. Type I (anaphylactic) depends on the release of vaso-active amines by antigen from mast cells previously sensitised by specific IgE class antibodies. Type II (cytotoxic) reactions are initiated by antibodies that directly damage the tissue that they react with. In Type III (immune complex) circulating complexes of antibody and antigen are precipitated in the walls of blood vessels and glomeruli and there excite an inflammatory reaction. Type IV reactions (cell mediated) depend on specifically sensitised lymphocytes becoming cytotoxic to the sensitising tissue. Type II reactions are considered responsible for some types of rapidly progressive nephritis and Goodpasture's syndrome, pemphigus and myasthenia gravis. Whilst Type III reactions are certainly responsible for many of the manifestations of systemic lupus erythematosus and probably for rheumatoid arthritis, polyarteritis nodosa and Wegener's granulomatosis, Type I reactions are probably rarely auto-allergic. The role of Type IV reactions though likely to be important is as yet uncertain. Immune complex disease has been reviewed by Cochrane and Koffler (1973) and anti-basement membrane antibody disease by Wilson and Dixon (1973) and Rees et al. (1978).

The inflammatory response

The damage that results from any type of immune reaction is amplified by the inflammatory response (Weissman, 1975). This response depends on the interaction of humoral factors like the complement, kallekrein, coagulation and fibrinolytic systems with cells such as neutrophils, eosinophils, macrophages and some types of lymphocyte. Platelets are probably also involved. The net effect is vasodilatation, increased vascular permeability and the migration of cells into the damaged area. It seems probable that drugs effective in the treatment of auto-allergy act initially by reducing the inflammatory response, thus reducing damage rather than by modifying the basic immunological event.

THERAPY

Introduction

As alluded to above the aim of therapy is to suppress the allergic reaction and its inflammatory consequences. The most commonly used drugs are steroids and the immunosuppressives, normally purine analogues like azathioprine and 6-mercaptopurine or alkylating agents like cyclophosphamide and chlorambucil. These drugs are particularly useful because they possess both immunosuppressive and anti-inflammatory properties. Recently their clinical pharmacology (Berenbaum, 1975), mode of action (Bach, 1975b) and dangers (Cameron, 1975) have been reviewed. Less frequently drugs with a particular action such as antilymphocyte globulin (A.L.G.), anti-coagulants and anti-platelet agents have been used.

Steroids (Bach, 1975a; Fauci et al., 1976)

Although there is inferential evidence that all the steroids do not possess identical anti-inflammatory and immunosuppressive properties, even when given in equivalent dosage (Wilson, 1974; Fauci, 1976), there are as yet no rational grounds for choosing a particular member of the group. Consequently most people use hydrocortisone and methylprednisolone for intravenous and prednisolone for oral use. There is no doubt that steroids reduce vascular permeability and inhibit the migration of cells into an inflamed area. This inhibition is the probable reason for the neutrophilia consistently seen in steroid-treated patients. More subtle changes in the distribution of cells is probably responsible for the lymphopenia that develops immediately after clinical doses of hydrocortisone or prednisolone because human lymphocytes are resistant to the lytic properties of steroids seen in some species (Clamen, 1972). Humoral immunity is also influenced by steroids in man and a four day course of 100 mg methylprednisolone will diminish immuno-globulin levels for at least a month (Butler and Rossen, 1972). In treating serious auto-allergic disease most people start with 60 mg prednisolone. This dose is maintained for about one week then cautiously reduced if there has been a clinical response. Thereafter the dose is reduced by about 5–10 mg every week until a relapse occurs or until 20 mg per day is reached. It is prudent to stay on this dose for about a month before reducing further. Occasionally 1 g boluses of methylprednisolone have been used but there is no evidence that they are more effective.

Purine analogues

Azathioprine is rapidly converted by the liver into 6-mercaptopurine (6 M-P) and the effects of these two compounds are identical (2 mg 6 M-P being equivalent to 3 mg azathioprine). They damage actively dividing cells and in clinical doses azathioprine will suppress both cell mediated and humoral immunity in man (Swanson and Swartz, 1967). These drugs are also anti-inflammatory (Currey, 1971). The usual dose is 3 mg/kg/day of azathioprine or 2 mg/kg/day 6 M-P.

Alkylating agents

Clinical experience with cyclophosphamide and to a lesser extent chlorambucil has led to the belief that they are more powerful drugs than the purine analogues. This impression gains some credance from the fact that they are also able to damage non-dividing cells. In man both cellular and humoral immunity are modified by 3 mg/kg/day cyclophosphamide (Hurd and Guiliano, 1975) and chlorambucil 0.2 mg/kg/day which are the doses normally used.

Less commonly used drugs

The currently available A.L.G. is raised in horses and is active against circulating thymus-dependent (non-antibody producing) lymphocytes. The dose is 30 mg/kg/day for one week after a test dose to check for allergy to horse serum. It has not yet found a place in the treatment of auto-allergy in man. The use of anticoagulants and antiplatelet agents has been largely restricted to the treatment of severe nephritis and will be discussed later. Experimental data suggest that defibrination with ancrod may be more powerful than other anticoagulants (Naish et al., 1972; Thomson et al., 1975). It is given in a dose of 2 units/kg/day as a single intravenous injection. Therapy is monitored by measuring the fibrinogen level which rises when antibodies formed to the ancrod make it ineffective. This takes about one month.

Plasma exchange (plasmapheresis) (Editorial, 1976)

This technique involves the removal of whole blood from a patient, separation of the cells from the plasma by centrifugation and retransfusion of cells together with plasma protein fraction with another plasma substitute. Thus specific antibody, immune complexes and humoral mediators of inflammation such as fibrinogen and complement can be removed. Originally the separation was laboriously achieved by centrifugation of single units of blood but the introduction of continuous or semi-continuous cell separators, such as the Aminco continuous-flow blood cell separator (American Instrument Company, Silverspring, U.S.A.) or the Haemonetics Model 30 cell separator (Haemonetics Corporation, Natick, Boston, U.S.A.) have made one to four litre exchanges a clinical possibility (Fig. 1). A four litre exchange can be effected in about an hour and a half with one of these separators if vascular access is via an arterio-venous shunt. A single four litre plasma exchange will remove approximately 95% of an intra-vascular marker,

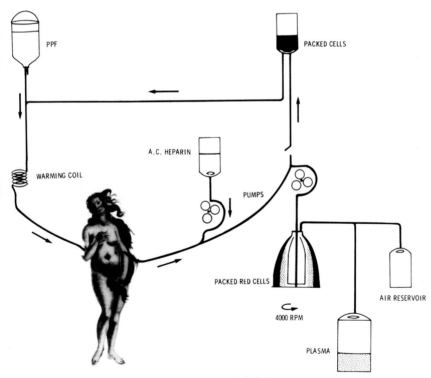

Fig. 1. Circuit diagram of a Haemonetics Model 30 Cell Separator.

and 75% of labelled IgG injected 48 h previously and daily 4 litre exchanges will reduce the level of complement (C3) to 30% of normal and fibrinogen to 75 mg/100 ml (Lockwood et al., 1976). Others have used 1 litre exchanges (Verrier-Jones et al., 1976) but no data are available on the amount of immuno-globulin removed.

The great benefit that has been claimed for plasma exchange is that it should be able to act more quickly than drugs and thus may prevent irreversible damage from ensuing before they are effective. For this reason, and because experiments have shown that the rebound in the level of specific antibody that follows plasma exchange may be abrogated by the concurrent administration of immunosuppressives (Bystryn et al., 1970, 1971), we routinely give prednisolone 60 mg and cyclophosphamide 3 mg/kg at the inception of a course of plasma exchange.

There are, as yet, no definite indications for plasma exchange except in Goodpasture's syndrome (Lockwood et al., 1977), but it should be considered in all patients with fulminant auto-allergic disease, especially when conventional therapy has failed. Controlled studies are urgently required to confirm this. The quantity of plasma best exchanged, the number of exchanges and the ideal solution to exchange are even less certain. Our policy is to do five daily four litre exchanges for plasma protein fraction before assessing the efficacy and thereafter to continue exchanges depending on the clinical progress.

MANAGEMENT OF SPECIFIC DISEASES

Introduction

Diseases caused by auto-allergy are heterogeneous and include the auto-allergic anaemias, thrombocytopenias and various skin diseases which are discussed in other chapters. The purpose of this section is to review the information available on the treatment of the collagen diseases and, since severe nephritis is often the life-threatening event in these diseases, to presage the discussion with an account of rapidly progressive nephritis.

Rapidly progressive nephritis (Kincaid-Smith et al., 1973; Heptinstall, 1974)

This form of nephritis which progresses to complete glomerular destruction in a matter of weeks has many causes. Most cases result from the deposition of immune complexes in glomeruli, a few from the destructive effect of an antibody directed against glomerular basement membrane (G.B.M.). It may occur in isolation sometimes following streptococcal or other infection; it may be superimposed on an underlying chronic nephritis or it may be a manifestation of systemic disease such as systemic lupus, polyarteritis, Wegener's granulomatosis, Henoch-Schonlein purpura or Goodpasture's syndrome. The clinical picture is inconstant; reflecting the systemic disease, infection, or uraemia if present. Proteinuria is invariable as is the presence of red cells and casts in the urine deposit, but both peripheral oedema and hypertension are inconstant and the level of serum complement reflects the original disease. The crucial investigation is a high dose intravenous program followed by renal biopsy which confirms the diagnosis. Immunofluorescence must be done on these biopsies to look for linear staining of the G.B.M. with anti-IgG which is indicative of anti-G.B.M. antibodies. Because many of these antibodies cross-react with lung basement membrane these patients are at risk from pulmonary haemorrhage (Goodpasture's syndrome). An outline of investigation and management is given in Tables 1 and 2 respectively. The use of specific treatment is controversial and no controlled data exist. Few, if any, patients who are anuric at presentation recover either with or without therapy (Harrison et al., 1964). Of those less severely affected,

Table 1. Investigation of severe nephritis

Initial
Full blood count and film
Blood urea, creatinine, electrolytes
Serum albumin
Urinalysis and microscopy
24 h urine protein. Creatinine chest X-ray

Confirmation
High dose I.V.P.
Renal biopsy with immunofluorescence

Ancillary
Immunoglobulins
Complement (CH_{50}, C_3)
A.N.F., D.N.A. binding, L.E. cells
Cryoglobulins
Coombs test
Australia antigen
Rheumatoid factor
Anti-G.B.M. antibody

Table 2. Management of severe nephritis

Hypertension
Diastolic > 105 mm Hg parenteral hydrallazine diazoxide
Diastolic < 105 mm Hg oral propranolol

Oedema
'Loop' diuretics (e.g. frusemide) hydrallazine
Sodium restriction (30 → 60 meq/24 h)
Water restriction (500 ml → 1500 ml)

Uraemia
Dietary protein restriction (40 → 60 g/24 h)
Dialysis

'Specific' therapy
1. Steroids – prednisolone 60 mg/day
        plus
2. Immunosuppressives – cyclophosphamide 3 mg/kg or azathioprine 3 mg/kg
   ?? plus
3. Anticoagulants – heparin 10 000 6 hourly or ancrod 10 units/kg/day
   ?? plus
4. Antiplatelet agent – dipyramidole 200 mg q.d.s.
        and
5. Consider plasma-exchange

Monitor progress
1. Blood urea + creatinine – daily
2. 24 h urea + creatinine excretion – twice weekly
3. Serum albumin – twice weekly
4. 24 h protein excretion – twice weekly
5. Full blood count – daily
6. Urine deposit – weekly

some with systemic disease (other than Goodpasture's) achieve useful recovery with immunosuppressives and steroids (usually prednisolone plus azathioprine or cyclophosphamide) (Sonsino *et al.*, 1972; Bacani *et al.*, 1968). Whilst recovery of renal function apparently as a result of a combination of steroids, immunosuppressives, anticoagulants and antiplatelet agents (for example heparin 10 000 six hourly plus dipyridamole 200 mg q.d.s.) have been reported even in those without systemic disease (Kincaid-Smith *et al.*, 1968; Kincaid-Smith *et al.*, 1970; Brown *et al.*, 1974), whether the benefits are greater than the dangers is still debated (Cameron, 1973). Despite the encouraging animal experiments cited above no clinical experience with ancrod has been reported.

We have plasma-exchanged thirteen patients with rapidly progressive nephritis not due to anti-basement membrane antibodies;

twelve improved with a fall in serum creatinine and a rise in creatinine clearance (Lockwood *et al.*, 1977). The case for intensive plasma exchange in anti-basement membrane antibody nephritis with lung haemorrhage (Goodpasture's syndrome) is perhaps stronger. Pulmonary haemorrhage was controlled in all seven patients in the series reported by Lockwood *et al.* (1976) and in the three patients with residual function the serum creatinine fell. Others have reported similar successes (Depner *et al.*, 1975; Rossen *et al.*, 1976). Bilateral nephrectomy in an attempt to reduce antibody stimulation has previously been advocated for control of life-threatening lung haemorrhage (Nowakowski *et al.*, 1971; Maddock *et al.*, 1967; Halgrimson *et al.*, 1971). There is no convincing evidence that it reduces either the stimulus to antibody production or lung haemorrhage (Wilson and Dixon, 1975); plasma exchange is the treatment of choice.

Systemic lupus erythematosus (Estes and Christian, 1971; Dubois, 1974)

Lupus is a disease of remissions and exacerbations which may present as an auto-allergic haemolytic anaemia or thrombocytopenia. Usually, however, there is evidence of an immune complex-induced small or medium sized vessel arteritis which produces life-threatening consequences, particularly if the cerebral or renal vessels are involved. The disease should be suspected in any patient who presents with fever, arthralgia and a rash, particularly when associated with alopecia or evidence of nephritis. There is usually a mild anaemia and often a

Table 3. Management of severe lupus

(*i*) Confirm diagnosis. A.N.F., D.N.A. binding, L.E. cells.
(*ii*) Define which organs are involved.
(*iii*) Manage nephritis as above.
(*iv*) 'Specific' therapy
    1. High dose steroids.
      consider
    2. Immunosuppressives e.g. cyclophosphamide or azathioprine 3 mg/kg.
      and
    3. Plasma-exchange.
(*v*) Monitor response
    1. Clinical – renal, cerebral.
    2. Immunological complement – weekly.
      D.N.A. binding – weekly.
      Cryoglobulins.
(*vi*) Developing psychosis is usually due to cerebral lupus.

lymphopenia; gamma globulins are raised and serum albumin low if proteinuria has been severe. The use of the L.E. cell phenomenon for laboratory confirmation has largely been replaced by the anti-nuclear factor (A.N.F.) and by D.N.A. binding, a test for antibodies to double stranded D.N.A. that are specific for lupus. When the disease is active the early complement components (C_4, C_3) are low, and cryoglobulins (globulin-anti-globulin complexes that precipitate in the cold) may be present. If there is any evidence of nephritis such as hypertension, proteinuria, abnormal urine deposit or impaired renal function, a renal biopsy is mandatory, and renal histology provides a guide to prognosis and therapy (Pollack et al., 1961).

The treatment of severe lupus is summarised in Table 3. Steroids in high dosage (the equivalent of 60 mg prednisolone per day) are the mainstay of the treatment for severe exacerbations. Patients with cerebral involvement are a special problem because the presentation is diverse and varies from the purely psychiatric, which may be difficult to distinguish from steroid-induced psychosis, to any form of organic brain syndrome (Johnson and Richardson, 1968; Bennett et al., 1972). Examination of C.S.F. is rarely diagnostic but should be done to exclude opportunistic infection and C.S.F. complement levels are not as helpful as was initially supposed (Handler, 1973). Brain scans, isotopic cerebral blood flow studies, and E.E.Gs. may demonstrate localised areas of vasculitis. Very high doses of steroids (greater than 100 mg prednisolone per day) may be necessary to control symptoms and even then may not be successful (Sergent et al., 1974). Verrier-Jones (1976) has reported the failure to control cerebral lupus by low intensity plasma exchange (3–5 litres per week) in two patients. Intensive plasma exchange has not been tried.

Severe lupus nephritis presents other problems. Hypertension requires vigorous treatment and diastolic pressures should be maintained below 90 mm Hg. A combination of a diuretic, β-blocker, such as propranalol, and hydrallazine (even though it can cause drug-induced lupus) is most suitable. Very high doses of frusemide (250 mg to 1 g daily), sometimes in conjunction with infusions of plasma, may be necessary to clear oedema. Dialysis should be used to treat uraemia if severe but it is important to remember that oliguric, malnourished patients, particularly when on steroids may have a disproportionately high plasma urea relative to creatinine. Under these circumstances dietary restrictions may exacerbate the situation. As with other manifestations of lupus, high dose steroids (prednisolone 60 mg/day) are helpful (Pollak et al., 1961; Holman, 1960). However, they do not halt the progression of the disease in some patients who have been documented to benefit from the addition of azathioprine (Lorenzen and Videback, 1965; Drinkard *et al.*, 1970; Hayslett *et al.*, 1972), chlorambucil (Amor *et al.*, 1972; Snaith *et al.*, 1973) or cyclophosphamide (Seah *et al.*, 1966; Cameron, 1973; Feng *et al.*, 1973). Controlled studies to date have been conflicting. With azathioprine some show benefit (Sztejnbok *et al.*, 1971; Cade *et al.*, 1973), others not (Donadio *et al.*, 1974; Hahn *et al.*, 1976). The reports on cyclophosphamide are equally confusing (Decker *et al.*, 1976). Methylprednisolone in 1 g doses has also been used (Cathcart *et al.*, 1976) as has low intensity plasma exchange (Verrier-Jones *et al.*, 1976). The general significance of these reports is impossible to judge. As a general policy most renal physicians treat severe lupus nephritis with steroids in combination with either azathioprine 3 mg/kg/day. We are instituting a controlled trial to see if plasma exchange gives additional benefit.

Polyarteritis nodosa (Rose and Spencer, 1957)

Polyarteritis nodosa is characterised by a widespread vasculitis reminiscent of the arthus reaction, a fact that encourages the belief that it is an immune complex disease. Many classifications have been proposed but are of little help prognostically. In some parts of the world polyarteritis is associated with chronic Australia antigen carriage (Gocke *et al.*, 1970; Trepo *et al.*, 1974; Sergent *et al.*, 1976) but this does not appear to be true in the United Kingdom. Drugs, usually antibiotics, have also been implicated as precipitants but it is difficult to know whether this is a true association or whether the symptom for which the drug was prescribed was the first of polyarteritis.

Despite the diversity of the pathological lesion, the clinical picture is surprisingly uniform; fever, weight loss, proximal muscle weakness and peripheral neuropathy being the most frequent presenting symptoms. Renal function may decline rapidly, either due to a severe glomerular nephritis in those with small vessel disease, or to renal ischaemia and infarction in those in whom larger vessels are involved. Proteinuria, numerous red cells and the absence of hypertension help to distinguish the former group from the latter who are usually hypertensive. Laboratory tests are unhelpful in confirming the diagnosis. Biopsy, even of an affected tissue often yields equivocal results (Maxeiner, 1954) and renal biopsy should probably be postponed until after angiography in those with hypertension for fear of entering an aneurysm. Angiography may be pathognomonic (Padovani *et al.*, 1974) and is the investigation of choice, both in making a diagnosis and in determining the site of a bleeding aneurysm.

The diagnosis and management of polyarteritis nodosa is summarised in Table 4.

High dose steroids and rigorous control of blood pressure are the cornerstones of therapy. No controlled data exist but many reports attest the effectiveness of steroids in controlling acute symptoms (M.R.C., 1957; Frohneurt and Sheps, 1967). It is hard to gauge whether immunosuppressive drugs confer additional benefit although many have been enthusiastic (Godeau *et al.*, 1972; Demis *et al.*, 1964). Our policy is to combine high dose prednisolone with cyclophosphamide with daily four litre plasma exchanges, and this pilot experience suggests that it may confer additional benefit (Lockwood *et al.*, 1977). A controlled study is now in progress.

Wegener's granulomatosis (Fauci and Wolff, 1973)

Wegener's granulomatosis is characterised by granulomas in the upper and lower respiratory tracts and in the kidneys. It presents either with respiratory symptoms, of which the most severe is massive pulmonary haemorrhage, or as a generalised disease with fever, weight loss etc. Renal involvement which may be severe is invariable with the latter presentation. There are no laboratory tests to confirm the diagnosis and chest X-ray may either show diffuse mottling or discrete lesions that may cavitate. Lung biopsy may reveal characteristic granulomas with vasculitis. Granulomas are rarely seen in renal biopsies which usually

Table 4. Management of polyarteritis nodosa

(*i*) Confirm diagnosis
    1. Visceral angiography.
    2. Biopsy of affected tissue.
    3. Australia antigen.
(*ii*) Define which organs are involved
(*iii*) Treat renal involvement.
(*iv*) Specific therapy
    1. Steroids – e.g. prednisolone 60 mg/day.
    2. Immunosuppressives.
      and consider
    3. Plasma-exchange.
(*v*) Monitor response
    1. Clinical.
    2. Immunological.

---

show a severe nephritis. Steroids appear to help pulmonary symptoms but not renal failure (Beidleman, 1963; Hollander and Manning, 1967) which does, however, appear to respond to azathioprine (Bouroncle *et al.*, 1967; Aldo *et al.*, 1970), methotrexate (Capizzi and Bertino, 1971) and particularly to cyclophosphamide (Fauci and Wolff, 1973; Reza *et al.*, 1975), which is the drug of choice and is given in the usual dose.

Scleroderma (Cannon *et al.*, 1974)

Scleroderma is a generalised disease characterised by thickening of the skin on the hands and face, thickening of the wall of the oesophagus and small intestine and sometimes of the heart. Aspiration pneumonia is common but the most severe complication is of irreversible renal failure associated with accelerated hypertension and a microangiopathic haemolytic anaemia. Renal angiography shows cortical necrosis and renal biopsy fibrinoid necrosis of the small vessels. Therapeutic regimes have included steroids, immunosuppressive drugs, anticoagulants including ancrod, but none is effective. Control of hypertension is all that can be offered.

Other conditions

Many other conditions presumed to be due to auto-allergic mechanisms occasionally present acutely to intensive care physicians. They include Henoch Schonlein purpura (Meadow *et al.*, 1972), polymyositis (Pearson, 1974), mixed cryoglobulinaemia (Meltzer and Franklin, 1966) and, occasionally, systemic rheumatoid arthritis. The principles of treatment are the same as those of the diseases discussed in detail (and the results just as uncontrolled!). The reader is referred to the original references for details.

CONCLUSION

This chapter has attempted to outline what is known about the origin of auto-allergic disease and what uncertainties persist, because it is only with a clear idea of these that new and more effective treatment regimes may be devised. There is a desperate need for such regimes to be evaluated by some form of controlled trial. These should aim to be more specific because at present opportunistic infection is a major cause of death in patients otherwise successfully treated.

REFERENCES

Aldo, M. A., Benson, M. D., Comerford, F. R. and Cohen, A. S. (1970). Treatment of Wegener's granulomatosis with Imuran. *Arch. Intern. Med.* **126**, 298.

Amor, B., Kahan, A., Pompidou, A. and Delbarre, F. (1972). Efficacité des immunodépresseurs dans la maladie lupique. *Nouvelle Presse Med.* **1**, 1699.

Bacani, T., Velasquez, F., Kanter, C., Pirani, C. L. and Pollack, V. E. (1968). Rapidly progressive (non-streptococcal) glomerulonephritis. *Ann. Intern. Med.* **69**.

Bach, J.-F. (1975a). Advances in steroid therapy. *In* 'Advances in Nephrology' (Ed. J. Hamburger, J. Crosnier and M. H. Maxwell). Year Book Medical Publishers, Chicago.

Bach, J.-F. (1975b). 'The Mode of Action on Immunosuppressive Agents.' Elsevier, New York.

Beidleman, B. (1963). Wegener's granulomatosis. Prolonged therapy with large doses of steroids. *JAMA* **186**, 827.

Berenbaum, M. C. (1975). The clinical pharmacology of immunosuppressive drugs. *In* 'Clinical Aspects of Immunology' (Ed. P. G. H. Gell, R. R. A. Coombs and P. J. Lachmann). Blackwell, Oxford.

Bennett, R., Hughes, G. R. V., Bywaters, E. G. L. and Hold, P. J. L. (1972). Neuropsychiatric problems in systemic lupus erythematosus. *Brit. Med. J.* **4**, 342.

Bouroncle, B. A., Smith, E. J., Cuppage, F. E. (1967). Treatment of Wegener's granulomatosis with Imuran. *Am. J. Med.* **42**, 334.

Brown, C. B., Wilson, D., Turn⌐⌐, D., Cameron, J. S., Ogg, C. S., Chantler, C. and Gill, D. (1974). Combined immunosuppression and anticoagulation in rapidly progressive nephritis. *Lancet* **2**, 1166.

British Medical Bulletin (1976). Immunological tolerance (Ed. D. W. Dresser). *Brit. Med. Bull.* **32**, 2.

Bystryn, J. C., Graf, M. W. and Uhr, J. W. (1970). Regulation of antibody by plasma exchange. *J. Exp. Med.* **132**, 1279.

Bystryn, J. C., Schenkein, I. and Uhr, J. W. (1971). A model for the regulation synthesis by antibody level. *In* 'Progress in Immunology' (Ed. B. Amos) p. 627. Academic Press, New York.

Butler, W. T. and Rossen, R. D. (1973). The effect of corticosteroids in Man: I Decreased serum concentrations of IgG caused by 3 or 5 days of high doses of methylprednisolone. *J. Clin. Invest.* **52**, 2629.

Cade, R., Spooner, G., Schlein, E., Pickering, M., Dequesada, A., Holcomb, A., Juncos, L., Richard, G., Shires, D., Leven, D., Hackett, R., Free, J., Hunt, R. and Fregly, M. (1973). Comparison of azathioprine, prednisolone and heparin alone or combined in treating lupus nephritis. *Nephron* **10**, 37.

Cameron, J. S. (1973). Are anticoagulants of value in the treatment of rapidly progressive nephritis? *In* 'Proceedings of the European Dialysis and Transplant Association' (Ed. J. F. Moorhead, C. Mion and R. A. Baillod) p. 57. Pitman Medical, Bath and London.

Cameron, J. S. and Boulton Jones, M. (1973). Lupus nephritis, long-term follow up. *In* 'Glomerulonephritis Part II' (Ed. P. Kincaid-Smith, T. H. Matthew and E. L. Becker) p. 1187. John Wiley, New York.

Cameron, J. S. (1975). Problems with immunosuppressive agents in renal disease. *In* 'Drugs and Disease' (Ed. S. Worlledge). Royal College of Pathologists.

Cannon, P. J., Hassar, M., Case, D. B., Casarella, W. J., Sommers, S. C. and LeRoy,

E. C. (1974). The relationship of hypertension and renal failure in scleroderma (progressive systemic sclerosis) to structural and functional abnormalities of the renal cortical circulation. *Medicine* (Baltimore) **53**, 1.

Capizzi, R. L. and Bertino, J. R. (1971). Methotrexate therapy of Wegener's granulomatosis. *Ann. Intern. Med.* **74**, 74.

Cathcart, E. S., Idelson, B. A., Scheinberg, A. and Couser, W. G. (1976). Beneficial effects of methylprednisolone 'pulse' therapy in diffuse proliferative lupus nephritis. *Lancet* **1**, 163.

Clamen, H. N. (1972). Corticosteroids and lymphoid cells. *New Engl. J. Med.* **287**, 388.

Cochrane, C. G. and Koffler, D. (1973). Immune complex disease in experimental animals and man. *In* 'Advances in Immunology 16' (Ed. F. J. Dixon and H. Kunkel) p. 185. Academic Press, New York and London.

Currey, H. F. L. (1971). A comparison of immunosuppressive and anti-inflammatory agents in the rat. *Clin. Exp. Immunol.* **9**, 879.

Decker, J. L., Klippel, J. H., Plotz, P. H. and Steinberg, A. D. (1975). Cyclophosphamide or azathioprine in lupus glomerulonephritis: a controlled trial: results at 28 months. *Ann. Intern. Med.* **83**, 606.

Demis, D. J., Brown, C. S. and Crosby, W. Y. (1964). Thioguanine in the treatment of certain autoimmune immunologic and related disorders. *Am. J. Med.* **37**, 195.

Depner, T. A., Chaffin, M. E., Wilson, C. B. and Gulyassy, P. F. (1975). Plasmapheresis for severe Goodpasture's syndrome. Abstracts. *Am. Soc. Nephrol.* 8th Annual Meeting, 13.

Donadio, J. V., Holley, K. E., Wagoner, R. D., Ferguson, R. H. and McDuffie, F. C. (1974). Further observations on the treatment of lupus nephritis with prednisone and combined prednisone and azathioprine. *Arthritis Rheum.* **17**, 573.

Donath, J. and Landsteiner, K. (1904). Über Paricysmale Hämoglobinorie. *Munch. Med. Wschr.* **51**, 1590.

Drinkard, J. P., Stanley, T. M., Dornfeld, L., Austin, R. C., Barnett, E. V., Pearson, C. M., Vernier, R. L., Adams, D. A., Latta, H. and Gonick, H. C. (1970). Azathioprine and prednisolone in the treatment of adults with lupus nephritis. *Medicine* (Baltimore) **49**, 411.

Dubois, E. L. (1974). 'Systemic Lupus Erythematosus.' University of California Press, Los Angeles.

Editorial (1976). Plasmapheresis and Immunosuppression. *Lancet* **1**, 1113.

Erlich, P. and Morgenroth, J. (1901). Über Hämolysine v. *Berl. Klin. Wschr.* **38**, 251.

Estes, D. and Christian, C. L. (1971). The natural history of systemic lupus erythematosus by prospective analysis. *Medicine* (Baltimore) **50**, 85.

Fauci, A. S. (1976). Mechanisms of corticosteroids on lymphoid sub-populations II Differential effects of *in vivo* hydrocortisone, prednisone and dexamethasone of *in vitro* expression of lymphocyte function. *Clin. Exp. Immunol.* **24**, 54.

Fauci, A. S., Dale, D. C. and Balow, J. E. (1976). Glucocorticosteroid therapy: mechanisms of action and clinical considerations. *Ann. Intern. Med.* **84**, 304.

Fauci, A. S. and Wolff, S. M. (1973). Wegener's granulomatosis: studies in eighteen patients and a review of the literature. *Medicine* (Baltimore) **52**, 535.

Feng, P. H., Jayartnam, F. J., Tock, E. P. C. and Seah, C. S. (1973). Cyclophosphamide in the treatment of systemic lupus erythematosus: 7 years experience. *Brit. Med. J.* **2**, 450.

Frohneurt and Sheps (1967). Long-term follow-up study of periarteritis nodosa. *Am. J. Med.* **43**, 8.

Gell, P. G. H. and Coombs, R. R. A. (1962). 'Clinical Aspects of Immunology.' Blackwell, Oxford and London.

Gershon, R. K. (1974). 'T' cell control of antibody production. In 'Contemporary Topics in Immunobiology Vol. III' (Ed. M. D. Cooper and N. L. Warner) p. 1. Plenum, New York.

Gocke, D. J., Hsu, K., Morgan, C., Bombardieri, S., Lockshin, M. and Christian, C. L. (1970). Association between polyarteritis and Australia antigen. Lancet 2, 1149.

Godeau, P., Sicard, D., Herreman, G., Imbert, J.-Ce. and Ghozlan, R. (1972). Aspects nosologiques et évoluties de la périartérite noueuse (à propos de 25 cas). Ann. Med. Interne 123, 967.

Hahn, B. H., Kantor, O. S. and Osterland, K. C. (1975). Azathioprine plus prednisone compared with prednisolone alone in the treatment of systemic lupus erythematosus. Ann. Intern. Med. 83, 597.

Halgrimson, C. C., Wilson, C. B., Dixon, F. J., Penn, I., Anderson, J. T., Ogden, D. A. and Starzl, T. E. (1971). Goodpasture's syndrome. Treatment with nephrectomy and transplantation. Archs. Surg. 103, 283.

Handler, N. M., Gerwin, R. D., Frank, N. M., Whitaker, J. N., Baker, M. and Decker, J. L. (1973). The fourth component of complement in the cerebrospinal fluid in systemic lupus erythematosus. Arthritis Rheum. 16, 507.

Harrison, C. V., Loughridge, L. W. and Milne, M. D. (1964). Acute oliguric renal failure in acute glomerulonephritis and polyarteritis nodosa. Quart. J. Med. 33, 39.

Hayslett, J. P., Kashgarian, M., Cook, C. D. and Spargo, B. H. (1972). The effect of azathioprine and lupus nephritis. Medicine (Baltimore) 33, 291.

Heptinstall, R. H. (1974). 'The Pathology of the Kidney', p. 371. Little, Brown, Boston.

Holman, H. (1960). Systemic lupus erythematosus: a review of certain recent developments in the study of this disease. J. Paediatr. 56, 109.

Hollander, D. and Manning, R. T. (1967). The use of alkylating agents in the treatment of Wegener's granulomatosis. Ann. Intern. Med. 67, 393.

Hurd, E. R. and Guiliano, V. J. (1975). The effect of cyclophosphamide on 'B' and 'T' lymphocytes in connective tissue disease. Arthritis Rheum. 18, 67.

Johnson, R. T. and Richardson, E. P. (1968). The neurological manifestations of systemic lupus erythematosus. Medicine (Baltimore) 47, 337.

Kincaid-Smith, P., Laver, M. C., Fairley, K. F. and Matthews, D. C. (1970). Dipyrimadole and anticoagulants in renal disease due to glomerular and vascular lesions: a new approach to therapy. Med. J. Aust. 1, 145.

Kincaid-Smith, P., Mathew, T. and Becker, E. L. (Ed.) (1973). 'Glomerulonephritis'. John Wiley, New York.

Kincaid-Smith, P., Saker, B. M. and Fairley, K. F. (1968). Anticoagulants in irreversible acute renal failure. Lancet 2, 1360.

Lachmann, P. J. (1975). Auto-allergy. In 'Clinical Aspects of Immunology' (Ed. P. G. H. Gell, R. R. A. Coombs and P. J. Lachmann) p. 859. Blackwell, Oxford and London.

Lockwood, C. M., Rees, A. J., Pearson, T. A., Evans, D. J. and Peters, D. K. (1976). Immunosuppression and plasma exchange in the treatment of Goodpasture's syndrome. Lancet 1, 711.

Lockwood, C. M., Rees, A. J., Pussell, B., and Peters, D. K. (1977). Experience of the use of plasma-exchange in the management of potentially fulminating glomerulonephritis and SLE. Exp. Hemat. 5, Supplement, 117–136.

Lorenzen, J. and Videback, A. (1965). Treatment of collagen diseases with cytostatics. *Lancet* **2**, 558.

Maddock, R. K., Stevens, L. E., Reemtsma, K. and Bloomer, H. A. (1967). Goodpasture's syndrome. Cessation of pulmonary haemorrhage after bi-lateral nephrectomy. *Ann. Intern. Med.* **67**, 1258.

Maxiener, S. R., McDonald, J. R. and Kirklin, J. W. (1952). Muscle biopsy in the diagnosis of periarteritis nodosa. *Surg. Clin. N. Amer.* **32**, 1225.

Meadow, S. R., Glasgow, E. F., White, R. H. R., Moncreiff, M. W., Cameron, J. S. and Ogg, C. S. (1972). Schönlein-Henoch nephritis. *Quart. J. Med.* **41** (N.S.), 241.

Medical Research Council (1957). Treatment of polyarteritis nodosa with steroids. *Brit. Med. J.* **1**, 608.

Meltzer, M. and Franklin, E. C. (1966). Cryoglobulinaemia: a study of twenty-nine patients. *Am. J. Med.* **40**, 828.

Naish, P., Penn, G. B., Evans, D. J. and Peters, D. K. (1972). The effects of defibrination on nephrotoxic serum nephritis in rabbits. *Clin. Sci. and Molec. Med.* **42**, 643.

Nowakowski, A., Grove, R. B., King, L. H. Jr., Antonovych, T. T., Fortner, R. W., Knieser, M. R., Carter, C. B. and Knepshield, J. H. (1971). Goodpasture's syndrome: recovery from severe pulmonary haemorrhage after bi-lateral nephrectomy. *Ann. Intern. Med.* **75**, 243.

Padovani, J., Kasbarian, M., Pollini, J., Faure, F. and Leynaud, D. (1974). Intérêt de l'arteriographie renale dans la periarterite noueuse. *Ann. Radiol.* (Paris) **17**, 141.

Pearson, C. M. (1974). Polymyositis and related disorders. *In* 'Disorders of Voluntary Muscle' (Ed. J. N. Walton). Churchill Livingstone, Edinburgh and London.

Pollak, V. E., Pirani, C. L. and Kark, R. M. (1961). Effect of large doses of prednisone on the renal lesion and life span of patients with lupus glomerulonephritis. *J. Lab. Clin. Med.* **57**, 495.

Rees, A. J., Lockwood, C. M. and Peters, D. K. (1978). 'Anti GBM Disease. Glomerulonephritis.' (Ed. A. d'Apice and P. Kincaid-Smith). John Wiley, New York.

Reza, M. J., Dornfeld, L., Goldberg, L. S., Bluestone, R. and Pearson, C. M. (1975). Wegener's granulomatosis: long-term follow-up of patients treated with cyclophosphamide. *Arthritis Rheum.* **18**, 501.

Rose, G. A. and Spencer, H. (1957). Polyarteritis nodosa. *Quart. J. Med.* **26** (N.S.), 43.

Rossen, R. D., Duffy, J., McCredie, K. B., Reisenberg, M. A., Sharp, J. T., Hersh, E. M., Eknoyan, G. and Suki, W. N. (1976). The treatment of Goodpasture's syndrome with cyclophosphamide, prednisolone and plasma exchange transfusions. *Clin. Exp. Immunol.* **24**, 218.

Seah, C. S., Wang, K. H., Chew, A. G. K. and Jayaratham, F. J. (1966). Cyclophosphamide in the treatment of systemic lupus erythematosus. *Brit. Med. J.* **1**, 333.

Sergent, J. S., Lockshin, M. D., Christian, C. L. and Gocke, D. J. (1976). Vasculitis with hepatitis B antigenaemia. *Medicine* (Baltimore) **55**, 1.

Snaith, M. L., Holt, J. M., Oliver, D. O., Dunnill, M. A., Holley, W. and Stephenson, A. C. (1972). Treatment of patients with systemic lupus erythematosus including nephritis with chlorambucil. *Brit. Med. J.* **2**, 197.

Sonsino, E., Nabarra, A., Kazatchine, M., Hinglais, N. and Kries, H. (1972). Extracapillary proliferative glomerulonephritis. *In* 'Advances in Nephrology II' (Ed. J. Hamburger, J. Crosnier and M. H. Maxwell). Medical Year Book, Chicago.

Swanson, A. M. and Swartz, R. S. (1967). Immunosuppressive therapy. The relationship between the clinical response and immunological competence. *New Engl. J. Med.* **277**, 163.

Sztejnbok, M., Stewart, A., Diamond, H. and Kapland, D. (1971). Azathioprine in the treatment of systemic lupus erythematosus. A controlled study. *Arthritis Rheum.* **14**, 639.

Thomson, N. M., Simpson, I. J. and Peters, D. K. (1975). A quantitative evacuation of anticoagulants in experimental nephrotoxic nephritis. *Clin. Exp. Immunol.* **19**, 301.

Trepo, C. G., Zuckerman, A. J., Bird, R. C. and Prince, A. M. (1974). The role of circulating hepatitis B antigen/antibody immune complexes in the pathogenesis of vascular and hepatic manifestations of polyarteritis nodosa. *J. Clin. Pathol.* **27**, 863.

Verrier-Jones, J., Cumming, R. H., Bucknall, R. C., Asplin, C. M., Frazer, I. D., Bothamley, J., Davis, P. and Hamblin, T. J. (1976). Plasmapheresis in the management of acute systemic lupus erythematosus? *Lancet* **1**, 709.

Weigle, W. O. (1973). Immunological unresponsiveness. *In* 'Advances in Immunology 16' (Ed. F. J. Dixon and H. G. Kunkel) p. 61. Academic Press, London and New York.

Wiessman, G. (ed.) (1974). 'Mediators of Inflammation.' Plenum, New York and London.

Wilson, C. B. and Dixon, F. J. (1973). Anti-glomerular basement membrane antibody induced nephritis. *Kidney Int.* **3**, 74.

Wilson, C. B. and Dixon, F. J. (1974). Diagnosis of immunopathologic renal disease. *Kidney Int.* **5**, 389.

Wilson, J. W. (1974). Cellular localisation of ^{3}H-labelled corticosteroids by electron microscopic auto radiography after haemorrhagic shock. *In* 'Corticosteroids in the Treatment of Circulatory Shock' (Ed. T. Glenn and A. Lefer) p. 275. University Park Press, Baltimore.

XIII

The Management of Dermatological Emergencies

J. S. Pegum

The skin is an organ of considerable size and extent. It has many functions (some vital): as a barrier to prevent fluid loss and dilution of the body's fluid in an aqueous environment; to guard against infection; the ability to pour out great quantities of sweat on to the largely hairless skin to promote cooling; the ability of the skin blood vessels to contract and conserve heat in the cold; and the sensory function which warns against hostile factors in the environment and which furnishes the brain with essential information. The widespread view that disease of the skin is not likely to prove fatal has enough substance in it to suggest that the organ is well adapted to its function in spite of the many maladies and abnormalities which may affect it.

Skin failure may lead to fluid, electrolyte or protein loss and failure to conserve heat so that a stable temperature cannot be maintained. The intact skin acts as a barrier against infection. The skin too can become widely and severely neoplastic.

EXFOLIATIVE DERMATITIS

Exfoliative dermatitis (E.D.) is not uncommon and it has been well

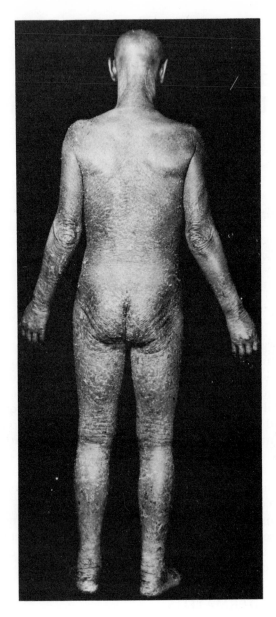

Fig. 1. Exfoliative dermatitis.

studied and documented. It is characterised by widespread or universal scaling, usually associated with redness (Fig. 1). The appendages, the hair, the nails and the glands of the skin may also be affected. Erythrodermia is a non-identical twin of E.D. It is a widespread or universal redness with little scaling. There is a large overlap in the causation and management of the two conditions.

Aetiology

Like other forms of dermatitis, E.D. has a number of causes. Drugs are the commonest cause according to Nicolis and Helwig (1973), accounting for 54 of their 135 cases. Any drug should be suspected, the commonest culprits varying from one society to another according to prescribing habits. The drugs which have most commonly been incriminated include penicillin, sulphonamides, gold, isoniazid, phenothiazines, para-aminosalicylic acid, chlorpropamide, barbiturates and phenylbutazone.

The extension of an existing dermatosis was the next commonest cause in Nicolis and Helwig's series and was the commonest in Wilson's series (1954).

Psoriasis may become universal either because an individual is naturally severely affected or as a result of injudicious treatment. Atopic eczema may be universal in an infant or in an older individual. Contact dermatitis, either of the allergic or the irritant variety, may proceed to E.D. Stasis dermatitis begins as a rash on one leg. It may spread by the auto-sensitisation mechanism of Whitfield (1921), or more likely because of allergy to applied medicaments (neomycin and soframycin are special culprits). Seborrhoeic dermatitis before the steroid era was a common cause – and still occurs particularly in infants. Other dermatoses which may proceed to E.D. include dermatomycosis (especially in warm humid climates and in those whose immune mechanism is defective from disease or medication), reticuloses, such as mycosis fungoides, Sezary's syndrome, leukaemia, reticulum cell sarcoma and Hodgkin's Disease, the skin manifestations of Reiter's disease, [thought by some to be a form of psoriasis (Baker et al., 1973)] and the rare pityriasis ruba pilaris. Idiopathic cases remain, middle-aged and elderly males occupy most of this group.

Clinical picture

The skin is universally red and scaly with swelling and oedema. Fissuring, pustulation and vesication may be features. Symptoms include itching, burning, fever, headaches and shivering. The lymph glands are often enlarged, either secondary to the inflamed and infected skin or related to a reticulosis. The scalp may be inflamed and the hair unseated leading to alopecia. The nails are often dystrophic, discoloured, pitted, ridged, thickened and separated from the nail bed (oncholysis) or generally shed. Secondary hyperpigmentation may be widespread and in men gynaecomastia is often a feature.

The widespread and intense nature of these events inevitably affects the body's economy. Heat loss can be enormous (and is the result of vasodilation of the skin vessels and hypermetabolism of the skin and internal organs). The basic metabolic rate may be raised to $+119\%$ and this is attributed by Zoon and Mali (1957) to evaporation of fluid; however convection and radiation must play a role. The pulse rate too is raised. Large quantities of water may be lost from the surface, as a result of an increased transepidermal water loss and may be complicated by hypothermia (Bettley and Grice, 1968). Hypothermia if severe may lead to cardiac dysrhythmias including ventricular fibrillation. Salts may also be lost in the fluid but the electrolyte barrier seems better preserved than the water barrier (Grice *et al.*, 1973; Grice, 1976). Paradoxically hyperthermia may also complicate E.D. because sweating is often much reduced.

The redness of the skin is due to vasodilation and as a result there is an increase in the circulating blood volume; it has been suggested (Shuster, 1963) that the raised jugular venous pressure, the hepatosplenomegaly, the oedema with warm extremities and the tachycardia with a full or collapsing pulse may be indicative of high output cardiac failure. Later work (Marks and Shuster, 1966) suggests that the high output failure may have been exaggerated but there seems little doubt that persons with impaired heart function can be forced into heart failure and collapse by the added load imposed by E.D. There is another danger too of an opposite nature. Increased vascular permeability leads to fluid and albumin leaking from the circulation into the tissues (and especially the skin) and this may produce depletion of circulating blood volume – the fall in plasma protein and hence a fall in intravascular osmotic pressure may possibly also be due to impaired liver function (Bauer, 1953). The net effect may be a rapidly developing and dangerous hypovolaemia. Weight loss is also a feature of E.D. Persons with dermatitis are more prone to skin infection because the skin is warmer and moister and the barrier of the horny layer may be broken, hence boils, cellulitis, lymphangitis and even septicaemia may occur, bronchopneumonia may be a terminal event.

Investigation

One or more biopsies of the skin may help in diagnosis. A lymph node should be removed for histology if a reticulosis is suspected. A blood count often reveals anaemia and eosinophilia. A marrow examination for leukaemia and skin scrapings for fungus infection may be required. Pulse, blood pressure, electrolytes, plasma proteins and temperature should be monitored. A low reading thermometer is essential. Skin swabs need to be taken frequently for bacterial culture and antibiotic sensitivity.

Management

1. Put the patient in bed in hospital in all those *suffering* from E.D. (A few tolerate chronic E.D. well and do not require hospitalisation.)

2. Stop all drugs unless it is quite clear that the E.D. is not drug-induced.

3. The room should be warm and the bed clothes adequate, especially in the winter months. Sweating and hypothermia are indications that the patient should be warmed (see Part 1, ch. VI, p. 133). A high body temperature should be corrected since it can place an added strain on the heart (Fox *et al.*, 1965).

4. The patient will need an ample and high protein diet to make good protein loss and calorie consumption. Abundant fluid by mouth is required. For further information regarding nutrition of hyper-catabolism, refer to Part I, ch. IX, p. 247.

5. A patient sufficiently ill to require intensive therapy will require right atrial pressure monitoring.

6. A sudden increase in the oedema, a rise in pulse rate, a fall in the blood pressure and central venous pressure, will require appropriate electrolyte replacement and volume replacement with plasma protein fraction or dried plasma.

7. A rising central venous pressure and increasing pulse rate generally signifies the onset of high output failure. Digitalis should be considered.

8. The skin should be cleaned in a bath at body temperature using Aqueous Cream B.P. as a cleanser or oatmeal 100 g may be added to the bath. If infection is present potassium permanganate should be added to the bath to give a concentration of 1 : 10 000. A steroid cream or ointment should be applied two or three times a day. An ointment is often more acceptable to the patient and reduces the heat and fluid loss. The steroid reduces the inflammation and helps to right the haemo- and thermo-dynamic upset. Hydrocortisone 2.5% may be used but stronger steroids may be required, e.g. clobetasol propionate 0.05% ointment

(Dermovate) diluted 1 in 5 with white soft paraffin (petrolatum). The use of topical steroids over an extensive area may lead to adrenal suppression.

9. If local steroid is ineffective prednisone 30–60 mg a day by mouth should be given for 1 to 2 weeks then reduced gradually to a maintenance dose as small as possible. In general, systemic steroids should not be given where the diagnosis is psoriasis as rebound is likely to occur when the steroid is reduced causing worsening of the psoriasis or even conversion into generalised pustular psoriasis.

10. It may be necessary to give methotrexate and azathioprine for psoriasis in the worst and most resistant cases. Liver and haematological function must be carefully monitored (Baker *et al.*, 1973).

11. Radiation and multiple chemotherapy may be needed for neoplasms or reticulosis.

12. *Infection.* The skin should be monitored bacteriologically and if a significant infection develops, systemic and local antibiotics should be used. Penicillin, streptomycin or sulphonamide should not be used as local applications. Neomycin and soframycin as local applications should be used with utmost discretion in view of the possibility of contact dermatitis. Oxytetracycline and clioquinol are safer and are often combined with steroids in ointments or creams. Barrier nursing should be used if necessary. Exfoliative dermatitis has a high mortality. Chest physiotherapy should be given to prevent a chest infection and leg exercises as a prophylactic against deep venous thrombosis.

13. It may be necessary to give an anti-histamine to help control skin irritation, e.g. brompheniramine maleate (Dimotane) 4 mg t.i.d. Sedation at night by nitrazaepam (Mogadon) 5–10 mg may be required.

GENERALISED PUSTULAR PSORIASIS (G.P.P.)

Aetiology and clinical picture

The presence of micro-abscesses in the epidermis is a histological feature of psoriasis. In G.P.P. there is a generalised macroscopically visible sterile pustulosis. G.P.P. may arise in those who have had ordinary psoriasis for many years and the stimulus to conversion may be an infection, pregnancy, hypocalcaemia or the administration of systemic steroids. It may occur also in those who develop late atypical psoriasis (Baker and Ryan, 1968). Clinically the patient has a fiery red skin associated with scaling and with flaccid superficial sterile pustules (Fig. 2). There is often fever, malaise, wasting and hair loss.

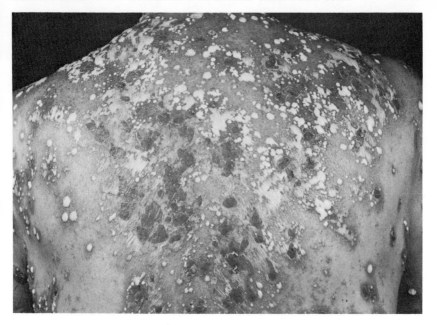

Fig. 2. Generalised pustular psoriasis.

Investigation

Skin biopsy may reveal the spongiform pustule of Kogoj (Lever, 1963) and perhaps the histology of psoriasis. The investigations are as for exfoliative dermatitis with special attention to the serum calcium.

Management

The general management will be as for exfoliative dermatitis as the metabolic consequences are similar. However, systemic steroids should be used only as a last resort. Some would consider it wise not even to use local steroids but to use calamine lotion alone at first. If spontaneous resolution does not occur methotrexate 10 mg intravenously every 4–5 days and later a once weekly oral dose of 15–25 mg may be given (Baker, 1975). Haemoglobin, W.B.C., platelet counts and liver function tests should be done. If there is intolerance to methotrexate, hydroxyurea 0.5 g once to three times a day or azathioprine 1.5 to 3 mg/kg daily may be substituted. The blood and liver function should be monitored.

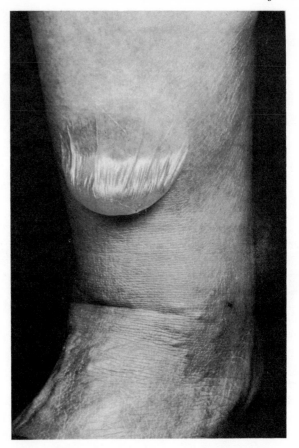

Fig. 3. Pemphigus, a flaccid bulla which is likely to rupture leaving a raw surface.

PEMPHIGUS

Aetiology and clinical picture

Pemphigus is a disease mainly arising in the 4th and 5th decades of life. It appears in both sexes. Untreated it has a very high mortality. The aetiology of the disease is uncertain, the incidence is high in the Jewish race. There are immunological changes *q.v.* and a replica of the condition occurs among some who are under treatment with penicillamine (Hewitt *et al.*, 1975).

Clinically flaccid blisters appear on normal skin; they break readily and leave erosions which spread and do not heal (Fig. 3). The lips and mouth are frequently affected by erosions.

Investigation

A biopsy of an early blister shows acantholysis (dissolution of the prickles of the prickle cells) and an intra-epidermal blister. The serum of the patient deposits IgG on the intercellular substance of stratified squamous epithelium; this is revealed by immunofluorescent techniques (Beutner *et al.*, 1968). The plasma albumin, sodium and chloride may be lowered.

Management

As soon as the biopsy and blood sample for immunofluorescence has been taken, treatment should be commenced. The earlier the treatment the less the difficulty in bringing the disease under control.

1. Prednisone should be given in a dosage of 120 mg daily in mild cases, 180 mg daily in severe cases. This dose should be maintained until healing has taken place (approximately eight weeks). The dose should then be reduced rapidly at first and later slowly to a maintenance level of 2.5 to 30 mg a day (Lever, 1965). Antacids should be given with each oral dose of steroid. If very high doses are required steroid sparing or even substitution may be achieved by giving azathioprine 1.5–3.00 mg/kg daily by mouth. The steroid takes effect in a few days whereas azathioprine takes approximately four weeks.

2. Anabolic steroids, e.g. methandienone (Dianabol) 5 mg and calcium 3 g per day may be given to counter osteoporosis, although there is no real evidence of their efficacy.

3. In diabetics, insulin requirements may be raised. Steroid-induced diabetes is generally mild and can usually be treated with diet alone or oral hypoglycaemics.

4. The blisters should be gently snipped and covered with paraffin gauze. Each blister should be counted as it is snipped and the number recorded daily on a chart to monitor the efficacy of the treatment.

5. The raw areas should be investigated for bacteria and if infected systemic and local antibiotics or antiseptics should be given.

6. Nutrition must be maintained. If the mouth is sore 2% lignocaine may be applied to the mouth 15 min before meals.

PEMPHIGOID (BULLOUS PEMPHIGOID)

This is a bullous eruption arising as a rule in an older age than pemphigus, in the 6th and 7th decades. It differs from pemphigus in that the blisters are tense and do not break easily (Fig. 4). The blisters tend to heal. The

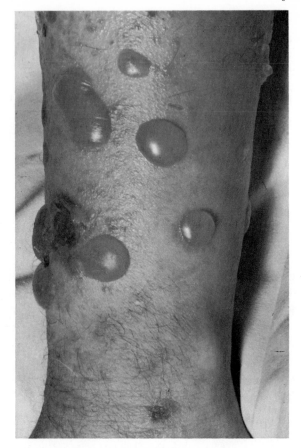

Fig. 4. Pemphigoid. Tense blisters which are less liable to rupture than pemphigus blisters.

lips and the mouth are infrequently affected. The histology of an early blister shows a dermoepidermal split without significant acantholysis. An immunofluorescent technique using the patient's serum shows a deposition of IgG on the basement membrane of stratified squamous epithelium (Beutner *et al.*, 1968).

Pemphigoid is less fatal and more easily brought under control than pemphigus. The treatment of pemphigoid is essentially the same as that of pemphigus, but the steroid dosage can be lower – commencing with 60–120 mg of prednisone per day and coming down to a lower dose more rapidly (Lever, 1965). The higher age group carries with it the risk of mortality from other causes.

EPIDERMOLYSIS BULLOSA

Classification, aetiology and clinical picture

Epidermolysis bullosa is a group of diseases, mostly genetically determined, in which blisters develop in response to minor trauma to the skin and mucous membranes. The types are as follows (Rook *et al.*, 1972):

1. Epidermolysis bullosa simplex (autosomal dominant inheritance).
2. Epidermolysis bullosa simplex of hands and feet (Cockayne-autosomal dominant).
3. Dystrophic epidermolysis bullosa (autosomal dominant).
4. Epidermolysis bullosa letalis (Herlitz-autosomal recessive).
5. Polydysplastic epidermolysis bullosa (dystrophic-autosomal recessive).

Types 1 to 3 are generally mild and hence only types 4 and 5 will be discussed here.

Epidermolysis bullosa letalis (Herlitz) is usually present at birth and the birth process often removes part of the epidermis leaving raw areas. Erosions and blisters start to develop and the nails tend to be lost. The mouth is also frequently blistered. In spite of the severity of the condition, scarring is seldom a feature due perhaps to the fact that the blister is at the plane of the dermoepidermal junction (Pearson, 1962). As the name implies, death occurs often in infancy, usually from sepsis. Some, however, may survive to adulthood (Ridley and Levy, 1968).

In recessive dystrophic epidermolysis bullosa, blisters and raw areas are often present at birth. The bullae may be haemorrhagic and when they heal leave scars (the blisters are deeper than in type 4, the outer dermis being affected as well as the epidermis). The mouth is often affected and lesions of the oesophagus may lead to stricture formation. The fingers and toes often join together as a result of adjacent blistering and the nails are usually deformed or lost.

Management

Soft clothing and bedclothes should be used. Soft food is indicated when there is oral or oesophageal involvement. The skin should be lubricated to lessen friction, more sensitive areas of skin should be protected. Pearson (1971) recommends covering the affected areas with an antibiotic ointment followed by a layer of zinc oxide paste and dressed with soft linen dressings. Moynahan (1975) states that such medications should be avoided since they cause blisters and recommends that babies and young children be nursed naked on parachute silk. A high room temperature promotes blistering and an incubator with too high a temperature and humidity can cause death, especially in the Herlitz type. Xenografts may be used as dressings, the technique is described by Hackett (1975). Systemic steroids have to be given in high dosage to achieve effects. They can be life saving in the Herlitz type especially in the vulnerable first year. Moynahan (1975) recommends prednisolone 60–200 mg a day for newborns and infants. Infection is minimised by giving pooled gamma globulin and by antibiotics. If cardiac failure sets in Moynahan (1975) insists steroids should be continued and digitalis given. In polydysplastic epidermolysis bullosa, steroids in large doses should be given intermittently in exacerbations and to help relieve (together with mechanical dilation by bougie) oesophageal obstruction. A steroid cover should be given for plastic surgery (to correct deformities) and at the time of oesophageal bouginage to inhibit blister formation.

Candidiasis of the mouth and oesophagus should be treated by local nystatin and amphotericin B. Syndactyly should be prevented in type 5 by using splints; physiotherapy is required in both types to prevent contractures. Anaemia and dietary deficiencies should be looked for and corrected.

TOXIC EPIDERMAL NECROLYSIS (LYELL'S DISEASE)

Aetiology and clinical picture

Toxic epidermal necrolysis (T.E.N.) is a condition in which the skin gives the appearance of having been scalded. There is redness, blistering and a tendency of the skin to come off when lightly touched (Lyell, 1956; Lang and Walker, 1956). It is a syndrome of multiple aetiology (Lyell, 1967). The factors producing this condition include:

1. Infection of the skin and/or throat with staphylococci phage type II (Types 3A, 3C, 52, 71). When it occurs in babies it is known as Ritter's disease. The disease can affect older children and even adults. The term staphylococcal scalded skin syndrome describes the disease in all age groups (Fig. 5). Conjunctivitis may be a feature.

2. Drug reaction. Many drugs may be responsible e.g. barbiturates, sulphonamides, phenylbutazone, phenolpthalein, hydantoins, penicillin and p-amino-salicylic acid. Stomatitis and eye involvement may occur in this type and in such cases the clinical picture may overlap with that of severe erythema multiforme (Stevens-Johnson syndrome).

3. Miscellaneous. These include infections (particularly viral infections), lymphomas, coma from barbiturates and carbon monoxide and external contact with paraffin (kerosene).

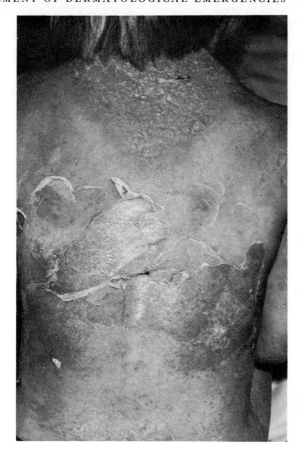

Fig. 5. The staphylococcal scalded skin syndrome (a type of Lyell's disease).

4. Idiopathic. This is most common in middle-aged and elderly females. There may be recurrent attacks.

Management

It is a disease with a high mortality, especially in groups 3 and 4 and to a lesser extent in group 2.

(a) As group 1 is due to resistant staphylococci systemic cloxacillin or erythromycin and local fucidin should be given. The response is rapid.

(b) It is wise to stop all drugs in case they are culpable but one should be careful in babies and children to substitute antibiotics mentioned above in (*a*), since these patients have often been treated with penicillin or tetracycline to which the staphylococci are resistant.

(*c*) Fluids and electrolytes may be lost in large quantities and should be replaced by mouth or parenterally.

(*d*) Tulle gras (vaseline gauze) or porcine xenograft may be used as local dressings.

(*e*) Nursing care is of great importance and a special bed which can be tested may be needed, e.g. the Emesay turning frame or the Stryker Circulo-electric hospital bed. The eyes and mouth need special attention. Tube feeding may be needed for nutrition and postural drainage to prevent chest complications.

(*f*) Antibiotics, both local and general may be needed to control secondary infection.

(*g*) Corticosteroids are usually administered in severe cases of groups 2, 3 and 4, although there is no proof of their efficacy, e.g. prednisone 60 mg per day with, if necessary, intravenous hydrocortisone (Lyell, 1973).

ERYTHEMA MULTIFORME

Clinical picture

Erythema multiforme (E.M.) is a clinical reaction pattern to a variety of noxae. E.M. presents clinically with target or iris lesions of the skin. The rings, which compose the lesions, are made of different shades of blue-red and red, and of blisters, which may mark the "bull's eye" or may also be in a ring form (Fig. 6). The mouth and lips may be affected with blisters which break to form erosions (Fig. 7), the eyes too may be inflamed. The average patient with E.M. does not require admission, much less intensive care. However, there is a specially severe form which is sometimes called the Stevens-Johnson syndrome (S.J.S.). The patient with S.J.S. is ill with high fever, ocular inflammation, haemorrhagic cheilitis and stomatitis. The skin lesions are often most marked around the orifices.

Aetiology

The known triggering factors are numerous (Lyell, 1971) and include:

1. *Infections.* Herpes simplex. Vaccinia. Atypical pneumonia. Histoplasmosis. Typhoid and other bacterial viral and fungal infections.

2. *Reactions to drugs.* The drugs are too numerous to mention but

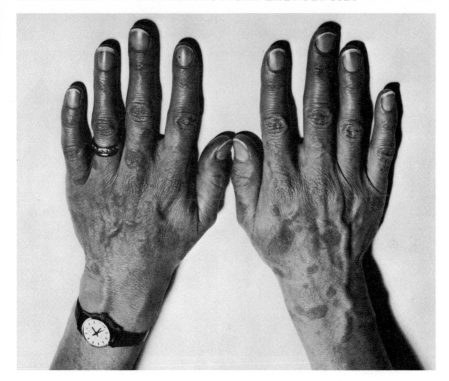

Fig. 6. Erythema multiforme, the target or iris lesions.

sulphonamides, co-trimoxazole (trimethoprin and sulphamethoxazole), phenylbutazone and barbiturates are common causes.

3. *Physical agents.* Exposure to cold, sunlight and X-radiation may trigger E.M.

4. *Idiopathic.* In some cases there is no detectable initiating factor.

Diagnosis

Erythema multiforme tends to come on acutely as a sharp attack lasting from two to six weeks. A triggering factor such as herpes simplex may precede the E.M. by one or two weeks but in other cases an upper respiratory tract infection may precede the rash by one or two days. E.M. is often recurrent. The characteristic skin lesions and the distribution on the extensor aspects of the arms and legs and also on the palms and soles, make the clinical diagnosis easy. In severe cases the lesions will be widespread and will also involve the trunk. The histology

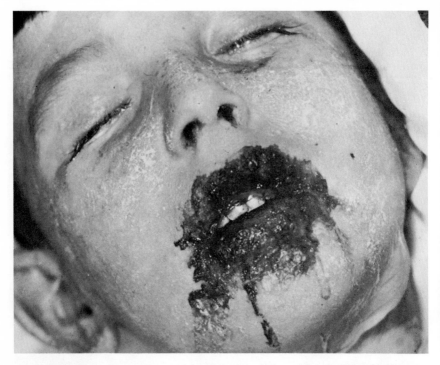

Fig. 7. Erythema multiforme (Stevens-Johnson syndrome) due to phenobarbitone in this case.

shows a sub-epidermal blister with necrosis of the epidermis. The immunofluorescent markers of pemphigus, pemphigoid and dermatitis herpetiformis are absent.

Management

Stop all drugs unless they can be exculpated with certainty. Mild cases are treated symptomatically as outpatients. Severe cases should be admitted to hospital and nursed with barrier precautions in a separate room. Systemic and local antibiotics should be given to prevent the superinfection of raw areas. The skin lesions should be cleaned with potassium permanganate 1 : 5000, the blisters should then be pricked and covered with paraffin gauze. The eyes should be bathed and antibacterial eye drops or eye ointments should be applied. The mouth should be rinsed with saline or with potassium permanganate 1 : 10 000. In severe cases, systemic steroids should be given beginning with prednisolone 60 mg daily for a week and then tapering the dose according to the response. If the mouth is very inflamed hydrocortisone 60 mg intravenously should be administered eight hourly. Nutrient fluids and electrolytes should be supplied intravenously if necessary.

REFERENCES

Baker, H. and Ryan, T. J. (1968). Generalised pustular psoriasis. A clinical and epidemiological survey of 104 cases. *Brit. J. Derm.* **80**, 771.

Baker, H., Fry, L. and Pegum, J. S. (1973). Psoriasis. *In* 'Recent Advances in Dermatology. No. 3' (Ed. A. Rook). Churchill Livingstone, Edinburgh and London.

Baker, H. (1975). Psoriasis: a review. *Dermatologica* **150**, 16.

Bauer, F. (1953). Generalised exfoliative dermatitis and liver function. *Aust. J. Derm.* **2**, 69.

Bettley, F. R. and Grice, K. A. (1968). A method of measuring the transepidermal water loss and a means of inactivating sweat glands. *Brit. J. Derm.* **77**, 627.

Beutner, E. H., Jordan, R. E. and Chorzelski, T. P. (1968). The immunopathology of pemphigus and bullous pemphigoid. *J. invest. Derm.* **51**, 63.

Fox, R. H., Shuster, S., Williams, R., Marks, J., Goldsmith, R. and Condon, R. E. (1965). Cardiovascular, metabolic and thermoregulatory disturbances in patients with erythrodermic skin diseases. *Brit. Med. J.* **1**, 619.

Grice, K., Sattar, H. and Baker, H. (1973). The cutaneous barrier to salts and water in psoriasis and normal skin. *Brit. J. Derm.* **88**, 459.

Grice, K. (1976). Personal communications.

Hackett, M. E. J. (1975). Preparation, storage and use of homografts. *Brit. J. Hosp. Med.* **13**, 272.

Hewitt, J., Benveniste, M. and Lessana-Leibowitch, M. (1975). Pemphigus induced by D. penicillamine 'an experimental pemphigus'. *Brit. J. Derm.* **93** (Suppl. 11) 12.

Lang, R. and Walker, J. (1956). An unusual bullous eruption. *S. African Med. J.* **30**, 97.

Lever, W. F. (1963). 'Histopathology of the skin', p. 124. Lippincott, Philadelphia.

Lever, W. F. (1965). 'Pemphigus and pemphigoid.' C. C. Thomas, Springfield, Illinois.

Lyell, A. (1956). Toxic epidermal necrolysis. An eruption resembling scalding of the skin. *Brit. J. Derm.* **68**, 355.

Lyell, A. (1967). A review of toxic epidermal necrolysis in Britain. *Brit. J. Derm.* **79**, 662.

Lyell, A. (1971). *In* 'Dermatology in General Medicine' (Ed. T. B. Fitzpatrick, K. A. Arndt, W. H. Clarke, A. Z. Eisen, E. J. Van Scott and J. H. Vaughan), p. 598. McGraw Hill, New York and London.

Lyell, A. (1973). Toxic epidermal necrolysis. *In* 'The skin and general medicine' (Ed. J. N. Agate), p. 22. Modern Medicine of Great Britain Ltd.

Marks, J. and Shuster, S. (1966). A method for measuring capillary permeability and its use in patients with skin disease. *Lancet* **2**, 88.

Moynahan, E. J. (1975). *In* 'Current dermatologic management' (Ed. Stuart Maddin). Second Edition, p. 148. C. V. Mosby, St. Louis.

Nicolis, D. and Helwig, E. D. (1973). Exfoliative dermatitis, a study of 135 cases. *Archs. Derm.* **108**, 788.

Pearson, R. W. (1962). Studies in the pathogenesis of epidermolysis bullosa. *J. Invest. Derm.* **39**, 551.

Pearson, R. W. (1971). The mechanobullous diseases. *In* 'Dermatology in general medicine' (Ed. T. Fitzpatrick, K. A. Arndt, W. H. Clark, A. Z. Esen, E. I. Van Scott and J. H. Vaughan), p. 640. McGraw-Hill, New York.

Ridley, C. M. and Levy, I. S. (1968). Epidermolysis bullosa and anyloidosis. *1968 Trans. St. John's Hosp. Derm. Soc. (Lond)* **54**, 75.

Rook, A. J. (1972). 'Textbook of dermatology' (Ed. A. Rook, F. J. G. Ebling and D. S. Wilkinson), p. 1299. Blackwell, Oxford.

Shuster, S. (1963). High output failure from skin disease. *Lancet* **1**, 1338.

Whitfield, A. (1921). Some points in the aetiology of skin diseases. *Lancet* **2**, 122.

Wilson, H. T. H. (1954). Exfoliative Dermatitis. Its Etiology and Prognosis. *Arch. Derm. and Syph. (Chicago)* **69**, 577.

Zoon, J. J. and Mali, J. W. H. (1957). The influence of erythroderma on the body. *Archs. Derm.* **75**, 57.

PART 3

Investigative Facilities and Drug Requirements in the I.T.U.

I

Laboratory Facilities

Section 1: Bacteriological Requirements and the
I.T.U.

B. Chattopadhyay

INTRODUCTION

Patients admitted to the Intensive Therapy Unit are usually more susceptible to infection because they are exposed to excessive hazards of cross-infection and contamination due to much more handling, prolonged and excessive antibiotic therapy and instrumentation, e.g. tracheostomy, mechanical ventilation, prolonged intravenous therapy, catheterisation of the bladder and treatment of major postoperative wounds. Also a proportion of these patients may be immunologically compromised.

Infection may be acquired from a hospital strain or from the patient's own bacteriological flora. They usually gain access either through the respiratory tract, gastrointestinal tract or the skin. The mode of transmission of micro-organisms may be:

1. By airborne dissemination, e.g. *Staphylococcus aureus* in small droplet nucleii.

2. By direct contact from personnel, e.g. *Pseudomonas aeruginosa* and Klebsiella species when not acquired from the patient's own flora (Lowbury *et al.*, 1975; Kominos *et al.*, 1972). Even *Staphylococcus aureus* can spread in this way (Speers *et al.*, 1969).

3. *Via fomites:* (*a*) instruments and equipment which come in direct contact with the skin and mucous membranes of the patient are liable to be contaminated with micro-organisms (Stark *et al.*, 1962). Cross-infection from ventilators (Phillips and Spencer, 1965) and self-inflating breathing bags (Cartwright and Hargrave, 1969) has now been established as a means of transmission of infection to patients (Joseph, 1952; Wyant and Nanson, 1957; Tinne *et al.*, 1967; Old *et al.*, 1972). (*b*) contaminated medicaments including intravenous infusion fluids have all been incriminated for causing outbreaks of infection with *Pseudomonas aeruginosa* (Phillips, 1966; Noble and Savin, 1966; Ayliffe *et al.*, 1966; Shooter *et al.*, 1969; Phillips *et al.*, 1972).

CONTROL OF INFECTION
Design

The unit should be divided into two or three bed wards with some isolation rooms bearing in mind the easy accessibility to the patient in an emergency. In the open section there should be adequate space between beds and washable partitions in between (Lowbury *et al.*, 1975). The isolation rooms should be so designed to nurse either the infected (source isolation) or the immunologically compromised patients (protective isolation) who are more susceptible to infection; otherwise the room for an infected patient to be exhaust ventilated (negative pressure) but separated from a corridor which is kept under positive pressure and for the susceptible patient to be plenum ventilated (positive pressure). The temperature and the humidity control should be incorporated into the ventilation system. The ideal isolation room (for source or protective) is 'plenum ventilated and separated from a plenum ventilated corridor by an exhaust ventilated vestibule which acts as an airlock' (Gaya, 1976).

There should be adequate space for an equipment room, clean and dirty utility rooms, store for C.S.S.D. supplies, changing room, staff room, waiting room for relatives and proper hand washing facilities. The taps on the hand wash basin should preferably be foot operated with built-in heated sink trap units.

Bacteriological monitoring of patients and environments

Routine culture of endotracheal aspirates, peritoneal dialysis fluid, catheter specimens of urine, rectal swabs, intravenous cannula site, postoperative wound site, fluid from drain site and intravenous catheters are to be done regularly (Gaya, 1974). Although the value of routine environmental swabbing is a debatable point, except for epidemiological purposes, they may also act as an indicator of the degree of bacterial contamination and, therefore, the ease of cross-infection. The build up of virulent micro-organisms may not be appreciated unless regular environmental swabbing is undertaken.

General

In order to maintain an efficient aseptic technique, members of staff handling patients in the unit should wash their hands with a chemical disinfectant, e.g. povidone iodine scrub. Disposable aprons and gloves should be used for those patients who are heavily infected or who are susceptible to infection. Aprons soiled with blood or excreta or pus to be changed at once. Hands to be washed thoroughly between patients and also before leaving the cubicles.

Disinfection policy (Table 1)

Heat is the best and cheapest way of killing micro-organisms and to be relied upon whenever possible. Chemical disinfectants to be reserved only for items where physical methods of sterilisation are not possible to apply. Useful agents for antisepsis will be povidone iodine tincture (e.g. Betadine) as skin preparation, hypochlorites (e.g. Milton) for surface disinfection and a phenolic (e.g. Clearsol) as a general purpose disinfectant (Maurer, 1974).

The floor of the isolation rooms and the ward should be cleaned twice daily or more if necessary with a phenolic disinfectant like Clearsol. The plastic cover of the mattress used by an infected patient should be wiped with Clearsol and allowed to dry. For handwashing and pre-operative wound cleansing povidone iodine is recommended. Seventy per cent isopropyl alcohol should be used prior to venepuncture, and for wound cleansing, either Eusol, or 1–5% acetic acid or Savlon.

Terminal disinfection

Thorough domestic cleaning with a detergent, followed by the use of a phenolic or a hypochlorite is all that is required. Fumigation of cubicles is normally recommended when a patient has left the cubicle and was known to harbour a highly resistant strain of organisms.

Special equipment

Although sterilisation is the penultimate goal for all types of equipment, because only this method will ensure the destruction of all living microbes, including bacteria, spores and viruses, this is far from

Table 1. The West Roding District Hospitals' antiseptic and disinfectant policy

Do not use these disinfectants for any purpose other than those described.
Non-appropriate use of disinfectants may be wasteful or dangerous.
Other problems concerning the use of disinfectants should be referred to the bacteriologist or pharmacist.

	Disinfectant	Further dilutions. These MUST be made up daily	Recommended uses	Notes
PHENOLIC	Clearsol 1 in 10	Either 1 in 8 (e.g. 1 pint to 1 gallon) or 1 in 10 (100 ml in 1 litre)	1. Disinfecting floors and surfaces where contamination with excreta or infected discharges has occurred. 2. Disinfection of mattress covers after use by each patient, wipe with disinfectant, then wash off with warm water. 3. Disinfection of bed pans containing excreta from patients with intestinal infection. (Leave in contact for *one hour*.)	Detergents, not disinfectants, should be used for normal ward cleaning. Pine disinfectant/deodorant may be used for its deodorant effect. Avoid the use of phenolics on rubber if possible, because they may be absorbed and cause irritation to skin.
CHLORINE	Sodium hypochlorite 1% (Milton)	1 in 80	1. Sterilisation of babies' feeding bottles. (Immerse for 90 min.) 2. Disinfection of baths, kitchen working surfaces. (After cleaning, swab with the disinfectant solution, leave for 5 min, then rinse and dry with a paper towel.) 3. Disinfection of crockery etc., after use for infected patients (rinse in separate sink then soak in disinfectant for 5 min).	Where heat sterilisation is not possible. Strong solutions of hypochlorite are corrosive to stainless steel, always wash off. A 1 in 4 solution of Milton is issued in place of Eusol for the treatment of ulcers, wounds, etc.
		Undiluted	Disinfection of surfaces, or materials contaminated by blood from patients with hepatitis (pour disinfectant over spilt blood, or soak material in disinfectant, leave for at least 30 min).	
IODINE	Povidone-iodine tincture ('Betadine', 'Disadine', 'Pevidine')	Undiluted	Disinfection of the skin before major and minor operations, including ward procedures such as lumbar puncture, cut-down, aspiration. (Allow at least 2 min.)	This is the only preparation that kills both spores and vegetative bacteria. Povidone-iodine is not irritant to the skin and may be used for

Category	Preparation	Dilution	Use	Notes
IODINE	Povidone-iodine scrub	Undiluted	For hand washing and scrubbing by nursing and medical staff – prior to surgery and ward procedures as above.	No preparation can be relied on to sterilise the skin of the hands, so there is no substitute for 'no-touch' technique.
CHLORHEXIDINE	Hibitane concentrate 5% sachet	One 10 ml sachet in 1 litre	Swabbing perineal area during labour.	This antiseptic is not suitable for any other purpose.
	Chlorhexidine and isopropyl alcohol 'Mediswab H' 'Sterets H'	—	Disinfection of skin prior to injections, venepuncture. (Rub for at least ½ min.)	Not sporicidal.
	Chlorhexidine 'Hibitane' 0.5% in 70% spirit	Undiluted	As alternative to Povidone-iodine for disinfection of skin before major or minor operative procedures. (Allow at least 2 min.)	
	Hibitane antiseptic cream	—	Application to the hands after washing (particularly if the skin becomes dry from frequent washing).	Although antiseptic it is issued mainly for cosmetic reasons.
CHLORHEXIDINE + QUATERNARY AMMONIUM COMPOUND	Mediprep swab (Cetrimide and Chlorhexidine)	—	Large area skin cleaning. (Allow at least ½ min.)	Discard after use on each patient.
	Savlon 1 in 30 (Cetrimide 0.5% and Chlorhexidine 0.05%)	Undiluted	Cleaning dirty wounds.	This preparation has excellent detergent properties but it is not suitable as a skin disinfectant. Discard unused solution one week after opening.
	Savlon hospital concentrate sachets 10 ml	One 10 ml sachet in 300 ml water	May be used as a substitute for Savlon 1 in 30 when this solution is not available. Make fresh solution on each occasion, and discard remainder.	

practicable. Disinfection, on the other hand, means the destruction of all potential pathogens which can cause disease and which are in the vegetative phase and does not usually include spores. Before the application of any of the above mentioned processes the equipment must be cleaned thoroughly to remove deposits of organic matter and to reduce the number of contaminating organisms (Ziegler and Jacoby, 1956). The cleansing can be done by soaking in disinfectant solution followed by cleaning under running water, in washing machines with a detergent solution or ultrasonic vibrations.

Equipment can be sterilised by autoclaving with moist steam under pressure at a temperature of 121°C and a pressure of 15 lb/in² for 20 min (the temperature may vary from 110 to 136°C). By this method all metal, heat resistant rubber and plastic materials can be sterilised. Low temperature (80°C) steam with formaldehyde for two hours can be used to sterilise heat sensitive materials. Care should be taken to avoid trapping of air within the chamber due to improperly packed material leading to inadequate sterilisation and a false sense of security (Lumley, 1976). Ethylene oxide sterilisation is another suitable alternative for bulky equipment or for heat sensitive materials.

Commercial firms use either Gamma-rays or a beta linear accelerator to sterilise disposable syringes, needles, endotracheal tubes, cannulae, etc. and both of them are highly effective (Artandi, 1972; Rainey, 1974). Provided the equipment is completely immersed in water, heating at 65–70°C for 10–15 minutes, i.e. pasteurisation, is an acceptable method of decontamination as this will destroy all vegetative forms on face masks, tubings, etc. where infection by spore bearers is not encountered in clinical practice (Jenkins and Edgar, 1964; Bennett et al., 1968; Craig et al., 1975).

Very few chemicals are suitable for this purpose because many of them are toxic to use or deteriorate on storage. Some are inactivated by plastic, organic matter, rubber, hard water, soap, detergents, etc. (Maurer, 1974). A 2% solution of glutaraldehyde has been used for this purpose and seemed to be satisfactory (Haselhuhn et al., 1967; Meeks et al., 1967) though rubber and plastic may adsorb it. Alcoholic chlorhexidine is quite active against most pathogenic organisms. It is to some extent inactivated by organic matter and plastics.

Hypochlorites are the best available disinfectants for disinfection of equipment soiled with blood from a patient with viral hepatitis. The effective concentration is 10 000 parts per million (p.p.m.) of available chlorine. They are inactivated by organic materials and a strong solution will corrode metals.

Ideally whenever possible presterilised disposable items should be used particularly for known infected patients. Although the cost may appear to be prohibitive this is the best way to prevent infection in patients and also to avoid cross-contamination.

ANTIBIOTIC POLICY (Table 2)

Routine pre-operative prophylactic use of antibiotics is not recommended and should be avoided except under the following conditions (three days treatment is the maximum that can be allowed):

1. Severe trauma or mid-thigh amputation for peripheral vascular disease where because of the presence of *Clostridium welchii* on the skin of the thigh and the perianal region, such patients are placed at risk from gas gangrene following surgery. Penicillin appears to be the drug of choice.

2. Open heart surgery (Darrell *et al.*, 1976).

3. Dental extraction or instrumentation on urethra for patients with valvular heart disease.

4. General surgery. Mechanical cleansing and avoidance of faecal contamination during bowel surgery are much more important than any other procedure. However the use of oral kanamycin and oral metronidazole has been recommended for colonic surgery (Goldring *et al.*, 1975). The use of total bowel perfusion may revolutionise the use of antibiotics for bowel surgery. Antibiotic cover may be necessary prior to prosthetic operative procedures and operations for septic abortions. Prophylactic antibiotics are recommended prior to delivery of a patient with valvular heart diseases.

Topical use of potentially life saving antibiotics, e.g. gentamicin, fusidic acid, etc. including ear drops and nasal application should be deprecated because of the danger of emergence of resistance and subsequent cross-infection. However chloramphenicol eye drops can be safely used.

For irrigation of cavities where infection is suspected, e.g. peritonitis, cystitis, an antiseptic like Noxythiolin would be a better choice instead of an antibiotic. Moreover many would prefer to use only a sterile infusion fluid like normal saline.

Tracheostomy
Whenever possible tracheostomy should be done in the theatre aseptically. Every care must be taken to prevent postoperative contamination of the wound. If necessary an antiseptic can be applied

Table 2. The West Roding District Hospitals' antibiotic policy

The indiscriminate use of antibiotics, especially as prophylaxis against infection must be very strongly deprecated, as it undoubtedly tends to lead to the emergence of antibiotic-resistant strains of organisms resulting in cross-infection.

This policy provides general guidelines and although not all-inclusive is intended to cover most situations. It will, of course, have to be revised from time to time as and when new antibiotics more effective than the present ones appear.

PROPHYLACTIC	Routine prophylactic antibiotics are NOT recommended except the following:
	1. Mid-thigh amputation – Benzyl penicillin 600 mg i.m. $\frac{1}{2}$ h before operation and every 6 h for 3 days postoperatively. If the patient is allergic to penicillin use erythromycin 100 mg i.m. every 12 h.
	2. Insertion of prosthesis or hip/knee replacement – Ampicillin 250 mg/Flucloxacillin 250 mg i.m. ('Magnapen') every 6 h for 3 days postoperatively.
	3. Sub-acute bacterial endocarditis:
	   (a) For dental extraction – Procaine penicillin 300 mg i.m. + Benzyl penicillin 600 mg i.m. $\frac{1}{2}$ h before extraction.
	   For penicillin sensitive patient – cephazolin 500 mg i.m. or erythromycin 100 mg i.m. $\frac{1}{2}$ h before extraction.
	   (b) For instrumentation on urethra – Ampicillin 500 mg i.m. $\frac{1}{2}$ h before instrumentation.
	4. Bowel surgery – mechanical cleansing and avoidance of faecal contamination during operation more important. Kanamycin 1 g orally + Metronidazole 200 mg orally every 6 h for 3 days pre-operatively. Antibiotic (Polymyxin, Bacitracin) or antiseptic (povidone-iodine) spray to the wound prior to primary closure.
	5. Pregnancy associated with heart disease – Ampicillin 250 mg/Flucloxacillin 250 mg i.m. ('Magnapen') at the time of delivery and every 6 h for 2 days postpartum.
	6. Prolonged rupture of the membranes – start antibiotics – same as in No. 5 within 24 h.
	7. Septic abortion – Benzyl penicillin 600 mg i.m. every 6 h + clindamycin 600 mg i.m. every 8 h.

TOPICAL	*Use of potentially life saving antibiotic (e.g. gentamicin) must be avoided* because of the risks of the emergence of gentamicin-resistant strains of *Staphylococci, Klebsiella* and *Pseudomonas* species.
	Antibiotics suitable for this purpose – Neomycin, Bacitracin, Framycetin, Polymyxin.
	It would be wiser to use an antiseptic instead – Chlorhexidine, povidone-iodine. Take extra care when using povidone-iodine on extensive areas of the body.
	  For cleaning dirty wounds – use centrimide 0.5% and chlorhexidine 0.05% ('Savlon').
	  For cleaning septic wounds – use Eusol or acetic acid 1–5%.
	  For irrigation of cavities – use Noxythiolin.

BLIND TREATMENT OR BEST GUESS ANTIBIOTICS

To be modified, if necessary, after receipt of the bacteriology report.

Postoperative

(a) Abdominal infection – Gentamicin 80 mg i.m. + Clindamycin 600 mg i.m. every 8 h. Clindamycin should be stopped at once should diarrhoea develop in a patient. (It is essential to control the dose of gentamicin according to peak and trough blood levels.)

(b) Chest infection – Ampicillin 250 mg/Flucloxacillin 250 mg i.m. every 6 h ('Magnapen').

(c) Urinary tract infection – Co-trimoxazole 2 tablets orally every 12 h or Cephalexin 500 mg orally every 6 h.

(d) Bone infection – Gentamicin 80 mg i.m. + Clindamycin 600 mg i.m. every 8h.

Medical

(a) Meningitis – Sulphadiazine 100 mg/kg/day i.v. + Benzyl penicillin 600 mg i.v. every 4 h + Chloramphenicol 75 mg/kg/day i.v.

(b) Septicaemic shock – Gentamicin 80 mg i.m. + Clindamycin 600 mg i.m. + Ampicillin 500 mg i.m.

(c) Chest infection – Co-trimoxazole 2 tablets orally every 12 h or Amoxycillin 250 mg orally every 8 h.

(d) Urinary tract infection – Co-trimoxazole 2 tablets orally every 12 h or Amoxycillin 250 mg orally every 8 h or Cephalexin 250 mg orally every 6 h.

Orthopaedics

(a) Osteomyelitis – Penicillin i.m. + Flucloxacillin i.m. or Erythromycin + Fucidin. Dose to be decided for each patient.

(b) Septic arthritis – Ampicillin 250 mg/Flucloxacillin 250 mg i.m. every 6 h ('Magnapen').

Paediatrics

(a) (i) Meningitis – Sulphonamide + Benzyl penicillin + Chloramphenicol. (ii) Neonatal meningitis – Benzyl penicillin + Gentamicin.

(b) General cover – Ampicillin + Flucloxacillin.

Accident and emergency

Routine use of antibiotics not necessary; where indicated – for boils, paronychia, etc. – Clindamycin 150 mg orally every 6 h or Flucloxacillin 250 mg orally every 6 h.

Abscesses are to be drained.

Burn – Framycetin ('Sofratulle') or Silver sulphadiazine ('Flamazine').

Ulcer – Framycetin ('Sofratulle') or Chlorhexidine tulle ('Bactigras') or Eusol packs.

For chest and urinary tract infections – see under *Medical* (c) and (d).

locally. Tracheal suction should be performed with presterilised disposable catheters. The tracheostome should be dressed at least once daily and cultures taken from the tracheostomy site 2–3 times weekly. Inspired air should be free from bacterial contamination with a high humidity (Gaya, 1974).

Urine drainage bags must be changed twice daily.

Staff
Since life is usually quite hectic in the I.T.U., in order to function smoothly and efficiently, and for the proper maintenance of a very high standard of patient care, the department must be adequately staffed by both medical and nursing personnel.

It is essential to maintain close co-operation and a direct link between the clinical and the laboratory staff in order to implement the antibiotic and disinfection policies, to prevent cross-infection, and to inform the I.T.U. at the earliest opportunity with results on the urgent specimens and antibiotics assays.

CONCLUSION

Whatever may be the isolation, antibiotic or disinfectant policy, it is the ultimate practice that matters. Therefore, all the basic principles laid down like the 'No-touch' technique, etc. must be strictly adhered to and practised rigidly and meticulously by everybody concerned be it medical, nursing or other categories of staff with access to the patient, in order to avoid both infection and cross-contamination in the intensive therapy unit.

REFERENCES

Artandi, C. (1972). Sterilization by ionizing radiation. *Int. Anesth. Clin.* **10**, 123.
Ayliffe, G. A. J., Barry, D. R., Lowbury, E. J. L., Roper-Hall, M. J. and Walker, W. M. (1966). Post-operative infection with *Pseudomonas aeruginosa* in an eye hospital. *Lancet* **1**, 1113.
Bennett, P. J., Cope, D. H. P. and Thompson, R. E. M. (1968). Decontamination of anaesthetic equipment. *Anaesthesia* **23**, 670.
Cartwright, R. Y. and Hargrave, P. R. J. (1969). Hazard of self inflating resuscitation bags. *Brit. Med. J.* **4**, 302.
Craig, D. B., Cowan, S. A., Forsyth, W. and Parker, S. E. (1975). Disinfection of anaesthesia equipment by a mechanized pasteurization method. *Can. Anaesth. Soc. J.* **22**, 219.
Darrell, J. H. and Uttley, A. H. C. (1976). Antibiotics in the peri-operative period. *Brit. J. Anaesth.* **48**, 13.

Gaya, H. (1974). The bacteriology of intensive care. *Brit. J. Hosp. Med.* **11**, 853.

Gaya, H. (1976). Infection control in intensive care. *Brit. J. Anaesth.* **48**, 9.

Goldring, J., Scott, A., McNaught, W. and Gillespie, G. (1975). Prophylactic oral antimicrobial agents in elective colonic surgery. *Lancet* **2**, 997.

Haselhuhn, D. H., Brason, F. W. and Borick, P. M. (1967). 'In use' study of buffered glutaraldehyde for cold sterilization of anaesthesia equipment. *Anesth. Analg.* (Cleve.) **46**, 468.

Jenkins, J. R. E. and Edgar, W. M. (1964). Sterilization of anaesthetic equipment. *Anaesthesia* **19**, 177.

Joseph, J. M. (1952). Disease transmission by inefficiently sanitized anesthetizing apparatus. *JAMA* **149**, 1196.

Kominos, S. D., Copeland, C. E. and Grosiak, B. (1972). Mode of transmission of *Pseudomonas aeruginosa* in a burn unit and an intensive care unit in a general hospital. *Applied Microbiology* **23**, 309.

Lowbury, E. J. L., Ayliffe, G. A. J., Geddes, A. M. and Williams, J. D. (1975). Special wards and departments. *In* 'Control of Hospital Infection', p. 229. Chapman and Hall, London.

Lumley, J. (1976). Decontamination of anaesthetic equipment and ventilators. *Brit. J. Anaesth.* **48**, 3.

Maurer, I. M. (1974). Choosing chemical disinfectants. *In* 'Hospital Hygiene', p. 60. Edward Arnold, London.

Meeks, C. H., Pembleton, W. E. and Hench, M. R. (1967). Sterilization of anesthesia apparatus. *JAMA* **199**, 276.

Noble, W. C. and Savin, J. A. (1966). Steroid cream contaminated with *Pseudomonas aeruginosa*. *Lancet* **1**, 347.

Old, J. W., Kisch, A. L., Eberle, B. J. and Wilson, J. N. (1972). *Pseudomonas aeruginosa* respiratory tract infection acquired from a contaminated anesthesia machine. *Am. Rev. Respir. Dis.* **105**, 628.

Phillips, I. (1966). Post-operative respiratory tract infection with *Pseudomonas aeruginosa* due to contaminated lignocaine jelly. *Lancet* **1**, 903.

Phillips, I. and Spencer, G. (1965). *Pseudomonas aeruginosa* cross-infection due to contaminated respiratory apparatus. *Lancet* **2**, 1325.

Phillips, I., Eykyn, S. and Laker, M. (1972). Outbreak of hospital infection caused by contaminated autoclaved fluids. *Lancet* **1**, 1258.

Rainey, H. B. (1974). Radiation sterilization and the anaesthetist. *Anaesth. Intensive Care* **2**, 48.

Shooter, R. A., Cooke, E. M., Gaya, H., Kumar, P., Patel, N., Parker, M. T., Thom, B. T. and France, D. R. (1969). Food and medicaments as possible sources of hospital strains of *Pseudomonas aeruginosa*. *Lancet* **1**, 1227.

Speers, R., Shooter, R. A., Gaya, H. and Patel, N. (1969). Contamination of nurses' uniforms with *Staphylococcus aureus*. *Lancet* **2**, 233.

Stark, D. C. C., Green, C. A. and Pask, E. A. (1962). Anaesthetic machines and cross-infection. *Anaesthesia* **17**, 12.

Tinne, J. E., Gordon, A. M., Bain, W. H. and Mackey, W. A. (1967). Cross-infection by *Pseudomonas aeruginosa* as a hazard of intensive surgery. *Brit. Med. J.* **4**, 313.

Wyant, G. M. and Nanson, E. M. (1957). Fulminating post-operative staphylococcal pneumonia. *Ann. Surg.* **145**, 133.

Ziegler, C. and Jacoby, J. (1956). Anaesthetic equipment as a source of infection. *Anesth. Analg.* (Cleve.) **35**, 451.

Section 2: Biochemical Requirements and the I.T.U.

A. M. BOLD

THE NEED FOR GOOD LIAISON

The intensive care of many types of critically ill patient requires a laboratory service that is reliable and rapid. Close cooperation is therefore essential between all the staff involved – medical, nursing and technical. Proximity of the I.T.U. to the laboratory is probably more important than for any other hospital unit. Effective communication places demands on I.T.U. and laboratory staff.

I.T.U.

Request precisely and with discrimination. To perform tests urgently is demanding in time and money; just because a patient is critically ill does not necessarily imply that every investigation is required urgently, unless immediate management will be different, depending on whether a requested test is high, normal or low. Telephone the laboratory to explain requirements, specifying what is really needed and the degree of urgency. For example, if a plasma potassium is needed, *ask* for plasma potassium, *not* 'U and E'; urea by some laboratory methods takes 20–30 min whereas plasma potassium can often be determined in 5 min or less.

Plan ahead where possible. If tests are required, say every 2 or 4 hours, let the laboratory know in good time. Do not repeatedly phone for results – it can be very irritating and slows down work.

Laboratory

Where a copy of the results cannot immediately be sent to the I.T.U., results must be telephoned, preferably to the requesting doctor, not an intermediary. In the Queen Elizabeth Hospital, Birmingham, a preprinted jotter is used on wards to record telephoned results (Fig. 1). This

Fig. 1. Example of a preprinted jotter, 50 sheets to a pad, for recording telephoned laboratory results.

802

URGENT LABORATORY RESULTS

For telephoned results – ALWAYS READ BACK TO CONFIRM

SURNAME........................FORENAME........................WARD.................

REG. No...................TIME & DATE OF SPECIMEN............h, ...

TEST	RESULT	REFERENCE RANGE (Rough guide only)
CLINICAL CHEMISTRY (Blood, Serum)		
a) Urea	............mmol/l	(3.0–8.0)
b) Sodium	............mmol/l	(135–146)
c) Potassium	............mmol/l	(3.5–5.2)
d) H^+	............nmol/l	(36–43)
e) Standard Bicarbonate	............mmol/l	(22–26)
f) PCO_2	............kPa	(4.7–6.0)
g) PO_2	............kPa	(11.3–14.0)
h) Bilirubin	.... µmol/l	(3–21)
i) Calcium	............mmol/l	(2.30–2.65)
j) Glucose	............mmol/l	(3.5–7.0) (non fasting)
(C.S.F.)		
k) Glucose	............mmol/l	(3.3–4.4)
l) Protein	............g/l	(0.15–0.40)
HAEMATOLOGY		
m) Haemoglobin (Hb)	............g/dl	(11.5–18.0)
n) White cell count	.... $\times 10^9$/l	(4.0–11.0)
o) Platelet count	.... $\times 10^9$/l	(150–400)
p) E.S.R.	............mm in 1h	(less than 7)
q) Prothrombin time	............s	—

OTHER TESTS (Specify both test and specimen)

....

....

MESSAGE RECEIVED BY...................................TIME...........................

DESTROY THIS RECORD WHEN OFFICIAL LABORATORY REPORT ARRIVES

minimises errors due to transcription, unfamiliar (S.I.) units, or complete loss of results written on a white coat sleeve! Results *must always* be read back to check.

I.T.U.-BASED LABORATORY EQUIPMENT

The need for a really rapid service for some investigations, together with improved technology, has led to the development of analytical instruments simple to use and maintain, designed for use by clinical staff.

One well established example is the use of 'dextrostix' which with a reflectance meter permits reasonably quantitative measurement of blood glucose in 2–3 min (Mazzaferri *et al.*, 1970; Percy-Robb *et al.*, 1972; Schersten *et al.*, 1974). This procedure is suitable for capillary blood, *not* for blood anticoagulated with fluoride-oxalate. A more recent example is the Radiometer ABL 1 blood gas analyser. Its high cost reflects a high degree of sophistication. It is designed for use with heparinised arterial blood, which is injected into a valved inlet. Thereafter analysis is completely automatic; after about 90 s pH, blood gases and various other parameters are printed out on a roll of paper (though the sophistication of the instrument is not matched in the printout). From experience this instrument is suitable for use by a variety of clinical staff. Similar instruments, such as the IL 613, the Corning 175 and Radiometer ABL 2 blood gas analysers have recently been introduced; these permit analysis using capillary blood as well as arterial blood specimens.

However, the use of such instruments is not without problems. Experience shows that in general, clinical staff lack the self-critical approach to analytical work that is drummed into laboratory workers. All laboratories should now employ quality control procedures for all routine and emergency work. The resulting constant and conscious search for errors, whether due to faults in the analyst, reagents, standards, or instruments, has revealed even in the best laboratories far more serious errors than were suspected previously. *A low standard of analytical reliability should not be countenanced for the critically ill patient.* In my opinion, whatever the test, as a routine procedure a quality control specimen must be determined in parallel with every test specimen, however urgent; the test result should only be accepted if the control result is within acceptable limits. Simulated blood products for testing glucose methods using dextrostix and reflectance meters (Eyetone) are produced by the Ames Division of Miles Laboratories. Quality control of blood gases is more difficult. Ideally whole blood specimens tonometered in the clinical chemistry laboratory should be analysed. Simpler though less satisfactory alternatives are gas controls produced by General Diagnostics and blood gas controls produced by Instrumentation Laboratories. These are tonometered buffer solutions which cannot behave exactly like blood. Regular exchange of specimens with the routine clinical chemistry laboratory is another valuable step to maintain quality of analytical work. Further problems are the need for adequate maintenance of the equipment (clinical staff are not notably good at this), and the need for back-up equipment. In times when money is short, it might be argued that to duplicate a service already provided by a routine laboratory is a luxury, however much clinical staff find it convenient.

There is no easy answer to these problems. I believe that ideally all analytical work, urgent or routine, should be performed by trained laboratory staff; to provide a fast service, I.T.U. and laboratory should be close together. Where this is not possible, some mechanical systems of conveying specimens rapidly to the laboratory have been employed – e.g. Lamson Airtube System. If I.T.U.-based analytical equipment is justified, analyses should be performed only by nominated staff, adequately trained and supervised. One consultant should be formally responsible for all analytical work performed by I.T.U. staff, medico-legally, and should actively monitor quality control procedures.

COMMONEST URGENT CLINICAL CHEMISTRY – SPECIMEN REQUIREMENTS

Guidelines only – check with your local laboratory:

Test	Specimen required	Reference interval (approx.)		Local comment
		S.I. Units	Conventional units	
Albumin	Clotted blood	33–48 g/l	3.3–4.8 g/dl	
Alcohol (ethanol)	Blood in fluoride oxalate bottle	–	–	
Ammonium	By arrangement with laboratory	Varies with method		
Amylase	Clotted blood	Varies with method		
Calcium	Clotted blood	2.2–2.7 mmol/l	8.8–10.8 mg/dl	
Catecholamines (as metanephrines)	Urine – acid preservative	<7.0 µmol/24 h	<1.3 mg/24 h	

(Cont.)

Guidelines only – check with your local laboratory:—(*Cont.*)

Test	Specimen required	Reference interval (approx.)		Local comment
		S.I. Units	Conventional units	
Cortisol (09.00 h) (24.00 h)	Clotted blood or heparinised blood	140–700 nmol/l <140 nmol/l	5–25 µg/dl <5 µg/dl	
Creatine kinase	Clotted blood	Varies with method		
Drugs (unknown)	Heparinised blood (20 ml + +) urine and gastric contents	–	–	
Globulin	Clotted blood	21–37 g/l	2.1–3.7 g/dl	
Glucose, plasma: random fasting	Blood in fluoride oxalate bottle	3.3–5.9 mmol/l 3.3–8.0 mmol/l	60–105 mg/dl 60–145 mg/dl	
pH H ion concentration PaCO$_2$ PaO$_2$* Standard bicarbonate	Anaerobic, heparinised arterial blood; Anaerobic, heparinised capillary blood	36–43 nmol/l 4.7–6.0 kPa 11.3–14.0 kPa 22–26 mmol/l	7.44–7.37 35–45 mmHg 85–105 mmHg 22–26 mEq/l	
Lactate	By arrangement with laboratory	410–1540 µmol/l	3.7–13.9 mg/dl	
Magnesium	Clotted blood	0.7–0.95 mmol/l	1.4–1.9 mEq/l	
Methaemalbumin	Clotted blood	–	–	
Methaqualone	Clotted blood or heparinised blood	–	–	
Osmolality	Clotted blood; Urine (no preservative)	278–294 mmol/kg 278–294 mosmol/kg depends on state of hydration		
Paracetamol	Clotted blood or heparinised blood	–	–	
Salicylates	Clotted blood or heparinised blood	–	–	
Sodium Potassium	Heparinised blood or clotted blood	134–146mmol/l 3.6–5.2 mmol/l	134–146 mEq/l 3.6–5.2 mEq/l	

*Capillary blood is not satisfactory for PaO$_2$ (see p. 808).

Guidelines only – check with your local laboratory:—(*Cont.*)

	Urine collection (24 h)	–	–
Transaminase, aspartate (GOT)	Clotted blood	Varies with method	
Urea	Heparinised blood or clotted blood	2.5–7.5mmol/l · 15–45 mg/dl (depends on age and diet)	

Volumes required depend on methods used in your laboratory. Whenever possible send more than the minimum required to permit repeat of what may be a crucial test, i.e. if possible send a full tube of blood, or for anti-coagulated specimen, to *the mark* (do not mix).

Comments

Albumin and globulin. With some analytical methods, errors may be caused by turbid serum – e.g. after intravenous lipid infusion.

Alcohol (ethanol). Avoid swabbing skin at venepuncture site with spirit or isopropanol impregnated swabs!

Ammonium. Unstable – only by prior arrangement with laboratory. In patients with portacaval anastromosis, values up to twice those found normally occur routinely. In hepatic encephalopathy, two- or three-fold rises may occur (Fenton, 1967).

Amylase. Apart from acute pancreatitis, high values may be found in other acute intra-abdominal conditions such as perforated peptic ulcer and afferent loop obstruction after gastrectomy (McGowan and Willis, 1964).

Calcium. Avoid prolonged venous stasis which may elevate serum calcium by up to 10%.

Catecholamine metabolites. Urine *must* be collected in acid preservative. Many hypotensive drugs affect catecholamine release, metabolism or analysis. In suspected phaeochromocytoma whenever possible collect urine *before* treatment is begun (even 1–2 h urine may be invaluable, related to creatinine excretion).

Cortisol. Serum cortisol is *normally* low in the evening. Blood values may be misleading if patient is receiving oral or even topical cortico-steroid therapy. In suspected Addison's disease, if in doubt measure cortisol before and 1, 4 and 5 h after intramuscular injection of 1 mg tetracosactrin (Synacthen). Normally a peak cortisol in excess of 1000 nmol/l occurs.

Creatine kinase. Rapid but relatively short-lived rise after myocardial infarction. Misleading rises may follow exercise or intramuscular injections (Scott *et al.*, 1974). Testing for the presence of the cardiac muscle specific MB isoenzyme is valuable in doubtful cases.

Drugs. Many drug assays are unnecessary for management of the patient.

(*a*) Note time after drug ingestion.

(*b*) Drug interaction may affect both analysis and interpretation. For example by some analytical methods, detection of barbiturates is difficult in the presence of other drugs. Coma may be caused by a combination of relatively innocuous amounts of say hypnotics, salicylate and alcohol. Let the laboratory know as much as possible about drugs that might have been taken.

(*c*) Identification of unknown drugs can be difficult and very time consuming. If really necessary provide the laboratory with 20 ml or more of blood, a full specimen of urine, *and* gastric contents (not washings).

pH, blood gases. In my experience, plastic syringes are better than glass syringes for arterial blood. Dead space of the syringe must be filled with *dilute* heparin (100 units/ml). Strong heparin is acidic. Dilute, with sterile precautions, 1 ml heparin (5000 units/ml) in 50 ml sterile saline. After collecting blood, stopper syringe or close with cork or bung on needle. Rotate syringe to mix blood with heparin.

Alternatively pH and $PaCO_2$ (but not PaO_2) and standard bicarbonate etc. may be determined on free flowing capillary blood taken into heparinised capillary tubes. In shocked or dehydrated patients, or those with cold extremities, when free-flowing capillary blood is not obtainable, an arterial blood sample is neccessary. To attempt to collect capillary blood in such circumstances is useless as the pH will be falsely low.

Lactate. Unstable. By prior arrangement with laboratory only – a carefully measured volume of blood must *immediately* after collection be mixed with a preservative (usually perchloric acid or trichloracetic acid). Avoid venous stasis and especially hand clenching (Braybrooke *et al.*, 1975).

Methaemalbumin. Its appearance in serum is thought to indicate the acute haemorrhagic form of pancreatitis (Northam *et al.*, 1965).

Paracetamol. Patients with severe overdose may be wide awake in the early stages. If treatment is contemplated, serum paracetamol is required as early as possible, and certainly not later than 12 h after ingestion (Prescott *et al.*, 1974). If blood level is greater than 200 mg/l at 4 h, or greater than 50 mg/l at 12 h after ingestion, liver toxicity is likely.

Salicylates. As with paracetamol, in early stages patients with severe overdose may be fully conscious. Aspirin is relatively slowly absorbed and if in doubt a second serum salicylate level 1–2 h later may be valuable. Serum salicylate levels greater than 500 mg/l suggest severe toxicity and possible need for treatment.

Sodium and potassium. Do not leave blood unseparated for hours, plasma or serum potassium rises markedly – refrigeration makes this *worse*.

Transaminase. For suspected myocardial infarction, note time after onset of chest pain. No significant rise is usually detectable in first few hours after myocardial infarction.

REFERENCES

Braybrooke, J., Lloyd, B., Nattrass, M. and Alberti, K. G. M. M. (1975). Blood sampling techniques for lactate and pyrurate estimation: a reappraisal. *Ann. Clin. Biochem.* **12**, 252.

Fenton, J. C. B. (1967). The plasma ammonium and liver disease. *Brit. J. Hosp. Med.* **1**, 491.

Mazzaferri, E. L., Skillman, T. G., Lanese, R. R. and Keller, M. P. (1970). Use of test strips with colour meter to measure blood glucose. *Lancet* **1**, 331.

McGowan, G. K. and Wills, M. R. (1964). Diagnostic value of plasma amylase, especially after gastric surgery. *Brit. Med. J.* **1**, 160.

Northam, B. E., Winstone, N. E. and Banwell, J. G. (1965). Biochemical aspects of pancreatitis. *In* 'Recent Advances in Gastro-enterology' (Ed. J. Badenoch and B. N. Brooke). Churchill, London.

Percy-Robb, I. W., McMaster, R. S., Harrower, A. D. B. and Duncan, L. J. P. (1972). Blood glucose assay using dextrostix and a reflectance meter. *Ann. Clin. Biochem.* **9**, 91.

Prescott, L. F., Newton, R. W., Swainson, C. P., Wright, N., Forrest, A. R. W. and Matthew, H. (1974). Successful treatment of severe paracetamol overdose with cysteamine. *Lancet* **1**, 588.

Schersten, B., Kuhl, C., Hollender, A. and Ekman, R. (1974). Blood glucose measurement with dextrostix and new reflectance meter. *Brit. Med. J.* **3**, 384.

Scott, B. B., Simmons, A. V., Newton, K. E. and Payne, R. B. (1974). Interpretation of serum creatine kinase in suspected myocardial infarction. *Brit. Med. J.* **4**, 691.

Section 3: Haematological Requirements and the I.T.U.

P. Jones

INTRODUCTION

The laboratory serving an intensive therapy unit has two broad functions – to supply facts for diagnosis and monitoring, and to supply advice. In this section are listed suggestions for a basic range of on-site haematological tests. With the modern trend to grouping of hospitals, and thus the more complex and expensive diagnostic procedures, every on-site laboratory should not be expected to provide a full range of text book investigations. Emphasis should be on tests relevant to the need for quick and accurate investigation and monitoring, and provision of commonly required blood products. It should be appreciated that the diagnosis of many haematological disorders, particularly the haemolytic anaemias, coagulopathies and malignant disease, may be extremely complex, and ease of access to both a reference laboratory and the Blood Transfusion Service is essential.

BASIC LABORATORY TESTS

Peripheral blood examination

Haemoglobin, red cell count, *haematocrit*, M.C.V., M.C.H., M.C.H.C., *reticulocyte count, white cell count* (total and differential), *examination of film*. Most laboratories will be equipped with a Coulter Counter with automatic print out of blood indices. Note that automatic (Coulter) calculation of haematocrit eliminates plasma trapping error of centrifugation methods and therefore M.C.H. is a better indicator of hypochromia than M.C.H.C.

810

Platelet count: when this is performed automatically an artificially low platelet count may result from clumping. A visual screen should therefore be performed in addition before thrombocytopenia is diagnosed. A more common fault is the finding of a small clot in the sample – in this case the white cell count may also be artificially low.

Erythrocyte sedimentation rate. An additional useful test, conveniently obtained in kit form*, is the *H.E.A. test* (horse erythrocyte agglutination test) for infectious mononucleosis.

Bone marrow

Although examination of marrow smears may conveniently be performed in another hospital there should be on-site provision for the expert collection and initial preparation of the sample. Marrow aspiration is by no means a painless procedure and poor technique will inevitably result in a request for repeat investigation.

Additional basic tests for the diagnosis of haemolysis (see also Table 1)

Urinary urobilinogen, bilirubin, haemoglobin and haemosiderin, and estimation of plasma haptoglobins and methaemalbumin.

Screening tests for haemoglobinopathies: Sickle cell disease may be conveniently detected with Sickledex^R test kit†, a qualitative tube test for the presence of haemoglobin S.

G-6-PD deficiency may be detected by using a qualitative test kit supplied by the Sigma Chemical Company‡. The technique requires long-wave U.V. light for the detection of fluorescence denoting normal blood. A similar test is available from Sigma for the qualitative detection of *pyruvate kinase* deficiency.

Tests for haemostasis

Bleeding time, one stage prothrombin time (P.T.), *partial thromboplastin time with kaolin* (P.T.T.K.), *thrombin time* (T.T.), *fibrinogen estimation, and fibrin(ogen) degradation products.*

---

* MONOSPOT^R Ortho Diagnostics, Raritan, New Jersey, 98869, U.S.A.
† Ortho Diagnostics.
‡ Sigma, P.O. Box 14508, Saint Louis, Missouri, 63178, U.S.A.

Table 1. Laboratory evidence of haemolysis

Haemoglobin	Decreased in uncompensated haemolysis
Reticulocyte count	Usually increased
Blood film	Normocytic or macrocytic
	Abnormalities of red cells in some disorders, for instance microspherocytes in hereditary spherocytosis, and fragmentation in microangiopathic haemolytic anaemia
Plasma haptoglobins	Decreased or absent
Haemoglobinaemia and haemoglobinuria	Present when haptoglobins are saturated
Methaemalbumin	Present following breakdown of free haemoglobin to haematin, plus albumin
Haemosiderinuria	Present after initial tubular reabsorption of haem
Bilirubin	Increase depends on hepatic function
Urinary urobilinogen	Increase depends on hepatic function and normality of gut flora. Often misleading

N.B. Findings depend on rate of haemolysis

Two rapid latex particle tests for the semi quantitative detection of F.D.Ps. are available*†. Note that the thrombin time is a convenient test for both heparin and streptokinase therapy as well as a rapid indicator of fibrinogen deficiency.

BLOOD PRODUCTS LABORATORY

Techniques

Antiglobulin tests (Direct and Indirect Coombs'), *detection of irregular antibodies, grouping and cross match procedures.*

Back-up tests

Necessary back-up tests include measurement of serum iron, folate and vitamin B_{12}; the Schilling test; detection of L.E. cells; special stains for the diagnosis of leukaemia; electrophoretic techniques for the detection of abnormal haemoglobins; estimation and differentiation of plasma bilirubin; measurement of cell survival, and red cell fragility; detection of paroxysmal nocturnal haemoglobinuria, coagulation factor assays and platelet function tests; hepatitis surface antigen (HBsAg) detection, and specific grouping and genotyping techniques. These

---

* Thrombo-Wellcotest, Wellcome Research Laboratories, The Wellcome Building, Euston Road, London NW1 2BP.
† Diagen F.D.P. test, Diagnostic Reagents Ltd. Thame, Oxford.

tests, which depend on the accuracy that can only be obtained by frequent practise on a large number of samples, are not essential on-site requirements.

Supply of therapeutic materials

The following products should be available on site: *Whole blood and red cells, fresh frozen plasma* (F.F.P.) *fibrinogen concentrate, albumin and plasma protein fraction.*

Laboratories in hospitals serving patients with hereditary coagulation disorders should also stock cryoprecipitate, factor VIII lyophilised concentrate, and II, (VII), IX, and X lyophilised concentrate.

Platelet concentrates should be obtainable via the laboratory from the Blood Transfusion Service on request, and IgG preparations from either the Regional Transfusion Centre or the Public Health Laboratory Service.

The storage requirements and approximate shelf life of products are given in Table 2.

Table 2. Storage and approximate shelf life of blood products

Product	Storage (°C)	Shelf life
Whole blood	4	21 days
Red cells	4	14–21 days
Platelet concentrate	4–20	48–72 h
Fresh frozen plasma	−30	6 months
Cryoprecipitate	−30	6 months
Factor VIII lyophilised concentrate	4	2 years
Factors II, (VII), IX, X lyophilised concentrate	4–20	2 years
Fibrinogen concentrate	20	5 years
Albumin	20	3 years
Plasma protein fraction	20	5 years

Exact criteria on label or in literature supplied with product, or from the Blood Transfusion Service. Blood products should be stored in the dark.

PREPARATION OF BLOOD PRODUCTS FOR USE

Whole blood and red cells should be used within six hours of issue from the bank. Drugs should never be added to the blood pack.

F.F.P. and cryoprecipitate should be used within one hour of thawing at 37°C. Cryoprecipitate may be pooled in the laboratory before issue.

Factor VIII and IX concentrates should be used within one hour of addition of diluent.

Advice on blood products

A function of the blood product laboratory should be to advise clinicians on the most appropriate blood product and its dose for clinical problems (Davison, 1976). The rapidly increasing demand for blood fractions, especially for factor VIII for the treatment of haemophilia A, means that clinicians have a major responsibility to prescribe *whole* blood only when really necessary.

Urgent request for blood

Modern techniques of ABO and Rhesus grouping and cross match have obviated the need for emergency transfusion of O Rhesus Negative ('universal donor') blood to ungrouped recipients, at least in the hospital setting. In extreme emergency ABO and Rhesus specific blood can be provided within 15 minutes of receipt of the patient's sample, and, in a large blood bank, fully compatible blood within 45 minutes.

Transfusion reactions

Full details of the side effects of blood transfusion are given by Tovey and Bird (1974). When a transfusion reaction is suspected the laboratory should be provided with the following specimens:

(*a*) Remains of blood product transfused in original packs or bottles.

(*b*) Two samples of blood from the patient, one into heparin and one into a plain tube.

(*c*) Samples of urine passed during or after transfusion.

ACKNOWLEDGEMENT

The author is grateful to the technical staff of the Department of Haematology, Royal Victoria Infirmary, for their help in the preparation of this article.

REFERENCES

Davison, J. F. (1976). A hospital blood products laboratory. Symposium on blood component therapy. British Society of Haematology, Glasgow.

Tovey, G. H. and Bird, G. W. G. (1974). Blood transfusion and the use of blood products. *In* 'Blood and its Disorders', pp. 1481–1506 (Ed. R. M. Hardisty and D. J. Weatherall). Blackwell, Oxford.

II

Radiological and Ultrasound Requirements and the I.T.U.

Section 1: Radiological and Ultrasound Requirements and the I.T.U.

J. PORTNOY

GENERAL

Most I.T.U. patients are helpless, immobile and breathless. They are attached by tubes and cables to monitoring and life-support systems, often with many attendant personnel (Fig. 1). This makes them less than ideal subjects for high quality radiography (Raphael, 1972; Mohr, 1971), see also Table 1.

Table 1

A PROBLEMS LIMITING X-RAY QUALITY IN AN I.T.U.
Problems relating to the patient
  I   Immobility and helplessness. *Need for assistants for lif ng patient onto the cassette.*
 II   Patient cannot hold breath for exposure duration. *A. mentary arrest of ventilator needed.*
III   Multiple tubes and cables attached to patient.
IV Anteroposterior projections only. *A P.A. film is not possible* (Fig. 1).

815

B   PROBLEMS RELATING TO SURROUNDINGS
  I   Bright ambient light. This obscures the light beam diaphragm. *Need for blinds and accessible switching.*
  II   Multiple personnel carrying out their functions (radiation hazard to personnel).
  III   Long lead to the machine from 13 amp socket, *big volt drop, so long exposure.*
  IV   Limited height of X-ray tube above supine patient (Fig. 1).

In short we are faced with an unhelpful combination of a low voltage and current, a long exposure, anteroposterior course of the rays to the film, a short focus to film distance and frequently a restless tachypnoeic patient all tending to produce a distorted blurred image. The size of the heart is not assessable because of variable magnification. These factors may vary from day to day with the patient's position (Fig. 2) (Mohr, 1971). The X-ray factors should be kept as constant as possible by recording them permanently. The best place for this is *on the film* (Table 2). Then the radiographer summoned to take an ensuing film automatically looks at the last films and adjusts the factors to get the best results. Putting the time on the film helps to ensure that the sequence of the films on the same day is obvious.

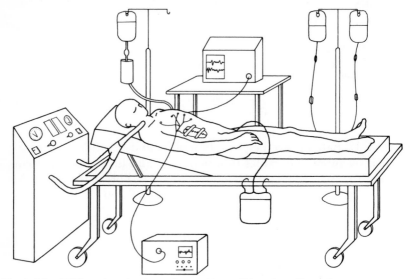

Fig. 1. The I.T.U. patient showing unfavourable conditions for radiography.

ORGANISATION IN THE I.T.U.

To ensure a good service to the I.T.U. the patient's films should be stored in separate compartments at or under a large four box viewer

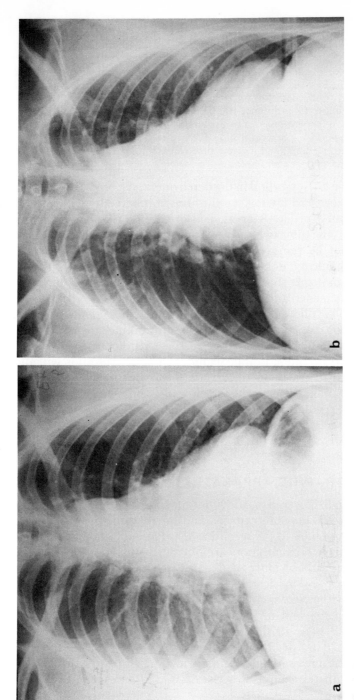

Fig. 2. Two X-ray films of the same patient to show the effect on the heart shadow, lungs and mediastinum, of the (a) erect and (b) supine positions.

Table 2. The factors to be written on the X-ray film taken in the I.T.U.

Name   First name   Age   Sequence number and time (using 24-hour clock)
kV   mA   Seconds (or mA seconds as appropriate)
A.P.   Film to focus distance (F.F.D.)
Inspiration or expiration   Erect or supine position
Grid or non-grid   Screens if special, e.g. rare earth
Any contrast medium, and if given, time elapsed from exhibition

---

near to the nurses station in the department. An X-ray clerk should visit the department daily to keep the films numbered in sequence and kept in sequential order. A great deal of confusion and time is saved by having all the films to hand and sorted, near to the viewing box. Films should not be removed from the ward and all documentation and sorting should be done on the spot.

The radiologist should be ready to discuss the films with the I.T.U. staff when needed and a daily visit by a radiologist to report on the films is valuable. The radiologist may be able to suggest other ways of checking on doubtful points of diagnosis by taking other views and using ancillary methods, e.g. contrast media, or other imaging techniques, such as ultrasound or isotope scanning. This consultation will allow the radiologist to check on the standard of work being produced and if necessary make suggestions for improvement.

A short regular meeting should be held between the I.T.U. staff and radiologists to discuss diagnostic difficulties and methods whereby they may be solved.

RADIOGRAPHIC APPARATUS

A very high-powered *mobile* X-ray unit is essential. It must be of 300 milliamps 150 kilovolts capacity and capable of taking a chest film with exposures of 0.04 to 0.1 second range. Patients who cannot hold their breath or are on ventilators are obviously unfavourable for obtaining clear films without movement blur.

An X-ray room close to the I.T.U. and on the same level in the hospital with a *fixed image intensifier* and high-powered machine could be of great value and might well be equipped with good resuscitation facilities (Schlag, 1976). It must be recalled that *high radiation doses* can be achieved by accumulated screening time (Ardran and Fursdon, 1973). The maximum screening time, e.g. for insertion of a cardiac pacing catheter should be set at 30 min at 1 mA and any one in the vicinity must wear lead aprons. Unprotected hands must never be in the primary beam of the X-ray tube. No member of the staff who is pregnant, or could be pregnant, should be within the area during X-ray exposure. There is an increasing awareness of the danger to staff by radiation during these screening procedures; the risk to the patients is usually small, since the cases that are screened are usually elderly and not generally repeated. Consideration should be given to the issue of *film badges* to assess the amounts of radiation being received by the staff. It must be recalled that distance is the best substitute for lead protection, *the quantity of irradiation being reduced by the square of the distance* between the subject and the X-ray tube.

RADIOGRAPHIC DIAGNOSIS

The chest X-ray in the I.T.U. (See Tables 4 and 5)

The most frequently needed X-ray view in the I.T.U. is necessarily the chest. Some features of technique and indications should be considered as the request is made, so that the film will give the required information. The degree of penetration used to take the film may influence the findings greatly or miss the lesion altogether (Fig. 3). For example, when checking the position of a tube or catheter, pacemaker electrode, or even a foreign body, a slightly greater penetration than usual will be required (Tager, 1942).

The indications for a fixed grid film with penetration are enumerated in Table 3. A grid film enables the voltage of the X-rays to be increased (thereby improving penetration), the resultant scatter being absorbed by the grid.

Fluid

If the patient is not fully erect when the film is taken (and this is not always possible or desirable), the usual signs of fluid – 'the Damoiseau

Table 3. Indications for a fixed grid film with penetration in the I.T.U.

Dense infiltrate	Foreign body
Heavy patient	For the trachea and carina
Dense pleural or pulmonary opacity	For cavities (Tager, 1942)
Calcification	Mediastinal structures
Air bronchogram	Pulmonary vascular markings, through
To elucidate some rib fractures, especially in the last 3 ribs (Felson, 1973)	an effusion

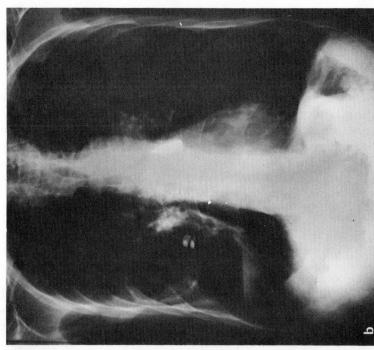

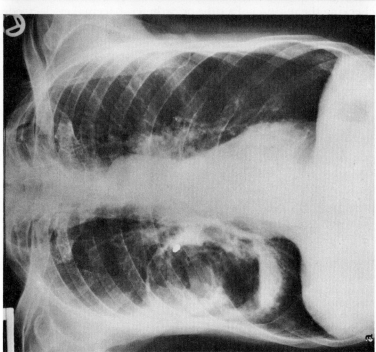

Fig. 3. Two films of the same patient to show the effect of degrees of penetration in establishing the full diagnosis. (a) Ordinary degree of penetration, two abcess cavities are shown in the right lung; (b) a more penetrated view reveals the bullet lodged in the mediastinum.

Table 4. Diagrams of chest X-ray signs

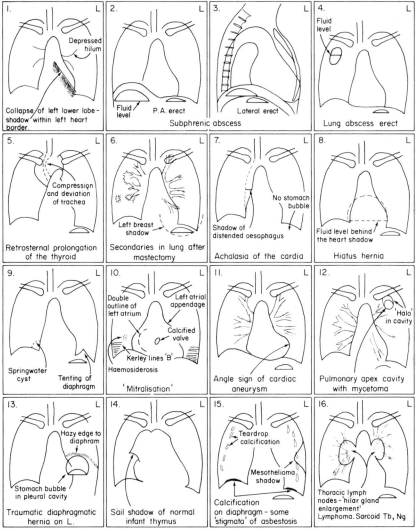

curve' – will not be seen. A homogeneous greyness above the diaphragm (Fig. 4) with loss of its silhouette on that side may be all that is shown. If the patient is lying flat the greyness spreads all over the affected lung field and is much reduced in density, so that only the careful comparison of the two sides will detect it. If it is not possible to take an X-ray in the erect position, a horizontal *lateral decubitus view*

Table 5. Diagrams of chest X-ray signs

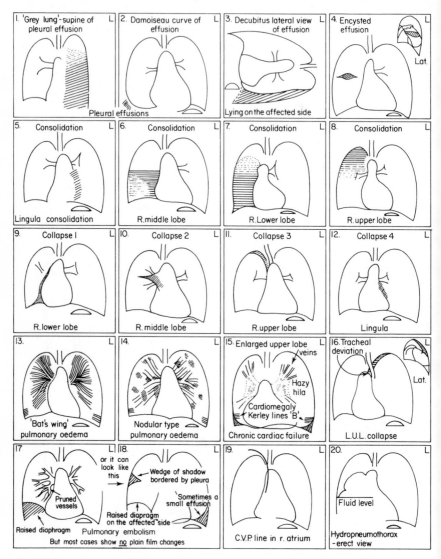

1. 'Grey lung'-supine of pleural effusion	2. Damoiseau curve of effusion	3. Decubitus lateral view of effusion	4. Encysted effusion
Pleural effusions		Lying on the affected side	Lat.
5. Consolidation	6. Consolidation	7. Consolidation	8. Consolidation
Lingula consolidation	R.middle lobe	R.Lower lobe	R.upper lobe
9. Collapse 1	10. Collapse 2	11. Collapse 3	12. Collapse 4
R.lower lobe	R.middle lobe	R.upper lobe	Lingula
13.	14.	15. Enlarged upper lobe veins / Hazy hila / Cardiomegaly / Kerley lines 'B'	16. Tracheal deviation
'Bat's wing' pulmonary oedema	Nodular type pulmonary oedema	Chronic cardiac failure	L.U.L. collapse / Lat.
17. Pruned vessels / Raised diaphragm	18. or it can look like this → Wedge of shadow bordered by pleura / Sometimes a small effusion / Raised diaphragm on the affected side / Pulmonary embolism / But most cases show no plain film changes	19. C.V.P line in r. atrium	20. Fluid level / Hydropneumothorax -erect view

should be taken with the patient lying on the affected side (Harris and Harris, 1975a). The fluid present then accumulates along the de-pendent chest wall (Barry, 1956), and shows as a denser band (Figs 5(a) and (b)). Ultrasound examination may also be used to demonstrate the presence of fluid in a body cavity.

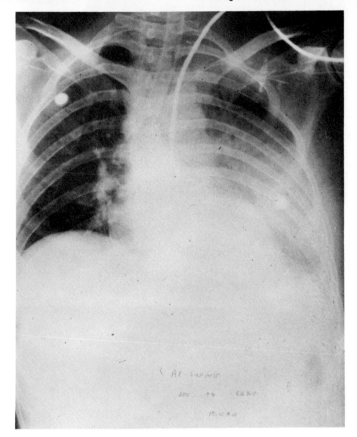

Fig. 4. Chest X-ray showing appearance of fluid in a pleural ethusion (left) when the patient is X-rayed in the supine position.

Position of intra tracheal tubes

A too-deeply placed tracheal tube may block a main bronchus if it reaches the carina and cause collapse of the affected lobe or lung (Figs 6(a) and (b)). A slightly penetrated view is then needed. The presence of long-standing indwelling cuffed tubes may lead to tracheal stenosis (Fig. 7).

Pneumothorax

The technique required to show this more clearly is to take an expiratory film, so that the rest of the lung becomes more dense as the air leaves it, while the trapped air in the pneumothorax remains lucent.

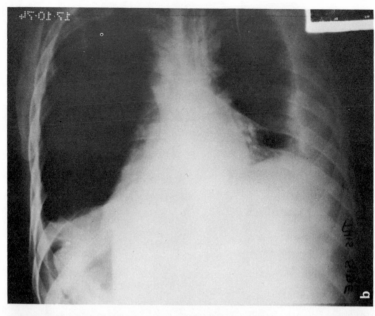

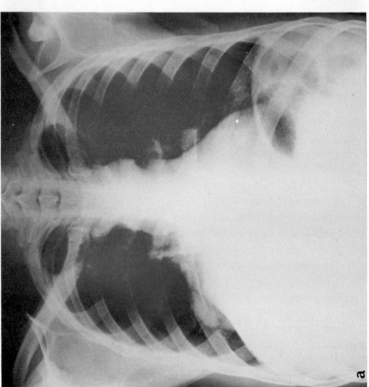

Fig. 5. (a) A right subpulmonary pleural effusion in the P.A. view. The fluid mimics a raised right diaphragm. (b) Right subpulmonary pleural effusion. After lying the patient on the affected side and taking the film with a horizontal ray, the lateral decubitus view, the fluid has flowed onto the paracostal margin as a denser layer. (Note the reverse position – patient lying on right side.)

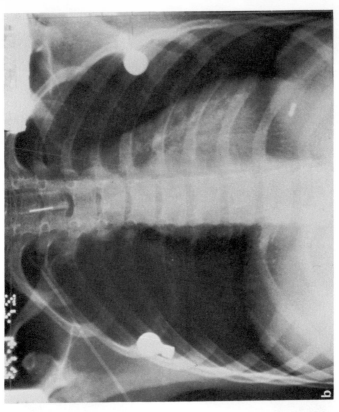

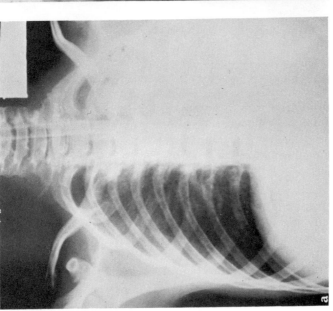

Fig. 6. (a) Total collapse of the left lung from blockage of the left main bronchus by an endotracheal tube. (b) Re-expansion of the lung following partial withdrawal of the tube.

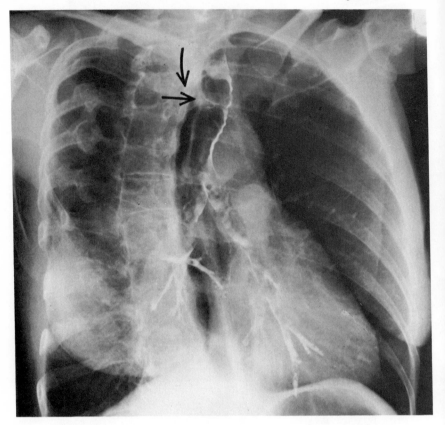

Fig. 7. Tracheal stenosis, from indwelling endotracheal tube with inflated cuff: an X-ray after a contrast medium introduced to produce a tracheogram.

The expiratory film can be obtained in patients on artificial ventilation by maintaining the patient in expiration during hand ventilation. It should be noted that a plaster or strapping dressing can obscure an area of pneumothorax and can simulate the lung markings in the air-filled zone of a pneumothorax.

Patchy consolidation

Patches of consolidation, so frequently seen in critically ill patients, are radiologically nonspecific and may be due to infection, collapse or patchy oedema. They must therefore be interpreted in the light of the clinical findings, other X-ray signs and the sequence of X-ray changes. The appearance of the adult respiratory distress syndrome, the 'wet lung' syndrome, the 'stiff lung' or 'shock lung' (Jaffe, 1974), may give rise to a radiological diagnosis of intra-alveolar pulmonary oedema. This may be seen as the familiar 'bat's wing' shadow (Fig. 8), but usually the shadowing is more patchy than confluent, and is often posture related. The appearances are often indistinguishable from the aspiration syndrome. The distribution of shadowing in uraemia, hypersensitivity pneumonitis, and following radiation therapy may also be posture related. Similar appearances may be seen in the fat embolism syndrome and following embolism of amniotic fluid (Wilkins *et al.*, 1976). In these latter conditions, there is no relationship to posture.

Subphrenic abscess
Free gas may be seen under the diaphragm, when the patient can be placed erect, the gas rising to lie under the hemidiaphragm, in the

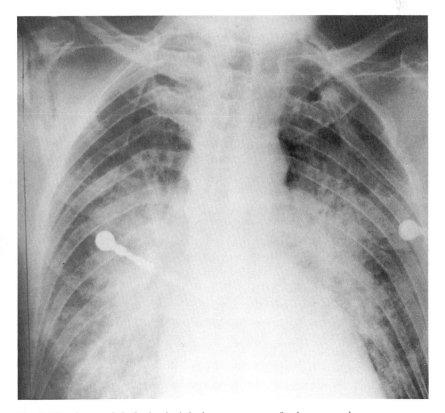

Fig. 8. The characteristic 'bat's wing' shadow appearance of pulmonary oedema.

anterior or posterior subphrenic space, with a fluid level. At first the diaphragm shows limitation of movement, but as the disease progresses the dome rises and becomes fixed. To demonstrate these features and avoid screening all that is needed may be a clear 'inspiration/expiration' set of two films. Often a small *pleural effusion* forms above the diaphragm, which obscures its outline; and when the abscess is on the left side, which is the less common site, the position of a gas bubble in the stomach fundus will define the position of the dome. If the patient is too ill for an erect film, a lateral decubitus view with a horizontal ray (as described for subpulmonary effusion) will show the gas and fluid level. Gas will also be seen for about 14 days after an operation, with perforations of any intestinal viscera, and during peritoneal dialysis. To show stomach displacement a *gastrografin swallow* (Fig. 9) can be done in the unit, the contrast medium being given direct or down the nasogastric tube, 100 ml will be adequate. The patient is laid onto his right side for 2 minutes and then the film is taken in the supine position, with the mobile X-ray machine, if possible with the head of the patient a little low. Sometimes the *liver shadow* may be seen to be displaced downwards by the abscess.

It is essential to use a water soluble medium when perforation or obstruction is suspected.

Fractured ribs

It is important to look for underlying lung damage, and pneumothorax or haemothorax are important findings. A series of 'double fractures' may be associated with a *flail segment*, and one may not see this on X-ray because fractures are through the costal cartilages. *Subcutaneous emphysema* may indicate a rib fracture (Fig. 10). Oblique views of the rib cage should be taken when rib fractures are suspected. A fracture of the sternum or dislocated costocondral junctions may be demonstrated by a lateral view. Fractures of the lower ribs may be associated with injury to the liver, kidney or spleen (Harris and Harris, 1975). A *penetrated bucky* or fixed grid film may help delineate the appropriate organ and demonstrate the site of rib fracture.

Pericardial effusion may be suspected on the chest X-ray, may be detected by ultrasound (p. 848) and the gamma camera can differentiate clearly between cardiomegaly and pericardial effusion. Clearly, these non-invasive techniques are better suited to the management of the critically ill than angiography, with its attendant hazards. The introduction of contrast medium by hand injection into the right atrium through a catheter or the C.V.P. line and a film taken at the end of the

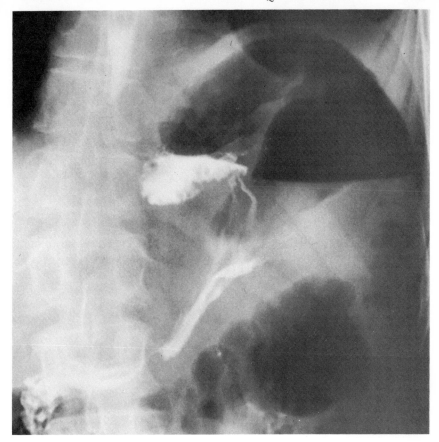

Fig. 9. Left-sided subphrenic abscess. Gastrografin to distinguish the stomach gas shadow from gas in the abscess.

injection will effectively demonstrate the widening of the distance between the ventricle and the lateral margin in effusion. It should be remembered that the very rounded shape of a pericardial effusion contrasts with the angle outline of the ventricular profile seen with cardiac aneurysm (Table 4, no. 11).

Contrast media and the gastrointestinal tract

Upper gastrointestinal tract
Always keep alert to the possibility that in the critically ill the contrast medium may be aspirated into the bronchus or may enter the lung via a

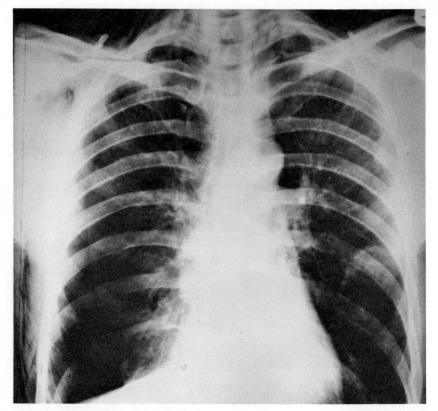

Fig. 10. Fractures of the right ribs with streaks of fine gas shadows in the subcutaneous tissues (surgical emphysema).

fistula. It is wise to use a bronchographic medium like Dionosil or Lipiodol, if there is this possibility, since gastrografin and other similar water soluble media are five times the osmolarity of plasma and hence are irritant and hypertonic. These media may cause severe hydroscopic reactions when inhaled. There are two types of Dionosil – aqueous and oily, the aqueous being most useful, since it is readily absorbed from the bronchial tree. Should barium enter the bronchus, its removal is difficult even by endobronchial suction.

Leaks from anastomoses
A leak from an anastomosis can be demonstrated by a gastrografin swallow examination (Figs 11(a) and (b)) which will adequately de-lineate the intestinal tract. Further down the gastrointestinal tract the

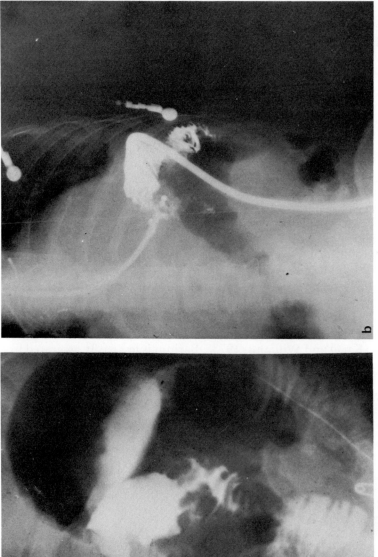

Fig. 11. (a) Gastrografin 'swallow' showing an anastomotic leak following a subtotal gastrectomy. (b) Gastrografin injected down the Ryles tube (same patient) showing the contrast medium leaking from the stomach into a left subphrenic drain.

gastrografin becomes diluted and structural outline is inadequately shown. A series of films taken at $\frac{1}{2}$ h intervals as the medium passes down the tract may, however, exclude the possibility of obstruction or perforation. It is essential to use a water-soluble medium when perforation or obstruction is suspected. For most other gastrointestinal tract examinations barium is to be preferred (Forrest and Finlayson, 1974).

Emergency 'meals'

A preliminary erect and supine film is taken in order to exclude obstruction, which would be indicated by multiple fluid levels and gaseous distension, with progressive increase in these signs in successive films. If an erect film is not possible, a lateral decubitus film with horizontal ray will be adequate (Fig. 12). Emergency barium or gastrografin meals are often useful in patients with bleeding from the gastrointestinal tract, while a higher diagnostic yield may be obtained by both endoscopy and barium meal. Before examination it is wise to aspirate the stomach to dryness in order to get a clearer view. Although barium gives a much clearer and detailed picture the double contrast barium meal is even more effective, being able to detect very small lesions (Kreel and Williams, 1973). Barium is less easily aspirated from

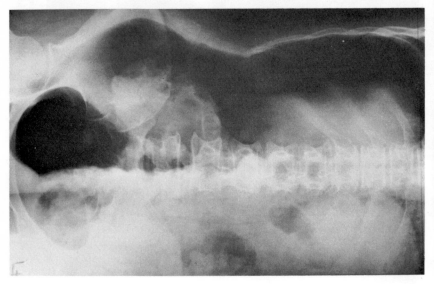

Fig. 12. The appearance of free gas in the peritoneum in a lateral decubitus view, with the patient lying on the left side.

the stomach than gastrografin, and should therefore be avoided immediately prior to anaesthesia. Gastrografin is very hypertonic and large amounts can cause dehydration and purgation in the very ill, especially in children. Radiology and endoscopy are not mutually exclusive in the critically ill patient, and both techniques may be needed (Stevenson *et al.*, 1976) and complement each other (Cumberland, 1975).

Water soluble contrast medium into the balloon of a Sengstaken tube (for control of bleeding from oesophageal varices) helps to visualise the level in the film, after a swallow examination has confirmed the position and extent of the varices (Parbhoo, 1975).

Contrast media and the urinary tract

Urography (I.V.U.)

Safer modern contrast media have increased the value of high dose urography. It may be necessary to use up to 2 ml per kilogram of body weight, using 420 Conray or similar media. Not more than 1 ml of 420 Conray should be used per kg/B.W. in children.

In patients with failing kidneys or oliguria much useful information can be obtained (Brown *et al.*, 1970), retrograde pyelography is now rarely necessary. Obstructive changes can usually be recognised, or excluded, and the site and cause of the obstruction can generally be demonstrated (van Waes, 1972). Assessment can be made of the size, shape and position of the kidneys. A prone film, to allow the contrast medium to flow forward and down to the site of an obstruction, or a late film to detect slow nephrogram formation, or its continuance, may be valuable (Kelsey Fry and Cattell, 1972). A calculus which might be missed on a plain film may be shown by plain film tomography. *Nephrotomography*, combined with an immediate 'cut' at the end of injection, is invaluable. The examination should be supervised by the radiologist (Fig. 13).

Renal trauma may be shown by extravasation of the contrast medium from tears in the renal parenchyma or collecting system: the perirenal tissue will be opacified by streaks of leaking medium. Subcapsular or extrarenal haematoma may displace or deform the kidney or the calyceal systems may be distorted by an intrarenal haematoma.

Selective renal angiography is the method of choice if a renal tumour is detected or suspected on I.V.U. Lesions such as cysts, vascular anomalies, and neoplasms can be conclusively identified and a 'flush' arteriogram can be done at the time which will identify renal artery

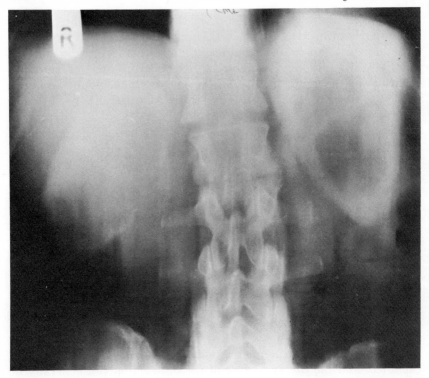

Fig. 13. The 'rim' sign in hydronephrosis. This shows the 'negative shadow' of dilated calyces against the opacified kidney substance (white), displayed by nephrotomography immediately at the end of the injection, of intravenous contrast medium.

stenosis. This will have been suspected on the intravenous pyelogram because of increased opacification on the affected side. A slow unilateral increase in the density of the nephrogram for 15 to 24 hours after injection might suggest that the examination be supplemented by selective renal venography to exclude or confirm renal vein thrombosis (Kelsey Fry and Cattell, 1972).

Needle nephrostomy may be needed in a few selected cases.

Renal scintigraphy using Gamma camera is discussed on p. 867.

Contrast media and the gallbladder and liver

Oral cholecystography will be the earliest contrast method of investigation in the majority of cases but when it fails to show the common duct, and/or the hepatic ducts (when visualisation is required), intravenous cholangiography, or slow drip cholangiography may be indicated; see the algorithm, Table 6.

Table 6. Algorithm of cholecystography in the I.T.U.

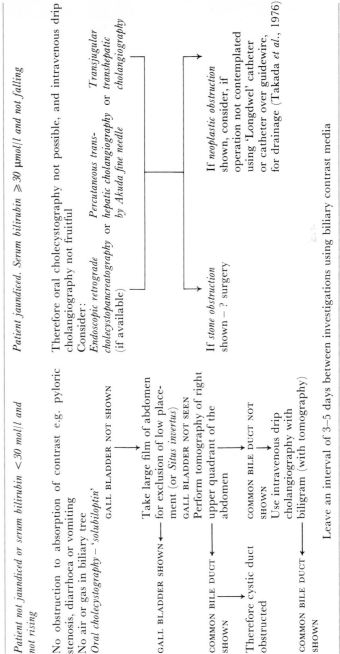

Patient not jaundiced or serum bilirubin <30 mol/l and not rising

No obstruction to absorption of contrast e.g. pyloric stenosis, diarrhoea or vomiting
No air or gas in biliary tree
Oral cholecystography – 'solubiloptin'

    GALL BLADDER NOT SHOWN
      Take large film of abdomen
GALL BLADDER SHOWN — for exclusion of low place-
      ment (or *Situs invertus*)
      GALL BLADDER NOT SEEN
      Perform tomography of right
COMMON BILE DUCT — upper quadrant of the
SHOWN   abdomen

Therefore cystic duct   COMMON BILE DUCT NOT
obstructed   SHOWN
          Use intravenous drip
          cholangiography with
COMMON BILE DUCT — biligram (with tomography)
SHOWN

      Leave an interval of 3–5 days between investigations using biliary contrast media

Patient jaundiced. Serum bilirubin ≥30 μmol/l and not falling

Therefore oral cholecystography not possible, and intravenous drip cholangiography not fruitful
Consider:
Endoscopic retrograde   *Percutaneous trans-*   *Transjugular*
cholecystopancreatography or *hepatic cholangiography* or *transhepatic*
(if available)   *by Akuda fine needle*   *cholangiography*

If stone obstruction
shown – ? surgery

If neoplastic obstruction
shown, consider, if
operation not contemplated
using 'Longdwel' catheter
or catheter over guidewire,
for drainage (Takada *et al.*, 1976)

In jaundice where the serum bilirubin is higher than 130 µmol (3.5 mgm %) further investigation may be performed by direct puncture of the liver by percutaneous transhepatic cholangiography. The transhepatic needle which was usually used was a 'Longdwel' needle with a covering catheter of Teflon, the needle being withdrawn after puncture. By this method only distended ducts were easily shown and entered and operation had to be immediately available (in case of leakage of bile), or the catheter left in the liver to drain. The advent of the very fine gauge 'Akuda' needle has made this a safer and less traumatic procedure. A summary of these hazards is given by Keighley and co-workers (1973).

The Burhenne technique for removal of gallstones from the common bile duct through the 'T' tube track should be considered in patients developing this complication following cholecystectomy. A 'T' tube can be replaced with this apparatus through the track. A simpler method using a Dormia Basket is possible (Magarey, 1971).

Endoscopic retrograde cholangiography and pancreatography with the injection of 60% sodium diatriazoate 'Hypaque') into the duct to visualise both the bile duct system and the pancreatic duct system is valuable of available and may be more helpful if combined with 75-selenomethionine scanning (Zimmon et al., 1974).

Unfortunately E.R.C.P. has a high failure rate (approximately 30% in experienced hands), a high complication rate and even some mortality (Bilbas et al., 1976).

Selective angiography of the coeliac axis and mesenteric vessels

This is an important technique for investigating disease of the liver, spleen and pancreas (Kreel and Williams, 1964). It is also of value in assessment of the extent of hepatic trauma (Nahum and Levesque, 1973).

In the I.T.U. its relevance will be mainly in order to predict the resectability of ischaemic bowel or malignancy. This method will also delineate the portal vein and can take the place of *splenoportography*. This is especially useful if the spleen has already been removed.

Angiography of the superior mesenteric artery, using this selective technique was originally used to identify the origin of a massive bleed in the lower G.I. tract but it has now proved even more useful for detection of small bleeds in any part of the intestine (Gray and Grossman, 1974). Selective arteriography of the coeliac and superior mesenteric artery can detect blood loss at a rate as small as 0.5 ml per minute. It is necessary that no contrast medium (barium or water soluble medium) is present in the bowel at the time and clearly the vessel must be bleeding at the time of the injection. Cineradiography or the videotape recorder is helpful in this rather difficult diagnostic area.

Contrast studies of the lung

The angiographic diagnosis of pulmonary embolism by catheterisation of the pulmonary artery may be hazardous in the critically ill patient but differential diagnosis is often of such importance (Bookstein and Silver, 1974) that with a full team of practised personnel and facilities immediately available for cardiopulmonary bypass (Stein *et al.*, 1975), it may be attempted with confidence (Bookstein and Silver, 1974; John *et al.*, 1974). Using small volumes of contrast, it may even be feasible at the bedside, with a 'P.A. seeking' catheter (Loups *et al.*, 1975). Selective small sections are opacified with small injections, using the mobile intensifier.

Angiography of the aorta and peripheral vessels
A definitive diagnosis of an aortic aneurysm can frequently be made using plain films in association with a history and careful clinical examination (Figs 14(a) and (b) ; Fig. 15). To detect early rupture of an aortic aneurysm and when there is uncertain diagnosis of aortic dissection, flush aortography using a pigtail catheter for the upper thoracic aorta, or a straight catheter for the lower aorta is often feasible (Hayaski *et al.*, 1974). Facilities must be available for resuscitation and the patient should be monitored throughout the procedure (Parsavand, 1974).

Peripheral studies of vessels in the upper and lower limbs are rarely hazardous and are not greatly disturbing to the patient. This technique can confirm the diagnosis of thrombosis or occlusion of embolism or arteriovenous fistula.

Venography and venacavography

Phlebography of the peripheral vessels and opacification of the inferior and superior vena cava to exclude or confirm occlusion, is technically possible in selected cases, can be done using a portable machine and although poor films may be obtained, the views are diagnostic. A long cassette system or a series of views will produce acceptable confirmatory phlebograms (Wilson, 1976).

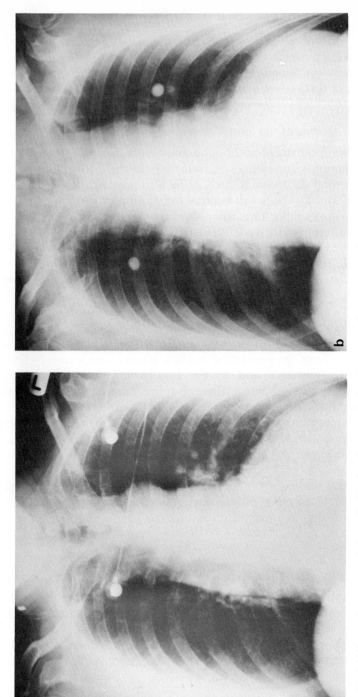

Fig. 14. (a) History of severe central chest pain. The film shows a normal mediastinal outline. (b) Twelve hours later, film of the same patient shows widening of the aortic outline confirming the diagnosis of aortic dissection.

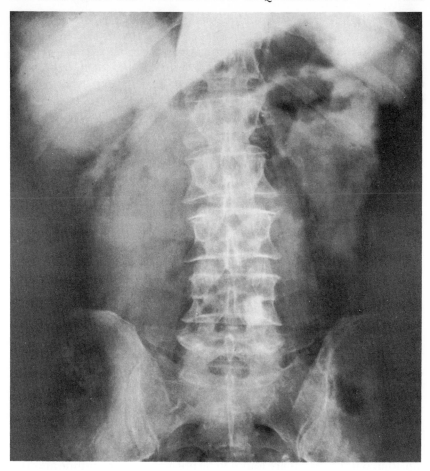

Fig. 15. Plain film of the abdomen showing bulging of the right psoas shadow due to a ruptured aortic aneurysm.

The skull

The value of specific views and projections of the skull

While the external suture line is serrated and usually easy to identify, the internal suture line which is straight and more difficult to differentiate from a fracture line, can usually be seen to lie superimposed. The films taken in the Accident and Emergency Department may be taken with a restless patient under poor conditions and in certain circumstances must be considered too poor for diagnosis (Jennett, 1976). Should there be a suspicion of a depressed fracture, or an apparent line crosses the middle meningeal vascular line (raising the possibility of extradural haemorrhage), then the X-rays should be repeated with first class radiography, preferably using a skull unit. Two lateral views are often helpful and if a fracture of the frontal or ethmoid region of the sinuses is suspected, a lateral 'brow-up' view with a horizontal ray of the X-ray beam may demonstrate unsuspected collections of air in the skull, which may be the only sign of a fine hairline fracture.

Severe brain injury however can occur without any visible fracture and quite severe fractures without any significant brain injury (Lewin, 1976).

Intracranial haemorrhage

Subarachnoid haemorrhage when it has been confirmed by lumbar puncture should be localised by angiography in order to define the cause and site. The majority are due to a ruptured aneurysm.

Intracranial haematomata

(a) An extradural haematoma is usually associated with a skull fracture. The diagnosis is established by arteriography showing displacement of the normal intracranial vessels away from the skull vault and sometimes displacement of the sagittal sinus downwards (Glickman et al., 1973).

(b) Subdural haematoma – the post-traumatic subdural haematoma is often unsuspected clinically. Indeed the injury may be so trivial that it may not be recalled by the patient. In up to 20% of cases they are bilateral. The possibility of a haematoma on the other side should be considered if the vessels are found to be normal and the midline anterior cerebral course is seen, or with only minimal displacement. The condition can accompany a subarachnoid haemorrhage, complicating the picture.

Computerised axial tomography when available can offer nontraumatic noninvasive methods for diagnosing accurately subdural, extradural and intracerebral haemorrhage with accuracy (Galbraith et al., 1976). This technique can even demonstrate small areas of contusion. When generally available these methods will become routine in the early diagnosis of head injury (Lewin, 1976).

Ultrasound scanning. The ultrasound scan for the midline is a coarse screening test of the deviation of midline structures and is of value when positive.

Facial bones. Special views are needed for fractures of the facial bones and the advice of the radiologist should be obtained to ensure that useful views of the area are taken. A 30° occipitomental view is essential. Tangential views are often needed, directed to a particular wound or haematoma to show a difficult fracture.

Tomography may be the only way to identify fractures in the orbit, e.g. 'blow out fractures' which might later produce diplopia (Editorial, 1975).

The cervical spine

This may be a very difficult region, oblique views and tomography may be helpful. A patient in whom damage to the atlanto-axial region is suspect may need tomography; transport of such a patient to the tomography room should be done only after consultation with the orthopaedic surgeons. X-ray views of C7/T1 are difficult, visualisation may be improved by depressing the shoulders while the X-rays are taken.

The 'straight' abdomen

Plain films of the abdomen should be scrutinised very carefully to assess the 'gas pattern', this often being informative. On rare occasions an X-ray of the patient in the supine position is sufficient (Fig. 16), but generally an erect film, or if this is not possible a film with the patient in the lateral decubitus position using a horizontal beam should be taken. Using these views and in cases where information to localise a lesion more fully is needed, a lateral view should be considered.

The gas pattern

In the critically ill patient free gas is best seen in the erect and lateral decubitus films. When these films are to be taken, the patient should lie with the lateral side up or be erect for about ten minutes before the film is taken to allow the gas to rise and accumulate under the flank or diaphragm. Free gas implies a perforation of the bowel or artificial entry of air (as in dialysis patients, or after abdominal section) and this may be associated with abscess formation. Free gas is determined when the lucent area which is darker on an X-ray film appears outside and separate from the normal bowel content shadows. Gas can be seen in pneumoperitoneum; when air enters the female abdomen through a

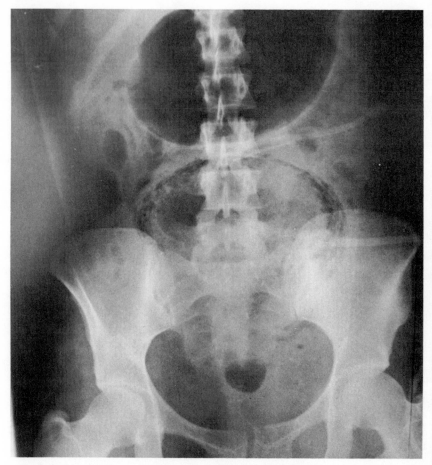

Fig. 16. Gas gangrene of the uterus. Curvilinear lucencies of gas shown in the uterine wall. Note the gas distension of the stomach.

patent fallopian tube, or in *Pneumatoides coli* secondary to obstructive airways disease, or diabetes.

Gas in the liver or bile duct and bowel

Gas seen in the gallbladder or bile ducts is an important finding and may be due to surgical connection of the biliary system to the gut, or surgery on the sphincter of Oddi. Rarely it occurs with infection by gas forming organisms, when gas will be seen in the gallbladder wall.

Gas in the portal venous radicles indicates gangrene of the bowel, it collects in the peripheral parts of the liver, thus differentiating it from biliary gas. The gas pattern in the small bowel is usually sparing and not more than two short fluid levels should be seen in the normal individual,

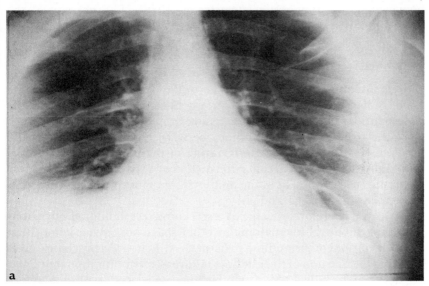

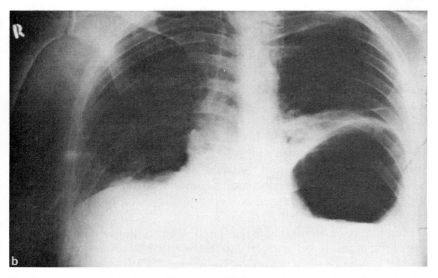

Fig. 17. (a) Rupture of the left hemidiaphragm. (b) Same patient – some hours later – showing how the stomach air 'bubble' has distended into the chest.

except after enemas or purgatives. Sentinel loops of small bowel denotes localised inflammatory disease of the small bowel, whereas 'a string of beads' appearance is consistent with generalised ileus. The distribution of the dilated loops of bowel and their distinction into small and large bowel are often diagnostic (Armstrong, 1976). The position of the gastric bubble may also be helpful, Figs 17(a) and (b).

ULTRASOUND IN THE I.T.U.

Mobile apparatus, that can be taken to the bedside, is of value in the I.T.U. The 'A' scan machine produces a linear oscilloscope trace of the time-relations between echoes returning from the two sides of the skull, with the echo from the 'midline' between them. The relationship between them is altered with deviation of the midline echo from the midpoint, due to a lateral collection of fluid or a space-occupying lesion. Computer techniques, as in the 'midliner' are more accurate and easier to perform (Figs 18(a) and (b)).

'A' scan is therefore of value as a screening test in finding but not in excluding subdural haematoma or other space occupying lesions that cause deviations of the midline structures. Although the procedure gives accurate localisation of the midline, failure to record midline shift by its use does not exclude a lesion. More elaborate procedures are therefore generally required if a space-occupying lesion is suspected.

The Mobile 'B' scan machine is less often available but can undertake many more investigations on the critically ill without any invasive procedure (Wells, 1976). Preparation is usually unnecessary and in the few cases where it is needed, it is simple, e.g. a well-filled bladder for the uterus/bladder interface to determine placental site and exclude placenta praevia, or a full fluid-filled stomach for visualisation of the spleen.

The kidney, thyroid, gall-bladder, liver (Figs 19(a) and (b)), spleen and the abdominal aorta (Figs 20(a) and (b)) are accessible to this examination (Barnett and Morley, 1972). Should percutaneous puncture be required to gain access to a cyst, the 'B' scan is most helpful. This technique can be used to aspirate a cyst or to inject contrast material in order to delineate by X-ray.

Biopsy may be facilitated using the 'B' scan technique, the depth and size of the organ to be biopsied can be obtained by using the electronic caliper system of the apparatus (Goldberg, 1975).

Abdominal fluid accumulations cannot be differentiated by ultrasound, aspiration being required to sample them. The future use of real

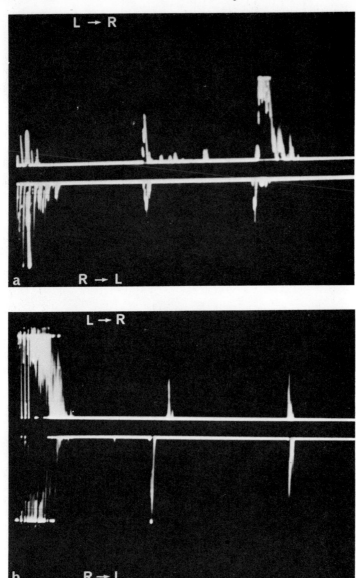

Fig. 18. (a) A normal ultrasound 'A' scan for the midline echo. The midline echo is of normal width and is central between the echoes from the two sides of the skull. (b) An abnormal 'A' scan. The midline echo is markedly deviated from the midline from the left towards the right, indicating space-occupying lesion on the left side. At operation a subdural haematoma was found and successfully drained.

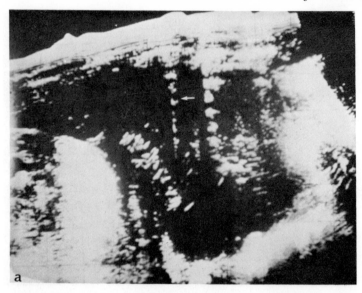

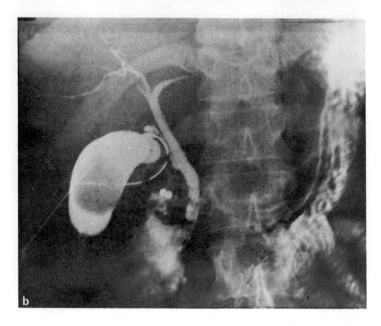

Fig. 19. (a) Ultrasound 'B' scan showing (arrowed) a ruptured liver. (b) Postoperatively (same patient) contrast medium was run into the drainage tube in the gall bladder. This showed a traumatic leak at the lower end of the common bile duct.

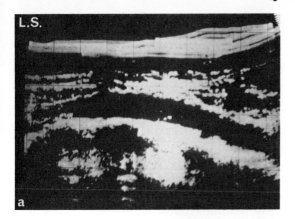

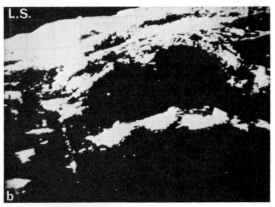

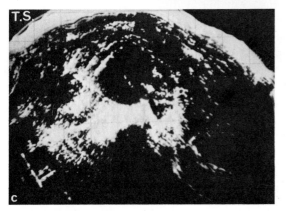

Fig. 20. (a) Ultrasound longitudinal 'B' scan of the normal aorta. (b) Longitudinal 'B' scan of an aortic aneurysm. (c) Transverse 'B' scan of an aortic aneurysm (same patient).

time display, and multiple head systems, and the additional facility for 'grey scale', perhaps supplemented by hard copy readout systems, will greatly increase the usefulness of these imaging techniques. Obstetric problems occasionally come to the I.T.U., amniocentesis is easy and safe under ultrasound guidance. On rare occasions a late pregnancy who has received anticoagulant therapy may require to have vitamin K correction of the coagulation factors in the foetus. In order to do this the injection must be given into the foetus under ultrasound guidance, the needle being directed through the amniotic cavity and into the buttock or thigh of the foetus.

The diagnosis of pericardial and pleural effusion can be made by ultrasound 'A' scan. Pericardiocentesis is made safer and facilitated by ultrasound guidance; this will become reliable and easier when multi-element and real time transducer systems are readily available (Feigenbaum, 1965).

The Doppler ultrasound method
This utilises the change in frequency of a reflected signal when the reflecting surface or boundary is moving. The audible beat frequency between the echo frequency and the original signal changes, lowering in frequency when the reflector moves away and rising when it moves towards the source. By this means occlusion or stenosis of vessels can be detected non-invasively.

In *venous thrombosis* the Doppler can be used on the femoral, popliteal and posterior tibial veins. Further valuable information of the obstruction of the iliac veins and femoral veins can be obtained by the loss of the normal respiratory variation of venous flow, which may be obscured at the point of detection at the femoral vein. Also, if valve action above this point is lost, Valsalva's manoeuvre produces a 'pistol shot' of refluxing blood under the probe. A continuous low pitched sound is heard if the vein is blocked, with no cessation when breath is held under pressure, with a rush of blood when breathing resumes. The method is of most use for *complete* occlusion and *phlebography* is the most useful and definitive test for venous thrombosis. The tiny hand-held 'doposcope' is a useful screening test, however. A compressed artery opens and closes to produce the audible signals for blood pressure estimation. The 'doppler' is a very sensitive method for operating automatic blood pressure mensuration, and can act as the end point for continuous blood pressure measurement.

Transaortic velography

This method provides a non-invasive technique for measurement of transaortic velocity.

Ultrasound is thus a most valuable noninvasive technique for the imaging and diagnosis of I.T.U. patients.

Wells (1976) stated that: 'Patients are seldom too ill to be brought to a fixed ultrasonic scanner. One cannot over emphasise how valuable a mobile "B" scanner would prove.' However, as he notes, the newest *'real time' scanners* are very easily portable, produce excellent views and can be brought to the patient's bedside. When these instruments are more universally available they will prove of the greatest value in the I.T.U., where their noninvasive and unobtrusive use will not disturb, significantly, the critically ill who may be put at risk by more invasive methods.

REFERENCES

Ardran, G. M. and Fursdon, P. S. (1973). Radiation exposure to personnel during cardiac catheterisation. *Radiology* **106**, 517.

Armstrong, P. K. H. C. (1976). The plain abdominal X-ray film in adults. *Brit. J. Hosp. Med.* **15**, 597.

Barnett, E. and Morley, P. (1972). Diagnostic ultrasound in renal disease. *Brit. Med. Bull.* **28**, 196.

Barry, W. F. J. (1956). Infrapulmonary pleural effusion. *Radiology* **66**, 740.

Bilbas, M. K., Dotter, C. T., Lee, T. G. and Kayton, R. M. (1976). Endoscopic fibreoptic retrograde chole-pancreatography. *Gastroenterology* **70**, 314.

Bookstein, J. J. and Silver, T. M. (1974). The angiographic differential diagnosis of acute pulmonary embolism. *Radiology* **110**, 25.

Brown, C. B., Glancy, J. J., Kelsey Fry, I. and Cattell, W. R. (1970). High dose excretion urography in oliguric renal failure. *Lancet* **2**, 952.

Cumberland, D. C. (1975). Fibre optic endoscopy and radiology in the investigation of the upper gastrointestinal tract. *Clin. Radiol.* **26**, 223.

Editorial (1975). Blackeyes and blow-out fractures. *Brit. Med. J.* **1**, 5949.

Feigenbaum, H. (1976). Ultrasound diagnosis of pericardial effusion. *JAMA* **191**, 9.

Felson, B. (1973). *In* 'Chest Roentgenology' (Ed. B. Felson). W. B. Saunders, Philadelphia, London and Toronto.

Forrest, J. H. and Finlayson, N. D. C. (1974). The investigation of acute upper gastrointestinal haemorrhage. *Brit. J. Hosp. Med.* **160**, 8.

Galbraith, S., Teasdale, G. and Blacklock, C. (1976). Computerized tomography of acute traumatic intracranial haematoma. *Brit. Med. J.* **2**, 1371.

Glickman, M. A., Macnamara, T. O. and Margolis, M. T. (1973). Arteriographic diagnosis of subtemporal subdural haematoma. *Radiology* **109**, 607.

Goldberg, B. B., Pollack, H. M. and Kellerman, E. (1975). Ultrasonic localization for renal biopsy. *Radiology* **115**, 167.

Gray, R. K. and Grossman, J. H. (1974). Acute lower gastrointestinal bleeding secondary to varices of the superior mesenteric venous system. Angiographic demonstration. *Radiology* **3**, 559.

Harris, J. H. and Harris, W. H. (1975). 'The Radiology of Emergency Medicine', (a) p. 209, (b) p. 226 and (c) p. 293. Williams and Wilkins Co., New York.

Hayaski, K., Meaney, T. F., Zelch, J. V. and Tarar, R. (1974). Angiographic analysis of aortic dissection. *Am. J. Roentgenol.* **122**, 769.

Jaffe, N. (1974). The adult respiratory distress syndrome. *Am. J. Roentgenol.* **122**, 719.

Jennett, B. (1976). Some medicolegal aspects of the management of acute head injury. *Brit. Med. J.* **1**, 1383.

John, B. A., Everett, J. J. A., White, J. and Robert, I. (1974). Oblique and selective angiography in the diagnosis of pulmonary embolism. *Radiology* **3**, 246.

Keighley, M. R. B., Wilson, A. and Kelly, J. P. (1973). Fatal endotoxic shock of biliary tract origin complicating transhepatic cholangiography. *Brit. Med. J.* **3**, 147.

Kelsey Fry, I. and Cattell, W. R. (1972). The nephrographic pattern during excretion urography. *Brit. Med. Bull.* **28**, 3.

Kreel, L. and Williams, R. (1964). Selective angiography for the liver, spleen and pancreas. *Brit. Med. J.* **2**, 1500.

Lewin, W. (1976). Changing attitudes to the management of severe head injuries. *Brit. Med. J.* **2**, 1234.

Loups, J. W., Archer, G. and Curtis, H. (1975). Bedside pulmonary angiography. *Radiology* **114**, 2.

Magarey, C. J. (1971). Non-surgical removal of retained biliary calculi. *Lancet* **1**, 1044.

Mohr, V. (1971). Radiography of a patient confined to the ward. *Radiography* **37**, 444.

Nahum, H. and Levesque, M. (1973). Arteriography in hepatic trauma. *Radiology* **109**, 557.

Parbhoo, S. (1975). Management of bleeding in liver disease. *Brit. J. Hosp. Med.* **13**, 1.

Parsavand, R. (1974). Angiographic demonstration of ruptured aortic aneurysm. *Radiology* **3**, 577.

Rapheal, M. J. (1972). Radiological investigation of ischaemic heart disease. *Brit. J. Hosp. Med.* **7**, 297.

Schlag, G. (1976). Planning and fitting out a shock room and its significance for traumatology. *Electromedica* **1**, 32.

Stein, M. A., Winter, J. and Grollman, J. H. (1975). The value of the pulmonary artery seeking catheter in percutaneous selective pulmonary arteriography. *Radiology* **114**, 299.

Stevenson, G. W., Cox, R. R. and Roberts, C. T. C. (1976). Prospective comparison of double contrast barium meal examination and fibre optic endoscopy in acute upper gastrointestinal haemorrhage. *Brit. Med. J.* **2**, 723.

Tager, S. N. (1942). Use of overpenetrated film technique in diagnosis of cavities. *Radiology* **39**, 389.

Takada, T., Hanyu, F., Kobayashi, S. and Uchida, Y. (1976). Percutaneous Transhepatic Cholangial Drainage: Direct Approach under Fluoroscopic Control. *J. Surg. Onc.* **8**, 83.

Van Waes, P. F. G. (1972). 'High Dose Urography in Oliguric and Anuric Patients.' Excerpta Medica, Amsterdam.

Wells, P. N. T. (1976). Choosing a 'B' scanner. *Brit. J. Clin. Equip.* **1**, 187.

Wilkins, R. A., de Lacey, G. J., Flor, R. and Taylor, S. (1976). Radiology in Mendelson's syndrome. *Clin. Radiol.* **27**, 81.

Wilson, J. (1976). Venography. The role of radiography in the management of deep vein thrombosis. *Radiography* **42**, 94.

OTHER REFERENCES OF INTEREST

Eaton, R. J., Senior, R. M. and Pearce, J. A. (1973). Aspects of respiratory care pertinent to the radiologist. *Radiol. Clin. N. Amer.* **11**, 93.

Flower, C. D. (1976). Radiology Seminars. *In* 'Hosp. Update', Vols 2, 4, 6 and 10.

Zimmon, D. S., Falkenstein, D. B. and Abrams, R. M. (1974). Endoscopic retrograde cholangiopancreatography (E.R.C.P.) in diagnosis of pancreatic inflammatory disease. *Radiology* **113**, 287.

Section 2: Nuclear Medicine and the I.T.U.

M. N. MAISEY

INTRODUCTION

Advances over the last few years in instrumentation and radiopharmaceuticals have increased the scope of clinical investigations using radioactive isotopes; particularly for organ imaging. Easy and rapid access to a nuclear medicine facility in the same way that we expect of X-ray facilities is now essential for the adequate care of patients. This is as true in the field of critical care as it is in the investigation and management of less acute illness. In this chapter, the various nuclear medicine techniques which may be of value in critical care with particular reference to the I.T.U. will be discussed.

INSTRUMENTATION

The only imaging instrument which will be considered is the Anger type gamma camera. This has now largely replaced the older rectilinear scanner particularly where emergency investigations are involved when speed and possibly mobility are required. The gamma camera consists of a detector head in which there is a lead collimator, a large flat sodium iodide crystal, and an array (usually 37) of photomultiplier tubes which transform into an electrical signal and then magnify the scintillations which result from photon interaction with the crystal (Fig. 1).

This detector system records the distribution of radioactivity within the organ under investigation and the data are transferred to the console consisting of the electronics required to process the signals and produce an image of the radionuclide distribution. The time intervals

852

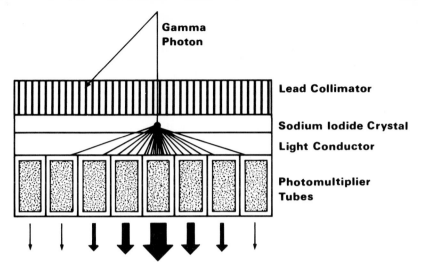

Fig. 1. Schematic representation of the detector from a modern gamma camera.

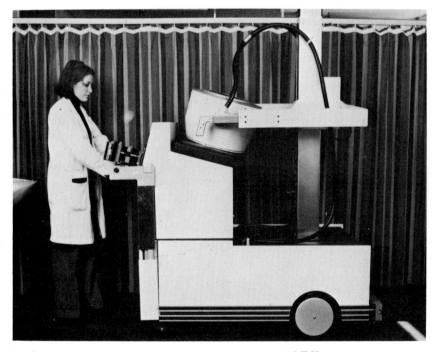

Fig. 2. A modern mobile gamma camera suitable for use in the I.T.U.

over which the images are produced may be very short (e.g. $\frac{1}{4}-\frac{1}{2}$ s in the case of cardiac dynamic studies) or several minutes (e.g. brain scan). The final image may be displayed on polaroid film, negative film (35 or 70 mm) or X-ray film. A recent development of particular importance to the intensive therapy unit (I.T.U.) has been the production of mobile gamma cameras which has permitted imaging to be performed at the bedside (Fig. 2). Most modern cameras have an interfaced digital data system which may either be a hardwired preprogrammed system or based on a programmable minicomputer. These are used to process and optimise the images and even more importantly enable quantitative numerical data to be obtained in addition to the qualitative images, thus adding a new and vitally important dimension to the investigation.

RADIONUCLIDES AND RADIOPHARMACEUTICALS

A major advance in radionuclide imaging took place with the introduction of ^{99m}Technetium (^{99}Tc^m) (Harper et al., 1964). This is a man-made radionuclide which has a short half-life (6 h) and decays to Tc^{99} with the emission of gamma photons with an energy of 140 KeV which is almost ideal for gamma camera imaging. These physical characteristics mean that large doses (10–30 mCi.) can be administered to patients permitting images with high statistical accuracy to be produced rapidly with a high resolution and resulting in only very low radiation doses to the patients. Fortunately, ^{99}Tc^m can be attached to various chemical compounds with high affinities for particular organs, which has enabled radionuclide images of most organs to be obtained with a high specificity (Table 1).

Table. 1. Commonly used ^{99}Tc^m compounds for radioisotope imaging

Compound	Use
Sulphur colloid	Liver, spleen, bone marrow
Human albumin microspheres	Lung perfusion, coronary perfusion
Diphosphonates	Bone, myocardial infarcts
DTPA (chelate)	Kidneys, brain
Dimercaptosuccinic acid	Kidneys
Red blood cells Albumen	Vascular cavities
^{99}Tc^m as pertechnetate	Brain, thyroid

METHODS WHEREBY RADIO-ISTOPES CAN BE USED IN DIAGNOSIS AND MANAGEMENT

The various ways in which these techniques can be used in the diagnosis and management of acutely ill patients will be discussed in the context of particular clinical problems rather than as a catalogue of techniques.

Coma

The causes of coma can very simply be considered in terms of systemic or metabolic causes (diabetes, poisoning, etc.) and focal intracranial causes. Brain scanning is a valuable, simple, non-invasive method of identifying the vast majority of focal intracranial lesions (Holman, 1973). The brain scan is obtained 1–2 h after the i.v. injection of $^{99}Tc^m$ pertechnetate, with perchlorate to block uptake into the thyroid and choroid plexus. Additional information is obtained by rapid sequence imaging performed in the vertex or anterior view during the first intracranial transit of tracer to assess regional cerebral blood flow through a hemisphere or a specific lesion (Cowan, 1973). Using this technique, typical findings are seen in subdural and extradural haematomas, intracranial tumours, abscesses and cerebrovascular accidents (Fig. 3). The overall accuracy rate of brain scanning is approximately 80–90% (Burrow, 1972; Hurley, 1972). This is not of course as high as that obtained with the newer C.T. scanning techniques (E.M.I. scanning); but when it is remembered that radionuclide brain scanning can be performed at the bedside, and the increased accuracy obtained using these new tomographic techniques is mainly in the area of cortical atrophy, it remains a valuable tool and is the investigation of choice in the unconscious undiagnosed patient especially when there is a reason to suspect a focal intracranial cause.

Chest pain

Chest pain is probably the commonest cause for admission to an I.T.U. Frequently the diagnosis is in doubt and there is a wide differential diagnosis. The intelligent use of radioisotope techniques can frequently make a firm diagnosis possible.

Pulmonary embolism

Perfusion lung scanning using $^{99}Tc^m$ labelled human albumin microspheres is the most sensitive method for diagnosing pulmonary

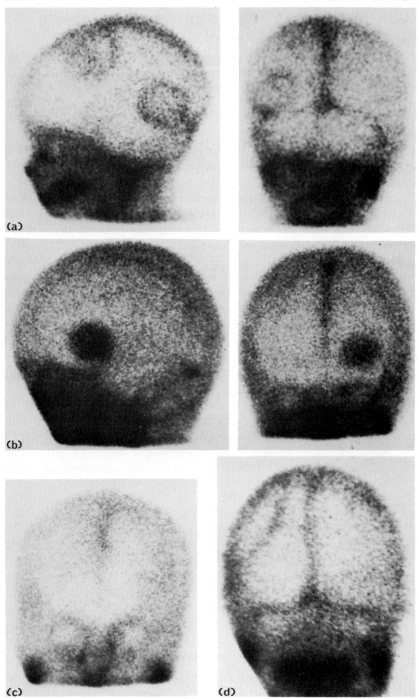

Fig. 3. (a) Lateral and anterior views of a patient admitted unconscious with multiple intracranial abscesses. (b) Lateral and anterior views of a patient with an intracranial tumour. (c) Anterior view of a patient in coma due to a subdural haematoma. (d) Anterior view of an acute extradural haematoma ('rim sign').

(e) Anterior view cerebral dynamic perfusion study and routine brain scan showing a highly vascular A.V. malformation. (f) Lateral and anterior views showing the classical changes of a left middle cerebral artery thrombosis.

(g) 0–4, 4–8, 8–12 s views from the cerebral dynamic perfusion study performed prior to the brain scan shown in (f). This shows delayed diminished flow through the left cerebral hemisphere. (h) Dynamic computer generated curves from the 'areas of interest' indicated in the last frame of (g). These confirm the delayed, diminished blood flow through the left hemisphere (see overleaf). (R, right; L, left.)

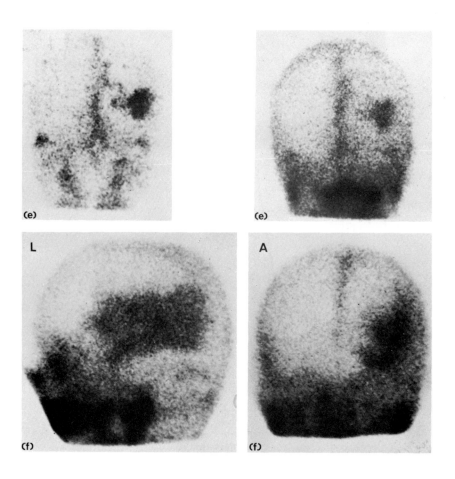

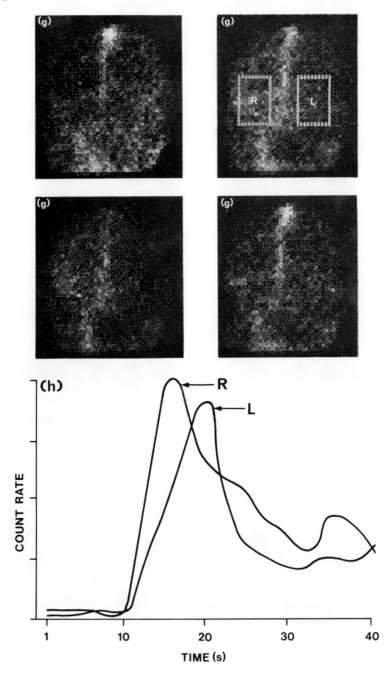

embolism (Mishkin, 1973; Tow, 1975). 100–150 000 labelled microspheres are injected intravenously with the patient supine and the scan is performed immediately. Areas of the lung which are underperfused due to pulmonary emboli are usually clearly demarcated as areas with no radioactive tracer. These usually correspond to specific anatomical lung segments but there is considerable variation in the appearances. The investigation is made more specific by repeating the lung scan during the inhalation of a radioactive gas (Xe^{133} or more recently $Krypton^{81m}$) (Loken, 1971; Fazio, 1975). Perfusion defects due to emboli are ventilated normally and those due to other causes (e.g. pneumonia, pulmonary oedema, emphysema, etc.) have ventilation defects which match the perfusion deficits. These scans are simple, safe and can be used in critically ill patients without moving them from the I.T.U. Therefore they can be used repeatedly to follow the progress or resolution of pulmonary emboli.

Figure 4 shows a series of scans in a patient with acute chest pain and a normal chest X-ray. The first scan shows several segmental perfusion defects. A ventilation scan performed at the same time demonstrates normal ventilation in the underperfused areas. When repeat scans were performed 2 weeks later, both the perfusion and ventilation scans had almost returned to normal.

Pericardial effusions

Chest pain followed by increasing heart size may be due to pericarditis with a pericardial effusion as well as myocardial infarction and cardiac dilatation. Blood pool scanning is a very simple method of differentiating (Staab, 1973). An agent which remains confined to the vascular space is used ($^{99}Tc^m$ labelled red cells, $^{99}Tc^m$ albumen or $Indium^{113m}$ transferrin) (Mahon, 1973). Figures 5(a) and (b) show a large pericardial effusion before and after aspiration of 300 ml of fluid. Figure 5(c) in contrast shows the scan of a patient with cardiac dilatation without effusion as the cause of cardiomegaly. This technique may also be used in the measurement of cardiac ejection fraction and for demonstrating myocardial akinesia and dyskinesia as may occur for example in a ventricular aneurysm following an acute myocardial infarct and be the cause of persistent cardiac failure (Rigo, 1975; Berman, 1975). The same blood pool agent is used and the Gamma camera is linked (gated) with the E.C.G. in such a way that the camera records for only a few milliseconds during each cardiac cycle (Fig. 6). Two images of the cavity of the heart in diastole and systole are

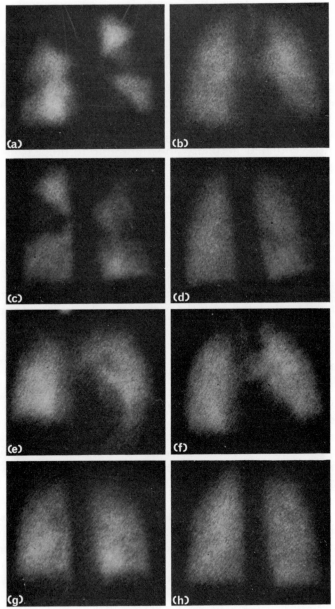

Fig. 4. (a) and (b) Anterior view of perfusion (a) and ventilation (b) scans in acute pulmonary embolism showing normally ventilated segmental perfusion defects. (c) and (d) Posterior views of the same patient at the same time. (e) and (f) Anterior view of perfusion (e) and ventilation (f) scans in the same patient showing almost complete resolution after 1 week. (g) and (h) Posterior views of the same patient at the same time as (e) and (f).

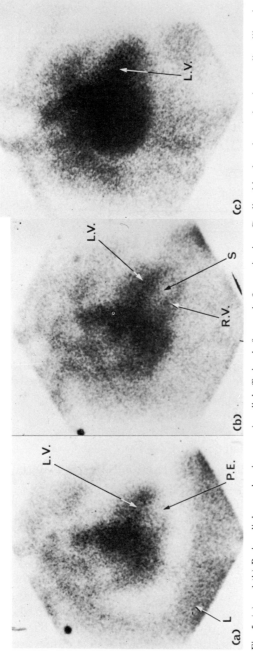

Fig. 5. (a) and (b) Pericardial scan showing a pericardial effusion before and after aspiration. Cardiac blood pool scan showing cardiac dilatation without an effusion. (L.V., left ventricle; P.E., pericardial effusion; L, liver; S, septum; R.V., right ventricle.)

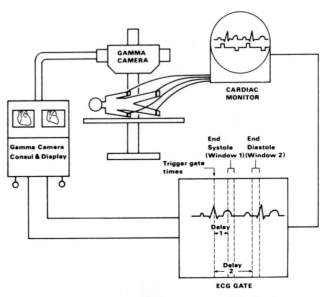

Fig. 6. Schematic diagram of the circuitry for producing gated cardiac images.

produced. From these two images, areas of poor contraction or paradoxical movement can be identified (Fig. 7) and if two views (anterior and L.A.O.) are obtained, the ejection fraction can be calculated. Using this method, there is a good correlation with standard cineangiographic methods; angiography is therefore only necessary for detailed anatomical investigation prior to surgery and not as the diagnosic procedure of choice.

Myocardial infarction

Recently it has been shown that some labelled materials concentrate in acute infarcted muscle (Bonte, 1975). Examples are $^{99}Tc^m$ pyrophosphate, $^{99}Tc^m$ tetracycline and $^{99}Tc^m$ glucoheptonate. Positive scans of infarcted myocardial muscle can be obtained after the injection of one of these agents (Rossman, 1975). In contrast to the positive images of infarcted muscle, radioactive analogues of potassium can be used to produce a scan of the normal myocardium with dead and ischaemic tissue appearing as cold spots (Bradley-Moore, 1975; Strauss, 1975) (Fig. 8). Although these techniques are in widespread use, particularly in North America, the exact place for them in the diagnosis and management of acute myocardial thrombosis has yet to be clearly defined. The prospects however for such techniques are very promising.

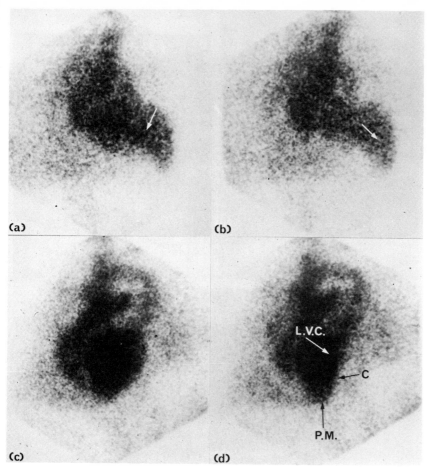

Fig. 7. Gated study of a patient with a ventricular aneurysm complicating a large myocardial infarction.

(a) Anterior view in diastole. (b) Anterior view in systole showing only limited contraction of the ventricle. (Arrows = left ventricular cavity with paradoxical movement.) (c) Left anterior oblique view in diastole. (d) Left anterior oblique view in systole showing poor contraction confined to the posterior wall and some paradoxical movement of the apex. (L.V.C., left ventricular cavity; C, contraction; P.M., paradoxical movement.)

Bone scans

Very occasionally acute chest pain may be caused by bony rather than cardiac or pulmonary causes. Bone scanning has been shown to be more sensitive than X-rays for detecting active bony lesions although it is less specific (Mall, 1975). Bone scanning is now usually performed with a

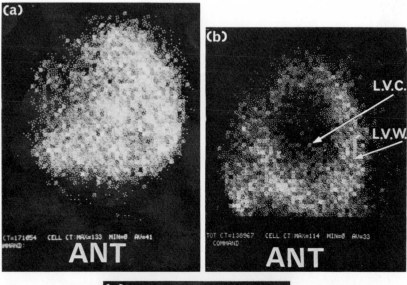

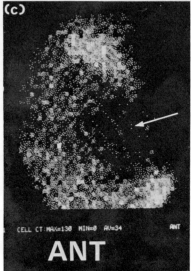

Fig. 8. (a) Normal anterior Thallium 201 cardiac scan. (b) Thallium 201 scan showing dilated left ventricular cavity. (L.V.C., left ventricular cavity; L.V.W., left ventricular wall.) (c) Thallium 201 scan showing a large myocardial ischaemic defect in the left ventricular wall. (Arrow indicates defect of thallium uptake in myocardium.)

^{99}Tc^m phosphate compound (e.g. ^{99}Tc^m E.H.D.P., ethylenehydroxy-diphosponate). Approximately 4 h after the injection of 15 mCi. of one of these compounds, the bones can be imaged. There will be increased tracer accumulation wherever there is active bony metabolism occurring (Merrick, 1975). Figure 9 shows the bone scan of a patient with chest pain. She has active lesions in T6 and the sternum which were subsequently shown to be due to metastatic deposits from breast cancer.

Hepatic failure

Usually the cause of liver failure is quite clear, e.g. fulminating hepatitis, end stage alcoholic disease, etc. However, when there is doubt the liver scan may be helpful particularly in differentiating diffuse parenchymatous hepatic failure from failure secondary to focal disease (usually metastatic deposits) (McCready, 1972; Drum, 1973). Liver scans are obtained following the intravenous injection of ^{99}Tc^m labelled sulphur colloid. This is extracted by the reticuloendothelial cells in the liver spleen and bone marrow, and forms the basis for imaging these organs.

Figures 10 and 11 show the different appearances of diffuse parenchymatous disease from focal tumour infiltration.

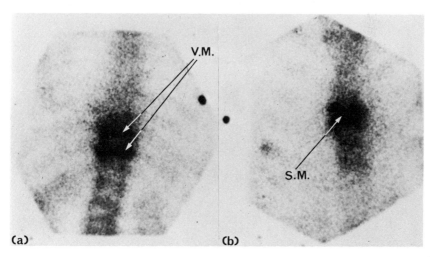

Fig. 9. (a) and (b) Thoracic spine and sternum showing metastatic deposits in a patient presenting with acute chest pain. (V.M., vertebral metastases; S.M., sternal metastases.)

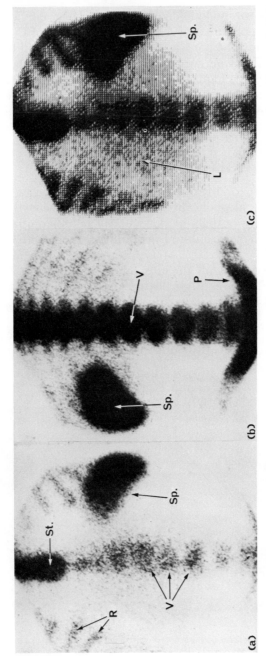

Fig. 10. (a) lateral, (b) posterior and (c) anterior computer enhanced images of the liver spleen and bone marrow in a patient with acute alcoholic hepatic failure. (R, ribs; St., sternum; Sp., spleen; V, vertebrae; P, pelvis; L, liver.)

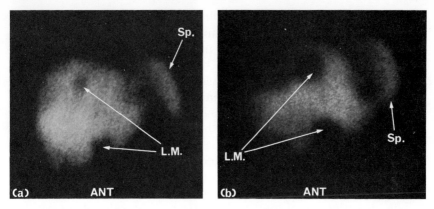

Fig. 11. Anterior liver/spleen scan in a patient with carcinoma of the colon showing progressive intrahepatic metastases. (Sp., spleen; L.M., liver metastases.)

Renal failure

Using $^{99}Tc^m$ D.T.P.A. (diethylenetriaminepentacetic acid) which is cleared by the kidneys in the same way as inulin (Klopper, 1972), useful information may be obtained about renal function in acute renal failure. A rapid bolus i.v. injection of 15 mCi. $^{99}Tc^m$ D.T.P.A. is given and the kidneys imaged during the first transit (vascular phase). During the next few minutes, the tracer concentrates in the renal parenchyma, and is subsequently excreted. Using this technique, the total and regional perfusion, function and excretion of the kidneys can be rapidly assessed. Typical patterns can be identified in acute renal failure (Hilson, 1976). For example, acute tubular necrosis is characterised by normal perfusion, normal tracer concentration at 2 min followed by rapid diffusion from the kidney back into the circulation; acute obstruction is characterised by poor perfusion, dilated calyceal system and progressive concentration in both renal parenchyma and collecting system. Many other patterns have also been described. This simple technique can be used to assist in the different diagnosis and management of acute renal failure.

Fluid and metabolic imbalance

Standard techniques are available for the evaluation of the volume of various body fluid compartments and the total body electrolyte concentration of sodium or potassium. The most important of these techniques include:

1. Red cell mass using Cr^{51} labelled red blood cells.

2. Plasma volume I^{131} labelled albumin. A combination of 1 and 2 accurately measures total blood volume, a measurement which can be made, but with inevitably errors, by using either measurement together with the P.C.V. The results must be interpreted with caution in a situation where there may be increased capillary permeability but these errors are usually small and not clinically important.

3. Extra-cellular fluid volume using bromine or more recently using stable bromine and measuring the bromine in the samples by X-ray excitation analysis;

4. Total body water using tritiated water;

5. Total exchangeable potassium using K^{43};

6. Total exchangeable sodium using Na^{24}.

The measurement of total body water may be valuable in patients with hyponatraemia particularly when the serum sodium is low. The total exchangeable sodium may be found to be normal in the critically ill in spite of a low serum sodium – such a finding would suggest the 'sick cell syndrome' (see Part 1, ch. VII, p. 170).

Potassium is a largely intracellular ion and movement between the intracellular and extracellular compartment is radically affected by metabolic changes and drugs (see p. 172). The indications for the estimation of total exchangeable potassium in the critically ill is yet to be assessed – but may prove useful where a high total body potassium is suspected in the presence of a normal or low serum potassium.

These investigations result in very low radiation doses and consequently can be repeated frequently, e.g. daily for blood volume or weekly for sodium space. The factors which limit the frequency are usually the availability of the isotope rather than those of radiation safety.

Trauma

Organ scanning particularly liver, spleen and renal scanning may be the simplest method of diagnosing trauma to these organs in the severely traumatised patient (Gilday, 1974; Berg, 1974).

Infection

The localisation of infection may be necessary when pyrexia complicates other problems, frequently postoperatively or as a complication of serious medical illness. Total body scanning using Gallium[67] which concentrates in areas of acute inflammation as well as tumours has been shown to be clinically valuable (Teates, 1975). Six hours or more following the intravenous injection of 1–2 mCi. Gallium[67], a total body scan is performed either with a rectilinear scanner capable of total body scans or by multiple gamma camera views. Tracer is concentrated in areas of acute inflammation particularly where there is pus. Figure 12 shows the gallium scan of a patient with an acute pyrexial illness following a ruptured appendix with peritonitis. There is an abnormal concentration of gallium under the left diaphragm. This was subsequently drained and shown to be a subphrenic abscess.

Thus, with the increasing availability of nuclear medicine departments, particularly when mobile gamma cameras are used, there is a great deal that radioisotopic techniques have to offer in the management of critically ill patients in the intensive therapy unit.

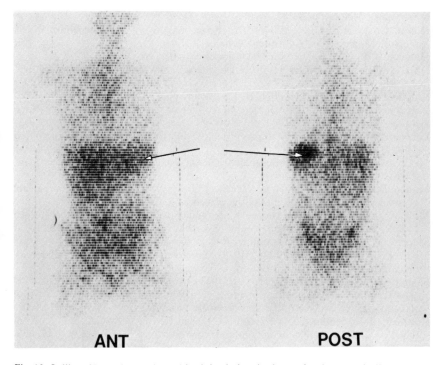

ANT   POST

Fig. 12. Gallium 67 scan in a patient with a left subphrenic abscess showing a markedly abnormal increased gallium accumulation. (Arrows indicate abnormal Ga 67 uptake.)

REFERENCES

Berg, B. C. (1974). Radionuclides after urinary tract injury. *Sem. Nuclear Med.* **4**, 371.

Berman, D. S., Salel, A. F., De Nardo, G. L., Bogren, H. G. and Masen, D. T. (1975). Clinical assessment of left ventricular regional contraction patterns and ejection fractions by high resolution gated scintigraphy. *J. Nuclear Med.* **16**, 865.

Bonte, F. J., Parkey, R. W., Graham, K. D. and Moore, J. G. (1975). Distribution of several agents useful in imaging myocardial infarcts. *J. Nuclear Med.* **16**, 132.

Bradley-Moore, P. R., Lebowitz, E., Greene, M. W., Atkins, H. L. and Ansari, A. N. (1975). Thallium 201 for medical use. *J. Nuclear Med.* **16**, 151.

Burrow, E. H. (1972). False negative results in brain scanning. *Brit. Med. J.* **1**, 473.

Cowan, R. J., Maynard, C. D., Meschan, I., Janeway, R. and Shigeno, K. (1973). Value of the routine use of the cerebral dynamic radioisotope study. *Radiology* **107**, 111.

Drum, D. E. (1973). Scintigraphy of the liver and spleen. *Post Grad. Med.* **54**, 118.

Fazio, F. and Jones, T. (1975). Assessment of regional ventilation by continuous inhalation of radioactive krypton 81m. *Brit. Med. J.* **2**, 673.

Gilday, D. L. and Alderson, P. O. (1974). Scintigraphic evaluation of liver and spleen injury. *Sem Nuclear Med.* **4**, 357.

Harper, P. V., Lathrop, K. A. and McArdle, R. J. (1964). The use of technetium 99m as a clinical scanning agent for thyroid, liver and brain. *In* 'Medical Radioisotope Scanning,' Vol. 2, pp. 33–45. IAEA, Vienna.

Hilson, A. J. W. and Maisey, M. N. (1976). Renal imaging in acute renal failure. British Nuclear Medicine Society Annual Meeting.

Holman, B. L. (1973). The brain scan. *Post Grad. Med.* **54**, (4), 143.

Hurley, P. J. and Wagner, H. N. (1972). Diagnostic value of brain scanning in children. *J. Amer. Med. Assoc.* **221**, 877.

Klopper, J. F., Hauser, W., Atkins, H. L., Eckelman, W. C. and Richards, P. (1972). Evaluation of 99mTc DTPA for the measurement of glomerular filtration rate. *J. Nuclear Med.* **13**, 107.

Loken, M. K. (1971). Camera studies of lung ventilation and perfusion. *Sem. Nuclear Med.* **2**, 229.

McCready, V. R. (1972). Scintigraphic studies of space occupying liver disease. *Sem. Nuclear Med.* **2**, 108.

Mahon, D. F., Subramanian, G. and McAfee, J. G. (1973). Experimental comparison of radioactive agents for studies of the placenta. *J. Nuclear Med.* **14**, 651.

Mall, J. C., Bekerman, C., Hoffer, P. B. and Gottschalk, A. (1975). A unified radiological approach to the detection of skeletal metastases. *Radiology* **118**, 323.

Merrick, M. V. (1975). Bone scanning. *Brit. J. Radiol.* **48**, 327.

Mishkin, F. S. and Johnson, P. M. (1973). The role of lung imaging in pulmonary embolism. *Post Grad. Med. J.* **49**, 487.

Rigo, P., Strauss, H. W. and Pitt, B. (1975). The combined use of gated cardiac blood pool scanning and myocardial imaging with Potassium 43 in the evaluation of patients with myocardial infarction. *Radiology* **115**, 387.

Rossman, D. J., Strauss, H. W., Siegel, M. E. and Pitt, B. (1975). Accumulation of 99mTc-glucoheptonate in acutely infarcted myocardium. *J. Nuclear Med.* **16**, 875.

Staab, E. V. and Patton, D. D. (1973). Nuclear medicine studies in patients with pericardial effusion. *Sem. Nuclear Med.* **3**, 191.

Strauss, H. W., Harrison, K. and Langon, J. K. (1975). Thallium 201 for myocardial imaging. *Circulation* **51**, 641.

Teates, C. D. and Hunter, J. G. (1975). Gallium scanning as a screening test for inflammatory lesions. *Radiology* **116**, 383.

Tow, D. E. and Simon, A. L. (1975). Comparison of lung scanning and pulmonary angiography in the detection and follow-up of pulmonary embolism. *Progress in Cardiovascular Disease* **17**, (4), 239.

III

Drug Requirements and the I.T.U

PATRICIA STONE

DRUG CHECKING AND MONITORING

Accurately documented prescribing is the key to successful drug therapy. All the effort which has gone into diagnosing the patient's condition and deciding on the treatment regime, which may have entailed battling along a jungle trail of laboratory reports, metabolic pathways and excretion data, will be wasted if the patient fails to receive the right drug at the right time. Several studies have measured the number of errors that can occur with hospital in-patient drug administrations. Vere (1965) showed that the error rate is likely to be higher when the number of drugs concurrently prescribed is high, and this is clearly important in the Intensive Therapy Unit where drug prescription is likely to be complex. Various prescribing systems have been developed to overcome the problems, notably at Aberdeen as described by Crooks *et al.* (1965, 1967) and at the London Hospital, outlined by Hill and Wigmore (1967). It is preferable to have a prescription sheet specially designed for I.T.U. use, based on one of the above designs, as the requirements are rather specialised. It should have separate sections for prescribing regular treatments, 'when required' drugs and adequate provision must be made for 'once only' drugs as these prescriptions are far more frequent in the I.T.U. than they are in an ordinary ward. All sections must have a corresponding section for

873

recording the administration of the dose to prevent accidental omissions and duplications. A separate sheet will be required for the prescription of intravenous therapy (see below).

DRUGS ON CLINICAL TRIAL

It may occur quite frequently that drugs not yet commercially available may be required for use in the Intensive Therapy Unit. It is important that prescribers are aware of the restrictions governing the use of such drugs. Clinical trials of drugs pass through a number of clearly defined stages. Before each new stage is begun, experimental evidence from the previous stage is submitted to the Committee on Safety of Medicines, which has statutory powers under the Medicines Act to regulate clinical trials. A clinical trial certificate is issued for each stage which defines the scope of use of the drug – from the earliest stage when perhaps one clinical centre in the country is trying the drug on a few closely monitored patients, through several stages up to the one immediately before marketing when the use has broadened and the number of doctors prescribing it may be large. Even at a fairly early stage it may be possible for a consultant to obtain an individual supply for a named patient. Clinical trial drugs are always issued for the use of a named consultant, who will have discussed the currently permitted applications of the drug with the maker. It is important that such drugs should be securely stored and access to them restricted to prescribers who are supervised by the original consultant. Only in this way can accurate and effective monitoring of use and any side effects be carried out. The Department of Health has prepared a number of leaflets explaining how the clinical trials regulations made under the Medicines Act affect doctors, see Department of Health and Social Security (1971, 1974a, b, c).

REFERENCE SYSTEM

The need has been recognised in recent years for readily accessible information about the actions and uses of drugs, and never before has this been so easily obtainable. New drugs are extensively documented before they can be released, and information on their absorption, metabolism, mode of action, and routes of excretion is collated and published. Strangely enough, it is sometimes the drug which has been established in use for many years which is less well documented. Useful sources of drug information are listed below.

In the Intensive Therapy Unit

Every I.T.U. should have available for immediate reference certain basic sources of drug information. A list which covers most day-to-day requirements is enumerated below.

(a) *British National Formulary* (current edition). In addition to the formulary section this contains much useful information about prescribing for adults and children, and also has lists of intravenously additive incompatibilities and drug interactions.

(b) *Data Sheet Compendium* (current edition). The Medicines Act requires manufacturers to publish Data Sheets giving fairly detailed information about all their non-Official drugs. Most manufacturers combine their Data Sheets to form this compendium which thus forms an excellent reference book about the majority of drugs in current use. It is published annually.

(c) *Martindale, The Extra Pharmacopoeia* (current edition). This invaluable book contains monographs on practically every drug in use, giving actions, uses, side effects, English and foreign trade names and literature references and abstracts.

In the hospital pharmacy

The therapeutic management of the critically ill is often difficult, for example oral absorption may not be possible, and the desired drug not available in a suitable form for parenteral administration. An experienced pharmacist, well-versed in therapeutics, can often contribute to the patient's treatment by advising about presentations of alternative drugs available. A comprehensive reference library including books on pharmacology, therapeutics for adults and children, and drug induced diseases and side effects is essential. The library should include the Committee on Safety of Medicines Register of Adverse Reactions. A file of manufacturers' literature must be kept, preferably under a pharmacological system of filing for ease of cross-reference, and additionally files of information about such specialised topics as intravenous additives and incompatibilities, drugs in pregnancy and lactation, drugs in neonates and data on tablet identification.

Outside the hospital

There are a number of outside agencies from which information may be obtained.

(a) *Drug information centres*. These centres, often based in a teaching hospital, run abstracting services and cross-indices and maintain comprehensive files of drug information. They are organised on a Regional basis in many parts of the country, and all hospital pharmacists are able to refer queries to them. They provide a valuable source of information which may be otherwise difficult to locate.

(b) *Poisons information centres*. These provide a comprehensive source of information about poisoning and its treatment, both by drugs and by household, industrial and agricultural chemicals. (See p. 613.)

(c) *Drug manufacturers' medical information departments*. Most drug manufacturers have such a department and their knowledge about their own and related products is usually second to none. Files of all references relating to the drugs made by the firm are maintained and a telephoned enquiry usually produces results very quickly. Information about the effects and treatment of overdosage is also available, and, indeed, some firms publish specialised literature on this subject.

INTRAVENOUS SOLUTIONS AND ADDITIVES

Since virtually all the patients in the I.T.U. will receive intravenous therapy, it is vitally important that prescriptions should be non-ambiguous in all particulars. Only then can the nursing staff be sure of correctly carrying out the prescriber's intentions. It must be re-membered that there are legal considerations involved when drugs are to be added to i.v. infusions, and whose responsibility it is to make drug additions to infusions must be clearly defined in each hospital to protect both nurse and doctor. Guidance on every aspect of the field of intravenous additives may be found in the circular 'Addition of Drugs to Intravenous Infusion Fluids', Department of Health and Social Security (1976).

The design and lay-out of the prescription sheet is all important. Listed below is the information which must appear if the prescription is not to be capable of misinterpretation:

1. Patient's name and hospital unit number.
2. The date and for how long the prescription is valid.
3. Name and strength of the i.v. fluid to be administered.
4. The volume to be given in a stated period of time.
5. The site of the i.v. infusion (particularly if there is more than one infusion running simultaneously).
6. The name and dose of any drug to be added.

7. The exact method of addition (i.e. to the bottle, via the drip tubing or by using a burette unit).

A chart should be designed with spaces for all these details and with ample space for the nursing staff to record administrations as they actually occur – it must be remembered that it is not always possible to adhere to the stated timetable and so it is important to record the actual starting and finishing times of each container. The temptation to speed up the drip to revert to the original time stated if delays have occurred must be avoided – the correct rate of fluid administration is more important than the total quantity of fluid given. To minimise errors, abbreviations should be avoided in prescriptions – in particular the use of chemical symbols, as many nurses have never studied chemistry and may therefore have to guess at their meaning.

Contamination of intravenous fluids

All i.v. bottles should be inspected for the absence of cloudiness (which would imply the presence of bacterial growth) and damage immediately before use. At the same time the expiry date must be checked. If a patient exhibits any unusual reaction to an i.v. infusion which it is thought might be due to bacterial contamination or other manufacturing problem, the infusion should be discontinued and the container and giving set retained for investigation. The procedures laid down in the two D.H.S.S. circulars on this subject (Department of Health and Social Security 1975a, b) must be followed without delay to protect other potential recipients of the same batch. It has been shown experimentally that prolonged use of a giving set, and/or the use of blunted giving sets (resulting in clumsy insertion), increases the risk of contamination. The sources of contamination in i.v. infusions have been surveyed by Woodside *et al.* (1975) and also in an Editorial (1974). Each change of giving set should be recorded by labelling, and no set should be in use for more than 24 hours.

Drug additions to i.v. infusions

It is very convenient to add drugs to i.v. infusions and insufficient attention is taken of the potential chemical interactions between drugs and i.v. fluids, for example:

The stability of many drugs is reduced by the acidity of dextrose solutions. As described by Lynn (1970) and Ashwin and Lynn (1975), this is particularly important with the semi-synthetic penicillins such as ampicillin and cloxacillin. The cephalosporins are similarly affected. Many drugs precipitate when mixed with sodium bicarbonate solutions, and it is advisable that no drugs be added to this injection. Drugs must never be added to i.v. fat emulsions. The packaging insert enclosed with injections usually supplies information about compatibilities; if not available, a pharmacist or the drug manufacturer should be consulted. In some cases it may be better to inject the drug into the drip tubing (i.v. bolus technique). The relative merits of the two methods are summarised in Table 1.

A useful compromise method may be to add the drug to a measured volume of infusion using a burette. Drug additions are better avoided on the ward or I.T.U. where possible as this saves nursing time and reduces the risk of contamination. Ready-mixed i.v. solutions of drugs such as potassium chloride and lignocaine are commercially available, and it may be possible to obtain others from the hospital pharmacy. Preloaded syringes are currently obtainable of certain drugs, e.g. lignocaine, and this simplifies additive procedures where pre-mixed solutions are not available. The use of excessive quantities of sodium bicarbonate is relatively common during resuscitation – a pre-loaded syringe containing 50 mmol of bicarbonate ions is to be preferred (Min-

Table 1. The addition of drugs to i.v. infusions

Advantages of adding drug to i.v. infusion bottle	Advantages of injecting drug into drip tubing
1. Constant blood level, provided that drip rate is constant 2. Dilutes irritant drugs, e.g. fusidic acid	1. Dose level not affected by changes in drip rate 2. Less time for drug to react chemically with diluting fluid
Disadvantages of adding drug to i.v. infusion bottle	Disadvantages of injecting drug into drip tubing
1. More time for contaminating bacteria to multiply 2. More time for drug to react with fluid and deteriorate 3. Variations in drip rate influence dosage 4. If more than one drug added, may react together chemically 5. Blood levels may be too low to be effective	1. Method not suitable for drugs which must be given slowly, e.g. potassium chloride 2. Any adverse reaction likely to be instantaneous 3. Not suitable for drugs needing constant blood level 4. Precipitated drug may enter vein unobserved

i-jet, made by International Medication Systems). It also obviates the risk of interaction involving a drug injected into the side arm of an infusion containing sodium bicarbonate.

Tables 2 and 3 summarise information about chemical interactions which will occur between a number of commonly prescribed drugs and infusion solutions.

Table 2. Drug incompatibilities in intravenous fluids

Drug	Incompatibility with	Reason
The penicillins (Na^+ or K^+ salts of benzyl-penicillin and the semi-synthetic penicillins)	Tetracyclines (HCl) Gentamicin	Precipitation Inactivation of gentamicin
Carbenicillin	Kanamycin	Inactivation of carbenicillin
	Colistin	Inactivation of colistin
	Gentamicin	Reduced activity of gentamicin
Tetracyclines (HCl)	Penicillin	Precipitation
	Sulphonamides (Na^+ salts)	Precipitation
	Hydrocortisone sodium succinate	Precipitation
	Calcium salts	Tetracycline chelate formed
	Sodium bicarbonate	Precipitation
Gentamicin	All penicillins	Reduced activity of gentamicin
Cephaloridine	Tetracyclines	Precipitation
Ampicillin	All other antibiotics	Loss of potency
	Hydrocortisone sodium phosphate	Loss of potency
Hydrocortisone sodium succinate	Tetracyclines (HCl)	Precipitation
Calcium salts	Tetracyclines (HCl)	Tetracycline chelate formed

Table 2. Drug incompatibilities in intravenous fluids (*Cont.*)

Drug	Incompatibility with	Reason

Amphotericin
Barbiturates
Frusemide
Heparin
Phenothiazines
  e.g. chlorpromazine
Phenytoin
Sulphadimidine and
  sulphadiazine
Vitamin B complex ±
  vitamin C
	These should not be mixed with
	any other drugs in solution	

No drugs should be added to bottles of:
Blood
Plasma
Parenteral amino acid preparations
Parenteral lipid solutions
Mannitol
Sodium bicarbonate solution

Table 3. Stability of drugs in intravenous fluids

Ampicillin	Loses 10% of its activity in 2 to 4 h in dextrose and dextrose/saline
Methicillin	Loses 10% of its activity in 5 to 6 h in dextrose, dextrose/saline, and saline
Carbenicillin Gentamicin	Adequate serum levels may not be achieved if given by continuous infusion and they are best given intermittently
Amphotericin	Must be given in dextrose solution of suitable pH (see manufacturer's literature)
Erythromycin lactobionate	Unstable in electrolyte solutions. Should only be added to 5% dextrose solution
Tetracyclines	Should not be added to solutions containing calcium ions, e.g. Hartmann's solution

Tables 2 and 3 have been reproduced from the British National Formulary 1976–1978, published by the British Medical Association and the Pharmaceutical Society of Great Britain.

DRUG INTERACTIONS

It is only since about 1965 that the potential clinical importance of pharmacological drug interactions has begun to be realised by prescribers. During the last ten years there has been an overwhelming number of publications devoted to this subject; in many cases the true position has been obscured by the publication of references to interactions of poorly documented clinical significance. The following notes give a very brief outline of the major potential sites of interaction. Further study of this interesting subject will prove rewarding, and some suggestions for further reading are included.

Absorption from the gastrointestinal tract

Many factors influence the absorption of drugs from the gastrointestinal tract, but it is not always easy to predict the effects of interaction on a particular drug. For example, Manninen *et al.* (1973) and Nimmo *et al.* (1973) have shown that metoclopramide and propantheline alter the amount and the rate of absorption of digoxin and paracetamol by influencing gastric motility, the effect of the alteration depending on the site of absorption in the tract, which differs with these two drugs. It is clear from this work that any drug which significantly alters gastric motility may affect the absorption characteristics of concurrently administered drugs. Adsorbent materials such as kaolin and food, and such diverse substances as silicone and cholestyramine resin have been known to interfere with drug absorption.

Transport in the plasma

Two drugs may compete for the plasma protein binding sites on which they depend for transport from the site of absorption to the receptor site. Bound drug is pharmacologically inert, and displacement by a competitor from the binding sites may result in a sudden enhancement of effect producing the symptoms of an overdose. Once again it is not easy to predict the effect of this type of interaction, as many other factors may influence the result, such as the distribution of the drug in the body tissues. These factors are summarised in the book by Smith and Rawlins (1973).

Metabolism and excretions

Since most drugs are metabolised by the liver prior to excretion by the kidney, competition for liver enzyme pathways is a common source of drug interaction. Likewise enzyme induction by one drug resulting in the enhanced rate of metabolism of a concurrently administered drug provides many interesting possibilities. For example, Neuvonen and Pentila (1974) showed that the half-life of doxycycline was reduced in patients simultaneously receiving phenobarbitone, and many workers have shown that barbiturates can affect the metabolism of such widely differing drugs as oral anti-coagulants and corticosteroid hormones. Kenwright and Levi (1973) showed that probenecid can interfere with the hepatic uptake of drugs; it can also interfere with the renal excretion of drugs, thus enhancing their blood levels. This may or may not be an advantage, according to the circumstances. It is known to have clinical significance in the case of the penicillins and cephaloridine.

There are many other factors which may alter the predicted effect of drugs. Some of these are summarised in the paper by Rawlins (1974). Others may be found in the many books now available. Some of the most helpful books about drug interactions are those published by the following authors: Stockley (1974), Hansten (1976) and also the American Pharmaceutical Association (1973 and 1974).

DRUG DOSAGE IN RENAL FAILURE

Certain drugs may cause renal damage; in the presence of renal impairment the dosage schedule of other drugs may require considerable amendment to avoid accumulation and consequent adverse reactions. In an excellent review, Bennett *et al.* (1974) have tabled many common drugs and suggested doses for use in varying degrees of renal impairment. Part of their table, selecting drugs commonly used in the I.T.U., is reproduced in Table 4. For the purpose of the table, qualitative degrees of renal failure have been arbitrarily defined as follows:

'Mild'   – creatinine clearance 0.8–1.3 ml/s
                (50–80 ml/min)

'Moderate' – creatinine clearance 0.2–0.8 ml/s
                (10–50 ml/min)

'Severe'   – creatinine clearance less than 0.2 ml/s
                ($<$10 ml/min)

The normal interval between maintenance doses is given in column 3. The number of times that this interval should be increased if necessary in renal failure is given on the second line in columns 4, 5 and 6 in brackets.

Table 4. A guide to drug therapy in renal failure (adapted and reproduced with kind permission from Bennett *et al.*, 1974)

A. ANTIMICROBIAL AGENTS

Drug	Route of excretion	Normal half-life (h)	Maintenance dose intervals				Significant dialysis of drug‡	Toxic effects *Remarks
			Normal	Renal failure				
				Mild	Moderate	Severe		
Cephalosporins*								*Agents in this group may be nephrotoxic in combination with aminoglycoside antibiotics and frusemide
Cephalexin	Renal	0.6–1	Q6 h	Q6 h (×1.5)	Q6 h	Q6–12 h (×2)	Yes (HP)	—
Cephalothin	Renal Hepatic	0.5–0.9	Q6 h	Q6 h	Q6 h	Q8–12 h** (×1.5–2)	Yes (HP)***	*Group toxicity **Uraemic patients more likely to get positive Coombs test ***Only moderate dialysis; if high blood level desired, add a maintenance dose after H, or add drug to P dialysate at desired serum level (e.g. 20 μg/ml)
Cefazolin	Renal	1.4–2.2	Q8 h	Q12 h (×1.5)	Q12–16 h (×1.5–2)	Q24 h (×3)	No (HP)	*Group toxicity
Chloramphenicol	Hepatic (Renal)	2.5	Q6 h	Unchanged	Unchanged	Unchanged	No (HP)	Bone marrow toxicity adds to uraemic marrow suppression
Clindamycin	Hepatic (Renal)	2	Q6 h	Unchanged	Unchanged	Unchanged	No (HP)	—
Colistin sulphomethate	Renal	1.5–2	Q12 h	Q24 h (×2)	Q36–60 h (×3–5)	Q60–96 h (×5–8)	Yes (P) No (H)	Nephrotoxic; peripheral neuropathy; respiratory paralysis; toxicity can be unrelated to dose
Erythromycin	Hepatic	1.5	Q6 h	Unchanged	Unchanged	Unchanged	?	—

† All agents in this group may cause excessive sedation. ‡ H indicates haemodialysis; P, peritoneal dialysis.

Table 4. Antimicrobial Agents (Cont.)

Drug	Route of excretion	Normal half-life (h)	Normal	Renal failure			Significant dialysis of drug‡	Toxic effects *Remarks
				Mild	Moderate	Severe		
Gentamicin	Renal	2	Q8 h	Q8–12 h (×1.5)	Q12–24 h (×1.5–3)	Q48 h (×6)	Yes (H) No (P)	Ototoxic; nephrotoxic; respiratory paralysis; incidence less than with colistin or kanamycin Toxicity enhanced by cephalosporins, frusemide
Kanamycin	Renal	3–4	Q8 h	Q24 h (×3)	Q24–72 h (×3–9)	Q72–96 h (×9–12)	Yes (HP)**	Nephrotoxic; ototoxic **May add to P dialysate at twice desired serum level
Lincomycin	Hepatic (Renal)	4.5	Q6 h	Q6 h	Q6 h	Q8–12 h (×1.5–2)	No (HP)	—
Penicillins*								*Agents in this group may cause allergic interstitial nephritis; convulsions may occur with high blood levels
Amoxicillin	Renal	1	Q8 h	Q8 h	Q12 h (×1.5)	Q16 h (×2)	Yes (H)	*Group toxicity
Ampicillin	Renal Hepatic	1.5	Q6 h	Q6 h	Q9 h (×1.5)	Q12–15 h** (×2–2.5)	Yes (H) No (P)	*Group toxicity **If high urine levels desired, normal intervals needed
Carbenicillin	Renal Hepatic	1.5	Q4 h	Q4 h	Q6–12 (×2–3)	Q12–16 h (×3–4)	Yes (H) No (P)**	*Group toxicity **May add to peritoneal dialysate at desired serum level (100 µg/ml) Coagulopathy; acidosis at high blood levels

Drug								Comments
Cloxacillin	Hepatic Renal	0.5	Q6 h	Unchanged	Unchanged	Unchanged	No (H)	*Group toxicity
Methicillin	Renal Hepatic	0.5	Q4 h	Q4 h	Q4 h	Q8–12 h (×2–3)	No (HP)	*Group toxicity
Penicillin G	Renal Hepatic	0.5**	Q8 h	Q8 h	Q8 h	Q12–16 h (×1.5–2)	No (HP)	*Group toxicity / Potassium salt has 1.7 mEq K^+ per 1 million units / **Half-life prolonged by many drugs
Streptomycin	Renal	2.5	Q12 h	Q24 h (×2)	Q24–72 h (×2–6)	Q72–96 h (×6–8)	Yes (HP)	Ototoxic; rare nephrotoxicity
Sulfamethoxazole trimethoprim (Co-trimoxazole)	Renal	10	Q12 h	Q12 h	Q24 h (×2)	Avoid*	Yes (H)	*May cause deterioration of renal function if serum creatinine greater than 2 mg/100 ml
Tetracyclines*								*Agents in this group may potentiate acidosis, increase catabolism and BUN level
Tetracycline	Renal Hepatic	6	Q6 h	Q12 h (×2)	Q12–24 h (×2–3)	Q48 h** (×8)	No (HP)	*Group toxicity / **Avoid
Doxycycline	Renal Hepatic	20	Unchanged	Unchanged	Unchanged**	Unchanged**	No (HP)	Group drug of choice for extrarenal infections in patient with renal disease / **Not useful in urinary tract infections
Minocycline	Hepatic	8	Q12 h	Q12 h	Q18–24 h** (×1.5–2)	Q24–36 h** (×2–3)	?	*Group toxicity / **Not useful in urinary tract infections

†All agents in this group may cause excessive sedation. ‡ H indicates haemodialysis; P, peritoneal dialysis.

Table 4. A guide to drug therapy in renal failure
B. ANALGESICS SEDATIVES AND TRANQUILLIZERS*

| Drug | Route of excretion | Normal half-life (h) | Maintenance dose intervals | | | | Significant dialysis of drug‡ | Toxic effects *Remarks |
| | | | Normal | Renal failure | | | | |
				Mild	Moderate	Severe		
Analgesics (non-narcotic)*								
Pethidine	Hepatic (Renal: <10%)	5.5	Q4 h	Unchanged	Unchanged	Unchanged	?	*may cause excessive sedation **Subgroup toxicity
Methadone	Renal 58%** (Nonrenal: 42%)	10–18***	Q6–8 h	Q8–12 h (×1.5)	Q12–16 h (×1.5–2)	Q16–24 h (×2–3)	?	*Subgroup toxicity **Excretion increased in acid urine ***Plasma half-life determined by protein binding
Morphine	Hepatic (Renal: <14%)	2–3 (part) 10–44 (part)**	Q4 h	Unchanged	Unchanged	Unchanged	?	*Subgroup toxicity **May be recirculating metabolites
Naloxone (Narcan)	Hepatic	1.5	i.v. boluses	Unchanged	Unchanged	Unchanged	?	*Subgroup toxicity
Pentazocine (Fortral)	Hepatic (Renal: <13%)	2(i.m.)	Q4–6 h	Unchanged	Unchanged	Unchanged	?	*Subgroup toxicity
Barbiturates*								*For drugs in this sub-group, haemodialysis at least two times more effective than peritoneal dialysis
Amylobarbitone (Amytal)	Hepatic	0.6 (part)** 15.8–21 (part)	i.m. or i.v. bolus	Unchanged	Unchanged	Unchanged	No (HP)*	†Group toxicity *Subgroup remarks; haemodialysis may be useful in poisoning **Biexponential pharmacokinetics
Phenobarbitone	Hepatic Renal 30%	37–96	Q8 h	Q8 h	Q8 h	Q8–10 h (×2)	Yes (HP)*	†Group toxicity *Subgroup remarks

Benzodiazepines

Drug	Metabolism	t½ (h)					Dialysis	Remarks
Chlordiazepoxide (Librium)	Hepatic	22–24	Q8 h	Q8 h	Q8–12 h (×1.5)	Q12–24 h (×1.5–3)	No (H)	†Group toxicity
Diazepam (Valium)	Hepatic	2–10 (part)** 48–192 (part)	Q8 h	Unchanged	Unchanged	Unchanged	No (H)*	†Group toxicity *May need supplemental dose if used as an anticonvulsant **Complex biexponential pharmacokinetics
Phenothiazines*	Hepatic		Q6 h	Q6 h	Q9–12 h (×1.5–2)	Q12–18 h (×2–3)	No (HP)	†Group toxicity; anticholinergic; may cause urinary retention, pigmentation, lactation *Prototype: chlorpromazine

C. CARDIOVASCULAR, ANTIHYPERTENSIVE AND DIURETIC AGENTS†

Drug	Metabolism	t½ (h)					Dialysis	Remarks
Antiarrhythmic agents*								*All agents in this subgroup: excretion enhanced in acid urine; blood levels best guide to therapy
Lignocaine*	Hepatic* (Renal: <20%)	0.1–2 (part)** 1.2–2.2 (part)	i.v. drip or boluses	Unchanged	Unchanged	Unchanged	?	*Subgroup remarks **Biexponential pharmacokinetics; clearance depends on hepatic blood flow; specific nomograms available
Procainamide* (Pronestyl)	Renal (60%)* (Nonrenal)	2.5–4.5	Q3 h	Q3 h	Q4.5–6 h** (×1.5–2)	Q6–9 h** (×2–3)	Yes (H)	*Subgroup remarks **Usual clinical practice to decrease size and frequency of dose

† All agents in this group may cause excessive sedation. ‡ H indicates haemodialysis; P, peritoneal dialysis.

Table 4. Cardiovascular, Antihypertensive and Diuretic Agents (*Cont.*)

Drug	Route of excretion	Normal half-life (h)	Maintenance dose intervals				Significant dialysis of drug‡	Toxic effects *Remarks
			Normal	Renal failure				
				Mild	Moderate	Severe		
Propranolol (Inderal)	Hepatic*	3.2 (PO)* 0.1 (part i.v.)** 2.8 (part i.v.)	Q6 h	Unchanged	Unchanged	Unchanged	No (H)	*Clearance depends on hepatic blood flow; threshold exists: PO dose < 30 mg completely extracted by normal liver **Biexponential pharmacokinetics (complex in uraemia); blood levels best guide
Quinidine*	Renal*	3–16	Q6 h	Unchanged	Unchanged	Unchanged	Yes (HP)	*Subgroup remarks
Antihypertensive agents*								*Blood pressure response best guide
Diazoxide*	Renal (Nonrenal: 20%)	22–31	i.v. bolus	Unchanged	Unchanged	Unchanged**	Yes (HP)	*Subgroup remarks **Decrease dose size if given very frequently; very rapid injection needed for therapeutic response
Guanethidine*	Nonrenal Renal (25–40%)	48–72 (part)** 216–240 (part)	Q24 h	Q24 h	Q24–36 h (× 1.5)	Q36–48 h (× 1.5–2)		*Subgroup remarks **Biexponential pharmacokinetics; tricyclic antidepressants decrease therapeutic effectiveness; may decrease renal blood flow
Hydrallazine* (Apresoline)	Hepatic** Gastrointestinal (? Renal)	2–7.8	Q8 h	Q8 h	Q8 h	Q8–16 h (× 2)	No (H)	*Subgroup remarks **Genetic variation in metabolism exists

Drug	Route of elimination	Half-life (h)					Dialysis	Remarks
Methyldopa* (Aldomet)	Renal* Hepatic	1.4–2 (part, 95%)** 5.2–8.1 (part, 5%)	Q6 h	Q6 h	Q9–12 h (× 1.5–2)	Q12–18 h** (× 2–3)	Yes (HP)	*Subgroup remarks **Biexponential pharmacokinetics; 5% part may increase to 50% in severe renal failure with retention of active metabolites Prolonged hypotension; hepatitis (HAA negative)
Reserpine*	Nonrenal	4.5 (part)** 48–168 (part)	Q24 h	Unchanged	Unchanged	Unchanged	No (HP)	Excessive sedation; gastrointestinal bleeding *Subgroup remarks **Biexponential pharmacokinetics for drug and metabolites
Cardiac glycosides*								*Add to uraemic gastrointestinal symptoms; blood levels best guide to therapy (about 12 h after dose). Usual clinical practice to decrease size and frequency of dose. Toxicity may be enhanced by dialysis K⁺ removal
Digitoxin	Hepatic** Renal: metabolites	72–144***	Q24 h	Q24 h	Q24 h	Q24–36 h** (× 1.5)	No (HP)	*Subgroup remarks **Converted to digoxin (8%); conversion increased in uraemia ***Blood level depends on plasma protein in concentration and drug binding
Digoxin*	Renal (Nonrenal: 15%)	36	Q24 h	Q24 h	Q36 h (× 1.5)	Q36–72 h** (× 1.5–3)	No (HP)	*Subgroup remarks **Decrease loading dose to ⅔ normal if using for inotropic purposes
Ouabain*	Renal (50%) Faecal (30%)	22	Q12–24 h	Q24 h (× 2)	Q24–36 h (× 2–3)	Q36–48 h (× 3–4)	No (HP)**	*No change in dosage size needed **15% of dose given during dialysis removed in 4 h

† All agents in this group may cause excessive sedation. ‡ H indicates haemodialysis; P, peritoneal dialysis.

Table 4. Cardiovascular, Antihypertensive and Diuretic Agents (*Cont.*)

Drug	Route of excretion	Normal half-life (h)	Maintenance dose intervals				Significant dialysis of drug‡	Toxic effects *Remarks
			Normal	Renal failure				
				Mild	Moderate	Severe		
Diuretics								
Ethacrynic acid	Hepatic Renal	? 2–4	Q6 h as needed for diuresis	Q6 h	Q6 h	Avoid*	?	Ototoxic; volume depletion; may augment antibiotic neprotoxicity *Use alternate if possible
Frusemide	Renal (Nonrenal)	Biphasic 0.4 and 2	Q6 h as needed for diuresis	Unchanged	Unchanged	Unchanged*	?	Rare ototoxicity; volume depletion; may augment *Has been used in large doses in renal failure
Mercurials	Renal	Biphasic 36 and 288	Q24 h	Q24 h	Avoid	Avoid	?	Systemic mercury accumulation; nephrotoxic
Metolazone	Renal	8	Q24 h	Unchanged	Unchanged	Unchanged*	No (H)	Volume depletion *Has been used in large doses in renal failure
Spironolactone	Hepatic	10 min but active metabolite to 20 h	Q6 h	Q6 h	Q6 h*	Avoid*	?	*Hyperkalaemia
Thiazides*	Renal	3	Q12 h	Q12 h	Q12 h	Avoid**	?	Hyperuricaemia; volume depletion *Prototype: chlorothiazide **Ineffective
Triamterene	Hepatic	2	Q12 h	Q12 h	Q12 h	Avoid*	?	*Hyperkalaemia Folic acid antagonist

D. MISCELLANEOUS AGENTS

Anticoagulants*								*All agents in this group: add to uraemic bleeding tendency
Heparin	Nonrenal (Renal)	1.5 but increases with increasing dose	Q4 h	Unchanged	Unchanged	Unchanged	No (H)	*Group toxicity
Warfarin	Nonrenal (Renal)	Biphasic** 12 and 40	Q24 h	Unchanged	Unchanged	Unchanged	?	*Group toxicity **Some metabolites with anticoagulant properties are excreted by the kidney
Corticosteroids*								*All agents in this group may increase azotaemia by enhancing catabolism
Cortisone	Renal excretion of metabolites	0.5–2	Q8 h	Unchanged	Unchanged	Unchanged	No (H)**	*Group toxicity **Half-life shortened but serum value unchanged
Dexamethasone	Renal excretion of metabolites	4	Q6 h	Unchanged	Unchanged	Unchanged	?	*Group toxicity
Hydrocortisone	Renal excretion of metabolites	1.5–2	Q8 h	Unchanged	Unchanged	Unchanged	?	*Group toxicity
Methylprednisolone	Renal excretion of metabolites	3.5	Q24 h	Unchanged	Unchanged	Unchanged	No (H)**	*Group toxicity **Some shortening of half-life ‡
Prednisolone	Renal excretion of metabolites	4	Q24 h	Unchanged	Unchanged	Unchanged	?	*Group toxicity

† All agents in this group may cause excessive sedation. ‡ H indicates haemodialysis; P, peritoneal dialysis.

Table 4. Miscellaneous Agents (*Cont.*)

Drug	Route of excretion	Normal half-life (h)	Maintenance dose intervals				Significant dialysis of drug‡	Toxic effects *Remarks
			Normal	Renal failure				
				Mild	Moderate	Severe		
Prednisone	Renal excretion of metabolites	1	Q8 h	Unchanged	Unchanged	Unchanged	?	*Group toxicity
Other drugs								
Atropine	Nonrenal	?	Q6 h	Unchanged	Unchanged	Unchanged	?	
Tubocurarine	Renal	0.5	i.v. boluses	Unchanged	Unchanged	Unchanged*	?	*Duration of action of large single or multiple doses prolonged

† All agents in this group may cause excessive sedation. ‡ H indicates haemodialysis; P, peritoneal dialysis.

REFERENCES

American Pharmaceutical Association (1973). 'Evaluations of Drug Interactions.'
American Pharmaceutical Association (1974). 'Evaluations of Drug Interactions' (Suppl.)
Ashwin, J. and Lynn, B. (1975). Ampicillin stability in saline or dextrose infusions. *Pharm. J.* **214**, 487.
Bennett, W. M., Singer, I. and Coggins, C. J. (1974). A guide to drug therapy in renal failure. *JAMA* **230**, 1544.
British National Formulary. Published by the British Medical Association and the Pharmaceutical Society of Great Britain every two years.
Crooks, J., Clark, C. G., Caie, H. B. and Mawson, W. B. (1965). Prescribing and administration of drugs in hospital. *Lancet* **1**, 373.
Crooks, J., Weir, R. D., Coull, D. C., McNab, J. W., Calder, G., Barnett, J. W. and Caie, H. B. (1967). Evaluation of a method of prescribing drugs in hospital, and a new method of recording their administration. *Lancet* **1**, 668.
Data Sheet Compendium. Published by the Association of the British Pharmaceutical Industry annually.
Department of Health and Social Security (1971). Medicines Act 1968. 'Notes on Applications For Clinical Trial Certificates.' MAL 4 August 1971.
Department of Health and Social Security (1974a). Medicines Act 1968 and 1971. 'Clinical Trials Using Marketed Products.' MAL 32 March 1974.
Department of Health and Social Security (1974b). Medicines Act 1968 and 1971. 'Clinical Trials Arranged by Doctors or Dentists.' MAL 31 October 1974.
Department of Health and Social Security (1974c). Medicines Act 1968 and 1971. 'A Guide to the Licensing Provisions Affecting Doctors and Dentists.' MAL 30 October 1974.
Department of Health and Social Security (1975a). 'Reporting of Infusion Incidents Involving Suspected Contamination.' Health Service Circular (Interim Series) HSC (IS) 118 March 1975.
Department of Health and Social Security (1975b). 'The Laboratory Investigation of Suspected Contamination of Infusion Fluids.' Health Service Circular (Interim Series) HSC (IS) 119 March 1975.
Department of Health and Social Security (1976). 'Addition of Drugs to Intravenous Infusion Fluids.' Health Circular, HC (76)9 March 1976.
Editorial (1974). Microbiological hazards of intravenous infusions. *Lancet* **1**, 543.
Hansten, P. D. (1976). 'Drug Interactions', Third Edition. Henry Kimpton.
Hill, P. A. and Wigmore, H. M. (1967). Measurement and control of drug-administration incidents. *Lancet* **1**, 671.
Kenwright, S. and Levi, A. J. (1973). Impairment of hepatic uptake of rifamycin antibiotics and its therapeutic implications. *Lancet* **11**, 1401.
Lynn, B. (1970). Pharmaceutical aspects of semi-synthetic Penicillins. *J. Hosp. Pharm.* **28**, 71.
Manninen, V., Apajalahti, A., Melin, J. and Karesoja, M. (1973). Altered absorption of digoxin in patients given propantheline and metoclopramide. *Lancet* **1**, 398.
Martindale – The Extra Pharmacopoeia. Published by the Pharmaceutical Press, London every five years.
Neuvonen, P. J. and Pentilla, O. (1974). Interaction between doxycycline and barbiturates. *Brit. Med. J.* **1**, 535.

Nimmo, J., Heading, R. C., Tothill, P. and Prescott, L. F. (1973). Pharmacological modification of gastric emptying: Effects of propantheline and metoclopramide on paracetamol absorption. *Brit. Med. J.* **1**, 587.

Rawlins, M. D. (1974). Variability in response to drugs. *Brit. Med. J.* **4**, 91.

Smith, S. E. and Rawlins, M. D. (1973). Variability in human drug response. Butterworths, London.

Stockley, I. (1974). 'Drug Interactions and Their Mechanisms'. Pharmaceutical Press, London.

Vere, D. W. (1965). Errors of complex prescribing. *Lancet* **1**, 370.

Woodside, W., Woodside, M. E., D'Arcy, E. M. and Patel, R. H. (1975). Intravenous fluids as vehicles of infection. *Pharm. J.* **215**, 606.

PART 4

Monitoring, Computer Applications and Instrumentation in the Intensive Therapy Unit

1

Monitoring in the Intensive Therapy Unit

J. P. Blackburn

INTRODUCTION

During recent years many instruments have become available for collecting signals from patients and for processing and displaying the information. Monitoring devices are used when the signals cannot be detected and recorded directly by the nurse and when readings must be taken continuously or at frequent intervals. Such equipment thus plays an important part in the clinical care of the acutely ill patient both in the operating theatre and in the intensive therapy, coronary care or other specialised unit. However, the use of monitoring equipment in the general ward has tended to be unsatisfactory (Rawles and Crockett, 1969; Rawles, 1969).

The information of interest in any particular case depends on the patient's clinical condition, but in general only a limited range of signals is recorded routinely. The electrocardiogram (E.C.G.) is the most commonly displayed variable, but instruments to record the arterial blood pressure, central venous pressure, temperature and respiration are likely to be required. Blood gas analysis, electrolyte and haematocrit estimations may also be important. Obtaining these signals reliably from a patient who may be hypotensive and restless is often unexpectedly difficult and the patient/sensor interface is usually the most troublesome point in any patient monitoring system (Crockett, 1970; Payne, 1975).

897

Much of the information which is used routinely in the assessment of the patient, such as his colour, level of consciousness, response to stimuli or degree of abdominal distension cannot be transduced easily or reliably and this is a serious drawback in any automatic or semi-automatic data acquisition and display system (Maloney, 1968).

Invasive techniques are obviously justified for obtaining essential information from patients who are acutely ill, but there are many instances where reliable non-invasive methods would be advantageous. Pulse rate can usually be obtained relatively easily, but automatic indirect methods for determining blood pressure are still somewhat unreliable, particularly in shocked and restless patients (Greatorex, 1971). However, recently both ultrasonic and subsonic methods of detecting arterial wall movement have been used to improve the performance of such instruments (Stegall *et al.*, 1968, Gordon and Ur, 1970).

The various transducers and monitoring devices will now be considered in more detail.

MONITORING SYSTEMS

Electrocardiogram

This is usually recorded as a single lead system and displayed on an oscilloscope for dysrhythmia detection. Conventional 12 lead electrocardiograms are recorded for diagnostic purposes as required. Heart rate is frequently displayed on E.C.G. monitors and may be charted by the nurse or recorded automatically. Portable battery operated E.C.G. monitors are now available which can be used easily under all conditions and are particularly useful for patients who are being transferred from the operating theatre to the intensive therapy unit. A number of d.c. defibrillators use the defibrillator electrodes to pick up the E.C.G., so that in an emergency ventricular fibrillation can be diagnosed and treated with the minimum delay.

There have been improvements in display oscilloscopes and 'memory scopes' are widely available which provide non-fade displays of the E.C.G. complexes. In addition, the trace may be 'frozen' so that abnormal complexes can be studied in detail and, in some equipment, slowly changing trends can be displayed at the same time as the E.C.G. signal (Fig. 1).

The use of electrically isolated E.C.G. monitors and other equipment contribute to patient safety and will be considered below.

Dysrhythmia monitors are available for the detection of beats which

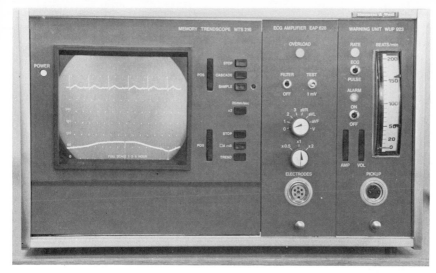

Fig. 1. Electrocardiogram monitor with rate meter and 'memory' oscilloscope showing conventional E.C.G. and two hour display of heart rate. (Courtesy of Simonsen and Weel Ltd.)

are premature or have a QRS complex of abnormal shape. The QRS complex may be compared with a previously stored 'normal' beat for that patient and the shape of the stored complex can be updated automatically if required. Artefacts such as excessive baseline wander or noise are detected and inhibit the feature recognition process (Bushman, 1967; Horth, 1969; Neilson, 1971). Dysrhythmia monitors are very complex internally but can be used easily at the bedside as they are largely self adjusting and have the minimum number of controls. Such monitors are usually used with recorders to display the number of abnormal beats and a signal delay system may be included, so that the abnormal beat which triggered the system can be recorded and examined in detail (Fig. 2).

A recent comparison of manual and automatic methods of dysrhythmia detection has been made by Vetter and Julian (1975). In the Group monitored by conventional means, 36% of dysrhythmias were successfully detected, while more than 99% of potentially serious ventricular dysrhythmias were recorded by the automatic system.

Pulse monitors

Peripheral pulse sensors are attached to the finger or the ear lobe and detect changes in light intensity reaching a photocell as a result of

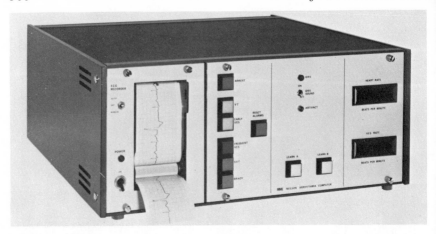

Fig. 2. Dysrhythmia monitor. (Courtesy of Reynolds Medical Electronics Ltd.)

capillary pulsations. The sensors detect pulse rate rather than heart rate and are unreliable in states of peripheral capillary shutdown. An approximate indication of the systolic blood pressure can be obtained by inflating the sphygmomanometer cuff until the pulse is no longer detected. Finger plethysmographs can be used for the same purpose.

Blood pressure

The measurement of blood pressure is obviously important in any severely ill patient. Blood pressure may be estimated either indirectly using an external pneumatic cuff and sensing device or directly using a pressure transducer connected to an intra-arterial catheter.

Indirect methods
Several techniques have been used to automate the detection of systolic and diastolic blood pressure. A microphone may be used to pick up the Korotkoff sounds and the flow of blood below the cuff may be detected by a second pneumatic cuff or by a variety of other transducers (Geddes, 1970; Greatorex, 1971). These methods tend to be unsatisfactory when patients are hypotensive or restless. Movements of the arterial wall beneath the cuff can be detected ultrasonically and show characteristic changes at systole and diastole (Ware and Laenger, 1967). The instrument is easy to use and is less affected by artefacts than most other methods (Stegall *et al.*, 1968). Another method depends on an observation by Gordon and Ur (1970) that if the pressure difference

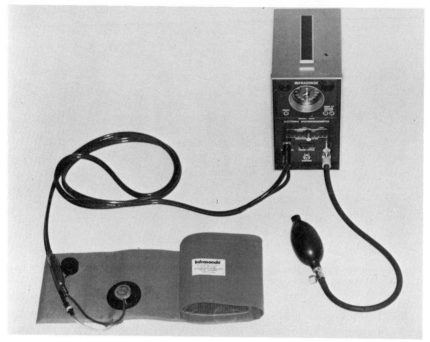

Fig. 3. Infrasonde blood pressure meter. (Courtesy of Kontron Instruments Ltd.)

across the wall of an artery is zero the wall oscillates at a subsonic frequency when fluid flows through the vessel. A microphone is used to detect the subsonic oscillations which occur for an instant in the cardiac cycle when the cuff is between systolic and diastolic pressure (Fig. 3). Good correlation has been shown between intra-arterial pressure and the infrasonde down to systolic pressures of 40 mm Hg.

Direct methods
Electromanometers are frequently used for measuring arterial pressure and if arterial puncture is justified then such measurements are more reliable than the indirect methods described above. Miniature transducers can be attached to the patient at the arterial puncture site (Fig. 4), thus eliminating the need for long fluid filled catheters, and small disposable continuous flushing devices delivering about 2 ml fluid per hour are commercially available (Shinebourne and Pfitzner, 1973). Electrically isolated pressure transducers are readily available and on some instruments the plastic dome is pre-sterilised, disposable and contains a flexible diaphragm which makes mechanical contact with the pressure sensing diaphragm of the electromanometer.

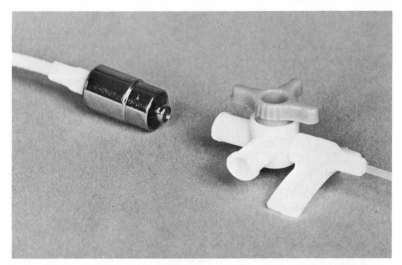

Fig. 4. Miniature pressure transducer. The diaphragm is situated in the tip of the male Luer connector. (Courtesy of Datascope Inc.)

Electromanometer tipped catheters have a wide frequency response and are useful for myocardial function studies involving left ventricular catheterisation. They cannot conveniently be calibrated *in situ* and are also relatively fragile and expensive. Such instruments are not in routine use for the measurement of blood pressure at the bedside.

Equipment for displaying the blood pressure trace is now reliable and simple to operate. Systolic, diastolic or mean pressures may be presented on analogue meters or in digital form.

Central venous pressure

Central venous pressure is frequently measured using a catheter passed into the right atrium and connected to a saline manometer. As the pressure is relatively low, errors in the hydrostatic reference level will substantially affect the measured pressure. This reference zero should be maintained at the phlebostatic axis of the patient (Latimer, 1971).

If an electrical output is required the catheter can be connected to a suitable electromanometer so that phasic or mean pressures may be recorded. A differential electromanometer (Fig. 5) for automatically correcting the reference level when the patient is tipped head-up or -down has been used (Blackburn, 1968; Corbett *et al.*, 1974).

Left atrial pressure may be measured in a similar fashion, particularly

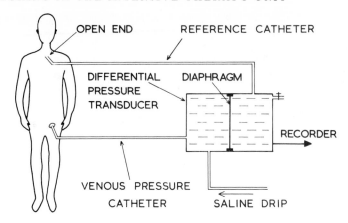

Fig. 5. A differential electromanometer used for measuring central venous pressure.

following open heart surgery when a suitable catheter is inserted at operation. It may also be estimated indirectly from the pulmonary capillary wedge pressure using a Swan-Ganz catheter (Swan *et al.*, 1970). For further comments on the clinical use of pulmonary capillary wedge pressure, refer to Part 2, ch. II, p. 319.

Temperature

The clinical thermometer tends to be unsatisfactory for use in the intensive therapy unit because it is fragile and difficult to use on unconscious patients. It is also unsuitable for continuous recording and cannot be used remotely. Thermistor or thermocouple probes are readily available and convenient to use in a variety of locations. The gradient between core and peripheral temperature has been used as a guide to the adequacy of peripheral perfusion (Joly and Weil, 1969). Further details on temperature monitoring in the clinical situation are described in Part 2, ch. II, p. 312.

Respiration

Quantitative information about the behaviour of the respiratory system is difficult to obtain unless the patient is receiving artificial ventilation when, on some machines, airway pressure, tidal volume and rate can be read directly. Pneumotachographs are difficult instruments to use clinically and are employed only in some highly specialised intensive therapy units (Grenvik *et al.*, 1966; Osborn *et al.*, 1968; Peters *et al.*,

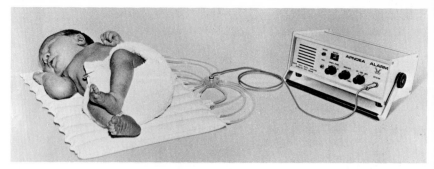

Fig. 6. Apnoea monitor. Respiratory movement is detected by alterations in the gas distribution within the mattress. (Courtesy of Vickers Medical Ltd.)

1974). An anemometer is particularly useful for measuring the patient's tidal and minute volume (Wright, 1955). The device is simple to use, sufficiently accurate for clinical purposes and instruments with an electrical output are available if required (Conway et al., 1974).

In many cases, particularly those without a tracheostomy or endotracheal tube, only qualitative information can be obtained. Changes in the diameter of the chest or abdomen can be sensed in various ways. A temperature sensor in the airway will detect changes in air temperature during respiration and impedance pneumography can be used to record changes in the electrical impedance of the chest (Baker and Hill, 1969). Respiratory rate has also been derived from central venous pressure (Meagher et al., 1966b). Temperature probes may become displaced or covered with secretions and the impedance pneumogram may continue to record respiratory efforts made by the patient even though complete respiratory obstruction has occurred.

Apnoea detection systems are of particular importance in neonatal intensive care units (Rolfe, 1975), where a high proportion of the children have respiratory distress syndrome. A number of mattress-type apnoea monitors (Fig. 6) have been developed (Lewin, 1969; Smith and Scopes, 1972), which have the advantage that no direct contact with the infant is required. They detect body movement rather than the specific effects of respiration and thus may be unreliable in certain circumstances.

Analysis of inspired and expired gases may be useful, particularly in an incubator when the inspired oxygen concentration should be monitored. A variety of oxygen analysers are available which are convenient to use in this situation. In addition, a rapid response carbon dioxide analyser is helpful in managing patients requiring artificial ventilation, while estimates of mixed venous PCO_2 by the rebreathing technique are useful if blood gas analysis cannot be performed.

Cardiac output

There are many techniques available for determining stroke volume and cardiac output, but many of them are relatively invasive and difficult to use in practice.

The Fick method involves measuring oxygen uptake (or carbon dioxide output) and arterial and mixed venous blood gas concentrations. These analyses are not easy to perform accurately in the intensive therapy unit in spite of the apparent simplicity of the technique.

The most widely used method for determining cardiac output is the indicator dilution technique using a bolus of indocyanine green dye or cold saline as the indicator. When green dye is used, arterial blood is usually withdrawn with a motorised syringe and the dye concentration estimated with a densitometer. Blood may be sampled and reinjected continuously using a roller pump (Cohn, 1969); alternatively, blood sampling is avoided if a fibre optic catheter is used (Monroe et al., 1965b; Taylor et al., 1972). This has the advantage that oxygen saturation may be estimated in vivo using the same catheter (Taylor et al., 1972; Woodroof and Koorajian, 1973).

Thermodilution methods are quite convenient to use when estimates of cardiac output are required at the bedside. A suitable thermistor catheter is placed in the pulmonary artery and a small volume of room temperature or ice cold dextrose injected into the right atrium. Cardiac output computers developed for this technique are easy to operate (Fig. 7) and the determination may be repeated at frequent intervals if required (Branthwaite and Bradley, 1968; Cowell and Bray, 1970.) Temperature fluctuations in the pulmonary artery and loss of indicator as it equilibrates in the body may limit the accuracy of the method (Wessel et al., 1971; Sanmarco et al., 1971).

Many attempts have been made to estimate cardiac output from analysis of the central aortic pressure waveform (Jones et al., 1966; Kouchoukos et al., 1969, 1970; Warner, 1966; Wesseling et al., 1974). Various assumptions are made in the application of pulse contour techniques and changes in heart rate, blood pressure and peripheral resistance are likely to alter the results (Starmer et al., 1973; Jurado et al., 1973).

Non-invasive methods for measuring stroke volume are particularly attractive. The mean minor axis of the left ventricular cavity can be

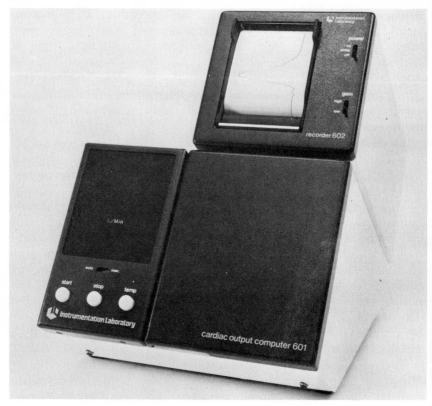

Fig. 7.   Thermal dilution cardiac output computer. (Courtesy of Instrumentation Laboratory Inc.)

measured by echocardiography and the cube of this dimension has been
shown to correlate well with left ventricular volume measured
angiographically (Feigenbaum *et al.*, 1969; Fortuin, 1971; Gibson,
1973). Stroke volume can thus be estimated from measurements taken
at end systole and end diastole. The assessment of volume from a single
measurement clearly implies a number of assumptions and the method
is unreliable in the presence of left ventricular dyskinesia or abnormal
cavity shape (Gibson, 1973). If left ventricular pressure can be
measured simultaneously, this technique can be extended to provide an
assessment of left ventricular function. Gibson and Brown (1976) have
plotted pressure dimension loops, the area of the loop expresses the
stroke work per unit area of myocardium in the direction of the scan.
This method has been used to investigate myocardial function in

patients after open heart surgery, but may be difficult to implement in the intensive therapy unit.

Ultrasonic techniques have also been used for measuring aortic blood velocity non-invasively. The ultrasonic beam is directed at the arch of the aorta from the suprasternal notch and the Doppler shift in the reflected frequency is related to the velocity of the blood. Stroke volume can be calculated if the arterial diameter is known and the mean blood velocity across the aorta averaged over one cardiac cycle.

The technique (transcutaneous aortovelography) has been described by Cross and Light (1974), Light (1976) and evaluated by Sequeira *et al.* (1976). The accuracy of stroke volume determinations compared with dye dilution measurements of cardiac output was poor, although changes in stroke volume could be followed easily. Peak velocity measurements obtained non-invasively correlated well with those obtained with an electromagnetic velocity probe. Transcutaneous aortovelography has also been used in the intensive therapy unit and may prove valuable as a non-invasive indicator of left ventricular function (Buchtal *et al.*, 1976), but the place of this investigation has yet to be established (see Part 2, ch. II, p. 323 for further details).

Electroencephalogram

The E.E.G. is a useful guide to the adequacy of cerebral perfusion and has been used in the assessment of brain death (Binnie *et al.*, 1970; Prior *et al.*, 1974). The array of electrodes is difficult to maintain and interference free signals are not easy to obtain under clinical conditions. Furthermore the records require expert interpretation. A cerebral activity monitor is shown in Fig. 8 (Maynard *et al.*, 1969; Prior *et al.*, 1971) which is considerably easier to use, requires only two electrodes and the records can be readily interpreted (Colvin *et al.*, 1974). The device is useful for monitoring patients with a wide range of disorders but focal disturbances cannot be detected and it is recommended that the cerebral function monitor is employed in association with intermittent E.E.G. traces using conventional apparatus.

Intracranial pressure

A water manometer is conventionally used to monitor intracranial pressure, but continuous records cannot be obtained by this method and it is difficult to maintain for long periods. Implantable extradural pressure transducers have been described by Richardson *et al.* (1970)

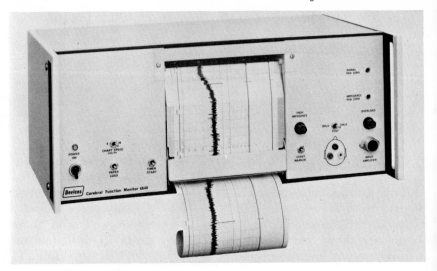

Fig. 8. Cerebral function monitor. This instrument processes the signals from a pair of parietal electrodes to provide a record of cerebral activity. (Courtesy of Devices Ltd.)

and Dorsch *et al.* (1971) which have remained *in situ* for several weeks. Some of the transducers can be zeroed and calibrated while they are implanted (Cooper, 1973). The clinical aspects of intracranial pressure monitoring are described in Part 2, ch. III, p. 406.

Fluid balance

The measurement of fluid balance plays an important part in the management of the seriously ill patient. Usually the rate of intravenous infusion is determined and adjusted manually by drop counting and the volume and type of fluid are recorded by hand. Urinary output and drainage from various sites are documented in a similar fashion. Semi-automated systems have been developed for measuring urinary output by means of an automatically emptying reservoir (Meagher *et al.*, 1966a) or using a load cell (North *et al.*, 1973). Chest drainage can be measured similarly (Sheppard *et al.*, 1972) or by an ultrasonic method (Blackburn *et al.*, 1974). Fluid administration may be accurately controlled using roller or syringe pumps and the volume infused can be continuously displayed. Details of fluid infusion systems are given in Part 4, ch. III, p. 940.

Blood gas and electrolyte analysis

Blood gas analysis is important in the management of patients with cardiorespiratory pathology and is particularly useful in the paediatric intensive therapy unit. Automatic blood gas analysers are now available which have considerably simplified the problems of obtaining reliable results.

Intravascular polarographic electrodes for the measurement of PO_2 are commercially available (Harris and Nugent, 1973; Meldrum et al., 1973; Dodd, 1975; Soutter et al., 1975), as are fibre optic catheters for the continuous determination of arterial or mixed venous oxygen saturation (Monroe et al., 1965a; Taylor et al., 1972). Clot formation affects the response of the catheters and may be troublesome if they are inserted for long periods of time.

Transcutaneous PO_2 can be estimated non-invasively using a heated polarographic electrode applied to the skin, but this measurement is likely to be influenced by variations in peripheral perfusion (Huch et al., 1974). The device is particularly suitable for paediatric use, but its place in clinical management has yet to be fully evaluated.

Some intensive therapy units have equipment for haematocrit or haemoglobin estimations and a flame photometer for blood and urine analysis. Biochemical requirements in the intensive therapy unit are discussed on p. 802 and local needs will depend on the work load of the unit and the availability of laboratory facilities.

ELECTRICAL SAFETY

It is important that all staff be aware of the electrical hazards which can arise when electromedical equipment is in use at the bedside (Bruner, 1967; Hopps, 1969; Loughman and Watson, 1971). There are two aspects of electrocution which must be considered.

Electric shock

Mains operated equipment may cause electric shock if faults develop within the instrument or associated wiring. The current which flows through the body will depend on the voltage applied between the contacts and the impedance of the pathway. Both of these factors may vary widely. The applied voltage will depend on the nature of the external circuit and skin impedance is very variable. Dry skin is a poor conductor, while electrode jelly may have been used to lower skin impedance. The area of contact will also alter the impedance of the circuit and will affect the current density which governs the response of the tissues. When surface electrodes are applied to the body only a small fraction of the current flows across the myocardium because of the multiplicity of available pathways. The current required to cause ventricular fibrillation is 30–200 mA when the 50 Hz a.c. mains is used.

The commonest undetected electrical fault in mains operated equipment is disconnection of the earth wire. The instrument may well operate normally, but a potentially hazardous situation now exists. A second fault can cause the equipment to become 'live' and electrocution may result.

Micro-electrocution

When there is a conducting pathway to the myocardium, such as is found when a pacemaker or saline filled catheter is used, all the current passes through the myocardium and the current density depends on the size and position of the electrode (Roy *et al.*, 1976). A current of 180 µA has been reported as causing ventricular fibrillation in man (Whalen *et al.*, 1964), but usually much larger currents are required. Green *et al.* (1972) found that the threshold for ventricular fibrillation in dogs with the electrode in the right ventricle was never less than 200 µA and usually a current of about 1 mA was required. In addition, ventricular fibrillation could not be produced with an atrial electrode using currents of up to 10 mA. A further study on normal dogs and animals with experimental myocardial infarction (Raftery *et al.*, 1975a) showed the threshold for minimal rhythm changes was 60 µA, while failure of pumping action without ventricular fibrillation occurred when a current of 100 µA was passed across the right ventricular wall. Similar thresholds were found in man (Raftery *et al.*, 1975b).

Small currents which can endanger the patient may occur particularly when combinations of equipment are used, even though the instruments are not faulty. Micro-electrocution may be difficult to detect, but currents large enough to produce pump failure or ventricular fibrillation will totally obscure the E.C.G. signal in 'mains hum' on the monitor screen or recorder.

Recommendations on the design and specification of electromedical equipment are available (Department of Health and Social Security, 1969). It is suggested that connections made to the patient should be isolated from earth as far as possible (Pocock, 1972a, b). Equipment used with intracardiac electrical connections (pacemaker, electro-manometer, intracardiac E.C.G. etc.), where there is a risk of microelectrocution, must be isolated from earth and should not allow mains frequency current of more than 10 μA (50 μA under fault conditions), to flow between any patient connections or between connections to the patient and earth. Equipment used with external electrodes only can pass up to 100 μA (500 μA under fault conditions) between the electrodes and earth. The d.c. current which can flow between connections to the patient should be less than 10 μA otherwise electrolytic skin reactions are likely to occur.

Isolated E.C.G. machines, pressure transducers, flow meters and other equipment conforming to these specifications are now readily available and should be used whenever possible. If the patient must be connected to earth, then if possible only a single earth connection should be made. This will reduce electrical interference affecting the E.C.G. as well as contributing to patient safety. Careful maintenance of equipment is important and needs consideration by those responsible for its use (Editorial, 1972; Monk and Shaw, 1975; North, 1975).

SELECTION AND INSTALLATION OF EQUIPMENT

The choice of equipment for an intensive therapy unit will depend to some extent on the types of patient to be treated. In the coronary care unit and thoracic surgical recovery unit every bed is likely to require an E.C.G. monitor. In the former situation a case can be made for a central nursing station, as the nursing load will be relatively light and the patients will benefit from being undisturbed as far as possible. The central station should contain large screen monitors for dysrhythmia surveillance and at least one pen recorder triggered either automatically or on demand to record abnormal complexes. Dysrhythmia computers should be included if appropriate and arterial and central venous pressure monitoring equipment may also be required (Hampton, 1972).

In all other types of intensive therapy unit the monitoring equipment should be at the bedside, with if necessary a few selected variables displayed centrally. Most critically ill patients require almost continuous nursing care and the information must be displayed at the bedside where there is no ambiguity about patient identification and where the nursing effort should be concentrated (Maloney, 1968).

Selection of the most appropriate equipment is not always easy. In many instances technical specifications of equipment from different manufacturers are comparable and consideration should be given to the suitability of the equipment to local needs, its reliability and the efficiency and convenience of servicing and maintenance arrangements. Many monitoring systems are modular in construction and this makes for convenience and flexibility in use. Ease of use is important and if possible the monitors should be compatible with existing equipment. Anticipated expansion and future developments also need careful consideration (Hayes and Healy, 1973; Hayes, 1974).

FUTURE DEVELOPMENTS IN MONITORING TECHNIQUES

As previously stated, the patient/transducer interface is the weak link in clinical data acquisition systems and developments which improve this aspect of patient monitors will lead to increased reliability.

Non-invasive methods are becoming more versatile and reliable. New techniques for the indirect measurement of blood pressure are now available and systolic time intervals derived non-invasively are contributing to the assessment of myocardial function (Diamont and Killip, 1970; Samson, 1970). The use of ultrasound for following changes in left ventricular function (Gibson and Brown, 1973, 1974) is likely to be particularly valuable. Bedside monitors are becoming easier to use, often as a result of considerable electronic complexity, and as digital computing techniques become cheaper and more widely available, dedicated mini-computers will be used increasingly for data processing and display.

REFERENCES

Baker, L. E. and Hill, D. W. (1969). The use of electrical impedance techniques for the monitoring of respiratory pattern during anaesthesia. *Brit. J. Anaesth.* **41**, 2.

Binnie, C. D., Prior, P. F., Lloyd, D. S. L., Scott, D. F. and Margerison, J. H. (1970). Electroencephalographic prediction of fatal anoxic brain damage after resuscitation from cardiac arrest. *Brit. Med. J.* **4**, 265.

Blackburn, J. P. (1968). Self-levelling venous pressure transducer. *Brit. Med. J.* **4**, 825.

Blackburn, J. P., Martindale, D. D. R. and Miller, J. (1974). Automatic measurement of chest drainage by an ultrasonic system. *Lancet* **2**, 698.

Branthwaite, M. A. and Bradley, R. D. (1968). Measurement of cardiac output by thermal dilution in man. *J. Appl. Physiol.* **24**, 434.

Bruner, J. M. R. (1967). Hazards of electrical apparatus. *Anesthesiology* **28**, 396.

Buchtal, A., Hanson, G. C. and Peisach, A. R. (1976). Transcutaneous aortovelography. Potentially useful technique in management of critically ill patients. *Brit. Heart J.* **38**, 451.

Bushman, J. A. (1967). Monitoring the E.C.G. waveform. *Biomed. Engng.* **2**, 106.

Cohn, J. D. (1969). A pump system for performing indicator dilution curves without blood loss. *J. Appl. Physiol.* **26**, 841.

Colvin, M. P., Scott, D. F., Prior, P. F., Maynard, D. E. and Simpson, B. R. (1974). A device for continuous monitoring of cerebral function. First World Congress on Intensive Care. *In* 'Scientific Abstracts'. (Ed. I. McA. Ledingham), p. 99.

Conway, C. M., Leigh, J. M., Preston, T. D., Walters, F. J. M. and Webb, D. A. (1974). An assessment of three electronic respirometers. *Brit. J. Anaesth.* **46**, 885.

Cooper, R. (1973). Measurement of intracranial pressure. *Brit. J. Hosp. Med. Equip. Suppl.* **10**, 18.

Corbett, G. A., Preston, T. D. and Bailey, J. S. (1974). A self-levelling central venous electromanometer. *Med. Biol. Engng.* **12**, 366.

Cowell, T. K. and Bray, D. G. (1970). Measuring the heart's output. *Electron. Power* **16**, 150.

Crockett, G. S. (1970). The patient-sensor interface. *Post Grad. Med. J.* **46**, 378.

Cross, G. and Light, L. H. (1974). Non-invasive intra-thoracic blood velocity measurement in the assessment of cardiovascular function. *Biomed. Engng.* **9**, 464.

Department of Health and Social Security (1969). Hospital Technical Memorandum No. 8, 'Safety Code for Electro-medical Apparatus.' H.M.S.O., London.

Diamont, B. and Killip, T. (1970). Indirect assessment of left ventricular performance in acute myocardial infarction. *Circulation* **42**, 579.

Dodd, K. L. (1975). Continuous monitoring of arterial oxygen tension in the newborn. *Brit. J. Hosp. Equip.* **1**, 35.

Dorsch, N. W. C., Stephens, R. J. and Symon, L. (1971). An intracranial pressure transducer. *Biomed. Engng.* **6**, 452.

Editorial (1972). Equipment maintenance. *Biomed. Engng.* **7**, 219.

Feigenbaum, H., Wolfe, S. B., Popp, R. L., Haine, C. L. and Dodge, H. T. (1969). Correlation of ultrasound with angiocardiography in measuring left ventricular diastolic volume. *Am. J. Cardiol.* **23**, 111.

Fortuin, N. J., Hood, W. P., Sherman, M. E. and Craig, E. (1971). Determination of left ventricular volumes by ultrasound. *Circulation* **44**, 575.

Geddes, L. A. (1970). 'The Direct and Indirect Measurement of Blood Pressure.' Year Book Medical Publishers Inc., Chicago.

Gibson, D. G. (1973). Estimation of left ventricular size by echo-cardiography. *Brit. Heart J.* **35**, 128.

Gibson, D. G. and Brown D. (1973). Measurement of instantaneous left ventricular dimension and filling rate in man, using echocardiography. *Brit. Heart J.* **35**, 1141.

Gibson, D. G. and Brown, D. (1974). Use of echocardiography in the evaluation of left ventricular function. *Proc. roy. Soc. Med.* **67**, 140.

Gibson, D. G. and Brown, D. J. (1976). Assessment of left ventricular systolic function in man from simultaneous echocardiographic and pressure measurements. *Brit. Heart J.* **38**, 8.

Gordon, M. and Ur, A. (1970). Origin of Korotkoff sounds. *Am. J. Physiol.* **218**, 524.

Greatorex, C. A. (1971). 'Indirect Methods of Blood Pressure Measurement'. *In* 'IEE Medical Electronics Monograph 1–6' (Ed. B. W. Watson). Peter Peregrinus Ltd., London.

Green, H. L., Rattery, E. B. and Gregory, I. C. (1972). Ventricular fibrillation threshold of healthy dogs to 50 Hz current in relation to earth leakage currents of electromedical equipment. *Biomed. Engng.* **7**, 408.

Grenvik, A., Hedstrand, U. and Sjögren, H. (1966). Problems in pneumotachography. *Acta Anaesth. Scand.* **10**, 147.

Hampton, J. (1972). The selection of equipment for coronary care units. *Brit. J. Hosp. Med. Equip. Suppl.* **8**, 4.

Harris, T. R. and Nugent, M. (1973). Continuous arterial oxygen tension monitoring in the newborn infant. *J. Pediat.* **82**, 929.

Hayes, B. (1974). Equipping the Intensive Care Unit. *In* 'Intensive Care' (Ed. A. R. J. Wise), p. 25. Health and Social Service Journal, London.

Hayes, B. and Healy, T. E. J. (1973). Equipment for intensive care. *Brit. J. Hosp. Med. Equip. Suppl.* **9**, 4.

Hopps, J. A. (1969). Shock hazards in operating rooms and patient-care areas. *Anesthesiology* **31**, 142.

Horth, T. C. (1969). Arrhythmia monitor. *Biomed. Engng.* **4**, 308.

Huch, r., Lübbers, D. W. and Huch, A. (1974). Reliability of transcutaneous monitoring of arterial PO_2 in newborn infants. *Archs. Dis. Child.* **49**, 213.

Joly, H. R. and Weil, M. H. (1969). Temperature of the great toe as an indication of the severity of shock. *Circulation* **39**, 131.

Jones, W. B., Russell, R. O. and Dalton, D. H. (1966). An evaluation of computed stroke volume in man. *Am. Heart J.* **72**, 746.

Jurado, R. A., Matucha, D. and Osborn, J. J. (1973). Cardiac output estimation by pulse contour methods: validity of their use for monitoring the critically ill patient. *Surgery* **74**, 358.

Kouchoukos, N. T., Sheppard, L. C., McDonald, D. A. and Kirklin, J. W. (1969). Estimation of stroke volume from the central arterial pressure contour in postoperative patients. *Surg. Forum* **20**, 180.

Kouchoukos, N. T., Sheppard, L. C. and McDonald, D. A. (1970). Estimation of stroke volume in the dog by a pulse contour method. *Circ. Res.* **26**, 611.

Latimer, R. D. (1971). Central venous catheterisation. *Brit. J. Hosp. Med.* **5**, 369.

Lewin, J. E. (1969). An apnoea-alarm mattress. *Lancet* **2**, 667.

Light, L. H. (1976). Transcutaneous aortovelography. A new window on the circulation? *Brit. Heart J.* **38**, 433.

Loughman, J. and Watson, A. B. (1971). Electrical safety in Australian Hospitals and proposed standards. *Med. J. Aust.* **2**, 349.

Maloney, J. V. (1968). The trouble with patient monitoring. *Ann. Surg.* **168**, 605.

Maynard, D., Prior, P. F. and Scott, D. F. (1969). Device for continuous monitoring of cerebral activity in resuscitated patients. *Brit. Med. J.* **4**, 545.

Meagher, P. F., Jensen, R. E., Pearcy, M. G., Weil, M. H. and Shubin, H. (1966a). Automatic urinometer for on-line monitoring of patients with circulatory shock. *Med. Res. Engng.* **5**, 38.

Meagher, P. F., Jensen, R. E., Weil, M. H. and Shubin, H. (1966b). Measurement of respiration rate from central venous pressure in the critically ill patient. *IEEE Trans. Biomed. Engng.* **13**, 54.

Meldrum, S. J., Watson, B. W. and Becker, G. A. (1973). A catheter tip transducer for continuous measurement of blood oxygen tension in neonates. *Biomed. Engng.* **8**, 470.

Monk, I. B. and Shaw, A. (1975). Medical equipment hazards – practical experience in a large region. *Biomed. Engng.* **10**, 132.

Monroe, R. G., Polanyi, M., Nadas, A. S., Gamble, W. J. and Hugenholtz, P. G. (1965a). The use of fibreoptics in clinical cardiac catheterisation. I. Intracardiac oximetry. *Circulation* **31**, 328.

Monroe, R. G., Polanyi, M., Gamble, W. J. and Hugenholtz, P. G. (1965b). The use of fibreoptics in clinical cardiac catheterisation. II. In vivo dye-dilution curves. *Circulation* **31**, 344.

Neilson, J. M. (1971). A special purpose hybrid computer for analysis of ECG arrhythmias. *Inst. elec. Eng. Conf. Publ.* **79**, 151.

North, R. (1975). Safety testing patient-connected electronic equipment. *Brit. J. Clin. Equip.* **1**, 29.

North, R., Watson, B. W. and Gay, P. (1973). An instrument for measuring urinary output volume. *Biomed. Engng.* **8**, 522.

Osborn, J. J., Beaumont, J. O., Raison, J. C. A., Russell, J. and Gerbode, F. (1968). Measurement and monitoring of acutely ill patients by digital computer. *Surgery* **64**, 1057.

Payne, J. P. (1975). Monitoring and the patient-sensor interface. *In* 'Bio-engineering in Britain' (Ed. A. R. J. Wise), p. 30. Health and Social Service Journal, London.

Peters, R. M., Shapiro, A., Wolfenson, L., Klein, C., Patitucci, P., Virgilio, R., Smith, D., Uhl, R. and Hogan, J. (1974). Respirator monitoring in ICU. First World Congress on Intensive Care. *In* 'Scientific Abstracts' (Ed. I. McA. Ledingham), p. 139.

Pocock, S. N. (1972a). Earth-free patient monitoring, Part I. *Biomed. Engng.* **7**, 21.

Pocock, S. N. (1972b). Earth-free patient monitoring. Part II. *Biomed. Engng.* **7**, 67.

Prior, P. F., Maynard, D. E., Sheaff, P. C., Simpson, B. R., Strunin, L., Weaver, E. J. M. and Scott, D. F. (1971). Monitoring cerebral function. *Brit. Med. J.* **2**, 736.

Prior, P. F., Scott, D. F. and Maynard, D. E. (1974). The EEG in assessment of brain death. First World Congress on Intensive Care. *In* 'Scientific Abstracts' (Ed. I. McA. Ledingham), p. 98.

Raftery, E. B., Green, H. L. and Gregory, I. C. (1975a). Disturbances of heart rhythm produced by 50 Hz leakage current in dogs. *Cardiovasc. Res.* **9**, 256.

Raftery, E. B., Green, H. L. and Yacoub, M. H. (1975b). Disturbances of heart rhythm produced by 50 Hz leakage currents in human subjects. *Cardiovasc. Res.* **9**, 263.

Rawles, J. M. (1969). Patient monitoring: A clinician's point of view. *Biomed. Engng.* **4**, 264.

Rawles, J. M. and Crockett, G. S. (1969). Automation on a general medical ward: Monitron system of patient monitoring. *Brit. Med. J.* **3**, 707.

Richardson, A., Hide, T. A. H. and Eversden, I. D. (1970). Long term continuous intracranial pressure monitoring by means of a modified subdural pressure transducer. *Lancet* **2**, 687.

Rolfe, P. (1975). Monitoring in newborn intensive care. *Biomed. Engng.* **10**, 399.

Roy, O. Z., Scott, J. R. and Park, G. C. (1976). 60-Hz ventricular fibrillation and pump failure thresholds versus electrode area. *IEEE Trans. Biomed. Engng.* **23**, 45.

Samson, R. (1970). Changes in systolic time intervals in acute myocardial infarction. *Brit. Heart J.* **32**, 839.

Sanmarco, M. E., Philips, C. M., Marquez, L. A., Hall, C. and Davila, J. C. (1971). Measurement of cardiac output by thermal dilution. *Am. J. Cardiol.* **28**, 54.

Sequeira, R. F., Light, L. H., Cross, G. and Raftery, E. B. (1976). Transcutaneous aortovelography. A quantitative evaluation. *Brit. Heart J.* **38**, 443.

Sheppard, L. C., Kouchoukos, N. T., Acton, J. C., Fincher, J. M. and Kirklin, J. W. (1972). Surgical intensive care automation. *J. Assoc. Advance. Med. Instr.* **6**, 74.

Shinebourne, E. A. and Pfitzner, J. (1973). Continuous flushing device for indwelling arterial and venous cannulae. *Brit. J. Hosp. Med. Equip. Suppl.* **9**, 64.

Smith, J. E. and Scopes, J. W. (1972). A new apnoea alarm for babies. *Lancet* **2**, 545.

Soutter, L. P., Conway, M. J. and Parker, D. (1975). A system for monitoring arterial oxygen tension in sick newborn babies. *Biomed. Engng.* **10**, 257.

Starmer, C. F., McHale, P. A., Cobb, F. R. and Greenfield, J. C. (1973). Evaluation of several methods for computing stroke volume from central aortic pressure. *Circ. Res.* **33**, 139.

Stegall, H. F., Kardon, M. B. and Kemmerer, W. T. (1968). Indirect measurement of arterial blood pressure by Doppler ultrasonic sphygmomanometry. *J. Appl. Physiol.* **25**, 793.

Swan, H. J. C., Ganz, W., Forrester, J., Marcus, H., Diamond, G. and Chonette, D. (1970). Catheterisation of the heart in man with use of a flow-directed balloon-tipped catheter. *New Engl. J. Med.* **283**, 447.

Taylor, J. B., Lown, B. and Polanyi, M. (1972). In vivo monitoring with a fiber optic catheter. *JAMA* **221**, 667.

Vetter, N. J. and Julian, D. G. (1975). Comparison of arrhythmia computer and conventional monitoring in the coronary care unit. *Lancet* **1**, 1151.

Ware, P. W. and Laenger, C. J. (1967). Indirect blood pressure measurement. Doppler ultrasound Kinetoarteriography, Proc. 20th Ann. Conf. on Engng. in Med. and Biol. (Boston). Wellesley Press, Mass.

Warner, H. R. (1966). The role of computers in medical research. *JAMA* **196,** 944.

Wessel, H. U., Paul, M. H., James, G. W. and Grahn, A. R. (1971). Limitations of thermal dilution curves for cardiac output determinations, *J. Appl. Physiol.* **30**, 643.

Wesseling, K. H., Smith, N. T., Nichols, W. W., Weber, H., deWit, B. and Beneken, J. E. W. (1974). Beat by beat cardiac output from the arterial pressure pulse contour. In 'Measurement in Anaesthesia' (Ed. S. A. Feldman, J. M. Leigh and J. Spierdijk), p. 150. Leiden University Press.

Whalen, R. E., Starmer, C. F. and McIntosh, H. D. (1964). Electrical hazards associated with cardiac pacemaking. *Ann. N.Y. Acad. Sci.* **111**, 922.

Woodroof, E. A. and Koorajian, S. (1973). In vitro evaluation of an in vivo fiber optic oximeter. *Med. Instrum.* **7**, 287.

Wright, B. M. (1955). A respiratory anemometer. *J. Physiol.* **127**, 25P.

II

Computer Applications in the Intensive Therapy Unit

J. P. BLACKBURN

INTRODUCTION

Computer assisted monitoring in the intensive therapy unit can be considered as a development of the various patient monitoring devices described in Part 4, ch. I. Indeed, some instruments such as dysrhythmia monitors and cardiac output computers are likely to contain analogue and digital processors. However it is customary to consider a computer-assisted intensive therapy unit as one where more or less continuous processing of patient data by computing techniques is used to help clinical personnel in the routine care of the patient (Glaeser and Thomas, 1975).

Conventional patient monitors, in spite of their limitations, can generate large amounts of data and the collection, analysis, editing and display of this information may be enhanced by computer processing. The success of the computer system will depend on the clinical relevance of the processed information and the adaptability of the system to deal with changing clinical situations and new developments in patient care. In addition, the availability of medical and nursing staff and their attitudes to computer monitoring must be considered when designing the system, as must the work load of the unit.

The various aspects of computer processing will now be considered in more detail.

917

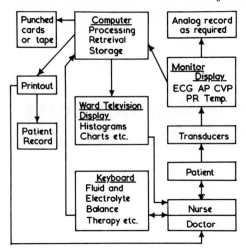

Fig. 1. Block diagram of a system for computer-assisted intensive therapy.

DATA COLLECTION, PROCESSING AND DISPLAY

The ease with which data can be entered into the computer is crucial in determining whether the system is clinically acceptable, as it is nurses and clinicians who are likely to be primarily concerned with data entry and display. Information may be obtained automatically from a variety of bedside monitors (Kouchoukos *et al.*, 1971; Shubin *et al.*, 1971; Lewis *et al.*, 1972; Osborn *et al.*, 1968; Preston *et al.*, 1974; Warner *et al.*, 1968) or entered by hand for processing and display (William-Olsson *et al.*, 1969; Ashcroft and Berry, 1974). A block diagram of one system is shown in Fig. 1. A small, simple numeric keyboard near the patient, with a code for identifying drugs, intravenous fluids and other manually entered information (Fig. 2) is preferable to a teletype which is likely to be at some distance from the patient. Raw or pre-processed data can be collected automatically from a wide variety of monitors. The use of analogue signal pre-processing at the bedside (e.g. systolic, diastolic and mean pressure derived from the arterial pressure waveform) not only reduces the load on the digital computer, but also ensures that clinically important information can still be displayed on monitors in the event of failure of the computer system.

There are a number of problems associated with automatic data collection. In particular, the computer must be informed when the signals are unreliable. Also when using conventional charts the act of measuring or recording data impresses on the nurse the state of the

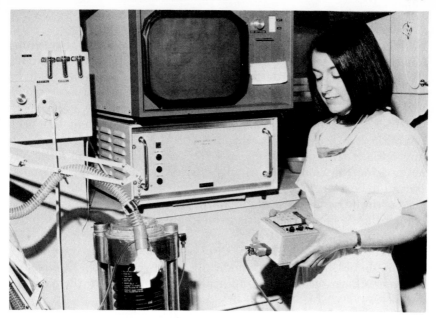

Fig. 2. Special purpose keyboard and visual display unit for presenting messages and graphs.

patient in a way which cannot easily be incorporated in a fully automated system.

Data processing

Complex signal processing and the analysis of long lengths of data may be required for research purposes. However, for routine clinical use most calculations performed by the computer are relatively simple, such as the determination of fluid balance or acid-base state. As previously mentioned, analogue pre-processors are often used for features recognition of waveforms and this greatly reduces the amount of digital signal analysis required. The digital computer is particularly well suited to correlate, edit and display information, but this feature may be of doubtful benefit unless the results are presented to the clinician in readily assimilable form.

The computer system can be linked to the operating theatres, clinical chemistry and blood gas laboratories, thus improving communications and enabling data to be added to the patient's record from various locations as required.

Data display

Computer driven oscilloscope displays should be situated at the bedside and capable of presenting messages and graphs. This information must be of immediate benefit to those using the system if the facility is to be used effectively. Conventional graphs of blood pressure, heart rate etc. with details of fluid balance should be displayed initially and manual charting abandoned as soon as confidence in the system has been established. More elaborate displays can then be provided if this is appropriate. In the first instance the computer system is merely automating the charting normally carried out by nurses, but it has proved to be acceptable in a number of intensive therapy units. About 10% of the nurses' time is taken up with manual chart keeping and 25% of their time is spent on activities which could be done by the computer (Drazen and Wechsler, 1973).

In addition to the oscilloscope display, a synopsis of the state of each patient should be printed periodically in case of system failure and summary charts, usually in graphical form, prepared for the patient's notes.

Computing requirements will vary depending on the clinical environment and we will now consider the different types of intensive therapy unit in relation to their needs for automatic data processing.

COMPUTER SYSTEMS IN INTENSIVE THERAPY

General purpose intensive therapy unit

The design of an effective computer system for a general intensive therapy unit is complicated by the wide range of clinical problems encountered involving a large number of different methods of investigation and treatment, different nursing activities and widely varying timescales.

Comprehensive systems for monitoring cardiovascular and respiratory variables have been described by Shubin et al. (1971) and Lewis et al. (1972). The computer controls the calibration and flushing of pressure transducers, cardiac output determinations using indocyanine green are automated and fluid infusion is also controlled by the computer. Computer-based monitoring of respiratory variables has been carried out in a small number of centres, where special techniques have been used to calibrate and maintain pneumotachographs and gas pressure transducers (Osborn et al., 1968; Peters et al., 1974; Hilberman et al., 1969; Wald et al., 1969; Turney and Blumenfeld, 1973).

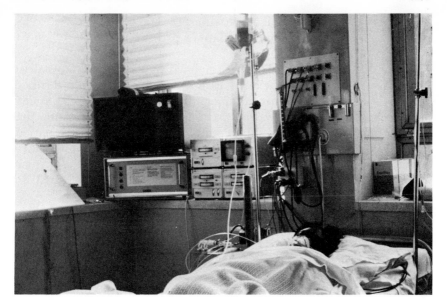

Fig. 3. One bed in a cardiac surgery recovery unit showing bedside monitors and visual display unit.

A computer based system for use in an intensive therapy unit is likely to be restricted and suitable for only a limited range of patients. Alternatively an immense amount of effort may be put into developing a general purpose system which is unwieldy and difficult to use in practice (Preston *et al.*, 1974).

Cardiac surgery recovery unit

Many of the computer based patient monitoring systems have been developed for use following open heart surgery (Osborn *et al.*, 1968; Kouchoukos *et al.*, 1971; Warner *et al.*, 1968; Mikolajczuk, 1974; Glaeser *et al.*, 1975). In this situation a restricted range of variables is monitored, postoperative care can be standardised to a large extent and the patient usually remains in the unit a relatively short time (Fig. 3). Consequently a suitable system is likely to be much easier to design compared with that required in a general purpose intensive therapy unit.

In addition to the automated measurement and display of cardiorespiratory variables, the measurement of fluid balance is of considerable importance in the management of the patient. Conventional fluid balance charts are often difficult to interpret and prone to error, so the automation of fluid balance calculations provides immediate benefits for nurses and medical staff.

If the decisions upon which treatment is based can be rationalised then the computer can be used to assist directly in some forms of therapy, such as the administration of intravenous fluids. Such a system has been implemented by Sheppard *et al.* (1974) who claim that developments of this kind result in improved and more uniform patient care and reduce the demands on skilled staff. Many clinicians are likely to view such developments with suspicion, particularly as clinical decisions are based on the assessment of many factors, some of which are unsuitable for computer processing.

Coronary care unit

A system for processing the E.C.G. waveform is likely to be the main requirement in the coronary care unit and stand-alone dysrhythmia detectors have been described on p. 898. These monitors may be connected to a digital computer to provide more comprehensive signal processing and display facilities. Alternatively, a small digital computer can be used to analyse the E.C.G. signals from a number of patients. A variety of feature recognition programmes has been developed for this purpose (Gerlings *et al.*, 1972; Oliver *et al.*, 1971; Rey *et al.*, 1971; Geddes and Warner, 1971; Feldman *et al.*, 1971; Haywood *et al.*, 1970; Frankel *et al.*, 1975). The range of dysrhythmias which can be identified is somewhat restricted as automatic P wave recognition is difficult to achieve, particularly if every beat is processed. The problem is somewhat simpler if an atrial lead is used, but this cannot be justified in most patients.

A comprehensive signal acquisition system, similar to that used in a general purpose intensive therapy unit, has been described by Russell *et al.*, (1972) and the advantages and limitations of such systems have been discussed by Macy and James (1971).

CONCLUSION

The prospect of using computing techniques in the management of the critically ill patient has its attractions and confident predictions were made that computers would be widely used in intensive care units. In general, the impact of computer-based monitoring has been disappointing and the problems of developing a system suitable for a general purpose intensive therapy unit have already been mentioned. It is important that the objectives of the system are clearly stated at the outset. There must be close collaboration between the medical, nursing and computer staffs and the nurses and clinicians must get immediate benefits from using the system. This means processing and displaying the variables which are normally recorded by the nurses in the first instance, before proceeding to more elaborate forms of analysis. Inevitably, automated computer-based intensive therapy systems are to some extent restricted since many clinical signs, such as the patient's degree of alertness, colour, abdominal distension etc. which are important for clinical management, cannot conveniently be fed into the system (Editorial, 1974). In addition, difficulties are likely to arise if the nurse is moved from the bedside to a central monitoring station (Maloney, 1968).

The evaluation of computer systems is unlikely to be easy. Intangibles like the quality of patient care are important but cannot be readily quantified. The installation, development and routine utilisation of the computer system are likely to affect patient management and invalidate accurate comparisons. Drazen and Wechsler (1974) have shown that although systems could not be considered cost effective, in some centres computer-based monitoring led to a reduction in the number of skilled nurses required and the patients spent a shorter time in the unit. Hilberman *et al.* (1975) however were unable to detect any difference between the patients monitored by computer and the control group.

In spite of these problems, the use of computers in intensive therapy units is likely to grow, particularly as conventional bedside monitors become more elaborate and expensive and computer systems become cheaper and more versatile. Methods of trend detection and predictive monitoring need to be developed, as do techniques for investigating and interpreting the complex interrelations between various physiological control systems using the limited range of signals which can be conveniently recorded from the critically ill patient. In the future, small dedicated computers, linked if necessary to a larger machine, may be used at the bedside to process, store and display information of direct clinical relevance leading to improvements in patient care.

REFERENCES

Ashcroft, J. M. and Berry, J. L. (1974). The introduction of a real-time patient data display system into the Cardio-Thoracic Department at Wythenshawe Hospital. *In* 'Medinfo 74' (Ed. J. Anderson and J. M. Forsythe), p. 101. North-Holland Pub., Amsterdam.

Drazen, E. C. and Wechsler, A. E. (1973). Evaluation of computer-based patient-monitoring systems. Report prepared for the Department of Health Education and Welfare by A. D. Little Inc.

Drazen, E. C. and Wechsler, A. E. (1974). Review of computer-based monitoring systems in the U.S. Report prepared for the Department of Health Education and Welfare by A. D. Little Inc.

Editorial (1974). Computers or nurses? *Lancet* **2**, 877.

Feldman, C. L., Amazeen, P. G., Klein, M. D. and Lown, B. (1971). Computer detection of ventricular ectopic beats. *Comput. Biomed. Res.* **3**, 666.

Frankel, P., Rothmeier, J., James, D. and Quaynor, N. (1975). A computerized system for E.C.G. monitoring. *Comput. Biomed. Res.* **8**, 560.

Geddes, J. S. and Warner, H. R. (1971). A P.V.C. detection program. *Comput. Biomed. Res.* **4**, 493.

Gerlings, E. D., Bowers, D. C. and Rol, G. A. (1972). Detection of abnormal ventricular activation in a coronary care unit. *Comput. Biomed. Res.* **5**, 14.

Glaeser, D. H. and Thomas, L. J. (1975). Computer monitoring in patient care. *Ann. Rev. Biophys. and Bioeng.* **4**, 449.

Glaeser, D. H., Trost, R. F., Brown, D. B., Kyle, A. C., Lenahan, M. S., Walker, C. K., Wilson, C. S. and DeBakey, M. E. (1975). A hierarchical minicomputer system for continuous post-surgical monitoring. *Comput. Biomed. Res.* **8**, 336.

Haywood, L. J., Murthy, V. K., Harvey, G. A. and Saltzberg, S. (1970). On-line real time computer algorithm for monitoring the E.C.G. waveform. *Comput. Biomed. Res.* **3**, 15.

Hilberman, M., Kamm, B., Tarter, M. and Osborn, J. J. (1975). An evaluation of computer-based patient monitoring at Pacific Medical Center. *Comput. Biomed. Res.* **8**, 447.

Hilberman, M., Schill, J. P. and Peters, R. M. (1969). On-line digital analysis of respiratory mechanics and the automation of respirator control. *J. Thor. Cardiovasc. Surg.* **58**, 821.

Kouchoukos, N. T., Sheppard, L. C. and Kirklin, J. W. (1971). Automated patient care following cardiac surgery. *Cardiovasc. Clinics* **3**, 110.

Lewis, F. J., Deller, S., Quinn, M., Lee, B., Will, R. and Raines, J. (1972). Continuous patient monitoring with a small digital computer. *Comput. Biomed. Res.* **5**, 411.

Macy, J. and James, T. N. (1971). The value and limitations of computer monitoring in myocardial infarction. *Prog. Cardiovasc. Dis.* **13**, 495.

Maloney, J. V. (1968). The trouble with patient monitoring. *Ann. Surg.* **168**, 605.

Mikolajczuk, A. (1974). Three years experience with computer-assisted patient monitoring. *In* 'Medinfo 74' (Ed. J. Anderson and J. M. Forsythe), p. 787. North-Holland Pub., Amsterdam.

Oliver, G. C., Nolle, F. M., Wolff, G. A., Cox, J. R. and Ambos, H. D. (1971). Detection of premature ventricular contractions with a clinical system for monitoring electrocardiographic rhythms. *Comput. Biomed. Res.* **4**, 523.

Osborn, J. J., Beaumont, J. O., Raison, J. C. A., Russell, J. and Gerbode, F. (1968). Measurement and monitoring of acutely ill patients by digital computer. *Surgery* **64**, 1057.

Peters, R. M., Shapiro, A., Wolfenson, L., Klein, C. Patitucci, P., Virgilio, R., Smith, D., Uhl, R. and Hogan, J. (1974). Respirator monitoring in I.C.U. First World Congress on Intensive Care. *In* 'Scientific Abstracts' (Ed. I. McA. Ledingham), p. 139. Bell and Bain, Edinburgh.

Preston, T. D., Bailey, J. S., Brown, D. J., Carrington, P. J., Jones, M. L., Leigh, J. M. and Mikolajczuk, A. (1974). Problems of computer assisted intensive care in a multidisciplinary environment. First World Congress on Intensive Care. *In* 'Scientific Abstracts' (Ed. I. McA. Ledingham), p. 138. Bell and Bain, Edinburgh.

Rey, W., Laird, J. D. and Hugenholtz, P. G. (1971). P-wave detection by digital computer. *Comput. Biomed. Res.* **4**, 509.

Russell, R. O., Hunt, D., Potanin, C. and Rackley, C. E. (1972). Hemodynamic monitoring in a coronary intensive care unit. *Arch. Intern. Med.* **130**, 370.

Sheppard, L. C., Kirklin, J. W. and Kouchoukos, N. T. (1974). Computer-controlled interventions for the acutely ill patient. *In* 'Computers in Biomedical Research' (Ed. R. W. Stacy and B. D. Waxman), Vol. IV, p. 135. Academic Press, New York.

Shubin, H., Weil, M. H., Palley, N. and Afifi, A. A. (1971). Monitoring the critically ill patient with the aid of a digital computer. *Comput. Biomed. Res.* **4**, 460.

Turney, S. Z., Blumenfeld, W. (1973). Online respiratory-waveform analysis using a digital desk calculator. Med. Biol. Eng. **11**, 275.

Wald, A., Jason, D., Murphy, T. W. and Mazzia, V. D. B. (1969). A computer system for respiratory parameters. *Comput. Biomed. Res.* **2**, 411.

Warner, H. R., Gardner, R. M. and Toronto, A. F. (1968). Computer based monitoring of cardiovascular functions in postoperative patients. *Circulation* **37** (Suppl. 2), 68.

William-Olsson, G., Norlander, O., Norden, I. and Petterson, S. O. (1969). A patient monitoring system with display terminals. *Opuscula Medica* **14**, 39.

III

Instrumentation for Patient Care

Section 1: Resuscitation Equipment – Defibrillators and Pacemakers

J. S. GEDDES

INTRODUCTION

The development of practical means of controlling the activity of the heart electrically, with the chest intact, less than a quarter of a century ago represented one of the most significant technological advances of our time.

The correction of ventricular fibrillation (V.F.) by external counter-shock was first documented by Zoll *et al.* (1956). Four years earlier Zoll had been the first to achieve successful cardiac pacing by repeated electric shocks applied to the chest. The relevance of the former discovery to the salvage of life was greatly increased by the demonstration by Kouwenhoven *et al.* (1960), that an artificial circulation could also be maintained through the intact chest, by external cardiac compression. Prolonged cardiac pacing became a practical proposition in 1958 when Furman and Robinson demonstrated that current passed from the tip of an electrode catheter inserted transvenously into the right ventricle could be used.

Continuing refinements in the design of defibrillators and pacing equipment are widening the applicability of these instruments, especially that of defibrillators. The logistics of preventing death from V.F. or asystole now differ only in detail from those of preventing a fatal outcome following haemorrhage or gastric perforation. If appropriate action is taken, survival of the stricken individual may be expected.

The selection of suitable equipment and its optimal development and maintenance are crucial to the success of resuscitation within the I.T.U., the hospital, and beyond. Defibrillators and pacemakers are found mainly in cardiac care areas. Many non-cardiac I.T.U.s are, however, equipped with defibrillators, and patients with external pacemakers are sometimes transferred to surgical or respiratory units. The staff of all varieties of I.T.U. may, therefore, need to acquaint themselves with these items of equipment.

DEFIBRILLATORS

Principles of defibrillation

Ventricular fibrillation is characterised by the presence of multiple depolarisation wave fronts in the ventricles. Defibrillation is achieved by causing simultaneous depolarisation of a critical mass of myocardium (Zipes et al., 1975). A powerful electrical discharge will depolarise all excitable fibres. Formerly, alternating current was used, but the superiority of direct current was demonstrated by Gurvich and Yuniev (1946) and again by Lown et al. (1962). The latter authors also demonstrated that the waveform of the defibrillatory pulse affected the incidence of post-shock dysrhythmias and of myocardial damage.

The optimal pulse waveform cannot be predicted theoretically. Many different configurations including multiple pulses of similar and opposing polarity have been tested (Schuder et al., 1964; Kugelberg, 1967; Resnekov et al., 1968). Less energy is, however, required to achieve defibrillation when a single pulse is employed (Schuder et al., 1970; McFarlane et al., 1971).

In animal studies with single pulse capacitor discharges, it has been found that voltage, current, and energy requirements are less with a critically damped monophasic pulse (Fig. 1) than with the pulse approximating a half sine wave employed by Lown (Anderson and Pantridge, 1971). Hardware weight is also minimised with the more efficient pulse. Peleska (1966) showed experimentally that the waveform illustrated in Fig. 1, with a duration of about 12 ms, was superior

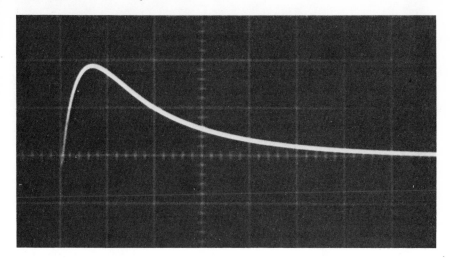

Fig. 1. Critically damped monophasic defibrillatory pulse (see text). This waveform is produced by the miniature defibrillator described. Time calibration: 2 ms.

to various other capacitor discharges. When the capacitor is discharged through the paddles (diameter 8.5 cm for adult defibrillation), the correct waveform is produced by a series inductance. The resistance of the thorax, usually about 50 ohms, also affects the waveform.

The maximum stored energy of most defibrillators currently available is 400 J. The energy delivered to the patient is of course a factor influencing the success of defibrillation. Most defibrillators deliver approximately 75% of the stored energy through a resistance of 50 ohms. The most effective use of the available energy is made by using adequate quantities of a saline-based electrode jelly to reduce skin resistance under the paddles, which are firmly applied below the right clavicle and over the cardiac apex.

Recent developments

Because of the conflicting requirements that defibrillators should defibrillate the hearts of even the heaviest subjects and that they should be as light and portable as possible, machines with various maximum stored energies have become commonplace. It has been suggested that 400 J will fail to defibrillate 35% of individuals weighing over 50 kg (110 lb) and will defibrillate only 50% of those weighing 82 kg (180 lb) (Tacker et al., 1974a). As a result, defibrillators with larger capacitors are being produced.

The wisdom of increasing the size of the capacitor may be questioned. It has yet to be established that the hearts of patients refractory to shocks from 400 J stored energy can often be restored to useful function when larger shocks are given. Furthermore, it is not universally accepted that heavier subjects often require high energy defibrillation. Indeed a 200 J capacitor discharge has been found effective even in heavier patients (Pantridge *et al.*, 1975a,b). One or more shocks of this magnitude were successful in 85% of 33 episodes of V.F. among patients weighing over 80 kg. Defibrillation was achieved in all but one of 27 episodes of primary V.F. occurring among patients within one hour of onset of myocardial infarction, when the energy required is significantly increased (Tacker *et al.*, 1974b).

In 1940, Wiggers noted that, when one defibrillatory shock was insufficient to correct V.F., a series of shocks might be successful, ventricular co-ordination increasing progressively after each shock. Mower *et al.* (1974) made similar observations. These experimental findings may explain the success of a second or third 200 J shock in correcting 13 out of 20 episodes of fibrillation when the initial shock had

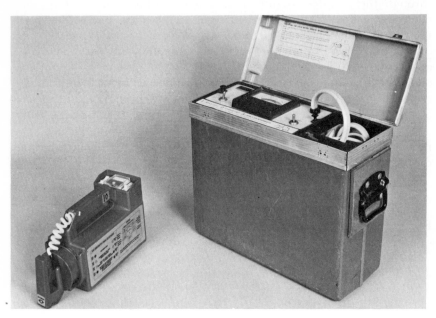

Fig. 2. A miniature defibrillator (left) beside an earlier battery operated defibrillator. (Manufactured by Cardiac Recorders Limited, England.)

failed. A decrease in impedance following the first shock (Geddes *et al.*, 1974) may also have contributed to the success of the later shocks.

High energy defibrillation may damage the heart (Dahl *et al.*, 1974; Ehsani *et al.*, 1976). Thus the traditional use of the highest energy setting on the defibrillator (Dunning, 1972) would have to be abandoned if shocks from a capacitor with maximum stored energy in excess of 400 J were used.

Smaller and cheaper defibrillators, which can be made widely available and perhaps eventually carried in the pocket, will be more relevant to the diverse situations inside and outside the hospital where ventricular fibrillation occurs than will machines that are large and static.

Significant miniaturisation has already been possible without reduction in stored energy (Figs. 2 and 3). The first portable defibrillation system consisted of a standard mains defibrillator powered by two 12 V motorcar batteries through a static invertor (Pantridge and Geddes, 1966). Early self-contained portable defibrillators weighed about 25 kg (55 lb). A battery operated defibrillator is now available weighing only

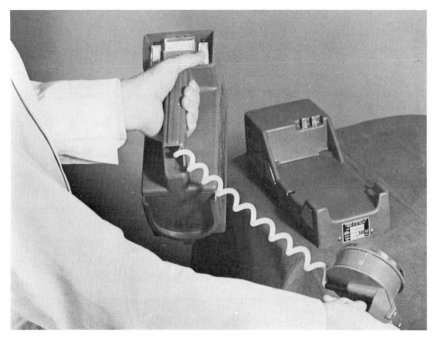

Fig. 3. Miniature defibrillator ready for use. Charging cradle on which defibrillator is stored is visible in the background.

3.2 kg (7 lb) (Pantridge *et al.*, 1975a,b). Part of the reduction in weight results from the incorporation of the components within the paddles. The pulse waveform is that depicted in Fig. 1, and 25 shocks of 400 J can be given from one battery charge.

Catheter defibrillation

Defibrillation has been accomplished in the experimental situation using electrodes mounted on a catheter and introduced into the heart transvenously (Mirowski *et al.*, 1972). The ultimate goal, an implantable automatic defibrillator, has not yet been realised. Nevertheless, catheter defibrillation, if adapted for clinical use, could find immediate application in the relatively pain-free correction of refractory recurrent V.F.

Determination of cardiac rhythm

In situations where all patients are not monitored a means of diagnosing V.F. is necessary. For this purpose combined defibrillators and monitoring oscilloscopes are available.

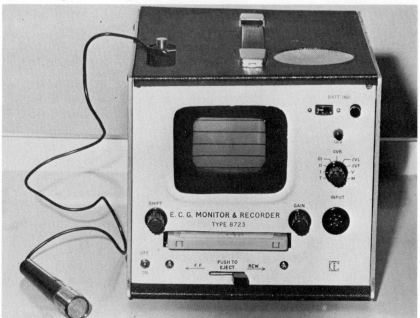

Fig. 4. Portable monitor/tape recorder for documentation of rhythm disturbance. Verbal comments are later transcribed on to the permanent chart record.

Documentary evidence of V.F. prior to d.c. shock is usually regarded as mandatory. Chart recorders are heavy and add unwanted weight to resuscitation equipment if this has to be carried. A relatively light-weight tape-recorder attached to an oscilloscope (Fig. 4), with a second recording channel for verbal comments, has proved especially valuable for the rapid monitoring of patients outside hospital (Pantridge et al., 1975b).

Power sources

Power for portable defibrillators is conveniently derived from recharge-able nickel-cadmium batteries. Where V.F. is liable to be frequent, as in cardiac care areas, a second defibrillator is substituted when V.F. is repetitive. Optional mains connection may be possible in the near future. Several hours must elapse before a fully discharged battery defibrillator is fully recharged.

PACEMAKERS

Pacemaker characteristics

Pacemakers intended for high voltage stimulation through external paddles are now obsolete. Immediate pacing may be achieved more conveniently by means of praecordial blows. Intracardiac electrodes are invariably employed for electrical pacing.

External pacemakers for emergency use deliver approximately rectangular stimuli of 1–2 ms duration. Stimulus strength is calibrated in volts or milliamps, with a maximum of about 10 volts (20 milliamps). A wide range of pacing rates is possible. Because of the hazard of V.F. precipitated by small leakage currents from imperfectly grounded equipment, only battery operated pacemakers are used (Whalen and Starmer, 1967).

Stimuli coinciding with the vulnerable period near the apex of the T wave may precipitate V.F. Pacemakers are therefore usually operated in a ventricle-inhibited, or 'demand' node, in which spontaneously occurring Q.R.S. complexes are sensed, and reset the timing mech-anism (Sowton, 1967). The form of the endocardial Q.R.S. complex is variable and in certain situations the amplitude may be of low voltage (Chatterjee et al., 1968), or the frequency may be inappropriate (Sutton et al., 1975). Sensitivity is therefore variable (e.g. 0.5–5 mV). The highest possible inhibit voltage (i.e. lowest sensitivity) is selected to minimise sensing of other signals (Escher et al., 1971; Barold, 1973).

Occasionally inappropriate sensing of signals generated by faulty connections, or extraneous noise necessitate operation of the pacemaker in asynchronous, or 'fixed rate', mode (Pickers and Goldberg, 1969; Sowton *et al.*, 1970). Diathermy equipment interferes even with fixed-rate operation, and the patient is 'weaned' from the pacemaker temporarily if diathermy must be used in the vicinity.

Most pacemakers include visible confirmation of each pacing and sensing event. A battery-check indicator is also provided.

Typical pacemakers are shown in Fig. 5. Relatively large instruments are intended for patients confined to bed, while the smaller pacemaker is suitable for ambulant patients.

Electrodes

When pacing is required following cardiac surgery, pacing electrodes attached to the epicardium intra-operatively are used. In the coronary care unit a number 5 or 6F bipolar electrode catheter is usually inserted transvenously and its tip positioned at the right ventricular apex under fluoroscopic control. The electrode at the catheter tip lies in close contact with the endocardium and is connected to the negative output of the pacemaker. The stimulation threshold is lower and the V.F.

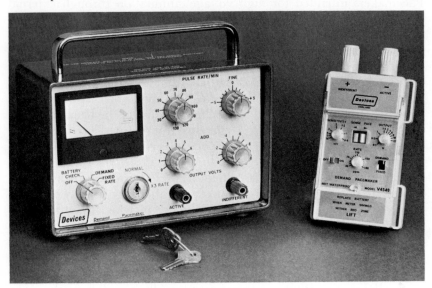

Fig. 5. Bedside and 'ambulatory' pacemakers. The bedside unit has a 'fast rate' facility. When the switch is operated with the key, the pacing rate is three times that indicated on the rate control. (Manufactured by Devices Limited, England.)

threshold higher with this configuration (Hoffman and Cranefield, 1960). The use of electrode catheters with an increase in the surface area of the proximal (ring) electrode, and the introduction of pacemakers which deliver pulses of about 0.5 ms duration will further reduce the risk of inducing V.F. Equipment with these characteristics is not, however, widely available.

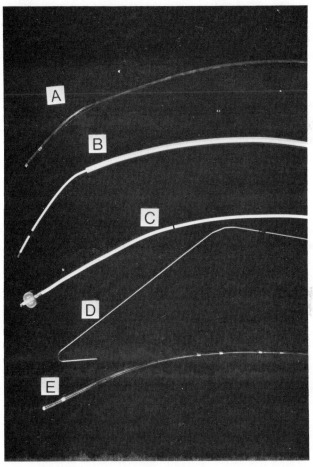

Fig. 6. Electrode catheters: A, bipolar 6F electrode; B, 4F electrode for cannula-introduction, with sleeving to facilitate sterile technique; C, balloon 'Swan-Ganz' electrode for 'blind' insertion; D, transthoracic pacing stylet, curve proximal to tip ensures endocardial contact after insertion; E, hexapolar Berkovits-Castellanos 6F electrode for sequential AV pacing; one of proximal electrode pairs is adjusted to achieve atrial capture after tip is positioned in ventricle. (Manufacturers: A and E, USCI, U.S.A.; B, Cordis Corporation, U.S.A.; C, Edwards Laboratories, U.S.A.; D, Electro-Catheter Corporation, U.S.A.)

Various electrode catheters are shown in Fig. 6. The 4F gauge electrode is particularly suitable for emergency insertion with a minimum of sterile preparation. It is inserted through a needle-cannula introduced percutaneously into an antecubital or subclavian vein (Macaulay and Wright, 1970).

Transvenous pacing is possible without fluoroscopic aid. The position of the electrode may be determined by recording an electrogram from the tip (Bay and Sivertssen, 1967). A balloon-tipped electrode catheter of the type introduced by Swan *et al.* (1970) may be used in conjunction with this method. The balloon is deflated when the electrogram indicates that the tip lies in the right ventricle and the electrode advanced to make contact with the endocardium.

Occasionally a chaotic heart rhythm warrants transthoracic electrode insertion. A fine electrode stylet with a central core insulated from a coiled spring sleeve is introduced into the right ventricle through a 15 cm (6 inch), 18 gauge needle directed posteriorly and slightly to the left from the fourth left intercostal space.

Special pacemakers

A higher cardiac output is obtained in the critically ill patient if a normal atrio-ventricular sequence is restored (Chamberlain *et al.*, 1970). When A–V block is present a hexapolar electrode is employed. One of two pairs of proximal electrodes is adjusted in the upper or lateral right atrium until stable atrial capture is achieved (Castellanos *et al.*, 1974). An atrio-ventricular sequential, ventricular demand, ('bifocal') pacemaker is connected to the appropriate poles of the catheter, and the sequential interval set at 100–150 ms. The pacemaker may also be used for control of re-entrant dysrhythmias associated with accessary atrio-ventricular pathways (Dreifus *et al.*, 1975).

Termination of tachycardia by programmed electrical stimulation

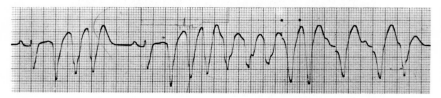

Fig. 7. Monitor E.C.G. lead from patient with ventricular irritability refractory to massive doses of procaine amide. Ventricular tachycardia corrected by two premature stimuli with intervals arbitrarily set at 280 ms. Timing of stimuli indicated by dots.

during electrophysiological studies is now commonplace (Wellens, 1975). Conversion of refractory recurrent ventricular tachycardia by this method (Fig. 7) is sometimes possible (Spurrell *et al.*, 1973). One or more stimuli are introduced via the pacing electrode at selected intervals after a detected R wave. The complicated stimulating device cannot be operated without significant preliminary experience and comparable results may be obtained by brief bursts of rapid unsynchronised stimulation at a rate slightly higher than that of the tachycardia. For this purpose a rapid-rate switch is provided on some pacemakers (Fig. 5).

REFERENCES

Anderson, J. and Pantridge, J. F. (1971). Unpublished.

Barold, S. S. (1973). Inapparent signals to demand pacemakers (editorial). *Chest* **63**, 467.

Bay, G. and Sivertssen, E. (1967). Intracardiac pacing as emergency treatment in Adams-Stokes syndrome. *Brit. Med. J.* **4**, 199.

Castellanos, A., Berkovits, B. V., Castillo, C. A. and Befeler, B. (1974). Sextapolar catheter electrode for temporary sequential atrioventricular pacing. *Cardiovasc. Res.* **8**, 712.

Chamberlain, D. A., Leinbach, R. C., Vassaux, C. E., Kastor, J. A., DeSanctis, R. W. and Sanders, C. A. (1970). Sequential atrioventricular pacing in heart block complicating acute myocardial infarction. *New Engl. J. Med.* **282**, 577.

Chatterjee, K., Sutton, R. and Davies, J. G. (1968). Low intracardiac potentials in myocardial infarction as a cause of failure of inhibition of demand pacemakers. *Lancet* **1**, 511.

Dahl, C. F., Ewy, G. A., Warner, E. D. and Thomas, E. D. (1974). Myocardial necrosis from direct current countershock: effect of paddle electrode size and time intervals between discharges. *Circulation* **50**, 956.

Dreifus, L. S., Berkovits, B. V., Kimibiris, D., Moghadam, K., Haupt, G., Walinsky, P., Thomas, P. and Brockman, S. K. (1975). Use of atrial and bifocal cardiac pacemakers for treating resistant dysrhythmias. *Eur. J. Cardiol.* **3**, 257.

Dunning, A. J. (1972). The treatment of ventricular fibrillation. *In* 'Textbook of Coronary Care' (Ed. L. E. Meltzer and A. J. Dunning) p. 371. Excerpta Medica, Amsterdam.

Ehsani, A., Ewy, G. A. and Sobel, B. E. (1976). Effects of electrical countershock on serum creatine phosphokinase (CPK) isoenzyme activity. *Am. J. Cardiol.* **37**, 12.

Escher, D. J. W., Furman, S., Parker, B. and Solomon, N. (1971). Malfunction in demand pacing (abstract). *Clin. Res.* **19**, 312.

Furman, S. and Robinson, G. (1958). The use of an intracardiac pacemaker in the correction of total heart block. *Surg. Forum* **9**, 245.

Geddes, L. A., Tacker, W. A. Jr., Cabler, P. S., Chapman, R. J., Rivera, R. A. and Kidder, H. R. (1974). Electrode-subject impedance with successive defibrillations. *Circulation* **50** (Suppl. 3) 99.

Gurvich, N. L. and Yuniev, G. S. (1946). Restoration of regular rhythm in the mammalian fibrillating heart. *Am. Rev. sov. Med.* **3**, 236.

Hoffman, B. F. and Cranefield, P. F. (1960). 'Electrophysiology of the Heart.' Blakiston Division of McGraw-Hill, New York.

Kouwenhoven, W. B., Jude, J. R. and Knickerbocker, G. G. (1960). Closed-chest cardiac massage. *J. Am. Med. Ass.* **173**, 1064.

Kugelberg, J. (1967). Ventricular defibrillation: a new aspect. *Acta chir. scand.* (Suppl. 372), 1.

Lown, B., Neuman, J., Amarasingham, R. and Berkovits, B. V. (1962). Comparison of alternating current with direct current electroshock across the closed chest. *Am. J. Cardiol.* **10**, 223.

Macaulay, M. B. and Wright, J. S. (1970). Transvenous cardiac pacing. Experience with a percutaneous supraclavicular approach. *Brit. Med. J.* **4**, 207.

McFarlane, J., Geddes, L. A., Milnor, W., Tacker, W. A., Bourland, J. and Coulter, T. W. (1971). Ventricular defibrillation with single and multiple half sinusoidal pulses of current. *Cardiovasc. Res.* **5**, 286.

Mirowski, M., Mower, M. M., Staewen, W. S., Denniston, R. H. and Mendeloff, A. I. (1972). The development of the transvenous automatic defibrillator. *Archs. Intern. Med.* **129**, 773.

Mower, M. M., Mirowski, M., Spear, J. F. and Moore, E. N. (1974). Patterns of ventricular activity during catheter defibrillation. *Circulation* **49**, 858.

Pantridge, J. F. and Geddes, J. S. (1966). Cardiac arrest after myocardial infarction. *Lancet* **1**, 807.

Pantridge, J. F., Adgey, A. A. J., Webb, S. W. and Anderson, J. (1975a). Electrical requirements for ventricular defibrillation. *Brit. Med. J.* **2**, 313.

Pantridge, J. F., Adgey, A. A. J., Geddes, J. S. and Webb, S. W. (1975b). 'The Acute Coronary Attack.' Pitman Medical, Tunbridge Wells.

Peleska, B. (1966). Optimal parameters of electrical impulses for defibrillation by condenser discharges. *Circ. Res.* **18**, 10.

Pickers, B. A. and Goldberg, M. J. (1969). Inhibition of a demand pacemaker and interference with monitoring equipment by radio-frequency transmissions. *Brit. Med. J.* **2**, 504.

Resnekov, L., Norman, J., Lord, P. and Sowton, E. (1968). Ventricular defibrillation by monophasic trapezoidal-shaped double-pulses of low electrical energy. *Cardiovasc. Res.* **3**, 261.

Schuder, J. C., Stoeckle, H. and Dolan, A. M. (1964). Transthoracic ventricular defibrillation with square-wave stimuli: one-half cycle, one cycle and multicycle waveforms. *Circ. Res.* **15**, 258.

Schuder, J. C., Stoeckle, H., Keskar, P. Y., Gold, J. H., Chier, M. T. and West, J. A. (1970). Transthoracic ventricular defibrillation in the dog with unidirectional rectangular double pulses. *Cardiovasc. Res.* **4**, 497.

Sowton, E. (1967). Clinical application of demand pacemakers. *Brit. Med. J.* **3**, 576.

Sowton, E., Gray, K. and Preston, T. (1970). Electrical interference in non-competitive pacemakers. *Brit. Heart J.* **32**, 626.

Spurrell, R. A. J., Sowton, E. and Deuchar, D. C. (1973). Ventricular tachycardia in 4 patients evaluated by programmed electrical stimulation of heart and treated in 2 patients by surgical division of anterior radiation of left bundle-branch. *Brit. Heart J.* **35**, 1014.

Sutton, R., Norman, J. and Briers, L. (1975). Sick sinus syndrome (letter). *Brit. Med. J.* **3**, 367.

Swan, H. J. C., Ganz, W., Forrester, J., Marcus, H., Diamond, G. and Chonette, D. (1970). Catheterisation of the heart in man with use of a flow-directed balloon-tipped catheter. *New Engl. J. Med.* **283**, 447.

Tacker, W. A. Jr., Galioto, F. M., Giuliani, E., Geddes, L. A. and McNamara, D. G. (1974a). Energy dosage for human trans-chest electrical ventricular defibrillation. *New Engl. J. Med.* **290**, 214.

Tacker, W. A. Jr., Geddes, L. A., Cabler, P. S. and Moore, A. G. (1974b). Electrical threshold for defibrillation of canine ventricles following myocardial infarction. *Am. Heart J.* **88**, 476.

Wellens, H. J. J. (1975). Contribution of cardiac pacing to our understanding of the Wolff-Parkinson-White syndrome. *Brit. Heart J.* **37**, 231.

Whalen, R. E. and Starmer, C. F. (1967). Electric shock hazards in clinical cardiology. *Mod. Concepts. Cardiovasc. Dis.* **36**, 7.

Wiggers, C. J. (1940). The physiologic basis for cardiac resuscitation from ventricular fibrillation – method for serial defibrillation. *Am. Heart J.* **20**, 413.

Zipes, D. P., Fischer, J., King, R. M., Nicholl, A. deB. and Jolly, W. W. (1975). Termination of ventricular fibrillation in dogs by depolarising a critical amount of myocardium. *Am. J. Cardiol.* **36**, 37.

Zoll, P. M. (1952). Resuscitation of the heart in ventricular standstill by external electric stimulation. *New Engl. J. Med.* **247**, 768.

Zoll, P. M., Linenthal, A. J., Gibson, W., Paul, M. H. and Norman, L. R. (1956). Termination of ventricular fibrillation in man by externally applied electric countershock. *New Engl. J. Med.* **254**, 727.

Section 2: Infusion Systems, Blood Warmers, Blood Pumps and Microfilters

H. F. SEELEY

In this section the principles governing the design and use of infusion systems, blood warmers, blood pumps and microfilters will be considered.

Medical instrumentation is developing at a pace which embarrasses the financial resources of most hospitals and in general the cheapest system which performs adequately and safely will have to be chosen. Prices and specifications change constantly and intending buyers should always check with manufacturers. A useful review of the principles involved in selecting equipment for intensive therapy, together with a list of names and addresses of suppliers, is given by Hayes and Healy (1973).

INFUSION SYSTEMS

A summary of the main features of various infusion systems is given in Table 1. Systems for the accurate control of infusion rate are required when potentially hazardous drugs are being administered intravenously or when the rate of infusion is to be governed by the patient's response. It is important to ensure that any drug infused over a period of hours will not deteriorate because of temperature changes or dilution with an unsuitable carrier solution. A further problem may be adsorption of the drug on to the plastic material of syringes and infusion sets (Sönksen, 1976).

Systems for controlled infusion may be divided into low volume and variable volume.

Low volume

These devices are accurate 'syringe pushers' and permit continuous infusion of 10–20 ml of fluid over 12–24 hours. The power is provided by an electric or clockwork motor; the latter allows the patient considerable mobility and is free from electrical hazard (Handley, 1970). Though originally introduced for cytotoxic drug therapy (Pegg et al., 1963) their uses have been extended to the infusion of heparin (Handley, 1967) and insulin (Page et al., 1974). A commercial infusor driven by clockwork is shown in Fig. 1.

A system which is useful for keeping arterial and venous lines open and yet infuses only 3 ml/h is described by Shinebourne and Pfitzner (1973).

Variable volume

Devices for controlling infusion rate over the range 1 ml/h to several litres/hour will be described in increasing order of sophistication.

Standard gravity-fed administration set
The behaviour and deficiencies of this system have been described by Flack and Whyte (1974). Nevertheless in experienced hands and with constant adjustment they are sufficiently accurate for administering parenteral feeding solutions.

Accurate gravity-fed administration set
Small drops whose size is less subject to variation are formed at the end of a fine metal tube. A plastic gate clip provides more reliable control than a roller clip. A graduated fluid reservoir allows drugs to be added to a small volume of fluid and guards against inadvertent over-transfusion if the gate clip is left open.

Electronic drop counter
Fluid is driven along the plastic tube of a standard infusion set by an electrically-powered peristaltic pump. A photoelectric detector is clamped to the drip chamber. The rate of infusion is determined by the drop-rate setting and the drop detector applies feedback control.

Though this system has proved very popular it is important to realise that it is a drop counter and variations in drop size will cause corresponding variations in volume infused. Though feedback control guards against an excessive number of drops it will not guarantee that the drops are equally spaced.

Roller pumps
Because of their simplicity and low cost these are becoming increasingly popular. The rate of infusion depends on the motor speed and the bore of the tubing beneath the rollers but can be accurately determined. Errors can arise if the wrong sized tubing is selected and since the pump

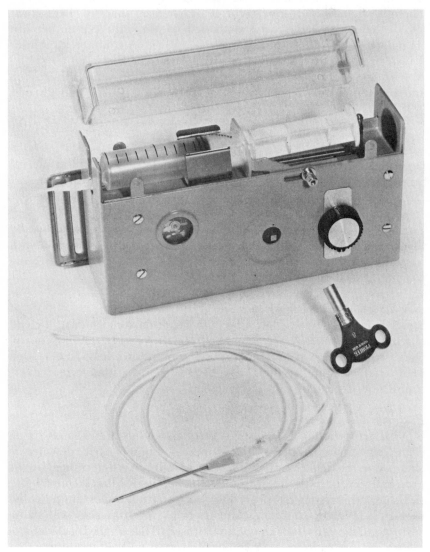

Fig. 1. Clockwork-powered infusor suitable for continuous drug administration.

is usually calibrated in revolutions/minute or divisions of a poten-
tiometer scale, a conversion table is usually necessary to determine
infusion rate in ml/h.

Volumetric infusion pump
This device is the logical successor to the electronic drop counter. The
disposable cassette consists of a pumping chamber, associated tubes to
allow fluid to be drawn into the chamber and then infused into the
patient, and a rotating valve.

The machine can be regarded as a self-filling 'syringe pusher' with a
wide range of infusion rates. Strictly speaking, infusion will not be
continuous as there will be a brief interruption whilst the syringe is
recharging; however, this is unlikely to be important in clinical
practice. A photograph of the pump with the cassette in place is shown
in Fig. 2.

Systems incorporating mechanical pumps are designed for both
arterial and venous infusion. It is important to check the cannulae at
frequent intervals to guard against extravasation of fluid since these
devices are capable of overcoming high pressures. Because of the risk of
entraining air and causing an embolus, a bubble detector should be
fitted which will switch off the pump if air enters the line.

Table 1 gives a comparison of various infusion systems.

BLOOD WARMERS

The problems which accompany rapid transfusion of stored blood are
well known (Burton and Holderness, 1964; Burton, 1968; Churchill-
Davidson, 1968). Though changes in biochemistry and cellular
function accompany storage of blood at 4°C, temperature appears to be
an important factor in the morbidity associated with massive transfusion (Mollison, 1972). This seems especially marked when the patient
is sick (Boyan and Howland, 1961; Ozinsky, 1963). In this context it is
worth remembering that on occasions the rapid infusion of fluids other
than blood may be necessary. The treatment of severe diabetic
ketoacidosis is one example.

Blood may be warmed before or during infusion. The simplest
method of warming blood prior to infusion is to stand the container in a
water bath at 37°C. However it takes at least 20 min to warm a bottle of
blood. Though there is some dispute over the temperature at which
significant haemolysis occurs in stored blood (Chalmers and Russell,
1973), it is generally agreed that heating above 40°C should not be

Table 1. Comparison of various infusion systems

Device	Advantages	Disadvantages
Syringe infusor	Electric or clockwork-powered. Patient can be fully mobile. Arterial or venous infusion. Fluid load can be made very small	Total volume infused limited by size of syringe, therefore used mainly for drug infusion
Standard gravity-fed administration set	Inexpensive	Needs constant adjustment. Infusion rate determined mainly by patient's venous pressure; some variation due to 'creep' in plastic
Accurate gravity-fed administration set	Fluid reservoir for adding drugs; also guards against over-transfusion. Drop size less variable; control clip more reliable	Still needs constant adjustment since rate determined mainly by patient's venous pressure
Electronic drop counter	Constant arterial or venous infusion. Usually fitted with bubble detector	Feedback circuitry complex and expensive. No allowance for change in drop size. Drops may not be equally spaced
Roller pump	Constant arterial or venous infusion. Relatively simple and inexpensive. Uses standard drip tubing	Bubble detector may not be supplied. Calibration depends on drip tube bore and sometimes on motor gearing
Volumetric pump	Constant arterial or venous infusion. Wide range of infusion rates directly calibrated. Price comparable with that of drop counter as electronic control relatively simple	Disposable cassettes. Expensive

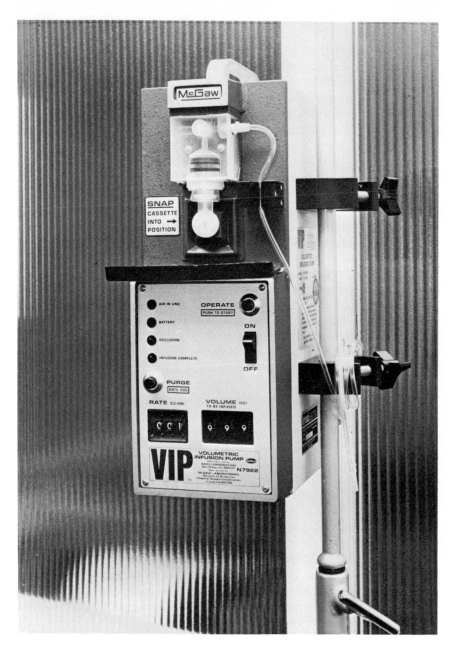

Fig. 2. Volumetric infusion pump with disposable cassette.

permitted. The temperature limits for the water bath are therefore narrow.

The second method of warming prior to infusion uses the energy of electromagnetic radiation. The original work was reported by Besseling *et al.* (1965). A unit of blood may be warmed to 37°C in 4 minutes but failure of mixing and the presence of any metal will give rise to localised overheating beyond the control of any heat sensor, which must necessarily remain outside the container. Severe haemolysis produced by a machine using this principle has been reported by Staples and Griner (1971), and McCullough *et al.* (1972). Restall (1974) suggests overcoming this problem by heating the blood to only 27°C.

Devices which warm during infusion pass blood through a long fluid path of narrow cross-sectional area. This path is in contact with a heat source thermostatically maintained at about 37°C; an additional alarm or cut-out system operates when the temperature reaches about 41°C. The heat source must have sufficient power to warm blood to an adequate temperature when the infusion rate is high.

The most common heat source is an electrically heated water bath. The addition of an agitator ensures uniform water temperature and improves the efficiency of heat transfer at high infusion rates. In one commercial instrument, the Fenwal 'dry heat' warmer, the heat source consists of two electrically heated metal plates, the fluid path being sandwiched between them.

The fluid path most commonly consists of a coiled plastic tube. Since the coil is immersed in a water bath adequate earthing is essential since any fault in the coil could allow an electric current to flow into the patient. The fluid path used with the Fenwal warmer consists of two rectangular plastic sheets welded together in a 'maze' pattern to provide one long continuous channel. A water bath warmer together with its infusion coil is shown in Fig. 3.

Plastic coils can be made from polyvinylchloride (P.V.C.) or polyethylene. P.V.C. coils are more flexible but polyethylene has a higher thermal conductivity (Xifaras and Healy, 1971). The Fenwal warming bag is made of P.V.C.

A long fluid path may offer significant resistance to flow. It is therefore important to establish the maximum blood flow which can be achieved with any coil using a standard giving set and gravity feed. Coils with low maximum flow may require an infusion pump for rapid transfusion.

A very comprehensive review of the problems of blood warmer design and comparison of some commercially available coils and warmers is

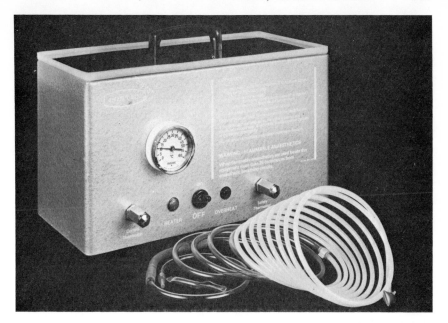

Fig. 3. Water bath blood warmer with disposable coil.

given by Russell (1974). A further comparison of the performance of four blood warmers is given by Harrison and Healy (1975).

A warming device must not introduce any unfavourable changes in the composition of blood. Manners and Mills (1968) described changes in plasma potassium and haemoglobin concentrations but most of the blood used in their study was at least 21 days old. Desmonts *et al.* (1975) investigated the effect of a 'dry heat' warmer on some components of stored blood. Warming resulted in no statistically significant changes in plasma potassium, sodium or pH after various periods of storage. Slight rises in plasma haemoglobin concentration observed were unlikely to be of clinical importance. However, as Dalili and Adriani (1974) have pointed out, investigations of this type do not show what happens to warmed blood once it has been infused into the patient.

BLOOD PUMPS

Many of the makeshift arrangements which have been devised for the rapid infusion of blood display considerable ingenuity but little regard for the problems of air embolism.

There are three principal methods for increasing the rate of infusion of blood: (*a*) modified administration set, (*b*) Martin's pump and (*c*) constant pressure bag.

The modified administration set has a valve incorporated into the drip chamber which allows 'milking' of blood along the tube by manual compression. Miyatake (1961) has shown that this system can cause appreciable haemolysis, particularly if the filtration and pumping chambers are combined.

The Martin's pump is a hand-operated roller pump which can be conveniently mounted on a drip stand. Clinical experience suggests that skill in its use and the degree of trauma inflicted on the blood are very variable. A review of the factors involved in selecting a roller pump for more specialised uses is given by Muir and Lewis (1972).

The constant pressure bag is made of tough material and can be inflated by a hand pump up to a pressure of 300 mm Hg; the pressure can be measured with the Bourdon gauge which is connected to the bag. A plastic infusion bottle can be placed in a pocket in the side of the bag and so subjected to high pressure. This system has the advantage that it releases an assistant and the infusion rate can be controlled solely by the clamp on the administration set.

du Plessis and Bull (1966) investigated the pressure bag as a means of rapid transfusion and found it caused less haemolysis than a modified administration set (Fig. 4). They also reviewed other likely causes of haemolysis during rapid transfusion and suggested ways of reducing it to a minimum.

BLOOD MICROFILTERS

Increasing interest has been shown recently in changes which occur in the cellular components of blood stored at 4°C. Swank (1961) reported that stored blood contains debris consisting mainly of platelet aggregates in which leucocytes, fibrin strands and occasional red cells become trapped. These changes could be observed after 24 h when A.C.D. was used as anticoagulant but after only 2 h when heparin was used. In general the amount of debris increased with storage time (Moseley and Doty, 1970). After one week of storage these aggregates may number $140 \times 10^6/l$ and range in size from 10 to 164 µm (Connell and Swank, 1973).

A study of combat casualties in Vietnam showed that cellular debris is filtered primarily by the lungs and secondarily by the systemic capillaries. The degree of postoperative hypoxaemia observed was

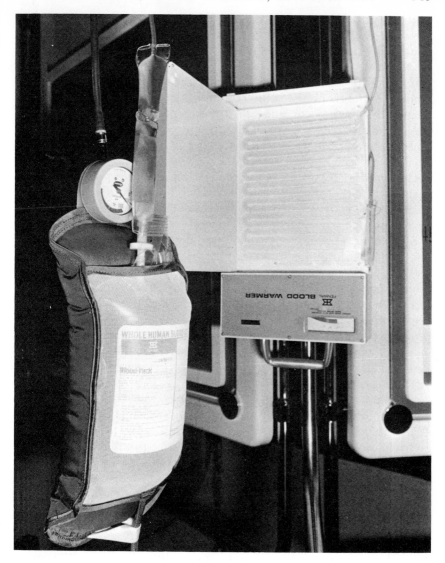

Fig. 4. Pressure infusor used in conjunction with Fenwal 'dry heat' blood warmer.

related to the volume of blood which had been transfused (McNamara *et al.*, 1970). It has been suggested that these microemboli may cause mechanical obstruction to the pulmonary vessels or release vasoactive substances which lead to ventilation – perfusion abnormalities (Blaisdell *et al.*, 1970).

However the requirements of any filter to remove these microemboli are stringent. Whilst filtering effectively they must not impede blood flow to any significant extent since patients most likely to benefit from microfiltration are those who are hypovolaemic and require rapid transfusion. The filter will begin to clog and reduce flow once a certain amount of debris has been filtered and if depth filtration is employed, channelling may occur and allow larger particles to pass. Red cells traversing microfilter are likely to be subjected to considerable pressure and it is important to establish that significant haemolysis does not occur.

Commercial blood microfilters have an effective pore size which varies in different models between 20 and 40 μm. Among the filtering elements used are pleated polyester mesh, randomly packed dacron wool, and polyester foam.

Studies on resistance have compared flow through various microfilters with flow through a standard giving set having a pore size of about 200 μm. Cullen and Ferrara (1974) and Buley and Lumley (1975) have shown that a 40 μm filter can permit a flow rate equivalent to that through a standard infusion set, even when up to 10 units of blood have been infused. Microfilters having a smaller pore size showed a progressive deterioration in flow as the number of units filtered was increased, and this effect was more marked with old blood. Cullen and Ferrara (1974) suggested that channelling occurs with a dacron wool depth filter.

The same pairs of investigators also studied the increase in plasma haemoglobin after blood had passed through various microfilters. The 40 μm filter gave increases comparable with those seen with a standard giving set whereas those with smaller pore size produced a significant degree of haemolysis, especially when several units of old blood had been infused.

Studies on the effect of microfiltration on the platelet count of fresh blood are conflicting. Cullen and Ferrara (1974) reported no change in count after passage through at 40 μm filter whereas Dunbar et al. (1974) reported a 25% fall. Neither group could detect any significant haemolysis. However, there is not yet any clinical evidence to suggest that patients benefit from microfiltration of fresh blood.

It has already been stated that stored blood will contain aggregates whose size ranges from 10 μm upwards. Since a 40 μm filter will pass appreciable quantities of smaller debris it is reasonable to ask whether use of a filter with pores this large results in clinical improvement. Clinical trials such as those of Goldiner et al. (1972) and Reul et al.

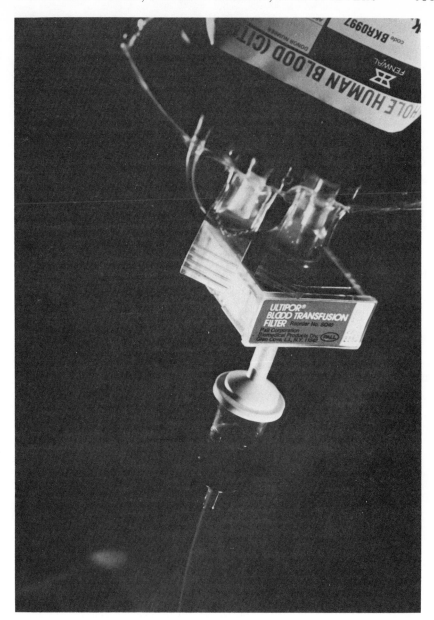

Fig. 5. 40 μm microfilter in use during blood transfusion.

(1973) suggest that the incidence of respiratory failure following massive blood transfusion can be very substantially reduced.

Firm indications for the use of microfilters in blood transfusion have not yet been established. Their use cannot eliminate the problem of platelet microemboli for Hissen and Swank (1965) have observed changes in the blood of dogs submitted to haemorrhagic shock and severe soft tissue trauma which parallel those in banked blood. Platelet microemboli have been observed in the lungs of patients dying from burns and injury even when no blood has been transfused (Sevitt, 1970). The use of a 40 μm filter does not seem to be associated with technical problems above those seen with simple transfusion. It would seem logical, therefore, to microfilter when large volumes of banked blood are transfused or when other factors are present which may contribute to the development of respiratory failure or the shock lung syndrome (Dowd and Jenkins, 1972; Stoddart, 1974).

A 40 μm microfilter using pleated polyester mesh as filter material is shown in Fig. 5.

REFERENCES

Besseling, J. L. N., Bull, A. B., du Plessis, J. M. E. and Mason, I. M. (1965). The rapid warming of blood for massive transfusion by radiofrequency induction. *S. Afr. Med. J.* **39**, 137.

Blaisdell, F. W., Lim, R. C. and Stallone, R. J. (1970). The mechanism of pulmonary damage following traumatic shock. *Surg. Gynec. Obstet.* **130**, 15.

Boyan, C. P. and Howland, W. S. (1961). Blood temperature: a critical factor in massive transfusion. *Anesthesiology* **22**, 559.

Buley, R. and Lumley, J. (1975). Some observations on blood microfilters. *Ann. roy. Coll. Surg.* **57**, 262.

Burton, G. W. and Holderness, M. C. (1964). On the management of massive blood transfusion. *Anaesthesia* **19**, 408.

Burton, G. W. (1968). Massive blood transfusion. *Proc. roy. Soc. Med.* **61**, 682.

Chalmers, C. and Russell, W. J. (1973). When does blood haemolyse?: a temperature study. *Brit. J. Anaesth.* **45**, 1237.

Churchill-Davison, H. C. (1968). Massive blood transfusion. *Proc. roy. Soc. Med.* **61**, 681.

Connell, R. S. and Swank, R. L. (1973). Pulmonary microembolism after blood transfusions: an electron microscopic study. *Ann. Surg.* **177**, 40.

Cullen, D. J. and Ferrara, L. C. (1974). Comparative evaluation of blood filters. *Anesthesiology* **41**, 568.

Dalili, H. and Adriani, J. (1974). Effects of various blood warmers on the components of bank blood. *Anesth. Analg. curr. Res.* **53**, 125.

Desmonts, J. M., Duvaldestin, P. and Henzel, D. (1975). The effects of a dry heat blood warmer on some components of stored blood. *Anaesthesia* **30**, 230.

Dowd, J. and Jenkins, L. C. (1972). The lung in shock: a review. *Can. Anaesth. Soc. J.* **19**, 309.

Dunbar, R. W., Price, K. A. and Cannarella, C. F. (1974). Microaggregate blood filters: effect on filtration time, plasma hemoglobin, and fresh blood platelet counts. *Anesth. Analg. curr. Res.* **53**, 577.

du Plessis, J. M. E. and Bull, A. B. (1966). Haemolysis occurring during pressure transfusion of stored blood. *S. Afr. Med. J.* **40**, 479.

Flack, F. C. and Whyte, T. D. (1974). Behaviour of standard gravity-fed administration sets used for intravenous infusion. *Brit. Med. J.* **3**, 439.

Goldiner, P. L., Howland, W. S. and Cole, R. (1972). Filter for prevention of microembolism during massive transfusions. *Anesth. Analg. curr. Res.* **51**, 717.

Handley, A. J. (1967). Heparin administration by a constant infusion pump. *Brit. Med. J.* **2**, 482.

Handley, A. J. (1970). Portable heparin injector. *Lancet* **2**, 313.

Harrison, M. J. and Healy, T. E. J. (1975). A comparison of four blood warmers. *Anaesthesia* **30**, 651.

Hayes, B. and Healy, T. E. J. (1973). Equipment for intensive care. *Brit. J. Hosp. Med.* **9** (Equip. Supp.) 4.

Hissen, W. W. and Swank, R. L. (1965). Screen filtration pressure and pulmonary hypertension. *Am. J. Physiol.* **209**, 715.

Manners, J. M. and Mills, K. L. M. (1968). Another blood warmer: some observations of blood changes using the 'Hemokinetitherm'. *Anaesthesia* **23**, 646.

McCullough, J., Polesky, H. F., Nelson, C. *et al.* (1972). Iatrogenic hemolysis: a complication of blood warmed by a microwave device. *Anesth. Analg. curr. Res.* **51**, 102.

McNamara, J. J., Molot, M. D. and Stremple, J. F. (1970). Screen filtration pressure in combat casualties. *Ann. Surg.* **172**, 334.

Miyatake, S. I., Ruesch, M. and Ballinger, C. M. (1961). Blood transfusion pumps: slight elevation in plasma hemoglobin levels following their use. *Anesth. Analg. curr. Res.* **40**, 199.

Mollison, P. L. (1972). 'Blood transfusion in clinical medicine,' Fifth Edition. Blackwell Scientific Publishers, Oxford.

Moseley, R. V. and Doty, D. B. (1970). Changes in the filtration characteristics of stored blood. *Ann. Surg.* **171**, 329.

Muir, W. M. and Lewis, B. (1972). Which blood pump? *Brit. J. Hosp. Med.* **7** (Equip. Supp.) 4.

Ozinsky, J. (1963). Hypothermia, ventricular fibrillation and halothane. *S. Afr. Med. J.* **37**, 110.

Page, M. McB., Alberti, K. G. M. M., Greenwood, R. *et al.* (1974). Treatment of diabetic coma with continuous low-dose infusion of insulin. *Brit. Med. J.* **2**, 687.

Pegg, D. E., Trotman, R. E. and Pierce, N. H. (1963). Apparatus for continuous infusion chemotherapy. *Brit. Med. J.* **1**, 1207.

Restall, C. J. (1974). Guest discussion following Dalili, H. and Adriani, J. (1974). *Anesth. Analg. curr. Res.* **53**, 130.

Reul, G. J., Greenberg, D. S., Lefrak, E. A. *et al.* (1973). Prevention of post-traumatic pulmonary insufficiency: fine screen filtration of blood. *Archs. Surg.* **106**, 386.

Russell, W. J. (1974). A review of blood warmers for massive transfusion. *Anaesthesia and Intensive Care* **2** (No. 2) 109.

Sevitt, S. (1970). Thrombosis and embolism after injury. *J. Clin. Path.* **23** (Suppl. (Roy. Coll. Path.) 4) 86.

954 H. F. SEELEY

Sönksen, P. (1976). Carrier solutions for low-level intravenous insulin infusion. *Brit. Med. J.* **1**, 151.

Shinebourne, E. and Pfitzner, J. (1973). Continuous flushing device for indwelling arterial and venous cannulae. *Brit. J. Hosp. Med.* **9** (Equip. Supp.) 64.

Staples, P. J. and Griner, P. F. (1971). Extracorporeal hemolysis of blood in a microwave blood warmer. *New Engl. J. Med.* **285**, 317.

Stoddart, J. C. (1974). Respiratory problems in intensive care units. *Brit. J. Hosp. Med.* **11**, 832.

Swank, R. L. (1961). Alteration of blood on storage: Measurement of adhesiveness of 'aging' platelets and leukocytes and their removal by filtration. *New Engl. J. Med.* **265**, 728.

Xifaras, G. P. and Healy, T. E. J. (1971). A comparative study of four blood warming coils. *Anaesthesia* **26**, 229.

IV

Organ Support Systems

Section 1: Mechanical Circulatory Support using Intra-aortic Balloon Counterpulsation

M. H. YACOUB

INTRODUCTION

The use of temporary mechanical circulatory support can favourably influence the outcome in a fairly well defined group of critically ill patients. In recent years intra-aortic balloon counterpulsation (I.A.B.C.) has proved to be a simple, safe and effective method of providing mechanical circulatory support (Moulopolos *et al.*, 1962; Kantrowitz *et al.*, 1968; Buckley *et al.*, 1970; Bregman and Goetz, 1971).

METHODS

I.A.B.C. can be initiated and maintained at the bedside without the need for radiographic screening. Constant monitoring of electrocardiogram, arterial tracing from one of the upper limbs, and the timing of balloon inflation and deflation in relation to the cardiac cycle is essential. Under local anaesthesia a special balloon-bearing catheter is introduced through a small graft attached to the femoral artery. The catheter is then advanced to the descending thoracic aorta and the

955

position of the balloon is adjusted simply by introducing a length of catheter equal to the distance between the femoral artery and the sternal angle (Fig. 1). The catheter is then attached to a special device which allows accurately timed rapid inflation and deflation of the

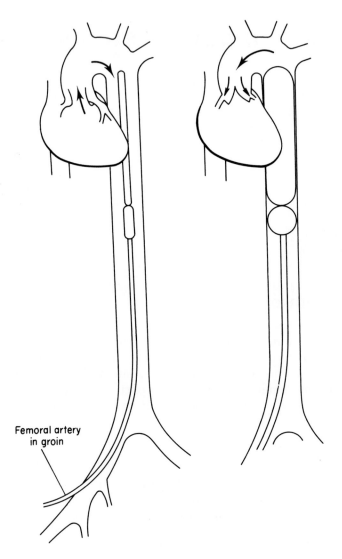

Femoral artery
in groin

Fig. 1. (a) Systole, active balloon deflation, ⟶, reduction of after load. (b) Diastole, active balloon inflation, ⟶, diastolic pressure augmentation; ⟶ increased coronary flow.

balloon using carbon dioxide or helium. Heparinisation is required to prevent clotting around the catheter and/or balloon. In addition, the balloon should not be left for any length of time without being moved (inflated and deflated). Balloon movements can be visualised by non-invasive echocardiography (Weir *et al.*, 1975).

PRINCIPLES

Rapid inflation of the balloon early in diastole produces augmentation of the diastolic pressure, which can reach levels higher than systolic pressure (Fig. 2). This produces marked increase in coronary flow (Fig. 3) due to the fact that coronary flow occurs mainly during diastole and is

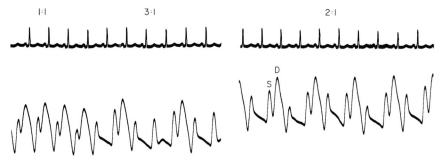

Fig. 2. Changes in systemic pressure with I.A.B.C. S, peak systolic pressure; D, peak diastolic augmentation.

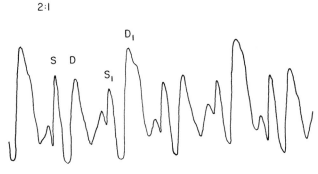

Fig. 3. Effect of I.A.B.C. on coronary flow. Every second beat is augmented. S, systolic coronary flow (measured by electromagnetic flow meter) without counterpulsation; D_1, diastolic coronary flow without augmentation; S_1, systolic coronary flow during counterpulsation; D_1, diastolic coronary flow during counterpulsation showing marked enhancement.

directly proportional to the mean diastolic pressure. Rapid deflation of the balloon at the beginning of the next ventricular systole, before the onset of ejection, reduces the after load (or systemic vascular resistance) and shortens the isometric ventricular systolic phase. This reduces cardiac work and myocardial oxygen consumption and minimises the amount of mitral regurgitation or left to right shunt at ventricular level should either of these haemodynamic disturbances be present. By increasing coronary flow and decreasing myocardial oxygen consumption, I.A.B.C. improves the myocardial oxygen supply/ demand ratio which tends to improve cardiac performance and enhance the chances of recovery of those parts of the myocardium which are damaged but still viable (Braunwald *et al.*, 1969; Powell *et al.*, 1970; Mueller *et al.*, 1971). Apart from its effect on the myocardium I.A.B.C. directly improves general tissue perfusion particularly in the upper parts of the body. Although some balloons are designed to produce a unidirectional impulse in an attempt to deliver maximal counterpulsation to the upper part of the body (Bregman and Goetz, 1971), we have found that the use of these balloons produces additional significant diastolic augmentation in the lower part of the body which could be of value in improving renal perfusion. However, the main improvement in tissue and renal perfusion following I.A.B.C. is due to enhancement of

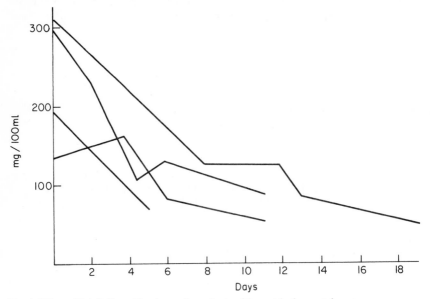

Fig. 4. Effect of I.A.B.C. on blood urea in patients with ventricular septal rupture.

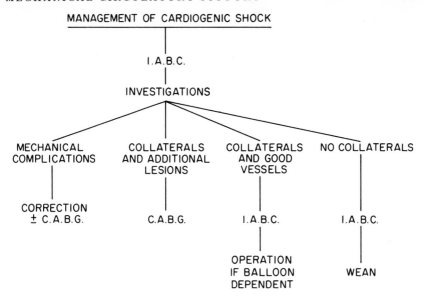

Fig. 5. Scheme for management of cardiogenic shock.

cardiac performance which results in increase of cardiac output (Fig. 4). The increased renal flow in patients with cardiogenic shock usually produces rapid sustained improvement of kidney function (Fig. 5).

INDICATIONS

The place of I.A.B.C. is now fairly well defined after passing through two stages, one of scepticism followed by another of over enthusiasm. The main current indications for I.A.B.C. are:

1. Postmyocardial infarction cardiogenic shock (Sanders *et al.*, 1972; Mueller *et al.*, 1971). This condition has been shown to carry a very high mortality in spite of vigorous medical treatment (Gunnar *et al.*, 1966, 1967). I.A.B.C. produces immediate clinical improvement in these patients and theoretically tends to limit the size of the infarct by maintaining viability of the peri-infarction zone, also it prevents irreversible multi-organ damage. To be effective I.A.B.C. should be started as soon as possible after the onset of cardiogenic shock. It has been shown, however, that counterpulsation alone produces only a modest improvement in long-term survival of these patients (Sanders *et al.*, 1972). To have maximum effect on the grave natural history of cardiogenic shock, I.A.B.C. should be combined with early coronary

and left ventricular angiography followed by myocardial revascular-isation or repair of mechanical lesions when indicated. A scheme for the management of patients with cardiogenic shock is shown in Fig. 5. Coronary angiography has been shown to be safe in patients under-going I.A.B.C. for cardiogenic shock (Leinbach et al., 1972). Revascularisation is only considered if the angiograms show distal filling of the blocked arteries by collaterals, thus suggesting the presence of viable myocardium in the territory of the blocked arteries. Early operation is considered if the patient is considered to be balloon dependant five days from starting I.A.B.C.

In patients with ruptured interventricular septum repair of the rupture with excision of the infarcted area and myocardial re-vascularisation should be performed. The timing of the operation depends on the anatomical type of rupture (Yacoub et al., 1975). In patients with antero- or posteroapical ruptures, repair should be per-formed one week after initiating I.A.B.C. In cases of central rupture, the optimal period of delay between I.A.B.C. and operation is two weeks whereas in posterobasal rupture this interval should be four.

In patients with mitral regurgitation secondary to myocardial infarction, the indication for and timing of operative correction depends on the clinicopathological type (Yacoub, 1972). In patients with massive mitral regurgitation secondary to complete rupture of the whole or major part of one papillary muscle, very early operation is indicated. In patients with subacute regurgitation due to progressive stretching of one papillary muscle in a developing aneurysm, I.A.B.C. should be continued as long as possible. In patients with mild to moderate regurgitation secondary to varying degrees of stretching or rupture of one of the minor heads of one papillary muscle attempts should be made to wean the patient off I.A.B.C. after one week and assess the haemodynamic lesion three months later. Patients with developing aneurysms should be weaned off, if possible, and considered for operation eight to twelve weeks later. If, however, they are balloon dependant I.A.B.C. should be continued for four weeks before considering mitral repair and excision of the aneurysm. This should be combined with revascularisation of ischaemic areas if required.

Acute infarctectomy alone has given disappointing results and should only be considered as part of other operations, e.g. revascularisation or repair of ventricular septal rupture.

2. Postpericardiotomy cardiogenic shock. In patients developing shock after cardiac operations or those who cannot be weaned off cardiopulmonary bypass, I.A.B.C. can be a life saving procedure (Berger et al., 1973; Bolooki et al., 1976). The rationale for its use is the

same as that for cardiogenic shock following myocardial infarction. I.A.B.C. is particularly effective in those patients who sustain myocardial injury just before or during operation, which constitutes a small but important proportion of the overall number of patients undergoing open heart operations.

3. Recurrent acute myocardial ischaemic episodes. I.A.B.C. is indicated in patients with recurrent episodes of prolonged ischaemic chest pain at rest which is not relieved by trinitrin and is associated with S.T. changes. Electrocardiographic and enzyme evidence of acute myocardial infarction may be present (evolving infarcts) or absent (unstable angina). In these patients I.A.B.C. produces immediate relief of pain which is due to increase in blood flow to the ischaemic areas through existing main channels and collaterals as well as decreasing myocardial oxygen consumption.

Within twenty-four hours of instituting I.A.B.C., coronary and left ventricular angiography should be performed. This usually reveals high grade obstructive lesions in the left main or anterior descending coronary arteries with or without lesions in other arteries in the majority of patients (Fig. 6). Revascularisation by bypass grafting all the

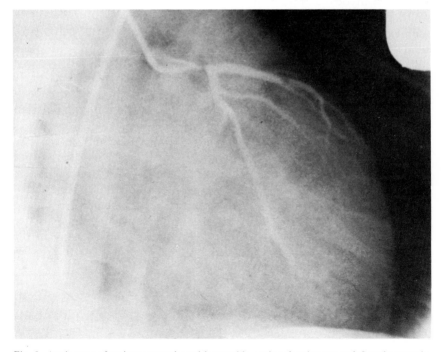

Fig. 6. Angiogram of patient presenting with unstable angina showing severe left main stenosis.

obstructed vessels, followed shortly afterwards by discontinuing
I.A.B.C. yields excellent results with preservation of myocardium and
improvement in left ventricular function (Fig. 7).

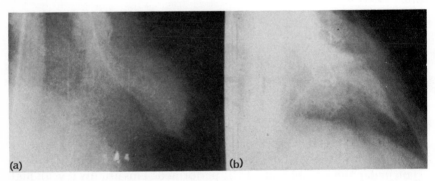

Figs 7(a) and 7(b). Pre- and postoperative left ventricular angiography (both showing end systolic
frames). Postoperative film (b) shows marked improvement in left ventricular segmental wall
motion, following myocardial revascularisation for acute ischaemic episode.

4. Post myocardial infarction, recurrent ventricular arrhythmia. A
small proportion of ventricular arrhythmias prove to be resistant to
medical treatment and could be life threatening. In these cases I.A.B.C.
tends to stabilise the rhythm.

5. Endotoxic shock. Shock as a complication of sepsis still carries a
mortality of 50–80% (Mclean *et al.*, 1967, 1971) in spite of early
diagnosis and intensive medical therapy. Recent clinical and experimental studies have shown that depressed myocardial function plays an
important role in the pathogenesis of septic shock (Clowes, 1971;
Hinshaw *et al.*, 1971; Wilson *et al.*, 1971). In addition sepsis creates an
increased metabolic demand which requires a higher cardiac output
(Clowes *et al.*, 1971; Grump *et al.*, 1970). If the myocardium is
incapable of meeting the extra demand, a vicious circle is created
whereby the inadequate cardiac output leads to metabolic acidosis
which produces further cardiac depression. Experimental evidence
suggests that mechanical circulatory support may be of value in the
treatment of septic shock (Dunn *et al.*, 1974).

REFERENCES

Berger, R. L., Saini, V. K., Ryan, T. J., Sokol, D. M. and Keeje, J. F. (1973). Intra-
aortic balloon assist for post cardiotomy cardiogenic shock. *J. Thorac. Cardiovasc. Surg.*
66, 906.

Bolooki, H., Williams, W., Thurer, R. J., Vargas, A., Kaiser, G. A., Mack, F. and Ghaharmani, A. R. (1976). Clinical and haemodynamic criteria for use of the intra-aortic balloon pump in patients requiring cardiac surgery. *J. Thorac. Cardiovasc. Surg.* **72**, 756.

Braunwald, E., Covell, J. W., Maroko, P. R. and Ross, J. R., Jr. (1969). Effects of drugs and counterpulsation on myocardial oxygen consumption. *Circulation* **39** (Suppl. 4) 220.

Bregman, D. and Goetz, R. H. (1971). Clinical experience with a new cardiac assist device. The dual chambered intra-aortic balloon assist. *J. Thorac. Cardiovasc. Surg.* **62**, 557.

Buckley, M. J., Leinbach, R. C., Kaster, J. A., Laird, C. A. and Austen, W. G. (1970). Hemodynamic evaluation of intra aortic balloon pumping in man. *Circulation* **41**, (Suppl. 2) 11.

Clowes, G. H. A., Jr. (1971). Oxygen transport and utilisation in fulminating sepsis and septic shock. *In* 'Septic shock in Man' (Ed. S. G. Hershey, L. R. M. Del Guerico and R. McGom) p. 85. Little Brown, Boston.

Dunn, J. M., Kirsh, M. M., Harness, J., Lee, R., Starker, J. and Sloan, H. (1974). The role of assisted circulation in the management of endotoxic shock. *Annals of Thorac. Surg.* **17**, 574.

Hinshaw, L. B., Archer, L. J., Greenfield, L. J. and Guenter, C. A. (1971). Effects of endotoxins on myocardial haemodynamics, performance and metabolism. *Am. J. Physiol.* **221**, 504.

Gunnar, R. M., Cruz, A., Boswell, J., Pretras, R. J. and Tobin, J. R., Jr. (1966). Myocardial infarction with shock. Haemodynamic studies and results of therapy. *Circulation* **33**, 753.

Gunnar, R. M., Pretras, R. J., Stavrakos, C., Loeb, H. S. and Tobin, J. R. Jr. (1967). The physiologic basis for treatment of shock associated with myocardial infarction. *Med. Clin. N. Amer.* **51**, 69.

Grump, F. E., Price, J. B., Jr. and Kinney, J. M. (1970). Whole body and splanchnic blood flow and oxygen consumption measurements in patients with intraperitoneal infection. *Ann. Surg.* **171**, 321.

Kantrowitz, A., Tjønnoland, S., Krakaver, J. S., Phillips, S. J., Free, P. S. and Butner, A. N. (1968). Mechanical intra aortic cardiac assistance in cardiogenic shock. *Archs. Surg.* (Chicago) **97**, 1000.

Leinbach, R. C., Buckley, M. J., Austen, W. G., Petchek, H. E., Kantrowitz, A. R. and Sanders, C. A. (1971). Effects of intra aortic balloon pumping on coronary flow and metabolism in man. *Circulation* **43** (Suppl. 1) 1.

Leinbach, R. C., Dinsmore, R. E., Mundthi, E. D., Buckley, M. J., Durkman, W. B., Austen, W. G. and Sanders, C. A. (1972). Selective coronary and left ventricular cine angiography during intra aortic balloon pumping for cardiogenic shock. *Circulation* **43**, 845.

Moulopoulos, S. T., Topas, S. and Kolff, W. J. (1962). Diastolic balloon pumping (with carbon dioxide) in the aorta. A mechanical assistance to the failing circulation. *Am. Heart J.* **63**, 669.

McLean, A. P. H., Duff, J. H. Groves, A. C., La Pointe, R. and McLean, L. D. (1971). Oxygen uptake in septic shock. *In* 'Septic shock in Man' (Ed. S. G. Hershey, L. R. M. Del Guerico and R. McGoon) p. 107. Little Brown, Boston.

McLean, L. D., Milligan, W. G., McGean, A. P. H. and Duff, J. A. (1967). Patterns of septic shock in man. A detailed study of 56 patients. *Ann. Surg.* **166**, 543.

Mueller, H., Ayres, S. M., Conklin, E. F., Gianelli, S., Maggara, J. R., Grace, W. T. and Nealon, T. F., Jr. (1971). The effects of intra aortic counterpulsation on cardiac performance and metabolism in shock associated with acute myocardial infarction. *J. Clin. Invest.* **50**, 1885.

Powell, W. J., Dagett, W. M., Magro, A. R., Branco, J. A., Buckley, M. J., Sanders, C. A., Kantrowitz, A. R. and Austen, W. G. (1970). Effects of intra aortic balloon counterpulsation on cardiac performance, oxygen consumption and coronary blood flow in dogs. *Circ. Res.* **26**, 753.

Sanders, C. A., Buckley, M. J., Leinbach, R. C., Mundth, E. D. and Austen, W. G. (1972). Mechanical circulatory assistance. Current status and experience with combining circulatory assistance, emergency coronary angiography and acute myocardial reviscularisation. *Circulation* **45**, 1292.

Wilson, R. E., Sever, E. J. and Riggs, J. (1971). Haemodynamic changes, treatment and prognosis in clinical shock. *Archs. Surg.* **102**, 21.

Weir, J., Yacoub, M. and Pridie, R. B. (1975). Echocardiography of the intra aortic balloon. *Brit. Heart J.* **37**, 1045.

Yacoub, M., Towers, M. and Somerville, W. (1972). Surgical treatment of mitral regurgitation secondary to myocardial in farction. (Abs.) *Brit. Heart J.* **34**, 965.

Yacoub, M., Fawzy, E. and Brennan, J. (1975). Post infarction ventricular septal rupture, clinicopathological study. *Brit. Heart J.* **37**, 552.

Section 2: Mechanical Support for the Treatment of Severe Pulmonary Failure, The Membrane Oxygenator

Keith D. Roberts

INTRODUCTION

Since the beginning of open heart surgery employing cardio-respiratory support apparatus ('heart lung' machines) a search was made for oxygenating equipment producing less damage to blood than bubbling or filming types (Kolff et al., 1956; Clowes and Hopkins, 1956; Dobel et al., 1965). It became apparent that fewer physical and chemical stresses were imposed on blood if direct contact between blood and gas was avoided by the use of a semi-permeable membrane between them. Landé developed an oxygenator consisting of a silicone rubber membrane, plastic membrane support plates and fluid distribution manifolds, in conjunction with Edwards Laboratories (Santo Ana, California) – the Landé-Edwards oxygenator (Landé et al., 1967). Much original work was done using this oxygenator but the membrane in the oxygenator was coated with dry powdered sodium chloride during manufacture to prevent the membrane envelopes from sticking together, and the sodium chloride had to be removed by thorough rinsing before use. The Landé-Edwards oxygenator was a free-standing unit requiring no pressure shim, clamping fixture or support equipment. It was available as 1.0 M², 2.0 M² or 3.0 M² modules, and multiples could be used in series or in parallel. Experience of the oxygenator revealed that, despite thorough washing prior to use, sodium chloride residues caused severe electrolyte problems in a high proportion of patients, and production of the Landé-Edwards oxygenator has been discontinued. Travenol Laboratories, Illinois have

965

developed the 'Modulung' membrane oxygenator with a surface area of membrane from 0.25 M^2 to 3.0 M^2, and this unit must be assembled prior to use with a universal bracket and an inflatable shim which *must* be pressurised to 150 mm Hg. More recently the Kolobow (Sci-Med Systems, Inc., Minneapolis, Minnesota) spiral coil membrane lung has become available in a range of from 0.2 M^2 to 4.5 M^2, and this has excellent oxygen and carbon dioxide gas transfer characteristics, with minimal blood trauma (Kolobow *et al.*, 1975). With both types of oxygenator the priming solution *must* be heparinised to avoid coagulation on the membrane and consequent poor gaseous interchange.

INDICATIONS FOR THE USE OF A MEMBRANE OXYGENATOR

Following the development of suitable membrane oxygenators it became logical to consider their use for organ-assist techniques in patients with respiratory disease causing acute respiratory failure, if the patient were not responding to the usual treatment. Extra-corporeal oxygenation of the blood in so called 'shock lung' was first successfully employed by Hill *et al.* (1972) and since then the same unit has reported a further three long-term survivors (two 'shock lung', one fat embolism syndrome) in a total series of twenty eight patients (Heiden *et al.*, 1975). Chang *et al.* (1974) described the successful support given to a young woman with postoperative pulmonary embolism, and the author's unit successfully managed severe acute respiratory failure due to post-operative acid aspiration syndrome in a woman of 35 years with $4\frac{1}{2}$ days of extra-corporeal oxygenation support (Browne *et al.*, 1977). In a review of patients reported from centres in the U.S.A., long-term survival was not high (15% of 130 patients, Hill *et al.*, 1974). The criteria for using the technique are therefore of fundamental importance.

Possible indications for the use of extra-corporeal oxygenation in cardio-respiratory conditions include:
1. Acute infections such as bacterial or viral pneumonias.
2. Chemical or inhalation pneumonitis.
3. Early pulmonary oxygen toxicity.
4. Multiple small pulmonary emboli (thrombotic or fat).
5. Neonatal respiratory distress syndrome.
6. Post-traumatic respiratory failure ('shock lung').
7. Cardiac failure and hypoxaemia following cardiac surgery.

To date the best results in long-term survival have been achieved in patients with 'shock lung' or pulmonary fat embolism. A prerequisite for the use of extra-corporeal oxygenation is the presence of a condition which is theoretically reversible, in a patient with absence of potentially irreversible complicating disease. Thus it would appear reasonable to keep the technique in mind in the case of relatively young patients where the prognosis appears otherwise hopeless. Many clinicians have seen death from acute respiratory failure within 24–72 h of the onset of a disease despite standard techniques of respiratory care. It is obviously essential to have criteria for the assessment of the individual patient's response to treatment, and warning signs (which may be too rigid and erring on the side of conservatism) have been stated as follows (*Anaesthesia and Intensive Care*, 1974):

1. An F_IO_2 of 100% for longer than 48 h.
2. A positive end-expiratory pressure in excess of 10 cm of water, at a high F_IO_2, for longer than 24 h.
3. A PaO_2 of less than 50 mm Hg for more than 24 h.

Other indications of progressive deterioration may be an increasing ventilatory pressure (especially in excess of 40 cm of water), a rising $PaCo_2$ despite an unchanged minute volume, or progressively deteriorating chest radiographs despite apparently adequate treatment.

It would seem reasonable to employ support by extra-corporeal oxygenation before the clinical condition has become desperate and the patient virtually moribund. It is undoubtedly preferable that it should be used in special centres familiar with extra-corporeal circulatory techniques (*British Medical Journal*, 1975).

TECHNIQUE AND OVERALL PATIENT MANAGEMENT

Prior to setting up extra-corporeal circulation it is preferable to place the patient on a weigh bed for the accurate control of fluid balance, hydration and nutrition. The apparatus is assembled in the Intensive Therapy Unit according to the diagram (Fig. 1). The definitive prime should be with fresh heparinised blood (400 i.u. heparin per 500 ml) rather than blood substitutes. Before adding the blood, the membrane is heparinised by circulating the appropriate volume of heparinised dextrose (400 i.u. heparin per 500 ml). The blood prime must not be allowed to stand in the oxygenator without circulating it. In the case of the Travenol 'Modulung' it is essential to adjust the shim pressure to 150 mm Hg before priming the circuit. With the Kolobow oxygenator the device must be flushed with filtered carbon dioxide prior to filling

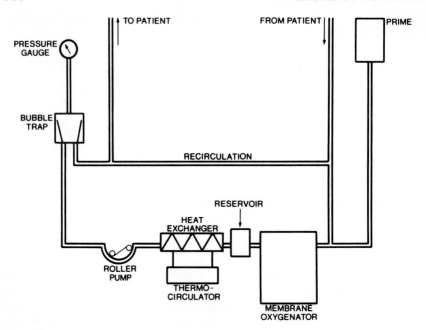

Fig. 1. The extra-corporeal circuit: prior to supporting the patient, the oxygenated blood is pumped through the recirculation line, the lines to and from the patient being clamped. When on patient support the latter two lines are unclamped and the recirculation line is occluded.

with heparinised dextrose, according to the manufacturer's recommendations. The definitive prime is again fresh heparinised blood.

The patient is transferred to the operating theatre for the necessary cannulations. An intravenous infusion allows necessary injections including heparin to be given, and arterial and central venous monitoring cannulae are inserted percutaneously. After the induction of anaesthesia and endotracheal intubation (the oral route is preferable because of the risk of bleeding from the nasal septum from trauma in the presence of heparinisation) the cannulation sites are exposed with the use of meticulous haemostasis. The incisions used will depend on the type of extra-corporeal oxygenation to be used. This may be veno-venous (Fig. 2a), veno-arterial (Fig. 2b) or a combination of these. The venous drainage and perfusion cannulae are preferably U.S.C.I. (United States Catheter and Instruments Corporation, Massuchusetts) armoured ones to avoid kinking.

In veno-venous perfusion the internal jugular vein is exposed in the neck for the return of oxygenated blood to the right atrium while venous blood is extracted from the femoral vein by a double cannulation –

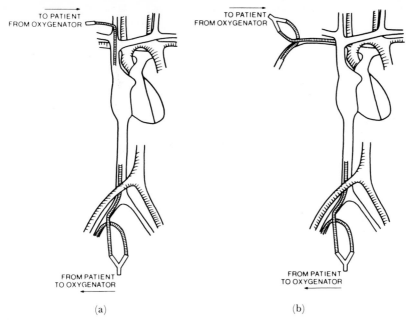

TO PATIENT
FROM OXYGENATOR

TO PATIENT
FROM OXYGENATOR

FROM PATIENT
TO OXYGENATOR

FROM PATIENT
TO OXYGENATOR

(a)   (b)

Fig. 2. (a) Veno-venous support: desaturated blood drains by gravity from the lower limb and inferior vena cava via a Y-connection and into the oxygenator, and is returned via a heat exchange (to maintain normal temperature) and bubble trap to the superior vena cava via the internal jugular venous cannula, the vein being ligated distal to the insertion site.

(b) Veno-arterial support: venous drainage is obtained as in (a), but the oxygenated blood is pumped into the axillary artery distally to maintain viability of the upper limb, and proximally into the ascending aorta for distribution to the rest of the body.

proximally the cannula is passed into the inferior vena cava, and distally into the femoral vein, the two cannulae being connected by a Y-tube, the remaining limb of this being temporarily occluded until connection is made to the extra-corporeal circuit. Prior to cannulation heparinisation is achieved by an intravenous dose of 1 mg per kg body weight (sodium heparin mucous 1 mg = 130 International Units), added to if necessary to maintain the clotting time between 20–30 min. The internal jugular vein is ligated distally and cannulated proximally, the cannula being occluded until junction with the oxygenator circuit is made. The wounds are carefully closed and the ends of the cannulae are covered with sterile gauze prior to return to the I.T.U.

In veno-arterial perfusion the femoral vein is used as before for drainage of venous blood, but the axillary artery is exposed for return of oxygenated blood, being cannulated proximally and distally with a Y-junction linking the two cannulae, two being necessary so that the upper limb (in addition to the aorta) is supplied with oxygenated blood. Axillary artery cannulation is preferable to the femoral artery because it is difficult with the latter to achieve a high enough PaO_2 in the aortic arch (and therefore in the myocardium and brain), unless a very long perfusion catheter is passed retrograde from the femoral artery to the aortic arch.

The patient is then taken to the I.T.U. and, with the greatest care to avoid the entry of air into the lines, connection is made to the extra-corporeal circuit. This has meantime been kept recirculating from time to time with oxygenated blood, and after the patient is joined to the circuit the recirculation line is clamped so that the patient is being supported. Careful watch must be kept on the reservoir and the oxygen flow rate into the oxygenator. The manufacturers' data concerning circulatory flow rates and gas transfer capacities must be carefully studied and applied in relation to the individual patient. The surface area of the membrane depends on the patient's metabolic requirements, but a rough guide is 0.5 M^2 for every 10 kg of body weight for partial replacement, and 1.0 M^2 per 10 kg for total replacement of respiratory function. If more than one module has to be employed they are better connected *in parallel* not in series, in order to avoid too great a resistance in the circuit.

Continuous monitoring of arterial and central venous pressure is essential. The efficacy of tissue perfusion is judged by measuring urine flow and the core-skin temperature gradient (oesophageal thermistor probe as a core temperature probe, a rectal probe is inaccurate because of the insulating effect of the faeces, and a skin probe on the medial aspect of the big toe). Temperature monitoring is discussed in greater detail in Part 2, ch. II, p. 312. Intravenous fluid maintenance therapy is essential until the bowel is active, with added electrolytes as required, and vitamin supplements. Sufficient heparin is added to the infusion to maintain the clotting time at 20–30 minutes, and this should be measured at least every 30 minutes. Blood chemistry investigations including sodium, potassium, calcium, PaO_2, $PaCO_2$ and base are made regularly as often as needed, but in any event at intervals no longer than four hours. Serum protein estimation is necessary twice daily and if necessary the appropriate fraction is transfused. Fresh frozen plasma or platelet concentrate may be necessary, and if the haemoglobin falls fresh heparinised blood transfusions are given.

Improvement of the patient in all parameters will be noted if the pulmonary lesion is recovering; thus the PaO_2 will steadily rise, the core-skin temperature gradient will decrease and the chest radiograph will show considerable clearing. If the patient has been unconscious hitherto, episodes of hypertension due to autogenous catechol-amine release will indicate returning awareness and require appropriate sedation (e.g. intravenous diazepam). As improvement continues the amount of support can be lessened until the extra-corporeal circulation can be discontinued (temporarily at first, the recirculation being employed, in case further support is needed). When a trial of non-support is being made any Y-drainage or perfusion tubes are clamped in such a way that, for example, femoral vein or axillary artery continuity is maintained through the Y-connection.

If extra-corporeal support can be discontinued the circuit is disconnected from the patient, who is then taken to the operating theatre for decannulation. Whenever possible vessels used for the perfusion are repaired rather than ligated. Intravenous protamine, calculated after titration may be needed in order to neutralise the effect of the residual free heparin.

COMPLICATIONS

The main complications arising from extra-corporeal respiratory support are related to inadequate control of heparinisation resulting in bleeding or in clotting (particularly a problem on the membrane, resulting in impaired gas transfer), loss of blood clotting factors particularly platelets, and the possibility of infection. Air embolism is an ever present danger which must carefully be guarded against.

CONCLUSION

The treatment is costly, time consuming, and involves a huge demand on supporting services, particularly biochemical. By analogy with renal transplantation, it would obviously be an invaluable adjunct if lung transplantation becomes a definitive treatment for irreversible respiratory failure. It cannot be too strongly stated, however, that success is only likely to result if it is practised in centres used to extra-corporeal circulatory techniques. If a suitable patient is passing beyond the control of conventional therapy for acute respiratory failure, thought should be given to moving him to a centre where extra-corporeal oxygenation can be carried out. This decision *must* be made before irreversible damage has occurred in vital organs, including the lung itself.

REFERENCES

Anesthesia and Intensive Care (1974). Editorial **2**, 106.
British Medical Journal (1975). Editorial **3**, 340.
Browne, C. H., Chew, H. E. R., Clark, E., Edwards, J. M., Hanson, G. C. and Roberts, K. D. (1977). The management of the pulmonary aspiration syndrome. *Intens. Care Med.* **3**, 257.
Chang, V. P., Harrison, G. A., Weston, M., Hickie, J., Benson, R., Wright, R., Shanahan, M. X. and Windsor, H. M. (1974). Acute respiratory failure managed by prolonged partial extra-corporeal oxygenation. *Med J. Aust.* **1**, 350.
Clowes, G. and Hopkins, A. (1956). Further studies with plastic films and their use in oxygenating blood. *Trans. Amer. Soc. Artif. Intern. Organs* **1**, 6.
Dobel, A., Mitri, M., Galva, R., Sarkozy, E. and Murphy, D. (1965). Biologic evaluation of blood after prolonged recirculation through film and membrane oxygenators. *Ann. Surg.* **161**, 617.
Heiden, D., Mielke, C. H., Rodivien, R. and Hill, J. D. (1975). Platelets, haemostasis and thrombo-embolism during treatment of acute respiratory insufficiency with extra-corporeal membrane oxygenation. *J. Thorac. Cardiovasc. Surg.* **70**, 644.
Hill, J. D., O'Brien, T. O., Murray, J. J., Dontigny, L. and Gerbode, F. (1972). Prolonged extra-corporeal oxygenation for acute post traumatic respiratory failure (shock lung syndrome). *New Engl. J. Med* **286**, 629.
Hill, J. D., Ratcliff, J. L., Fallat, R. J., Tucker, H. J., Lamy, M., Dietrich, H. P. and Gerbode, F. (1974). Prognostic factors in the treatment of acute respiratory insufficiency with long term extracorporeal circulation. *J. Thor. Cardiovasc. Surg.* **68**, 905.
Kolff, W. J., Effler, D. B., Groves, L. K., Peereboom, M. D. and Moraca, P. P. (1956). Disposable membrane oxygenator (heart-lung machine) and its use in experimental surgery. *Cleveland Clin. Quart.* **23**, 68.
Kolobow, T., Stool, E. W., Sacks, K. L., Vurek, G. (1975). Acute respiratory failure: survival following 10 days support with a membrane lung. *J. Thorac. and Cardiovasc. Surg.* **69**, 947.
Landé, A. J., Dos, S. J., Carlson, R. G., Pershau, R. A., Lange, R. P., Sonstegard, L. T. and Lillehei, C. W. (1967). A new membrane oxygenator-dialyzer. *Surg. Clin. N. Amer.* **47**, 1461.

Section 3: Equipment for the Treatment of Acute Renal Failure

H. A. LEE

INTRODUCTION

This section deals with equipment requirements that are specific for the management of acute renal failure patients. Since many of these patients present as intensive care problems, it is obvious that renal units will carry pieces of apparatus common to general intensive therapy units, such as cardiac monitors, facilities for cardiac pacing and ventilators. My choice of ventilator for a renal unit is the Cape-Bristol Ventilator which has simple controls and easily read dials.

PERITONEAL DIALYSIS

One of the virtues of peritoneal dialysis is its simplicity, both from a practical standpoint and for the simplicity of equipment required. Although there are a number of automatic peritoneal dialysis machines now available, the first of which I introduced in the U.K. in 1965 (Lee, 1965), I believe they all have limitations. The individual efficiency of all these machines is dependant upon the placement and patency of the peritoneal dialysis catheter. Even with simple peritoneal dialysis there is little cost difference with conventional haemodialysis. The advent of automatic peritoneal dialysis machines has considerably increased the cost of peritoneal dialysis. Furthermore, their introduction has taken away one of the principal advantages, that of simplicity. Whereas, many nurses are capable and confident of managing conventional peritoneal dialysis, those who are less mechanically minded become apprehensive of the modern machinery introduced with these automatic dialysers. (See Table 1 for peritoneal dialysis equipment.)

973

Table 1. Peritoneal dialysis equipment

Item	Specification	Manufacturer
Catheter Semi-rigid {	Trocath adult size V4900	McGaw Labs
	Trocath paediatric size V4901	McGaw Labs
	Dialaflex Mk 2	Allen and Hanburys Ltd
	Diacath	Baxter Labs (Travenol)
Flexible {	Adult	Braun-Melsungen
	Paediatric	
Administration set	Dianeal Y-Type Set	Baxter Labs (Travenol)
	Dialaflex giving Set	Allen and Hanburys Ltd
Dialysis solutions (all in plastic bags)	Dialaflex 61 (Dex. 1.36%)	
	Dialaflex 62 (Dex. 6.36%)	Allen and Hanburys Ltd
	Dialaflex 63 (Dex. 1.36%) (Na^+ 130 mmol/l)	
	Dianeal A5204 (Dex. 1.5%)	Baxter Labs
	Dianeal A5254 (Dex. 1.5%) (Na^+ 130 mmol/l)	(Travenol)
	Hartmann Sol. (Na^+ 131 mmol/l) (K^+ 5.0 mmol/l)	
	5% Dextrose	
Drainage bags (both 3L)	Aldon Type CV with non-return valve	Aldington Labs, Ltd
	Drainage bag	Baxter Labs (Travenol)

An example of a peritoneal dialysis chart is shown in Fig. 1. This chart is meant to be a guide both to the nurse and to the doctor and should not be signed by either until full understanding has been reached about the patient management requirements.

Patients receiving either peritoneal or haemodialysis are ideally managed on a weigh bed. Although weigh beds are expensive pieces of apparatus, I consider them a very vital part of any acute renal failure unit, or intensive care unit. The weigh beds with automatic alarms for set limits of weight gain or loss need careful nursing management so that alarms are not set off inadvertently.

Intravenous infusions are commonplace in the management of acute renal failure patients and mandatory for those with gastrointestinal failure and requiring nutritional support. The modern pumps which work on a principle of constant volume infusion and are not dependant upon external compression have been a great advance. The infusion pump referred to in Table 3 has proved extremely reliable and has many safeguards incorporated. Instructions are carefully printed on the side of this pump and in our unit it has received a high nurse

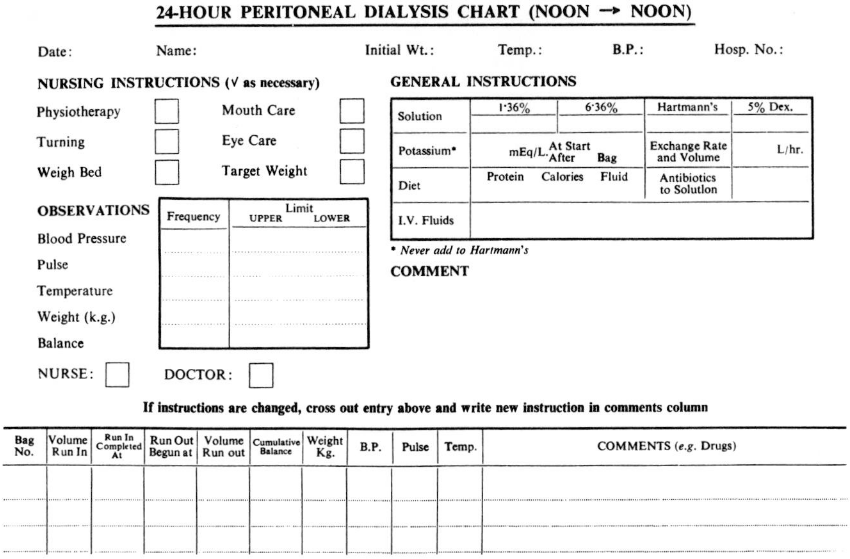

24-HOUR PERITONEAL DIALYSIS CHART (NOON → NOON)

Date: Name: Initial Wt.:   Temp.:   B.P.:   Hosp. No.:

NURSING INSTRUCTIONS (√ as necessary)   **GENERAL INSTRUCTIONS**

Physiotherapy	☐	Mouth Care	☐
Turning	☐	Eye Care	☐
Weigh Bed	☐	Target Weight	☐

	1·36%	6·36%	Hartmann's	5% Dex.
Solution				
Potassium*	mEq/L At Start After Bag		Exchange Rate and Volume	L/hr.
Diet	Protein Calories Fluid		Antibiotics to Solution	
I.V. Fluids				

OBSERVATIONS

	Frequency	Limit UPPER LOWER
Blood Pressure		
Pulse		
Temperature		
Weight (k.g.)		
Balance		

* Never add to Hartmann's

COMMENT

NURSE: ☐   DOCTOR: ☐

If instructions are changed, cross out entry above and write new instruction in comments column

Bag No.	Volume Run In	Run In Completed At	Run Out Begun at	Volume Run out	Cumulative Balance	Weight Kg.	B.P.	Pulse	Temp.	COMMENTS (e.g. Drugs)

Fig. 1. Upper part of peritoneal dialysis record chart.

acceptability. For patients who require a glucose insulin regimen, which has to be given either by one-hourly boluses or careful constant infusion, such a pump is not only a great asset to nursing management, but relieves the nurses of considerable time otherwise spent in 'drip fiddling'.

Table 2. Haemodialysis equipment

Item	Specification	Manufacturer
Heparin pump (clockwork)	Handley syringe injector (20 ml syringe)	Wheathampstead Sales Service Ltd, Caversham
Blood pump	MHRE 3 Mk III flow inducer	Watson and Marlow Ltd, Falmouth, Cornwall
Monitor	Bedside monitor (V.P., dialysate flow temp.). Cut out alarm	Watson and Marlow
Conductivity meters	Dialysis bath conductivity. Meter model D1	Baxters Ltd (Travenol)

Table 2. Haemodialysis equipment (*cont.*)

Item	Specification	Manufacturer
	Type MC9	Electronic Switch-Gear (London) Ltd, Hitchin
Pumps	Transfer and recirculating. Type 16 (stainless steel body)	Stuart Turner Ltd, Henley-on-Thames
Dialysate tank	Fibreglass 320 L. Free standing	Porter Plastics, Waterlooville, Hants
Cabinet	Houses coil and recirculating pumps	Made by hospital workshop
Coil housing	Stainless steel pail (optional)	Baxters Ltd (Travenol)
Water softener	Culligan soft no. 7	Culligans Ltd
Dialysers	Cuprophane ultra-flo II 1.5 m (ultrafiltration) Cuprophane ultra-flo II 1.4 m (high dialysance) Cuprophane ultra-flo II (standard 1 m filtration and dialysance) Cuprophane ultra-flo II 0.64 m (paediatric)	Baxters Ltd (Travenol)
	Dialyser cartridge 0.7 m, Ex. 21 (low ultrafiltration) Dialyser cartridge 1.0 m, Ex. 25 (high dialysance) Dialyser cartridge 0.8 m Ex. 23 (standard filtration and dialysance) Paediatric dialyser cartridge, Ex. 20 0·3 m	Extracorporeal SA
Arterial lines[1] with blood pump inserts	R 313 SP 200D	Avon Medicals Ltd Sandoz Ltd
Venous lines[1]	R 314 SP 201E	Avon Medicals Ltd Sandoz Ltd
Blood level detector	BLM 1	Sandoz Ltd
Dialysate conc.	QE (130 Na^+) (up to 50 different solutions available)	McCarthy's Ltd, Romford

[1] Can be adapted for Kiil- or coil-type dialysers.

Table 3. General items

Item	Specification	Manufacturer
Infusion set	Metriset V1428	McGaw Labs
Infusion catheters	Abbot flexible drum-cartridge catheter (peripheral insertion 70 cm long)	Abbott Labs
	Intramedicut catheter kit (no. 14 gauge, 30 cm long)	Sherwood Medical Industries Ltd
C.V.P. manometer	Non-autoclavable manometer adjustable zero arm no. 3488	Use B-P
	Manometer line	Portex Ltd
Weigh beds	Non-mobile, tare adjustable	C.M.S. Weighing Equipment Ltd
	'Seca' 780 electronic bed weighing system. Automatic alarm for max. $\pm$ 9.9 kg	Sandoz Ltd, Rugby Works
	Datex patient weighing system	Instrumentarium, Finland
Urine vol. measurer	Urimeter MM10 (up to 1500 ml)	Mediplast, Sweden
Blood sugar measurement	Ames 'Eyetone' meter	Ames Company, Miles Labs Ltd, Slough
Blood pump	VIP^{tm} constant volumetric T92	Tekmar Medical Ltd, Abingdon
Blood pump lines and insert	Accuset^{tm} V 1800	McGaw Labs

Table 4. Haemodialysis – vessel access requirements

Shunts (adult)
Silicone rubber cannula left standard
Silicone rubber cannula right standard
Etched Teflon vessel tips size 13 (large) – 22 (small)
Shunts (paediatric)
Silicone rubber cannula universal standard no. S-350P   } Extracorporeal SA, Medical Specialities
Etched Teflon T414–T220
Etched Teflon connectors 00-31-0502
Paediatric shunt adaptors DA-24
Fistula
Arterial outflow lines
Venous return lines   } Avon Medicals Ltd

Table 4. Haemodialysis – vessel access requirements (*cont.*)

Set connector PTFE
Shunt connections
Long adaptor R90 (male and female luer)   } Avon Medicals Ltd
Injection site insert R85

Central venous pressure monitoring may be a very important monitoring aspect of patients in acute renal failure, particularly those who have central venous lines. The simple manometric device referred to in Table 3 is very useful and easily used.

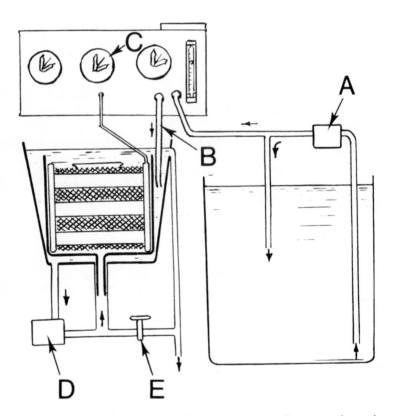

Fig. 2. Schematic diagram of Portsmouth coil/tank system. A, supply pump to the monitor and recirculator of tank dialysate. B, supply to pail assembly. C, central dial of monitor now free as modern coils (Table 2) are encased and need neither cuff or steel pail assembly. They fit directly into nozzle at base of dialyser compartment. D, recirculation pump for dialyser compartment. E, drain valve.

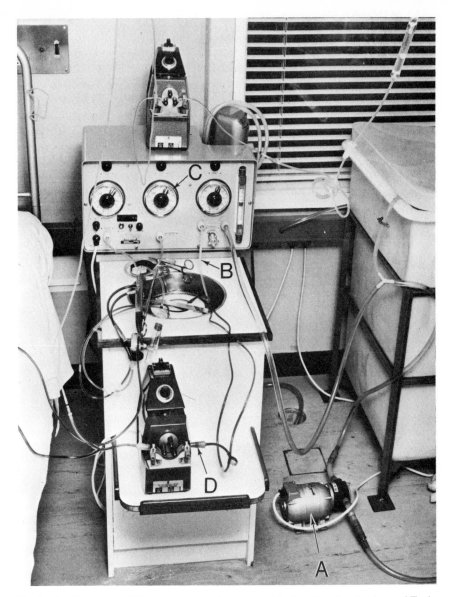

Fig. 3. The Portsmouth Coil system. A, supply pump to Monitor C and recirculator of Tank Dialysate. The current tanks are free standing and do not require metal frame support. D, this pump insert is now integral part of blood lines as supplied. The Heparin Pump atop main Monitor has now been replaced by small clockwork syringe pump. Dialysate heated by Tecam Temp-Unit behind right hand side of Monitor. B, supply to pail assembly.

HAEMODIALYSIS

There are many types of haemodialysis machines available. The one illustrated in Figs 2 and 3 is a very simple design and requires the minimum of maintenance (Down *et al.*, 1970). It has been designed on a modular basis so that any part can be readily replaced. Another point about this machinery is that it is relatively cheap. The items of equipment referred to in Table 2 apply mainly to the Portsmouth coil system shown in the figures. The range of dialysers (coils, layered types, capillary fibre models), blood lines and pumps is considerable but a selection that I have found most useful and allowing of flexibility are shown in Tables 2 and 4. Part of a haemodialysis record chart used in our unit is shown in Fig. 4.

Although there is a bewildering array of models for haemodialysis being used for regular dialysis treatment patients, there is little need for such variation in acute renal failure haemodialysis treatment. The apparatus referred to in Figs 2 and 3 has been thoroughly tested over eight years and found to be completely satisfactory for all types of acute renal failure patients.

DAILY HAEMODIALYSIS RECORD

	Temp.	Pulse	L	B/P	S	Weight
Before dialysis						
After dialysis						

Shunt condition:

General health:

Dialysis conductivity at machine:

Volume of saline given during dialysis:

Name:

Date: Dialysis No:

Starting Time: Finishing Time:

Shunt site No: Revision No:

Dialyser: Kiil / 145 Coil / 100 Coil.   Use No:

Bath: Standard / Low Sodium / Low Calcium

Wash-back: Volume: Dextrose/Saline

1) **Heparin:** Initial:

          Infusion:

          Total:

2) **Hypotensives:** Yes/No   Dose:

3) **Antibiotics:**   Yes/No   Name:

Fluid allowance

24-hour urine volume

Salt intake

Anticoagulation

Time	To	Pulse	B.P.	Wt.	Blood Flow	Art. Pump	Vein Press	Vein Clamp	Cuff or Neg. Press	Heparin	COMMENTS
				TARGET WEIGHT							

Fig. 4. Upper and lower parts of haemodialysis record chart.

REFERENCES

Down, P. F., Farrand, D. E., Wood, S. E. and Lee, H. A. (1970). Comparison of coil and Kiil dialysers. *Brit. Med. J.* **4**, 517.

Lee, H. A. (1965). Peritoneal dialysis in the management of acute renal failure. *In* 'Second Symposium on Advanced Medicine' (Ed. J. R. Trounce) p. 107. Pitman Medical Publishing Co. Ltd.

Section 4: Equipment for the Treatment of Hepatic Failure

P. N. Trewby and Roger Williams

INDICATIONS FOR THE USE OF LIVER SUPPORT SYSTEMS

To date the use of liver support systems has been largely confined to patients with fulminant hepatic failure rather than hepatic failure due to chronic liver disease. This is because of the much higher initial mortality in fulminant hepatic failure (when treated conservatively the mortality is 80–90%) (Benhamou *et al.*, 1972) and the excellent outlook if the patient survives. In the vast majority of cases both liver function and architecture return to normal (Gazzard *et al.*, 1974) with only the very occasional case progressing to cirrhosis.

In fulminant hepatic failure the aim of a liver support system is to provide sufficient time for the patient's own liver to regenerate and to provide a more favourable environment for this to occur.

Though largely untried in chronic liver disease, there remains considerable scope for the use of liver support systems in this situation. They may hasten the return of consciousness when coma has been precipitated by a potentially reversible event, such as gastrointestinal haemorrhage or electrolyte imbalance. They may also be used as a prelude to transplantation in cirrhotic patients to improve their general condition and to keep the patient alive until a donor organ becomes available. The greatest use for artificial liver support systems in the future may be the treatment of these patients with chronic liver disease.

LIVER SUPPORT SYSTEMS AVAILABLE

An ideal liver support system would replace both the synthetic function of the failing liver as well as its detoxification and excretory function. Techniques such as extracorporeal animal liver perfusion, cross-circulation and exchange transfusion can theoretically fulfill these criteria but they are expensive in terms of time and personnel, each is associated with technical problems, and none has survived the test of time.

Pig liver perfusion frequently exacerbates the patient's bleeding tendency by precipitating disseminated intravascular coagulation within the animal liver (Winch *et al.*, 1972). No controlled trial of pig liver perfusion has been carried out, but of the 130 pig liver perfusions reported in the world literature there are only 10 long-term survivors (Williams, 1974). In our unit there have been no long-term survivors with this treatment, although improvement in conscious level during perfusion was observed in some cases.

Exchange transfusion in one controlled trial (Redeker and Yamahiro, 1973) was not associated with increased survival. Very large amounts of blood are required and there is the risk of transfusing HBsAg. Again, temporary improvement in conscious level may occur. Cross-circulation using a healthy volunteer is limited to non-infectious cases and even then the volunteer is at risk and frequently develops abnormalities of liver function. Cross-circulation using an animal donor has been hampered by the danger of transmission of animal virus (Burnell *et al.*, 1967).

The technical difficulties associated with these methods, together with the poor survival figures, has led to a search for a purely artificial system of liver support which would be safe to apply and could be used on a daily basis. Such systems aim only to reproduce the excretory and detoxification function of the liver. The available evidence suggests that it is the accumulation of those compounds normally cleared by the liver which is responsible for coma in hepatic failure, although some authors have suggested that failure of the liver to synthesise essential compounds necessary for normal cerebral function may also be important (Opolon *et al.*, 1975b). The failure of the liver's synthetic function can be corrected at least in part by infusions of albumin, dextrose, and clotting factors.

For the sake of clarity toxic compounds known to accumulate in hepatic failure have been divided into water soluble substances, such as ammonia, fatty acids, mercaptans, and amino acids and false neuro-transmitters (e.g. octopamine), and lipid soluble protein-bound sub-stances such as bile acids and bilirubin (Gazzard *et al.*, 1974). Artificial liver support systems at present in use aim to remove the water soluble compounds, as it is these which have been most implicated in the pathogenesis of hepatic coma (Zieve, 1975).

Charcoal haemoperfusion

Activated charcoal is a very effective adsorbent for a wide range of water soluble substances including molecules in the middle molecular weight range (300 to 2000) (Gazzard *et al.*, 1974). Early attempts to use charcoal haemoperfusion were hampered by severe loss of platelets and by the embolisation of small particles of charcoal into the circulation. To improve biocompatibility Smith and Nephew Research Ltd developed an acrylic hydrogel coating for the charcoal, and with a 4% coating platelet damage and charcoal embolisation were found to be reduced with little loss of adsorptive capacity. The coated charcoal is packed in a specially designed column and is primed with saline and sterilised before use (Fig. 1).

An alternative solution to the biocompatibility problem was developed by Becton Dickinson who immobilised the carbon particles on a supporting polyester film which is then wound into a spiral and packed in polycarbonate housing.

Charcoal haemoperfusion was first tested in an animal model of hepatic failure when it was found to significantly prolong survival and to delay the rise in blood ammonia (Weston *et al.*, 1974).

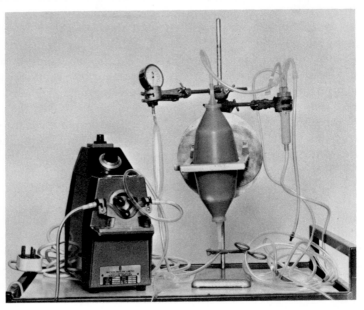

Fig. 1. The Watson-Marlow roller pump, Smith and Nephew charcoal column and connections for haemoperfusions.

In humans most experience of charcoal haemoperfusion has been obtained from its use in fulminant hepatic failure at King's College Hospital, London. Patients are admitted to a purpose-built liver failure unit with 24 h resident medical cover. When in grade IV coma and not responding to full supportive therapy, a daily 3–4 h period of charcoal haemoperfusion is performed until recovery or death occurs (Gazzard *et al.*, 1974). A Scribner arteriovenous shunt is inserted at the wrist and blood is pumped via a Watson-Marlow roller pump through the column of coated activated charcoal and returned via a bubble trap to the venous side of the shunt (Fig. 2). Systemic heparinisation is important and is achieved by an initial bolus plus intermittent doses to maintain a Lee-White clotting time of 20 to 30 min. Severe thrombocytopenia ($<30\,000/mm^3$) and persistent hypotension are the two contraindications to perfusion.

Simultaneous arteriovenous sampling across the column showed significant removal of amino acids, lactic acid, bile acids, and short-chain fatty acids (Fig. 3), and other workers have shown *in vitro* removal of mercaptans.

Charcoal haemoperfusion may also remove substances that inhibit liver regeneration. Hughes *et al.* (1975) have demonstrated in the serum

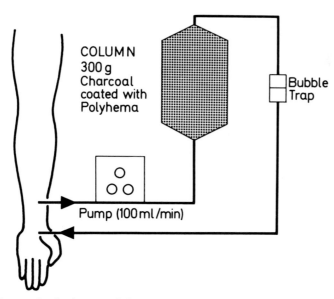

COLUMN
300 g
Charcoal
coated with
Polyhema

Bubble
Trap

Pump (100 ml/min)

Fig. 2. Diagram showing haemoperfusion circuit in man.

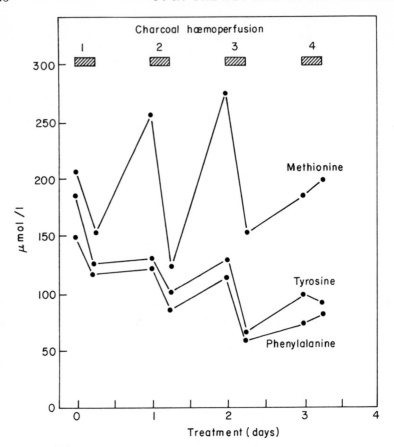

Fig. 3. Fall in methionine, tyrosine, and phenylalanine during successive charcoal haemoperfusions.

of patients with fulminant hepatic failure a heat-labile compound that is cytotoxic to isolated rabbit hepatocytes. Significant reduction in the cytotoxicity of the patients' serum was demonstrated following charcoal haemoperfusion.

Initial results showed improvement in survival rates from 13% to 35% in the first 49 patients treated with charcoal haemoperfusion at King's College Hospital. Subsequent results have not been as encouraging and have tended to emphasise the importance of biocompatibility associated with the use of extracorporeal systems in these very sick patients.

Charcoal haemoperfusion and biocompatibility

The main problems are platelet depletion, platelet aggregation, and hypotension. Weston *et al.* (1975) have demonstrated that in fulminant hepatic failure there is not only an absolute thrombocytopenia, but also a selective decrease in the large haemostatically more active platelets. Because of their increased adherence to charcoal this deficiency of large platelets is exacerbated during charcoal haemoperfusion, and the effect of this can be demonstrated by noting a disproportionate prolongation of the bleeding time following perfusion.

In addition charcoal haemoperfusion may result in the formation of platelet aggregates which may embolise to the patient's circulation. Using the Swank screen filtration pressure technique the formation of aggregates during perfusion has been demonstrated in some, but not all, perfusions. In those perfusions in which aggregates were detected there was a greater than average reduction in platelet count, and also profound hypotension. The latter may have been due to release of vasoactive amines from the platelet aggregates.

Hypotension during charcoal haemoperfusion can also occur in the absence of aggregation formation, when it may be due to an inability to compensate for the volume changes that occur in extracorporeal circulation. Alternatively, the charcoal may adsorb pressor compounds such as angiotension and this has been demonstrated *in vitro* (Wernze and Brachtel, 1975).

The importance of biocompatibility when liver support systems are used in fulminant hepatic failure is illustrated by our survival figures. Of the first 49 patients treated with charcoal haemoperfusion the overall survival was 35%, and the majority of these had uneventful perfusions with few side-effects. In the following 18 patients many of the perfusions had to be terminated prematurely because of hypotension and there were no survivors from these 18. Hopefully the use of standardised charcoal preparations and a better understanding of the problems associated with extracorporeal systems in these very sick patients will enable the earlier results with charcoal haemoperfusion to be obtained once again.

Haemodialysis with polyacrylonitrile membrane

Cumulative evidence from reported cases (Benhamou *et al.*, 1972) suggests that neither haemodialysis with standard cuprophan membranes nor peritoneal dialysis are of benefit in hepatic coma, apart from in the treatment of the associated renal failure.

However, haemodialysis with a polyacrylonitrile membrane allows a faster transfer of middle molecular weight molecules than a cuprophan membrane (Opolon et al., 1975a) and in addition it is permeable to compounds of molecular weight greater than 5000 while a cuprophan membrane is relatively impermeable to compounds of molecular weight above 2000. The effectiveness of haemoperfusion with a polyacrylonitrile membrane would be expected therefore to be similar to that found with charcoal haemoperfusion.

In a pig model of hepatic failure, improvement in both the electroencephalogram and the length of survival was demonstrated in those animals haemodialysed with a polyacrylonitrile membrane.

In humans Opolon et al. (1975a) has reported recovery of consciousness in 5 out of 9 patients with fulminant hepatic failure who were dialysed for 3–4 hours per day with a polyacrylonitrile membrane. We are currently evaluating the technique, but of the first 24 patients so treated 9 fully recovered consciousness and 8 (33%) left hospital (Silk et al., 1977).

REFERENCES

Benhamou, J. P., Rueff, B. and Sicot, C. (1972). Severe hepatic failure: a critical study of current therapy. In 'Liver and Drugs' (Ed. F. Orlandi and A. D. Jegevel) p. 213. Academic Press, London and New York.

Burnell, J. D., Dawborn, J. K., Epstein, R. B., Guttman, R. A., Leinbach, G. E., Thomas, E. D. and Volwiler, W. (1967). Acute hepatic coma treated by cross-circulation or exchange transfusion. New Engl. J. Med. 276, 935.

Gazzard, B. G., Weston, M. J., Murray-Lyon, I. M., Flax, H., Record, C. O., Portmann, B., Langley, P. G., Dunlop, E. H., Mellon, P. J., Ward, M. B. and Williams, R. (1974). Charcoal haemoperfusion in the treatment of fulminant hepatic failure. Lancet 2, 1301.

Hughes, R., Cochrane, A. M. G., Thompson, A. D., Murray-Lyon, I. M. and Williams, R. (1975). Plasma inhibitory factors. In 'Artificial Liver Support' (Ed. Roger Williams and I. M. Murray-Lyon) p. 263. Pitman Medical, Tunbridge Wells.

Opolon, P., Huguet, C., Granger, A., Gallot, D., Bloch, P. and Bidalier, M. (1975a). Comparison of single and cross haemodialysis with a donor through cuprophan and a new polymer membrane. In 'Artificial Liver Support' (Ed. Roger Williams and I. M. Murray-Lyon) p. 186. Pitman Medical, Tunbridge Wells.

Opolon, P., Lavallard, M. C., Crubille, C., Gateau, P., Nusinovici, V., Granger, A., Darnis, F. and Caroli, J. (1975b). Encephalopathie au cours de l'atrophie hepatique aigue. Effet de l'epuration des moyennes molecules. Resultats preliminaires. La Nouvelle Presse Medicale 4, 2987.

Redeker, A. G. and Yamahiro, H. S. (1973). Controlled trial of exchange transfusion therapy in fulminant hepatitis. Lancet 1, 3.

Silk, D. B. A., Hanid, M. A., Trewby, P. N., Davies, M., Chase, R. A., Langley, P. G., Mellon, P. J. and Williams, R. (1977). Treatment of fulminant hepatic failure by polyacrylonitile membrane haemodialysis. *Lancet* **2**, 1–4.

Wernze, von H. and Brachtel, D. (1975). Hypotension in hepatic failure. *Lancet* **1**, 287.

Weston, M. J., Gazzard, B. G., Buxton, B. H., Winch, J., Machado, A. L., Flax, H. and Williams, R. (1974). Effects of haemoperfusion through charcoal XAD-2 resin on an animal model of fulminant hepatic failure. *Gut* **15**, 482.

Weston, M. J. and Williams, R. (1975). Extracorporeal detoxification. *In* 'Proceedings of the first international symposium on gastrointestinal emergencies.' Pergamon, Oxford.

Williams, R. (1974). Fulminant viral hepatitis. *Clinics in Gastroenterology* **3**, 2, 414.

Winch, J., Kolthammer, J., Hague, R., Fleisher, R., Shilkin, K. B. and Williams, R. (1972). Haemorrhage as a complication of dextrocorporeal pig liver perfusion. Studies on mechanism and prevention. *Brit. Med. J.* **2**, 735.

Zieve, L. (1975). Metabolic abnormalities in hepatic coma and potential toxins to be removed. *In* 'Artificial Liver Support' (Ed. Roger Williams and I. M. Murray-Lyon) p. 11. Pitman Medical, Tunbridge Wells.

Index